45.00

The Handbook of International Adoption Medicine

D0131694

THE HANDBOOK OF INTERNATIONAL ADOPTION MEDICINE

A Guide for Physicians, Parents, and Providers

Laurie C. Miller, MD

OXFORD
UNIVERSITY PRESS

2005

Colorado Christian University
Library
180 S. Garrison
Lakewood, Colorado 80226

OXFORD
UNIVERSITY PRESS

Oxford   New York
Auckland   Bangkok   Buenos Aires   Cape Town   Chennai
Dar es Salaam   Delhi   Hong Kong   Istanbul   Karachi   Kolkata
Kuala Lumpur   Madrid   Melbourne   Mexico City   Mumbai
Nairobi   São Paulo   Shanghai   Taipei   Tokyo   Toronto

Copyright © 2005 by Oxford University Press, Inc.

Published by Oxford University Press, Inc.
198 Madison Avenue, New York, New York, 10016
www.oup.com

Oxford is a registered trademark of Oxford University Press

All rights reserved. No part of this publication may be reproduced,
stored in a retrieval system, or transmitted, in any form or by any means,
electronic, mechanical, photocopying, recording, or otherwise,
without the prior permission of Oxford University Press.

Library of Congress Cataloging-in-Publication Data
Miller, Laurie C.
The handbook of international adoption medicine:
a guide for physicians, parents, and providers / Laurie C. Miller.
p. ; cm.   Includes bibliographical references and index.
ISBN 0-19-517681-2; 0-19-514530-5 (pbk.)
1. Adopted children—Medical care—United States.
2. Adopted children—Health and hygiene—United States.
3. Adopted children—Diseases—United States.
4. Intercountry adoption.
5. Interracial adoption.   I. Title.
DNLM: 1. Adoption.   2. Child Welfare.   3. Internationality.
4. Physician–Patient Relations.
WS 105.5.F2 M648h 2004   RJ101.2.M54 2004   618.92—dc22   2003069102

The science of medicine is a rapidly changing field. As new research and clinical experience broaden our knowledge, changes in treatment and drug therapy do occur. The
author and publisher of this work have checked with sources believed to be reliable in
their efforts to provide information that is accurate and complete, and in accordance
with the standards accepted at the time of publication. However, in light of the possibility of human error or changes in the practice of medicine, neither the author, nor
the publisher, nor any other party who has been involved in the preparation or publication of this work, warrants that the information contained herein is in every respect
accurate or complete. Readers are encouraged to confirm the information contained
herein with other reliable sources and are strongly advised to check the product information sheet provided by the pharmaceutical company for each drug they plan to
administer.

2 4 6 8 9 7 5 3 1

Printed in the United States of America
on acid-free paper

To all children of the world
who wait for families—
you are not forgotten

PREFACE

It has been an extraordinary pleasure of my professional life to care for internationally adopted children and their families. Every pediatrician recognizes the surprising ability of children to overcome illness and misfortune. Nowhere in pediatrics is the incredible resilience of children so obvious as in international adoption. Although it is disheartening to see children live (or in some cases subsist) in orphanages, their transformation after adoption is miraculous. Abandoned children who have suffered multiple adversities change into happy, healthy, thriving kids by the "simple" act of adoption. The metamorphosis is sometimes visible within days.

The opportunity to work with prospective adoptive parents has also been a privilege. Most prospective parents deeply yearn for a child. It is a joy to behold the fulfillment of these dreams as a family is created or enlarged. The energy, devotion, and love of pre- and post-adoptive parents is unsurpassed.

When I visit orphanages, I often find myself wishing I could write "orders" for each child who lives there. I'd love to write a prescription for each child to have a loving, attentive family. No amount of medical care, education, interventions, or special activities can replace family love. For children from difficult backgrounds, adoption is the perfect remedy.

The medical model sometimes overlooks the importance of this fundamental human need. When I show colleagues the phenomenal growth recovery charts or "before-and-after" photos of recently arrived international adoptees, I'm often asked what was done to evoke such a transformation. Did the child have a medical problem that had been missed? Was a surgical procedure performed? Was some particular medication prescribed? Mistakenly, credit is given to a medical therapy, rather than the most profound intervention of all: adoption. Adoption allows children to belong to a family. It is no news to pediatricians that children need caring, attentive adult(s) in their lives, but nowhere is this more dramatically illustrated than in international adoption.

This book is primarily intended for pediatricians and other physicians who care for internationally adopted children. It is not intended as a comprehensive text covering every topic that might affect an international adoptee. Rather, it is meant to provide basic information for the practitioner caring for these children and to minimize the need to seek other sources to guide management of common problems. Some topics are covered in more detail than others, either because of their relative importance to the field of adoption medicine or because pediatricians may lack readily available resources about them. Some sections of this book will also be applicable to immigrant children, especially those from less privileged backgrounds (see Chapters 3, 8, 10–28, 31, 32). Some sections relate to children living in foster care in the United States (see Chapters 2, 5–9, 12, 13, 29, 30, 32, 34, 35). Some chapters may assist physicians caring for children in difficult congregate settings such as refugee camps or orphanages (see Chapters 2, 3, 8, 10–35); some are applicable to children living in poverty anywhere (see Chapters 5–8, 10–22, 24–26, 28, 32).

Although written with physicians in mind, I hope that social workers, other adoption professionals, health, therapy, and educational providers who work with adopted kids and their families, and adoptive parents also find this book a useful reference. Conversations over the years with adoptive parents and adoption professionals persuaded me that complex medical details and sometimes dense terminology would not hinder those interested in these subjects. Readily available material on the Internet offers the reader useful introductions to less familiar topics and explanation of terminology. Suggested sites are (1) Centers for Disease Control and Prevention, "A–Z" index of health topics, available at: http://www.cdc.gov/az.do for introductions to infectious diseases, (2) Medline-

plus Health Information Medical Encyclopedia, available at: http://www.nlm.nih.gov/medlineplus/encyclopedia.html for general medical topics, and (3) National Institute of Mental Health "For the Public," available at http://www.nimh.nih.gov/publicat/index.cfm for information on specific mental developmental disorders, and the related site http://www.nimh.nih.gov/publicat/childmenu.cfm which specifically addresses child and adolescent mental health.

A word about structure. The book is divided into seven sections that follow an introductory chapter. These sections are designed to introduce topics of importance to international adoption medicine. Most chapters end with Key Points for Internationally Adopted Children. Many chapters have case vignettes as sidebars. It should be emphasized that these vignettes are composites of cases from clinical practice fabricated to illustrate important points. The names were chosen arbitrarily and do not identify actual children. The book ends with a list of resources. This duplicates items listed elsewhere in the book, but is consolidated for the convenience of the reader. Additional information on all topics addressed in this book is available in many standard texts as well as on the Internet. Every effort has been made to ascertain the accuracy and availability of cited Web sites. However, these sites frequently change, move, or are updated. It is hoped that sufficient information has been provided to allow the reader to find the cited sources when desired.

Photographs are used throughout this book. Many were taken in orphanages throughout the world. Because of the sources of these photos, there was no mechanism to obtain explicit permission for the use of these images. I include these photographs to illustrate important points about orphanage life for children, with enormous respect and compassion for each of them. Some of these children may subsequently have been adopted. If so, I hope that they and their adoptive families accept the spirit in which these images were used.

This book is based on my experience in international adoption medicine for the past 15 years. As such, I am certain my biases and idiosyncrasies are apparent. For many years, there was no field of "international adoption medicine." From an initial focus on infectious diseases, international adoption medicine has expanded to include a wide variety of pediatric concerns, including growth delay, child development, behavior, school performance, and family adjustment. Today, the field is emerging and dynamic. Most children's hospitals are establishing clinics devoted to international adoptees. The corresponding influx of new enthusiasm, ideas, and investigations is a welcome addition to the field.

Boston, Massachusetts   L.C.M.

ACKNOWLEDGMENTS

I owe debts of gratitude to many who work with adopted children and their families. I am particularly grateful to my colleagues and friends from the early days of international adoption medicine, especially Drs. Jerri Jenista, Dana Johnson, and Peggy Hostetter. They provide inspiration to all of us who have followed and continue to contribute to the field. Without these pioneers, there would be no international adoption medicine.

Closer to home, I am deeply indebted to colleagues and friends Anne O'Keeffe Gordon, Kathleen Comfort, P.T., M.H.A., and Linda Grey Tirella, O.T.R., M.H.A., respectively the Coordinator and Developmental Therapists for our International Adoption Clinic at New England Medical Center. Their extraordinary devotion and dedication to children and families are unsurpassed. Their energy, intelligence, compassion, enthusiasm, and hard work have improved the lives of families and children throughout the world. I am honored and deeply grateful to have them as colleagues.

One of the pleasures of working in adoption medicine has been the opportunity to interact with professionals in a variety of disciplines within and beyond medicine. I've learned greatly from conversations with and the writings of adoption experts Elizabeth Bartholet, Mary Carlson, Ron Federici, Boris Gindis, Daniel Hughes, Steven Nickman, M.D., Joyce Maguire Pavao, and Adam Pertman. My admiration and gratitude are also owed to legislative aide Mark Agrast and Massachusetts Congressman William Delahunt for their work on behalf of adoptive families in Massachusetts and everywhere.

Very special thanks go to Sharon Cermak, whose pioneering work on sensory integration disorder in institutionalized children in Romania has been a model for applied research in this area. Her dedication to improving the lives of children residing in orphanages is an inspiration. Her knowledge and skills have made our collaborations and projects a pleasure.

Special gratitude is also due to Thais Tepper and Lois Hannon, cofounders of the Parent Network for the Post-Institutionalized Child. Their work has been instrumental in raising awareness in the medical and adoption communities of the specialized issues of children who have resided in institutions. They deserve widespread recognition for their efforts to improve diagnostic acumen, therapy, and support for these children and their families. Their ability to promote research collaboration, conversation, and interaction among diverse professionals is truly monumental.

Other valued colleagues include Nancy Hendrie, M.D. (The Sharing Foundation), Sandy Iverson and Kay Dole (University of Minnesota International Adoption Clinic), fellow members of American Academy of Pediatrics Section on Adoption and Foster Care (Sarah Springer, M.D., Chairman), subscribers to the listserv "Adoptmed", and colleagues and friends from the Joint Council for International Children's Services for insights and helpful discussions over recent years. Appreciation is also due to Joan Clark, Executive Director of the Open Door Society in Massachusetts, for all she has done to disseminate adoption education and information in New England. Thanks also go to the Open Door Society of New Hampshire for their ongoing support. I'm also grateful to the many fine adoption agencies in New England that have supported our work and found homes for so many children. Their ability to balance the desires of families and requirements of sending countries while maintaining a primary focus on the needs of the child is truly amazing. Particular thanks are owed to Mercy Marchuk, Karen Stager, and Stephanie Mitchell (all of Maine Adoption Placement Services) for their material and logistical support of our "Big Sisters" project in Murmansk, Russia.

Special thanks go to Dr. Arkady Rubin, Dr. Irina Rubina, and Dr. Aina Litvinova for helpful discussions, for hosting many visits to the orphanages in Murmansk, Russia and for our ongoing research collaborations. Thanks are also due to the staff of many orphanages in Kazakhstan, Guatemala, Russia, Nepal, and Romania for allowing me to visit, observe, and ask questions. Their care and concern for children under difficult circumstances is an inspiration.

Special thanks go to colleagues who helped review sections of this manuscript, including Elizabeth Barnett, M.D., Jeffrey Biller, M.D., Sharon Cermak, Ed.D, OTR/L, Lynne Karlson, M.D., Munir Mobasseleh, M.D., Steven Nickman, M.D., Roy McCauley, M.D., Abdollah Sadeghi-Nejad, M.D., and Lawrence Wolfe, M.D. Thank you also to Peter H. Pfund for his helpful review of Chapter 1. Any errors are my own responsibility and not that of these zealous reviewers. Thanks also to Victor Sloan, M.D., for providing the reference on complications of measles and to Jerri Jenista, M.D., for making me aware of Chuvash polycythemia. I also thank Jane Schaller, M.D., Chairman Emeritus of the Department of Pediatric at New England Medical Center and current President of the International Pediatric Association for her encouragement and support in the development of our international adoption program.

My heartfelt gratitude is owed to my husband, David Sherman, and my family for their support and encouragement throughout this and many other projects.

This book would not have been possible without the logistic help and support of Niko Pfund and Debbie Staab of Oxford University Press, and Wilma Chan, who ably organized all the permissions for use of figures and photographs. Nicholas Guerina, M.D., masterfully prepared electronic versions of all the illustrations and graphics. His good humor and extraordinary skill are gratefully acknowledged. I also thank Lauren Enck of Oxford University Press for inviting me to submit this manuscript. The support of many contributors to the International Adoption Research Fund at New England Medical Center is deeply appreciated. The Sirkin Family is gratefully acknowledged for their wonderful generosity to our international adoption research program.

CONTENTS

Part VI
Other Medical Conditions

Part VII
Neurocognitive and Behavioral Issues

1

INTERNATIONAL ADOPTION MEDICINE

Why a Special Book on International Adoption?

Since 1989, American families have adopted more than 167,000 children from other countries. These children usually reside in institutional care prior to adoption. Some have been exposed prenatally to alcohol, drugs, tobacco, or other substances. The children live in crowded conditions, sometimes with poor hygiene, inadequate nutrition, and limited numbers of caregivers. They come from countries with many endemic infectious diseases. At adoption, the children are frequently malnourished, developmentally delayed, and show signs of previous emotional and physical neglect. After arrival in the United States, children may not receive the recommended specialized medical attention for international adoptees. Some practitioners fail to recognize the unique needs of this group of children and are unaware of the recommendations to address these needs. Although many children thrive and do well after adoption (Figs. 1–1 to 1–3), some children have behavior problems, learning disabilities, psychological disorders, or emotional disturbances. Management of these problems must address the child's possible prenatal exposures, early experience in institutional care, and the emotional impact of being adopted.

The unique medical and developmental needs of internationally adopted children, and their rising numbers, have prompted considerable interest among pediatricians in the specialized care of this group of children. The growing body of literature in pediatric and other specialty medical journals reflects burgeoning interest in international adoption medicine. About 40 pediatricians in the United States now designate themselves "adoption medicine specialists." These pediatricians formed the core group of the newly constituted Subsection on Adoption and Foster Care of the American Academy of Pediatrics. More than 160 pediatri-

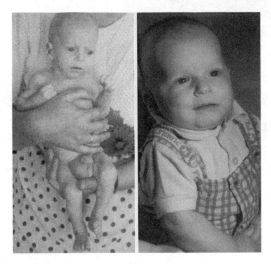

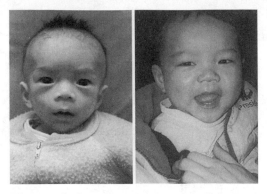

Figure 1-2 *Remarkable growth and change in mood after adoption. (With permission.)*

A   B

Figure 1-1 *Amazing transformation after adoption from Russia (A, age 5 months, B, age 12 months). (With permission.)*

cians have joined the Subsection in the past 2 years.

Concurrent with these changes in pediatrics, more parents of international adoptees are seeking international adoption medicine specialty care for their children, both pre- and post-adoption. Parents hope to find practition-ers who are knowledgeable about international adoption, the conditions their child might have experienced prior to adoption, and how these factors may affect their child. This text compiles the information needed by physicians to care for these children and guide their families—before, during, and after the adoption. It may also serve as a resource for adoptive parents, adoption professionals, and others who work with inter-nationally adopted children and their families.

The text is arranged in seven sections: Before the Adoption, Prenatal Exposures, Travel

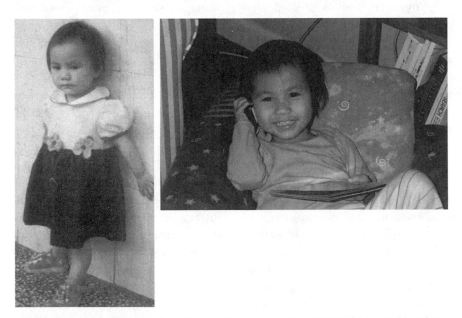

Figure 1-3 *The transformation to a "regular American kid." (With permission.)*

and Transition, Growth and Development, Infectious Diseases, Other Medical Conditions, and Neurocognitive and Behavioral Issues. Each section is divided into chapters. Topics found in standard pediatric texts and references are not reviewed exhaustively; rather, key points for internationally adopted children are highlighted. References, resources, and selected Web sites for more information are listed at the end of each chapter. Some chapters include a series of Frequently Asked Questions (FAQs) and/or Sidebars to illustrate important points for the practitioner. A general resource guide is found in the appendix at the end of the book. Abundant information and resources on many of these topics are also readily available on the Internet.

Most pediatricians already know that caring for internationally adopted children is one of the most gratifying parts of pediatric practice. The rapid recovery from growth and developmental delays, improvement in general health, and emotional blossoming of the children are all an astonishing testament to their resilience. It is a great pleasure to witness the emergence and consolidation of attachment between parent and child after adoption. The special delight of adoptive parents in the accomplishments of their child is contagious. But these children add another dimension to daily pediatric practice. Caring for internationally adopted children connects us to children outside of our practices, our communities, and our country. Internationally adopted children remind us of our obligation as pediatricians to provide care and advocacy for the world's needy children—especially those without families.

Adoption: An Introduction

Adoption is the process by which a child legally joins a family. There are many kinds of adoptions (Table 1–1). Most international adoptions are also intercountry adoptions; the former term is commonly used to indicate both (as in

Table 1–1 Types of adoptions

By Citizenship
- Domestic adoption: adoption of child by parents of the same nationality and country of residence
- Intercountry adoption: adoption in which child changes country of residence (regardless of nationality of adoptive parents; e.g., Brazilian child adopted by Brazilian parents residing in Italy)
- International adoption: adoptive parents and child have different nationalities; e.g., Brazilian child adopted by Italian parents residing in Brazil
  Thus, adoption of a Brazilian child by Italian parents residing in Italy is an intercountry *and* international adoption

By intermediary[a]
- Adoption through private child welfare agency
- Adoption through public child welfare agency
- Adoption via private attorney
- Private adoption via other adoption professional

By Amount of Information Shared
- Traditional/closed adoption: all identifying information is confidential; no social contacts
- Semi-open adoption: information is shared directly or through an intermediary; adoptive and birth parents meet at least once; letters and photos may be exchanged but there is agreement for ongoing connection; acknowledgment that, as a late adolescent or adult, the child will probably search for birth parent(s)
- Open adoption: identifying information is exchanged; one or more face-to-face meetings occurs, and ongoing contact is maintained to variable extent (letters, photos, phone calls, visits)

[a] Restrictions on these practices vary among states.
Source: Data From Spencer,[1] Pavao,[2] and Cantwell.[3]

this book). Most international adoptions are closed adoptions in which the birth parents are unknown to the adoptive family. Usually, the birth parents are also unknown to the agency mediating the adoption; most children are foundlings, or only minimal information is available about the birth parents. Occasionally, semi-open international adoptions occur. Usually the contact is limited to a brief meeting between the birth parents and adoptive parents at the time of placement. Long-term contact between these families is distinctly unusual, in part because of barriers of language and distance.

Historical Aspects of Adoption

Adoption has always been a part of human history. Adoption is mentioned in the Babylonian code of Hammurabi (2285 BC) and the Hindu Laws of Manu (200 BC), and was practiced by the ancient Romans, Greeks, Egyptians, Assyrians, Chinese, and Japanese.[4] Moses is perhaps the most famous adopted person in history. Adoption has served different purposes at different times in history. In some ancient cultures, unrelated boys or young men were adopted to safeguard inheritances, preserve family names, and allow participation in religious ceremonies. Throughout history, orphaned or abandoned children often were informally adopted by relatives. The heritage of such children was known to the adoptee as well as to the community.[5] In the 1600–1700s, children who could not be cared for by their families lived alone on the streets, in almshouses or foundling hospitals, or were indentured as servants or apprentices (see Chapter 2). The composer Handel donated all the royalties from his work *The Messiah* to help fund one of the first foundling hospitals in England.[4]

In precolonial America, almshouses and indenture continued, although a few charitable organizations promoted adoption as an alternative practice. The industrial revolution by the end of the 19th century resulted in increased urbanization. The incidence of pregnancies among single women increased. Adoption expert Lois Melina writes, "Children needed families not because their mothers had died but because their mothers were single in a culture that attached enormous stigma to both the unwed mother and the illegitimate child."[5] The first U.S. adoption law was passed in Massachusetts in 1851, requiring mandatory court approval for adoptions. Similar laws were eventually passed by all states in the United States.

Nonetheless, in the early part of the 20th century, indenture contracts were still in use in some states, and adoption remained popular as a method to supplement the household labor supply.[6] In 1921, a 6-month survey of newspaper advertisements in New York City concluded that one baby was sold or casually given away every single day.[6] Thus, adoption was a means to satisfy the needs of society or a family. The adopted person often benefited but this was generally a "happy accident"[4] rather than part of the adoption plan.

Such practices are a stark contrast to modern adoption, in which the needs and interests of child are paramount. In 1891, Michigan became the first state to require investigation of potential adoptive parents. The modern adoption era began in 1912 with the formation of the U.S. Children's Bureau. This organization promoted research, conferences, and legislative reforms related to adoption. The Child Welfare League of America (CWLA), formed in 1921, provided further impetus for reform and oversight of adoption practices. Over 1000 organizations now belong to the CWLA, and its adoption standards have recently been revised for the fifth time.[7] During this era, social work emerged as a profession. In the mid-1940s adoption agencies began to charge fees for adoptive placements.[6]

Around that time, secrecy became entrenched in the world of adoption. After World War II, adoption records were sealed to preserve the privacy of the birth parents, adoptive parents, and the child. Adoption practice was characterized by attempts to match physical and religious characteristics of the child and the new parents.[8] Adoption was a secret—often a shameful one—for all involved.

Gradually, transparency began to enter adoption practices. As Korean adoptions increased the visibility of adoption in the United States, adult adoptees began to demand information about their birth families.[9] Books such as Jean Paton's *Orphan Voyage*[10] and B.J. Lifton's *Lost and Found*[11] and organizations such as the Adoptee Liberty Movement Asso-

Table 1–2 Famous Adoptees

Mark Acre (baseball player)	Jesse Jackson (political activist)
Edward Albee (playwright)	Brent Jasmer (actor)
Louisa May Alcott (writer)	Steve Jobs (cofounder of Apple Computer)
Alexander the Great	Matthew and Patrick Laborteaux (actors)
Aristotle (philosopher)	Dalai Lama
John J. Audubon (naturalist)	John Lennon (musician)
Freddie Bartholomew (actor)	Representative Jim Lightfoot (R-Ohio)
Shari Belafonte-Harper (actress)	Art Linkletter (TV personality)
Ingrid Bergman (actress)	Ray Liotta (actor)
Les Brown (motivational speaker)	Greg Louganis (diver)
Richard Burton (actor)	Malcolm X (civil rights leader)
Senator Robert Byrd (D-West Virginia)	Nelson Mandela (leader and politician)
George Washington Carver (inventor)	James Michener (writer)
President Bill Clinton	Sarah McLachlan (singer)
Nat King Cole (singer)	Marilyn Monroe (actress)
Christina Crawford (writer)	Moses (Biblical leader)
Crazy Horse (Lakota war chief)	Dan O'Brien (decathlete)
Daunte Culpepper (football player)	Jim Palmer (hall-of-fame baseball player)
Faith Daniels (TV personality)	Edgar Allen Poe (poet and writer)
Ted Danson (actor)	Priscilla Presley (actress)
Charles Dickens (writer)	Nancy Reagan (First Lady)
Eric Dickerson (football player)	Eleanor Roosevelt (First Lady)
Clarissa Pinkola Estes (writer)	Jean Jacques Rousseau (philosopher)
President Gerald Ford	Buffy Sainte-Marie (musician and actress)
Melissa and Sara Gilbert (actresses)	Dave Thomas (founder of Wendy's restaurants)
Scott Hamilton (figure skater)	Leo Tolstoy (writer)
Langston Hughes (poet and writer)	Mark Twain (writer)

Source: Data from ref. 15.

ciation (ALMA) were influential in opening debate and discussions about adoption.[5] In 1972, the legal rights of birth fathers were recognized. Organizations such as Concerned United Birthparents formed to support and advocate for birth family members. In 1975, the Children's Act allowed adopted people the right of access to their birth records (although this law is not always upheld).[8] Concurrently, behavioral researchers started to suggest that greater honesty helped children develop trust and abetted their development.[9] Research in grief and loss, such as the work done by Elisabeth Kübler-Ross, was applied by members of the adoption triad—child, birth and adoptive parents—to their own experiences. Recognition spread that adoption does not annul birth family or heritage, nor cure infertility in adoptive parents, nor induce amnesia in birth parents. Acceptance of these realities has enabled triad members to address their respective losses without shame, and has introduced much needed compassion into adoption. (More details about the history of adoption may be found in Adamec and Pierce.[4])

Adopted people are now able to access original birth records and in some cases to search for birth parents (see Chapter 34). Openness has influenced the prevailing wisdom about international adoptions as well. Whereas families were once advised to ignore their child's country of origin and ethnic heritage (even to the extent of raising Korean children as "white"), now families are encouraged to incorporate some aspects of their internationally adopted child's culture, language, and customs into daily life.

Despite these developments, more work must be done to improve the image of adoption, reduce remaining stigmas, and educate the public about the venerable place of adoption in human culture. In a survey conducted in 1997 (quoted in Pertman[9]), 90% of Americans viewed adoption positively and 95% agreed it serves a useful purpose. However, 50% stated that adoption is not quite as good as having one's own child, 25% said it is sometimes harder to love an adopted child, and nearly 33% doubted children could love adoptive parents as much as birth parents.

This study highlights our cultural biases about adoption. The American or Western conception of adoption differs from that found in many other parts of the world. For example, Pacific Islanders consider adoption a particularly revered form of family. In Tahiti, 25%–40% of all children are adopted, and families hope "to establish between parents and natural children relationships which coincide as nearly as possible with those between parents and adopted children."[12] Other cultures view adoption as a generous gesture of communal solidarity rather than a shameful act.[13] Adoption is viewed as a practice to promote societal needs rather than to fulfill the desires of individual parents. On the southwest Pacific atoll Sikaiana, about half of the children live long-term with foster parents rather than with their biologic parents.[14] Culturally, this fosterage reflects love and compassion rather than pathology and misfortune. Families prefer children to move between different households. Furthermore, many African societies do not view parenting as something exclusive to biologic parents. Thus, Western customs that emphasize exclusive care of children by one conjugal couple, preferably the biologic parents, are not universal. Western views that involvement of unrelated adults is undesirable or deviant are also culture-specific. Some anthropologists question the possible connections of these idealized Western standards to conceptions of capitalism and exclusive possession,[14] and point out the paradox of these views

in a society in which a substantial majority of young children receive out-of-home day care.

Demographics of Adoption

It is estimated that there are somewhere between 5 and 6 million adoptees in the United States today, triple the number just a few years ago.[6, 9] Counting birth parents, adoptive parents, biologic and adoptive siblings, and extended family, tens of millions of Americans are directly connected to adoption. Some experts place the number much higher, as some individuals do not know that they are adopted.[9] The Evan B. Donaldson Adoption Institute recently found that an amazing 6 out of 10 Americans have a personal connection to adoption.[9,16] This was defined as being adopted, having a family member or a close friend who was adopted, or placing a child for adoption.

Adam Pertman's lively and informative book *Adoption Nation* details how adoption is becoming deeply interwoven into our culture. Aptly subtitled *How the Adoption Revolution Is Transforming America*, this book describes the pervasive effects of adoption on all aspects of American society. As adoption has changed, so has America. The rising trend of international adoption has been an important theme in this transition. Pertman writes, "It's getting increasingly difficult to find a playground without at least one little girl from China, being watched lovingly by a white mother or father.[9] The increased visibility of multiracial families is just one way in which adoption is changing America. Recent advertisements by Kodak, Land's End, Weight Watchers, and American Express feature Caucasian parents with Chinese children.

Adoption crosses some unusual bridges: culture, race, religion, and socioeconomic status. Due to the costs and other factors, most adoptive parents are middle class or above. In a survey conducted by the U.S. General Accounting Office in 1991, the income distribution of adoptive parents (domestic adoptions) was skewed toward middle- and high-income families.[17] However, most adoptees, whether domestic or international, come from less privileged backgrounds.

Author and adoptive mother Elizabeth Bartholet, a former civil rights lawyer and current law professor, writes

My initial reaction to the adoption world was one of shock. I was familiar with a world increasingly governed by the principle that such factors as race, religion, sex, age, and handicap should not be determinative. In the adoption world, just such factors are central in deciding who gets to parent and be parented. . . . Prospective parents are rated in terms of desirability *primarily* by race, religion, marital status, age, handicap, and sexual orientation. Children are similarly rated, with race, religion, age, and handicap being key.[12]

Prospective adoptive parents are usually asked to complete a form listing disabilities they are willing to accept in their child-to-be. Bartholet wonders if this "act of discrimination" is the same as or different than excluding such an individual from employment or housing.[12] Although ethical questions remain about many adoption practices, there is no argument about the benefits of adoption for children in need of homes.

Nearly one-third of adoptive parents in the United States in 2002 were single women, according to the Children's Bureau of the U.S. Department of Health and Human Services.[18] Many adopted internationally; countries such as China, Russia, Kazakhstan, India, Romania, and Peru accept single parents of either gender (although this is subject to change). Single African American women are more likely to adopt domestically. At one agency in Oakland, 40% of placements are to single black women.[18]

Domestic Adoption

Domestic adoption statistics are surprisingly hard to find. No records of formalized adoptions are kept by any national organization or branch of government, and states vary greatly in the statistical information collected. Many adoptions occur as informal arrangements among family members—for example, grandparents assuming responsibility for their grandchildren. The numerical high point for domestic adoptions was the 1970s, when approximately 175,000 adoptions per year were legalized.[6] The National Council for Adoption Survey counted 23,537 domestic infant adoptions in 1996 out of a total of 108,463 domestic adoptions.[19] Adoptions were split equally between relatives and nonrelatives. There were 6.4 infant adoptions per 1000 live births.[19] Thus, adoption plans are made for fewer than 1% of children born in the United States and only 2% of infants born to single mothers.[12] Of more than 31,000 public adoptions monitored by the Department of Health and Human Services in 1998, nearly one third crossed racial or cultural lines—fivefold more than just a few years earlier.[9] Even more striking has been the increase in special-needs adoptions, which have more than doubled between the 1980s and 1990s (to ~20,000/year). This may reflect new classifications to determine special needs, as well as the increased availability of subsidies for these adoptions. Pertman describes "special needs" as a "euphemism applied to a range of concerns—race, age, behavioral problems, and physical disabilities—that can diminish a child's prospects for adoption.[9]" Adoptions from foster care have also increased recently, to about 50,000 in 1998. However, more than 100,000 children in foster care still await adoption.[20]

International Adoption

In comparison to domestic adoption, the annual number of international adoptions is far less: 21,666 children arrived in 2003. However, the impact of international adoption may exceed the number of children involved, partially because these adoptions are often more visible. International adoptions are increasing annually: more than 150,000 internationally adopted children have arrived in the United States since 1995, more than 120,000 of them since 1998. Trends in international adoption are easy to track; all children receive an entry visa through the Department of Immigration and Naturalization Services, which designates their status as adoptees. The numbers of such visas issued has increased drastically in the past 15 years, and countries of origin have also changed substantially (Figs. 1–4 and 1–5). The Census Bureau recently reported that 13%, or 200,000, of the nation's 1.6 million adopted children, were born outside the United States.[21,22]

International adoption by Americans has its roots in the aftermath of World War II and the Korean War. Between 1948 and 1953, Americans adopted 5814 children from Germany, Italy, Greece, and other war-torn countries of Europe, along with 2418 Asian children, mostly from Japan.[3,9] Harry and Bertha Holt, residents of Oregon, provided further impetus for international adoption. Dismayed by the plight of biracial children left in Korea by American soldiers, the Holts not only adopted eight homeless Amerasian children (to add to their family of six birth children) but also successfully lobbied Congress to establish uniform procedures for adopting from other countries. Those laws, established in 1955, remain the legal basis for international adoption by Americans today.

Trends in country of origin reflect global and national political and economic changes. In general, as economic circumstance improve in individual countries, adoption by foreigners diminishes. Pertman succinctly states, "Countries don't like to give up their children any more than parents do. . . . increases in the outflow of children from a particular country [are] a strong hint that something has gone wrong."[9] Among the examples he cites are civil strife in Central America and Africa, the devaluation of girls in China, and overpopulation in India. One author links patterns of U.S. international adoption to the consequences of U.S. covert operations and Cold War activities.[23]

In most sending countries, international adoption is tolerated at best. The practice of international adoption may be viewed as an odd form of colonialism in which wealthy Westerners rob poor countries of their children and thus their resources.[12] In efforts to preserve national pride or to remove real or perceived abuses and corruption, international adoption is sometimes halted. Such political maneuvers may indeed benefit waiting children if local families are encouraged to adopt, and if waiting children receive better care and supervision. However, reducing or delaying international adoptions more often prolongs the wait of children for families.

Worldwide, the United States is the largest receiving country for international adoptees. Canada and European and Scandinavian countries also receive children from other countries (Table 1–3). The Scandinavian countries re-

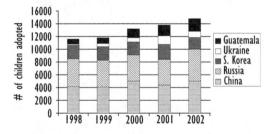

Figure 1–4 *Numbers of children adopted from the "top 5" sending countries, 1998–2002. (Data from www.travel.state.gov/orphan.)*

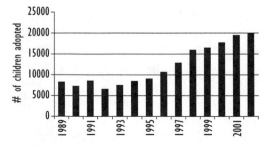

Figure 1–5 *Trends in international adoption by American families, 1989–2002. (Data from www.travel.state.gov/orphan.)*

Table 1-3 Numbers of internationally adopted children arriving 1993-7

Receiving country	1993-97
Canada	9670[a]
France	16,080
Italy	10,237
Netherlands	3199
Sweden	4530
Switzerland	3804
United States	50,349
Total	97,869

[a]Estimate; total is thought to be higher.

Source: Data from Cantwell.[3]

ceive disproportionate numbers of internationally adopted children (Table 1–4). In Norway, about 1% of the annual birth rate consists of children adopted transnationally, the highest rate in the world.[24] In Sweden, with a population of 8.8 million people, 40,000 children have been adopted from other countries since the 1960s.[3] Canadians adopt about 2000 children a year, roughly the same proportion of international adoptions for the population as in the United States,[25] Interestingly, most Canadian international adoptions take place in Quebec, where the rate is threefold that in the United States. Although not often discussed, about 100 American children are adopted by Canadians every year.[25] These children, mostly boys, are

Table 1-4 Adoption rate per 100,000 population (1999)

Country	Rate
Norway	14.6[a]
Denmark	13.0
Sweden	11.5
New Zealand	10.0
Iceland	8.3
Switzerland	8.0
France	6.0
United States	5.9
Netherlands	5.8
Italy	3.8
Finland	2.9
United Kingdom	0.5

[a]1998.[28]

Source: Data from Adoption/Medical News.[27]

often of mixed race and have physical or other special needs. The United States ranks sixth among countries sending children to Canada. In addition, a small number of healthy white American infants are placed each year with wealthy Western Europeans.[9] Although no statistics are kept (as exit visas are not required), it is estimated that about 500 American children each year are adopted in Australia, Europe, and Canada.[3]

Other major receiving countries include Austria, Ireland, Germany, United Kingdom, Israel, and Belgium, but in these nations detailed, centralized data about international adoptions are not collected. All receiving countries report annual increases in the numbers of intercountry adoptions. Some special links exist between sending and receiving countries. For example, adoptive parents in Spain choose children from Colombia, India, and China, Italian parents prefer children from Romania, Brazil, or Russia, and Malaysian parents tend to adopt Thai children.[3]

Legally, Europe has followed the lead of the United States in adoption. In England, the first adoption laws were passed in 1926. In 1959, adopted children in Sweden first acquired legal rights of full-fledged family members. Germany did not pass modern adoption laws until 1977.[4] Trends in international adoption in Europe also appear to follow experience in the United States.

In Finland from 1985 to 1998, 1259 children were adopted internationally, including 356 from Russia, 244 from Colombia, and 189 from Thailand.[24] In Spain there were 3022 international adoptions in 2000, from Colombia, China, India, Romania, and Nicaragua.[26] Children from Guatemala and Russia are being adopted with increasing frequency in Spain.[26]

Recently, the number of girls adopted internationally in the United States exceeded boys by nearly twofold (e.g., 4077 males and 7236 females in 1996), likely reflecting the large proportion of children arriving from China (see Chapter 3).[29]

International adoption has become firmly established in America. Every year, more families embrace multicultural and multinational heritages (Fig. 1–6). Most families welcome this role and see themselves as "bridge-builders between the nations."[12] Or as an adoptive parent in Pertman's book states, "We've become, unwittingly, educators in adoption and tolerance."[9] Cheri Register[30] writes that internationally adopting families find "deeper roots than we knew, an enlarged sense of family, another place in the heart." Thus, a dual heritage is seen "not as confusing, but life-enhancing."[12]

International adoption appeals to prospective parents with a wide variety of backgrounds, including single parents, couples with primary or secondary infertility, or parents with birth children who wish to expand their families. Some parents turn to international adoption after the death of birth children. Brian Rohrbough, whose son was killed in the shootings at Columbine High School, said, "Even as Columbine made us think that we lost a child and it cost us this much pain, we knew it would be just as hard for a child who has lost a parent."[31] The Rohrboughs adopted two children from Ukraine. Another family whose 14-year-old daughter died of leukemia adopted 8- and 10-year old brothers from Russia. "We wished to honor our daughter by this adoption; she taught us how much we enjoyed being parents" (personal communication). Particular reasons for selection of international adoption are discussed below (Process of International Adoption for Parents, Ethics and International Adoption).

Legal Aspects of International Adoption

The Hague Convention on Intercountry Adoption

The legal aspects of international adoption are complex and arcane (reviewed in Cantwell,[3] Herman,[6] Masson,[32] and Varnis[33]). Adoptive parents, like Elizabeth Bartholet, may feel that "the law is something that functions primarily to prevent good things from happening."[12] The cumbersome, outdated, nonstandardized legal process of international adoption has ample room for improvement in both sending and receiving countries. President Clinton's signing of The Hague Convention on Protection of Children and Co-operation in Respect of Intercountry Adoption on October 6, 2000, represented a major step toward redressing some of the legal problems in international adoption in the United States. This document, on which work began in 1988, was adopted unanimously by all 66 states attending The Hague Convention in 1993 and possesses full force of international law. The indisputable tenets of the Convention are to ensure (1) that the interests of the child are foremost in the adoption process, (2) that intercountry adoption is only considered in the case of a child for whom a suitable family cannot be found in his or her state of origin, and (3) that abuses associated with intercountry adoption are eliminated. The Convention man-

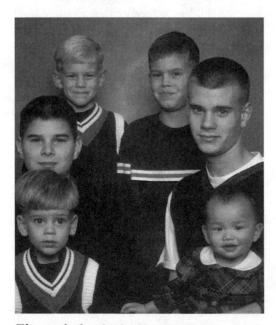

Figure 1–6 *After five birth sons, a Chinese daughter joins the family. (With permission.)*

dates that each signatory nation designate a central authority to oversee international adoption. In the United States, this authority is the Office of Children's Issues in the Consular Affairs Bureau of the State Department.[34] This office is instructed to reduce bureaucratic and legal barriers to adoption, prevent exploitation of birth parents, oversee the accreditation of agencies and individuals offering or providing adoption services, prevent improper financial gains, protect the rights of children, make annual reports to Congress, and maintain a registry of incoming and outgoing adoptions. It is expected that at least some aspects of the Hague Convention will be implemented in the United States sometime in 2004.[35] Full legal compliance with the Hague Convention may eventually incorporate provisions to extend immediate citizenship to children adopted by American parents, ending the need for specialized visa processing for these children.

In Europe, Hague-imposed regulations have promoted the emergence of networks (such as Euradopt) that facilitate international adoptions. In the United Kingdom and The Netherlands, only licensed adoption agencies may oversee international adoptions.[32] In anticipation of or in compliance with Hague Convention regulations, some sending countries now require that follow-up reports be submitted by adoptive families, for 10 years by Sri Lanka, 4 years by Peru, 3 years by Paraguay, and 2 years by Romania.[36]

Critics of the Hague Convention point out that the new bureaucratic requirements and associated costs may actually decrease the number of adoptions and will not reduce the number of children without families.[33] Furthermore, reliance on a central authority to oversee adoptions will not forestall all difficulties: similar government organizations did not halt corruption and delays due to judicial strikes in Peru, weak enforcement and abuse in Brazil, involvement of senior government officials in baby-selling schemes in Honduras, and inadequate government supervision in Sri Lanka.[33]

As with other codes of international law, enforcement is problematic. For example, Human Rights Watch reports that the Russian Federation, a signatory of the United Nations International Convention on the Rights of the Child, violates 20 of the first 41 articles of this document in its policies dealing with abandoned children.[33]

International Adoptees and U.S. Citizenship

On February 27, 2001, at Boston's historic Fanueil Hall, a celebration was held to mark the passage of the Child Citizen Act of 2000. This legislation, sponsored by leaders of the Congressional Coalition on Adoption, grants automatic U.S. citizenship to all international adoptees as they enter the United States as lawful permanent residents. For those who enter the United States on IR-4 visas (to be adopted in the United States), citizenship is bestowed when the adoption is finalized in an American state court. The Child Citizen Act was developed in part to prevent problems like those experienced by John Gaul, who was adopted at age 4 years from Thailand.[9] After conviction as a teenager for car theft and credit card fraud, Gaul was deported to Thailand under a 1996 law requiring deportation of any noncitizen found guilty of a felony. His parents had mistakenly neglected to apply for his U.S. citizenship after the adoption. Although he did not speak the language and knew no one in Thailand, Gaul was deported there in 1999. Similarly, non-citizen adoptees are theoretically liable for military service in their birth countries if they have not become naturalized U.S. citizens.

Entry into the United States for International Adoptees

Visas for entry to the United States are overseen by the Bureau of Citizenship and Immigration Services (formerly Immigration and Naturalization Services).[34] These visas are granted to internationally adopted children after approval of an Orphan Petition form, known as either an I-600 or I-600 A (described in INS Document M249Y and Form M-349). The I-600 is used when a specific child has been identified by the parents; the I-600A is used when a specific child has not yet been identified or the parents plan to travel overseas to identify a child (once the child is identified, an I-600 form must be approved). For purposes of this petition, a foreign child is considered an orphan if the parents have died or disappeared, if they have unconditionally abandoned or deserted the child, or if he or she is separated or lost from them. Abandonment normally involves permanent placement in an orphanage. An orphan immigrant visa petition must by filed before the child is 16 years of age. After consular review, an entry visa will be issued. Either an IR-3 (adopted abroad and then brought to the United States) or IR-4 (brought to the United States for the purpose of adoption) visa permits the child to enter the United States. Under unusual circumstances, children who do not qualify as orphans may be adopted. These nonorphan adoptees may not enter the United States until they have resided abroad with the adoptive parents for at least 2 years.

Some countries simply grant guardianship to the adopting parent(s) and permit the child to depart with the understanding that the adoption will be completed after arrival in the receiving country. A few countries allow adoptive parents to adopt through a third party without actually traveling to that country. Most countries, however, require a formal court hearing to approve the adoption of the child by foreigners.

In most cases, the formal adoption of a child in a foreign court is legally acceptable in the United States. It is strongly recommended, however, that the child adopted abroad be re-adopted in a court of his or her state of residence in the United States after arrival. Following this re-adoption, parents may request that a state birth certificate be issued. In some instances, re-adoption of the child in the United States is required, for example, if the adoptive parent (or one of a married couple) did not see the child prior to or during the adoption proceedings abroad. The child must be re-adopted in the United States in such circumstances, even if a full final adoption decree has been issued in the foreign country (for more information and country specifics, see ref. 34).

Ethics and International Adoption

Ethical concerns are paramount in adoption; the involvement of another country intensifies these complexities. Some American parents prefer international adoption because of perceptions of insurmountable obstacles and delays in domestic adoption, humanitarian impulses to "rescue" a child, and less stringent eligibility requirements.[33] However, international adoption has become a lucrative profit-making business: at roughly $20,000 per adoption, it is worth more than $300 million annually. As a business, children may come to be treated as commodities.[3] In the sending country, national (economic) interest rather than the needs of the child propels the process.[33] Countries may view their ability to satisfy the foreign demand for children as a means to garner needed cash resources from abroad.[33]

With large sums of money involved, abduction, baby-selling, trafficking, bribery, and corruption may occur (Table 1–5). These criminal activities and other abuses have been documented in many circumstances related to international adoption. Other high-risk situations for adoption malpractice include periods of emergencies (e.g., Operation Babylift in Vietnam—many children were mistakenly considered orphans),[3] armed conflict, disasters, economic crisis, and sociopolitical upheaval. Ethical concerns relate to disregard for children's rights as established in the United Na-

Table 1–5 Abuses in intercountry adoption

Circumventing the law
Illegally obtaining children for adoption
    Abduction of infants
    Pressuring vulnerable birth mothers
    Falsely informing the mother about stillbirth or death
        of her infant
    Exchange of child for financial or material rewards
    Offering women financial incentives to conceive
    Providing deliberately misleading information to
        birth families
    Providing false information to prospective adoptive
        parents
Illegally securing permission to adopt
    Falsifying certificates to adopt
    Corruption of judges and officials to accept false
        documents
Illegally avoiding the adoption process
    Making false maternity declarations
    Taking a child through a third country

Source: Data from Cantwell[3]

tions (UN) charter, questionable legalities, an absence of choice for birth parents, an often flagrant disregard of what is known to be best for children, and the absence of an ethical base for adoption practices.[37]

    Many philosophical and practical objections to the practice of international adoption have been proclaimed. Some individuals believe that international adoption is unacceptable under any conditions, as it undermines the development of local resources that would benefit large numbers of children to focus on a few children whose adoptions generate excessive remuneration.[32] Another argument against international adoption is that it discriminates against less privileged local families who might wish to adopt.[32] For example, in Guatemala, local families have difficulty "competing" with the material resources of foreigners who wish to adopt.[3] Concerns about "neocolonialism," the exploitation of the human capital of poor countries, loss of national assets, and implied admission of national failure[33] have also been raised. Finally, some have expressed concern about

possible racial and ethnic discrimination against the children in their new country.[33] Those in favor of international adoption simply state that it aids individual children in desperate need of families.

    In the middle ground are those who recognize the pressing need for improvements in international adoption practices, as well as the validity of arguments both for and against international adoption. Few disagree that far more needs to be done in countries of origin to prevent abandonment, to develop a range of child care and family support services, and to improve the quality of institutional care.[32] It is imperative to address the economic and educational levels of impoverished populations, to reverse the devalued status of women and girls, to promote responsible paternity, to decrease the stigma of a disabled child, and to augment structures within communities to support families and children (especially those with disabilities).[3] Alternative care arrangements should be explored; institutionalization should not be sustained to preserve the economic livelihoods of caregivers and other orphanage staff. Rather, substitute employment opportunities should be developed.

    Unfortunately, many countries lack adequate structures, financial means, personnel, and trained professionals to support families in crisis. Nonetheless, family reintegration should be supported, or domestic adoption promoted.[3] As mandated by the Hague Convention on Intercountry Adoption, national solutions should be sought. India provides a successful example of this: the Central Adoption Resource Center requires that at least 50% of children assigned to adoption agencies must be placed domestically. This policy has increased domestic adoption fourfold.[3] Sending and receiving countries should recognize that an expanding demand for adoption does not increase the number of children for whom adoption overseas is necessarily the best solution.[32]

    For those children placed in international adoptions, ethical criteria for adoption practices must be strengthened and enforced.[3] Agencies need to make long-term commitments to children whose adoptions they arrange, the adults who adopt them, and the parents who relinquish them.[32] All may need support for many years. Preeminent among these goals is the need—or right—of all children for a family life rather than institutional existence. Unfortunately, validation of this need has not yet attained international recognition.[33]

Legalities and the Pediatrician

Pediatricians and other care providers should be aware of the legal status of internationally adopted children. Disagreements about needed medical care are rare between parents and pediatricians. However, in the unlikely event of such a disagreement, the care provider should ascertain the legal status of the adoption. Depending on the country of origin, (one or both) parents may not have completed adoption proceedings in the birth country, or re-adoption in the United States may be incomplete. Children from India, Korea, and occasionally Romania and other countries may enter the United States without being adopted; some arrive via escorts. In these cases, the prospective adoptive parents or the adoption agency is awarded guardianship until the adoption is finalized in the United States. Gay or lesbian couples usually designate one partner to complete initial adoption proceedings; the second parent may later choose to adopt the child as well, gaining equal legal authority.

The Process of International Adoption for Families

The process of international adoption is circuitous, laborious, and complex. Virtually every family experiences difficulties, delays, frustrations, and uncertainty. The process may take years longer than anticipated. For some

parents, this follows a lengthy and discouraging period of infertility treatment. Eventually children and parents join as a family, but many describe the procedure as "excruciating," "torture," or "Byzantine" (Fig. 1–7). For some families, the process is smooth, but these are the exceptions. The expectant adoptive parent must be treated with sensitivity and compassion. The pediatrician's empathy for the prospective parent's frustration and anxiety prior to and during the adoption can be a source of comfort and provide a solid basis for an ongoing therapeutic relationship after the child arrives (see Chapter 4).

The process of international adoption begins when prospective parents identify a state-licensed adoption agency or independent adoption facilitator. (Residents of four states, Colorado, Delaware, Connecticut, and Massachusetts, are only permitted to use agencies). Careful selection of the agency or individual facilitator is of utmost importance. Ethical values and practices, honesty, moral values, experience, and reputation are crucial points for prospective clients to consider. The agency or facilitator's personal approach, ability to communicate, and openness to parental questions and concerns are vital during the often arduous and stressful process of international adoption.

Agencies or facilitators may provide various services; sometimes certain activities are provided by supplementary agencies or individuals. The general purpose of the agencies is to match available children to carefully screened, suitable parents. There are hundreds of agencies in the United States that place children by international adoption. Agencies vary vastly in their experience: in a survey of agencies that placed a randomly selected group of 200 children in 1991, the number of annual international adoptions facilitated by the agencies ranged from 0 to 540 (median 21, mean 42).[17]

Some agencies specialize in particular countries, others offer programs in multiple countries. In addition to placement of the child, agencies may also provide home studies (see below), parent support groups, in-country support services for parents who travel to collect their child (including in some cases an accompanying physician, see Chapter 9), and other pre- and post-adoption services. Fees vary widely depending on country, program, and other factors (Table 1–6). It is difficult to compare agency fees, as included services vary enormously. Adoption costs may be offset for some families with employee benefits such as adoption subsidies and tax credits ($5000–$6000 depending on adjusted gross income).

Families who wish to adopt internationally quickly realize that their personal characteristics limit their choices regarding their prospective child's country of origin and other characteristics (such as age). State of residence determines whether a private adoption is possible or if an agency must be involved. Age, marital status, religion, financial status, and other factors determine which countries and which programs will accept the prospective international adoptive parents' application.

Table 1–6 Sample fees for international adoption

Service or Agency	Fee ($ U.S.)
"Home study" or pre- and post-adoptive counseling for adoptive parents, including reporting for country of origin	3600
Legal fees (U.S. and abroad)	1000–3000
Travel and related costs	2000–10,000
Translation, government fees, etc.	500–1000
Fees to foreign agencies, governments	500–5000
U.S. agency direct costs	2000–5000
Direct costs (range)	9600–27,600
Indirect costs (range)	3840–11, 040
Total costs (range)	13,440–38,640

Source: From Marshner (1999).[38]

Prospective adoptive parents must participate in a "home study," an important part of the dossier needed in an international adoption. The home study is a detailed document prepared by a licensed social worker. This may by prepared by the same placing agency, a specialized home study agency, or a different professional.

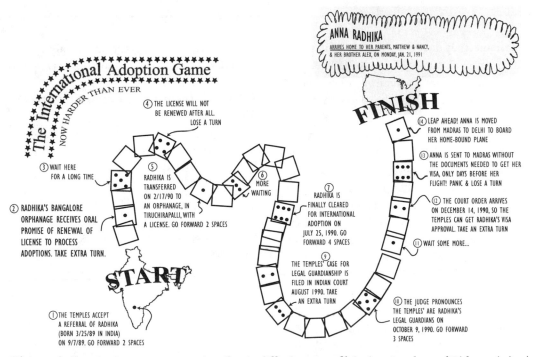

Figure 1–7 *Adoption announcement describes the difficult process of bringing Anna home. (With permission.)*

Andrea's parents fell in love with the cute 3-year-old Romanian with big brown eyes and a serious expression when they saw her face on a Web site listing waiting children. The listing stated that Andrea was healthy except for "typical developmental delays of a child living in an orphanage." They immediately claimed her as their daughter and arranged, for an additional fee of $50/week, to transfer her to foster care. Their facilitator assured them that the foster care was excellent. The family began to become alarmed about Andrea and her situation when they viewed a 20-minute video of their daughter-to-be, now 3½ years old, in her foster home. Andrea appeared extremely busy and unable to focus on any offered toys or activities for more than 5 seconds. She made no vocalizations other than grunting. She showed no signs of affection and minimal eye contact with the foster mother, although they had now lived together for nearly 6 months. The foster mother admitted, when pressed, that Andrea had some difficult behaviors, but adamantly stated that she was showing many signs of improvement and indeed had started to talk, show affection, and make good eye contact. The prospective parents maintained their commitment to Andrea as the legal process to complete her adoption dragged on. More positive reports arrived, along with a new video showing a "transformed Andrea" playing quietly with dolls and chatting in short phrases with her foster mother. A few months later, adoptions in Romania were halted to "correct abuses" in the system. After several more months, the adoption agency advised the family that they were ceasing operations in Romania, and that it would no longer be possible to support Andrea in foster care. She returned to a new orphanage, where she resided in horrendous conditions for the next 2 years. When the ban on adoptions was finally lifted, her parents were amazed to get a call from another agency who had located Andrea and found their name in her files. Did they still want her? They did, and within a few weeks they traveled to get her. When they met her, their hearts broke. Though still the beautiful child with big brown eyes, Andrea, now 6 years old, had regressed to worse condition than she'd been in at age 3. She had no language except grunts, would frequently bite or scratch herself so severely that she drew blood, and bang her head on the floor or wall at the slightest stress. She would frequently "space out" and appear to be hallucinating. She seemed to have no awareness of people around her or her environment. Her parents seriously questioned whether to proceed with the adoption, but felt unable to leave her in the orphanage. "She improved before," they reasoned, "we hope she can improve again. But why did she have to wait for so long and in such bad conditions when we were ready to receive her 3 years ago?"

The home study document extensively describes the prospective family (Table 1–7). The document is prepared after several visits between the prospective parent(s) and the social worker, including home visits to inspect the premises. Official documents often include sections to verify that the prospective family has running water and indoor plumbing, as well as an adequate physical environment for child-rearing. During the home study, prospective parents must also assemble a wealth of personal information (Table 1–8).[39] These documents must all be notarized in the state in which they were issued, and the notary's seal must also be authenticated. Some countries require federal authentication of documents. A psychiatrist must attest to the mental health of the prospective parent(s), a physician must attest to physical health, and clergy, colleagues, and friends must provide general recommendations of the prospective parent(s) capabilities. Becoming an adoptive parent requires

Table 1–7 Documents required for most home studies

Birth certificate
Marriage certificate, if applicable
Divorce/death certificate, if applicable
Statement from local police and from FBI
Psychiatrist's statement
Physician's report
Recommendations of clergy
Recommendations of community members
Financial statement
1040-front two pages
Verification of employment
Child abuse clearance
Police certificate
Fingerprint clearance
Photographs of the family

Source: Data from Hostetter and Johnson.[39]

Table 1–8 Topics addressed in home study

Motivation for adoption
Capacities and attitudes
Personal relationships and personality
Marriage
Health, age, nationality, race
Employment, finances, financial net worth
Religious, moral, and ethical beliefs and practices
Education
Environment
Child-rearing practices
Family interactions
Cultural issues

Source: Data from Hostetter and Johnson.[39]

a trip to the local police station to provide fingerprints, which are forwarded to the FBI. Although difficult, cumbersome, and lengthy, these procedures are intended to screen the prospective parent(s) for obvious physical, emotional, or practical difficulties that would impair their ability to provide a loving home for the child and to provide safeguards for the well-being of the adopted child. It has been suggested that all prospective parents (not just adoptive parents) should undergo such a screening process prior to being allowed to receive a child!

As prospective parents collect the necessary documents and participate in the home study, they select a country and sometimes also a particular program for their adoption. After the dossier of documents is completed, notarized, authenticated, and translated, it is forwarded to the appropriate authorities in the chosen country. The dossier is reviewed and, eventually, after a period from weeks to years, a "referral" is offered to the prospective parent(s) (see Chapter 4). Once the child is accepted by the prospective parent(s), travel arrangements are made. Children from India or Korea (or rarely Romania) may be escorted to the United States after the adoptive parent(s) are designated legal guardians in the country of origin. Most parents, however, travel to receive their child (see Chapters 4 and 9). Some parents are told to travel with large amounts of cash (as

much as $20,000), which is then distributed to various individuals and institutions connected with the adoption in their child's birth country. Accounts of hair-raising trips abound in the adoption literature.[9, 12] Many parents report uneasy feelings and suspicions that some of these transactions are illicit and illegal. (See "The Money's the Problem" in Pertman's[9]) for a full discussion of this important issue.)

Adoption Terminology

Adoption language has evolved over the past decade to reflect the growing recognition that labels matter (Table 1–9). Previous terminology was often "subtly hurtful to individuals involved in adoption."[1] Although arguments may be made about some of these distinctions, such a list may stimulate useful and enlightening discussion. As other authors have done[40] the term *adoptee* is used in this book for its brevity and not in any way to demean or depersonalize the adopted individual. Furthermore, the terms *abandonment* and *abandoned child*, and *foundling* are sometimes used. Sadly, this is the very real situation for many internationally adopted children, in contrast to most domestic adoptions in which a careful plan is made.

Adoption and the Internet

The Internet has revolutionized the availability of information and, consequently, many aspects of adoption as well. Use of the Internet affects the way in which adoptions take place, families' preparation for adoption, and communication and awareness after adoption.[41] A Google search resulted in more than 7.5 million matches for the term *adoption* and nearly 2 million matches for the term *international adoption*. As broad categories, these sites include information on the adoption process, adoption agencies (including photolistings of thousands of children in need of adoption), media reports,

Liza's parents hoped to receive a court date to travel to Kazakhstan to collect their daughter in October. They received no word from their agency until after New Year's. They were distraught to learn that the court in Liza's region had put all international adoptions on hold. The agency shared their pessimism that the region would open again soon. Sadly, the family tried to put Liza out of their hearts, and indeed adopted Jill from Russia. Two years later, their agency called with the news that the region was reopened, and they had located Liza. This time the adoption was completed within a few weeks, and she returned to the United States. She had barely grown in the intervening 2 years. They learned that she had spent several months in a hospital with respiratory infections and had received multiple parenteral medications and blood transfusions. Blood tests in the United States showed that Liza had active hepatitis B and hepatitis C infections.

and countless reports of individuals' experiences with adoption. Although the power of sharing information via the Internet and the importance of publicizing the needs of waiting children are unquestioned, it is disquieting to view Web sites with subtitles such as "Your source for children" or "See photolistings of available children." Education of prospective adoptive families about the complexities of adoption and other necessary parent preparation may be bypassed or minimized if crucial stages of the process are relegated to impersonal contact via the Internet. A considerable amount of solid factual information is available on-line, but incorrect, misleading, and even fraudulent material may also be published. Prospective parents anxious to receive a child may be susceptible to unscrupulous individuals who promise quick "delivery" of a child and short-cuts to completion of an adoption.

International adoptions have been particularly affected by the Internet. Technology is evolving rapidly; what was once unthinkable is now commonplace. Use of e-mail has accelerated communication between prospective parents, adoption agencies, and facilitators and orphanage staff in birth countries. Digital images

and videos may be sent easily. Many parents frequently communicate via the Internet with medical professionals or other advisors when meeting their prospective child, asking for analysis of medical and developmental information, and review of photos or videos. This technology continues to emerge; future prospects include real-time interactive video assessments, among other possibilities.

International Adoption and Health Insurance

It is unusual to address health insurance in a medical textbook. However, some special issues related to internationally adopted children should be described. Many children may arrive with "pre-existing" conditions, including such problems as congenital heart disease, neurobehavioral disturbances, or chronic hepatitis B. It is illegal for health insurance providers and other third-party payors to discriminate against these children after a legal adoption has been accomplished. It is nonetheless sensible for parents to verify the extent of coverage of their prospective child with their individual insurance carrier prior to completion of the adoption, especially if special medical needs have been identified.

Federal law mandates that states must provide consistent health care to all children within their borders. This includes internationally adopted children as well. Some parents sign a Bureau of Citizenship and Immigration Services waiver prior to receiving a visa for their child to speed the visa process. This waiver releases the state, however, from financial liability for the health care for the child. For children who are severely disabled or infected with human immunodeficiency virus (HIV), the adoptive family must provide certain documents to the Centers for Disease Control Office of Quarantine. This includes an affidavit that parents understand the medical condition of their child, proof of adequate financial resources (health insurance), and an affidavit of

Table 1–9 Adoption Vocabulary

Type of Term	Preferred	Discouraged
Terms for members of adoption triad	Adoption triad (signals relatedness of all parties) Adoption circle Adoption family tapestry	Adoption triangle (negative connotations—"love triangle," "three's a crowd")
Terms for parents	Birth parents, birthgivers, genetic parents, first parents Parents of the adopted child Adoptive parents	Biological parents Real parents Natural parents (are adoptive parents unnatural?) Blood relative Not the real parents
Terms for adopted individuals	Son, daughter, person, or individual who was adopted "My son is an American of Korean descent"; "I'm an American, I was born in Korea" Children in need of adoption Child born outside of marriage Child who has special needs Orphan	"Korean son" or "Colombian daughter" (would we say "my Austrian wife" or "my Irish husband"?) Children available for adoption Illegitimate child Hard-to-place child; special needs child Abandoned child, foundling (some feel the latter term is acceptable as it emphasizes the kindness of the person who found the child)
Type of adoption	International or intercountry adoption	Foreign adoption
Terms for decision-making process	Retain/transfer parental rights and obligations Move in, join, come to be part of Unplanned Release parental rights Make an adoption plan, agree to adoption	"To keep" or "not to keep" Placed, put up for adoption Adopt out Unwanted Relinquish, surrender
Terms for communication	Sharing information Seeking contact, requesting information Meeting Adoptive family	Telling Search (connotes illegal, daring, exciting activity) Reunion (misleading if child was adopted as a newborn) Adoptive home (much more than a home is provided)

Source: Modified from Spencer.[1]

The N family received an e-mail from their agency with the exciting news that a child in Russia had been assigned to them. Attached were several photos of the infant. They forwarded the information to Dr. J., who offered a list of suggested questions and a request for more photos to assess the child for features of fetal alcohol syndrome. A few days later, the N family received the information, which they again forwarded to Dr. J. Everything looked promising, so the referral was accepted. Updated photos were sent by the facilitator a month later. Several months later, the family was invited to travel to Russia to begin the adoption process. While there, they again sent information and photos to Dr. J to review, and daily (or more frequent) e-mails were exchanged as new information was provided and the family had more time with the infant. A short video clip was also sent. The Ns returned home to wait for the final court date. During the 3-month wait, they received four sets of treasured photos of their daughter and frequent short updates about her condition.

a U.S. physician promising to treat the child. Parents who sign the waiver may be haunted by that decision when their insurance coverage and savings run out.[42,43]

An additional consideration relates to billing codes for services provided to internationally adopted children in the United States. At present, there are no specific ICD-10 codes that adequately capture the complexity of services required by this special population of children. It is hoped that the insurance industry will recognize the medical and developmental evaluations needed by this group of children and will provide appropriate billing codes to allow physician reimbursement for services.

References

1. Spencer M. Adoption vocabulary: a guide to correct terminology. In: Marshner C, Pierce WL, eds. Adoption Factbook III. Waite Park, MN: National Council for Adoption, 1999: 12–17.

2. Pavao JM. Kinds of Adoption. Cambridge, MA: Center for Family Connections, 1997.

3. Cantwell N. Intercountry Adoption. Innocenti Digest, Vol. 4. Florence, Italy: UNICEF International Child Development Centre, 1998: 1–24.

4. Adamec C, Pierce WL. The Encyclopedia of Adoption. New York: Facts on File, 1991.

5. Melina L. Recent history of adoption practices. Available at: http://www.parentsplace.com/fertility/adoptioncentral/articles/0,,166265_253077-1,00.html.

6. Herman E. The paradoxical rationalization of modern adoption. J Soc Hist 2002; 36:339.

7. Child Welfare League of America. Available at: http://www.cwla.org/.

8. Pavao JM. The Family of Adoption. Boston: Beacon Press, 1998.

9. Pertman A. Adoption Nation: How the Adoption Revolution is Transforming America. New York: Basic Books, 2000.

10. Paton JM. Orphan Voyage. New York: Vantage Press, 1968.

11. Lifton BJ. Lost and Found: The Adoption Experience. New York: Dial Press, 1979.

12. Bartholet E. Family Bonds: Adoption, Infertility, and the New World of Child Production. Boston: Beacon Press, 1993.

13. Leon IG. Adoption losses: naturally occurring or socially constructed? Child Dev 2002; 73:652.

14. Donner WW. Sharing and compassion: fosterage in Polynesian society. J Comp Fam Stud 1999; 30:703.

15. National Adoption Awareness Month Guide: North American Council on Adoptable Children, 1999/2000. Available at: http://www.nacac.org

16. Evan B. Donaldson Adoption Institute. Benchmark Adoption Survey: Report on Findings. New York: Evan B. Donaldson Adoption Institute, 1997.

17. Smith C. Intercountry adoption experiences of Americans. In: Marshner C, Pierce WL, eds. Adoption Factbook III. Waite Park, MN: National Council for Adoption, 1999: 524–428.

18. Gardner M. One plus one makes a family. Christian Science Monitor. March 19, 2003: 15–9.

19. Placek PJ. National Adoption Data. In: Marshner C, Pierce WL, eds. Adoption Factbook III. Waite Park, MN: National Council for Adoption, 1999:

20. Child Welfare League of American. Foster care. Fact and Figures. Available at: http://www.cwla.org/programs/fostercare/factsheet.htm.

21. Peterson K. Census counts adoptee: 1.6 million kids. USA Today, August 22, 2003:1A.

22. U.S. Census Bureau. U.S. Census 2000. Available at: http://www.census.gov/population. 2002.

23. Gailey CW. Race, class, and gender in US international adoption. In: Rygvold A-L, Dalen M, Saetersdal B, eds. Mine–Yours–Ours and Theirs. Oslo: University of Oslo, 1999: 52–81.

24. Howell S. Biologizing and de-biologizing kinship. In: Rygvold A-L, Dalen M, Saetersdal B, eds. Mine—yours—ours and theirs. Oslo: University of Oslo, 1999: 32–51.

25. Cavanaugh D. The emerging relationship between the US and Canada. In: Marshner C, Pierce WL, eds. Adoption Factbook III. Waite Park, MN: National Council for Adoption, 1999: 549–552.

26. Allué X. Adopciones transnacionales. Cuestiones médicas y éticas. Anal Esp Pediatr 2000; 53:21–4.

27. Intercountry adoptions per capita. Adoption/Medical News 2003; 9:11.

28. Selman P. The demography of intercountry adoption. In: Rygvold A-L, Dalen M, Saetersdal B, eds. Mine—Yours—Ours and Theirs. Oslo: University of Oslo, 1999: 230–46.

29. U.S. Immigration and Naturalization Service. Statistical yearbook of the INS, 1996. Washington, DC: U.S. Government Printing Office, 1997: 59.

30. Register C. Are Those Kids Yours? American Families with Children Adopted from Other Countries. New York: Free Press, 1991.

31. Associated Press. 3 families adopt after Columbine. Newsday. Sept 29, 2003: A2

32. Masson J. Intercountry adoption: a global problem or a global solution? J Int Affairs Aff 2001; 55:141.

33. Varnis SL. Regulating the global adoption of children. Society 2001; 38:39.

34. U.S. Department of State, Office of Children's Issues. International adoptions. Available at: http://travel.state.gov/int'ladoption.html.

35. Hague Convention on Intercountry Adoption. Available at: http://travel.state.gov/hagueinfo2002.html.

36. Jacot M. Adoption: for love or money? UNESCO Courier 1999: 37–41.

37. Triseliotis J. Inter-country adoption: global trade or global gift? In: Rygvold A-L, Dalen M, Saetersdal B, eds. Mine—Yours—Ours and Theirs. Oslo: University of Oslo, 1999: 14–31.

38. Marshner C. The expenses of adoption. In: Marshner C, Pierce WL, eds. Adoption Factbook III. Waite Park, MN: National Council for Adoption, 1999: 452–54.

39. Hostetter M, Johnson DE. International adoption. An introduction for physicians [see comments]. Am J Dis Child 1989; 143:325–32.

40. Brodzinsky DM, Schecter MD, Henig RM. Being Adopted. New York: Anchor Books, 1993.

41. Adamec C. Adoption and the Internet. In: Marshner C, Pierce WL, eds. Adoption Factbook III. Waite Park, MN: National Council for Adoption, 1999: 405–7.

42. Nicholson LA. Adoption medicine and the internationally adopted child. Am J Law & Med 2002; 28: 473–91.

43. Jenista JA. The visa medical examination: the facts. Available at: http://www.fwcc.org/visamedical.html.

I

BEFORE THE ADOPTION

2

THE EFFECTS OF INSTITUTIONALIZATION ON CHILDREN

[T]he collecting of many little children under one roof is not good for them, no matter how well managed the institution.[1]

The unit of civilization is the family which offers the healthiest physical environment. The most susceptible member of the family to all external conditions is the infant . . . the little ones quickly droop and suffer most. . . . The best conditions for the infant require a home and a mother [or parent].[1a]

—Henry Dwight Chapin
1908 and 1915

Most internationally adopted children are placed with their families after residing for months or years in orphanages or other institutions. Many of the problems seen in these children after arrival in the United States have been attributed, rightly or wrongly, to institutional care during critical early phases of development. The adverse effects of institutionalization on young children have been recognized for many years.[2,3] However, many factors contribute to outcome,

including prenatal exposures, genetics, the reasons that the child was consigned to the institution, and the individual experience of the child within the institution prior to adoption. Although institutions are never optimal settings for children, in some cases they may be preferable to other local alternatives. In this chapter, the background of children placed in institutions, the history of institutions for abandoned children, the risks of institutionalization, and the outcome of children raised in orphanages will be reviewed (see Chapter 8 for a review of critical periods during development).

Who Are the Children?

Very few residents of orphanages and baby homes throughout the world are truly orphans, that is, children whose parents are deceased. Most children living in institutional care have been abandoned by their families. Abandonment occurs

From court documents terminating the rights of Elena's parents:

"The father did not take part in the upbringing of the daughter since her birth. The girl lived with her relatives while her parents abused alcohol. Father lived separately, didn't care for the daughter, didn't work. Since 1996, he's been serving his sentence in prison for torturing the relatives. The mother also didn't care for her daughter, didn't go for a walk with her, didn't treat her, thrashed her head and face, left her alone in the apartment, didn't work, didn't support the child financially. Therefore, the child was taken and placed in the social orphanage and then the baby home (where she is presently). The mother hasn't changed her behavior and attitude toward her daughter."

"Under such circumstances, the court comes to the conclusion that the respondents kept aloof from education, were very cruel to the child, and therefore their parental rights are hereby terminated."

for many reasons, including parental illness (mental or physical), inability of the parent(s) to care for the child because of family discord, drug and/or alcohol use, mental retardation, imprisonment, or lack of emotional, financial, or other resources (Table 2–1). Some children are placed in orphanages after parental rights have been terminated, often because of abuse or neglect. As in the United States, poverty, single parenthood, parental psychiatric disease (especially maternal depression[4]), and/or drug or alcohol abuse increase the likelihood of abandonment[5,6] (Tables 2–2 and 2–3). Political and economic constraints (such as the "one child policy" and preference for boys in China) may also lead to abandonment. Thus, children enter institutional care because of "stark human misery."[7]

Few surveys have analyzed the characteristics of abandoned children (see Chapter 3 for information about the sociology of abandoned children in China). In 2001, Shaginian reviewed the birth records at two hospitals in Moscow: an ordinary maternity hospital and a hospital specializing in infectious diseases.[4] In the former,

Table 2–1 Reasons for abandonment in Bangladesh[8]

Born "out of wedlock" (unmarried mother or born to married woman of extramarital union)
Mother "cannot return home" with child
Mother "cannot manage the child"
Poor economic conditions
Child might die

Source: Data from Wilson.[8]

15 children out of 2531 deliveries were abandoned. Seven of these children were healthy, six had prematurity and/or intrauterine growth retardation, two were said to have disorders of the central nervous system (although no objective findings were described; see Chapter 4 for further explanation of the unusual diagnostic categories used in Russian neonatology), and two were considered to have intrauterine infection (a "social diagnosis," made without supportive diagnostic tests but on the basis that there was no prenatal care and the birth mother was thought to be at risk for sexually transmitted disease). In the infectious disease hospital, 305 newborns out of 2910 live births were abandoned. Twenty-six newborns were studied in detail: six had prematurity/intrauterine growth retardation, one had malformation. All children in this group were also diagnosed with intrauterine infection (as above), "excitability syndrome," and "insufficiency of the cerebral circulation" (poorly defined entities, again without objective supporting data).

Table 2–2 Possible characteristics of some birth mothers (Latin America)

Ages 14–18 years
1–2 years of primary school
Functionally illiterate
Live below poverty line
Unemployed or street vendors, beggars, or prostitutes
Come from broken homes
Histories of neglect, abuse, abandonment
Live in "macho" societies
No access to sexual education
Totally unprepared for responsibilities of motherhood

Source: Data from Cantwell.[9]

Table 2–3 Survey of birth mothers in Moscow who abandoned their children (*n* = 41)

Factor	*n*
Age	
16–20 years	12
21–25 years	17
26–30 years	7
31–38 years	5
Gravidity	
First pregnancy	11
Second to seventh pregnancy	30
Pregnancy	
Desired	7
Desired until second half	6
Undesired	28
Reasons for Abandonment[a]	
Social and/or economic	41
No responsibility from father	32
Alcoholism in family	13
Rape	1

[a]Some mothers list more than one reason.

Source: Data from Shaginian.[4]

Care of Abandoned Children

Although living in orphanages and other institutions may adversely affect children, it may be far preferable to the alternatives. In some countries, infanticide, especially of females, is practiced. Unwanted children may lead stark and dangerous lives alone on the streets, may be "sold" into servitude as laborers, servants, or even as child sex workers, or may be neglected, exploited, or abused by family members. Thus, when reviewing the ill effects of institutional life, it is important to remember the bleak alternatives that abandoned children may face if such facilities did not exist.

Abandoned children have existed throughout human history. Throughout much of history, society paid little heed to abandoned children, offering no support and no organized response to their needs. In Western culture,

From court documents terminating the rights of Sergei and Anna's parents:

"The parents neglect their children (age 6 and 7), abuse alcohol, do not work, have no registered place of residence. The children do not attend school. They need to be bathed, they are infested with lice, are hungry, and walk unattended in the village. The children were taken to the orphanage, and the parents never inquired about them. . . . During the court hearing, the parents appeared under the influence of alcohol . . ."

orphanages were first established in the mid-19th century as a humanitarian response to the horrific conditions faced by abandoned children.[10,11] Previously, such children were left to fend for themselves on the streets, or were placed in "almshouses" along with the "poor, feeble-minded, criminal, crippled, and idiotic."[11] About 15% of the residents of these institutions were children, but no efforts were made to separate the children from the other populations. Orphanages were thus established to provide a "more appropriate" environment for children, and in some instances to provide education. In 1729, the first orphanage in the New World was founded by Ursuline nuns in New Orleans, after an Indian attack left many children without parents.[12] Religious groups supervised many orphanages.[10] Children suffered alarmingly high death rates in their first year of institutionalization. Mortality rates at some foundling homes were in excess of 75%.[11] Mortality rates were as high as 90% in Baltimore and 100% at Randall's Island Hospital in New York City, even as recently as the early 20th century.[13] "Orphan trains" and other schemes evolved during the latter half of the 19th century to address some of the deficiencies of the orphanage system.[14]

In early 20th century America, foster care was popularized and eventually replaced orphanages. Foster care was sparked by the White House Conference on the Care of Dependent

Children, in 1909. In the summary of the conference, Theodore Roosevelt stated, "Home life
is the highest and finest product of civilization.
Children should not be deprived of it except for
urgent and compelling reasons." [11] Foster care
theoretically offers considerable advantages
over institutional life but is not without problems as currently practiced.[15] Unfortunately,
children in American foster care often experience multiple placements with attendant emotional, psychological, and educational disruptions.[16] Furthermore, these children suffer from
lack of routine health care, immunizations,
dental care, and vision/hearing screening.[17]
These deficiencies are especially egregious, as
this population has considerable medical needs,
including emotional handicaps (33%), serious
physical illnesses (13%), mental retardation
(19%), and multiple handicaps (15%).[17] Children residing in foster care may not be as well
supervised as those in attentive, loving group
homes; unfortunately, neglect and abuse may
occur. Government-supervised foster care is
not widely practiced throughout the world, but
the practice is growing. A small proportion of
international adoptees reside in private foster
care prior to adoption, including most from
Korea, and some from Romania and Guatemala.

The Risks of Institutionalization

Institutional care presents many risks to growing children. Frank and colleagues described
some common themes of potential "biologic
and psychological risk to infants and young
children in orphanage care"[17a] (Table 2–4).

Table 2–4 Risks of institutionalization

Lack of medical care
Exposure to infections
Inappropriate medical care
Poor nutrition/growth
Physical neglect
Delayed cognitive development
Emotional neglect
Physical or sexual abuse

Source: Adapted from Frank.

Lack of Medical Care

Lack of medical care is a grave concern for
many institutionalized children. Children's
medical problems may be unrecognized by inattentive, overburdened caregivers, or, if recognized, there simply may be no money to pay for
needed medications, surgeries, or other treatments. Morbidity and mortality rates are not
reliably available but likely exceed that in the
general population. Orphanages throughout
the world are filled with children with treatable
or correctable medical conditions, even under
local standards of care. These children may be
consigned by their families to a lifetime of institutional care because of lack of resources to
address their problems. For example, cleft lip/
palates or club feet are not repaired, and hearing or other adaptive aids are not available.

Exposure to Infections

Children living in group settings are also at
higher risk for exposure to infectious diseases,
greater severity of illness, and acquiring resistant
organisms.[18] Respiratory (pneumonia, tuberculosis) and intestinal (bacteria, parasites) infections are particularly commonplace (see Chapters
14 and 17). In settings with faulty immunization
practices, vaccine-preventable diseases (diptheria, measles, hepatitis B) may occur (see Chapter
21). Care in many orphanages may be "over-
medicalized," resulting in increased needle and
medication exposures compared with children
living with their families. For example, in many
parts of the former Soviet Union, institutionalized children are routinely given series of injections of vitamins or other agents—more than 200
injections in some children prior to age 3 (see
sidebar in Chapter 15 and Fig. 9–3). In Romania,
needle exposures may also be frequent[19]—HIV-
negative children received ~142 needle exposures
by age 4 years. In some settings, institutionalized
children may be exposed to blood products such
as intravenous gamma-globulin (used to boost
the immune system of ailing children).

Screening of orphanage staff for health
problems varies greatly in different settings. The

health risks of the staff reflect the endemic infectious diseases. For example, a health survey of 18 caregiver applicants for a new private orphanage in Cambodia revealed intestinal parasites (18), salmonella (7), reactive tuberculin skin tests (18), hepatitis C (1), and HIV (1).[20]

Inappropriate Medical Care

Although not documented, it is certainly possible that children living in institutional care may be at risk of inappropriate medical care as well. Sedatives or other medications may be given to improve sleep or modify behavior that cannot be managed in the group setting. Conceivably, children may be used in "experimental" research protocols without proper oversight.

Growth

Growth delays are common among institutionalized children for many reasons (Table 2–5). Wasting and stunting have been reported among 35%–64% of orphanage residents in Malawi, Kenya, and India[21–23] and among post-institutionalized children from Russia, China, Romania, and other countries[24–29] (see Chapters 10 and 12). Children may suffer from deficiencies of calories, fat, protein, and micronutrients (vitamins, iron, iodine; see Chapter 11). At arrival, height, weight, and head circumference are less than the fifth percentile in nearly 50%, 35%, and 40% of post-institutionalized children[29] (Fig. 2–1). The actual number of children with growth delays is considerably greater: many children at the fifth, tenth, or even higher percentiles show rapid recovery after adoption, which suggests that earlier measurements did

Table 2–5 Reasons for growth delays

Insufficient food
Improper feeding techniques (Fig. 2–3)
Lack of nurturing physical contact
Depression, poor appetite
Poor absorption or utilization of calories
Illness
Medications

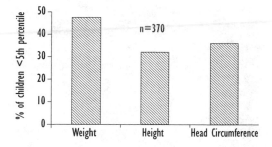

Figure 2–1 *Percent of internationally adopted children with height, weight, and head circumference measurements < 5th percentile on arrival to the United States (n = 370). Children were adopted from 29 countries. (L.C. Miller, unpublished data.)*

not reflect their true biologic potential. Poor growth may have a neuropsychiatric component.[17a] Depression, probably the most underdiagnosed condition among institutionalized children, may cause poor appetite. Furthermore, lack of tactile stimulation results in an inefficient use of ingested nutrients.[30] Many children residing in orphanage care have true "psychosocial dwarfism," that is, disproportionate delays in linear growth. Intriguingly, linear growth delays are quite consistent among several distinct populations of international adoptees. Data derived from children adopted from China, Russia, and Romania produce nearly identical curves (Fig. 2–2)[27] demonstrating that for every

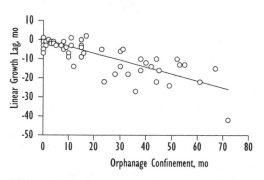

Figure 2–2 *Duration of orphanage confinement was inversely proportional to linear growth lag (height age – chronological age) for children adopted from Romania. mo, months (Johnson DE, Miller LC, Iverson S, et al. The health of children adopted from Romania. JAMA 1992; 268:3449. Copyright © 1992 American Medical Association. All rights reserved.)*

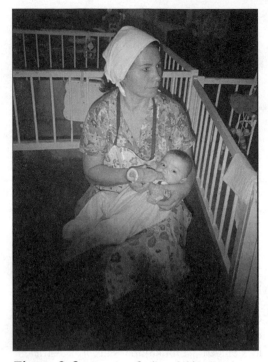

Figure 2–3   *Caregiver feeding child in Russian orphanage. Fourteen other infants were awaiting their turns to be fed.*

~3 months in institutional care, children lose ~1 month of height age.

Physical Neglect

Children in orphanages may also suffer from physical neglect. In some settings, basic hygiene is not maintained. Lack of nurturing physical contact is common and is particularly harmful during infancy. Bottle propping is commonplace in orphanages, as an understandable response to the need to feed many hungry infants with too few staff. In addition to the recognized risks of otitis media and dental caries, children miss out on the loving food-related human interactions that are critical for early emotional development. Lack of physical attention increases self-stimulatory behaviors as infants and young children seek to restore the

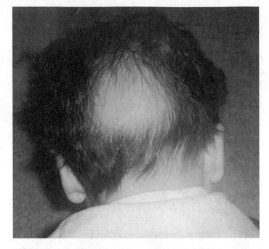

Figure 2–4   *A bald occiput in a child adopted from Romania. Prolonged supine position and self-stimulatory head shaking may result in this finding. (With permission.)*

sensory input necessary for normal brain development (see Chapter 33; Figs. 2–4 to 2–7).

Other physical risks of institutional life may include toxic exposures (such as lead; see Fig. 24–1 and Chapter 24), and the lack of exercise and opportunity to play. Many institutionalized children have never been outdoors:

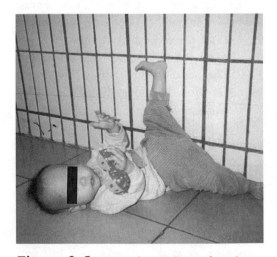

Figure 2–5   *Unusual posturing and staring at hands may occur in children living in understimulating environments. (With permission.)*

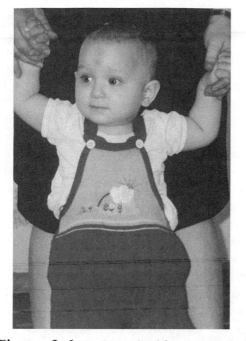

Figure 2–6 *Persistent head-banging resulted in forehead bruising in this Romanian girl. (With permission.)*

adoptive parents often report the wonderment their child displays on seeing the sun, moon, clouds, and sky for the first time.

Developmental Delays

Delays in cognitive development are also common among institutionalized children[21,31–33] (see Chapter 13). Because cognitive function in young children is critically dependent on experience, it is not surprising that most children display significant developmental delays (Table 2–6). Even children in clean, well-kept orphanages with lots of toys and games suffer from a paucity of experiences of the outside world. Most have never been off the grounds of the orphanage (except perhaps for frightening trips to the hospital where they may be

Table 2–6 Reasons for delayed development

Swaddling (Figs. 2–8 and 2–9)
Lack of nurturing physical contact
Lack of stimulation and novelty (Figs. 2–10 to 2–13)
Long naps
Ill health
Malnutrition
Lack of one-to-one attention
Medications

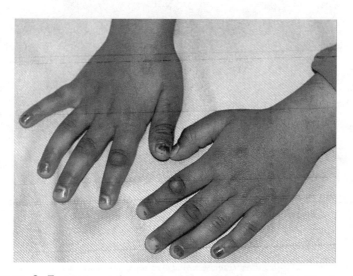

Figure 2–7 *Thickened finger joints from self-inflicted trauma (chewing and banging) in 7-year-old recently adopted from Romania. (With permission.)*

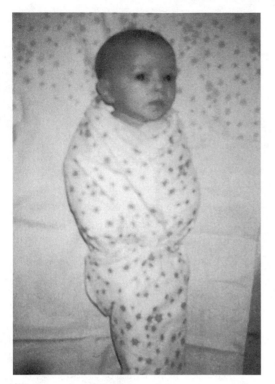

Figure 2–8 *Swaddling is common in orphanages. Infants like this child in a Russian orphanage spend many hours each day tightly swaddled, with little opportunity to practice gross or fine motor skills, or to experience proprioceptive input, varied visual stimulation, or nurturing physical contact. (With permission.)*

abandoned without familiar caregivers for weeks or months). Children lack the experience of going to parks, stores, and different homes and of the life of their village or town. Indeed, many exist as virtual prisoners of the orphanage.

Perhaps the most critical risk faced by institutionalized children is emotional neglect. Caregivers of young infants may all wear masks, depriving children of the experience of seeing human faces (Fig. 2–14). Depression is common in orphanages.[34] In virtually all institutional settings, children lack a one-to-one or "primary" caretaker. A common schedule for caregivers is a 24-hour shift every 3 to 4 days. Thus, each day the child is faced with a different caregiver's style of feeding, baths, bedtime, and emotional responses. As a result, the child experiences inconsistent responses to his or her needs. The problem is exacerbated by the common practice in most orphanages of moving children from group to group, depending on age and developmental skills. Thus, when the child learns to sit, he is taken from caregivers he has known and loved for many months. When the child walks, he is moved again. In well-staffed orphanages in the United Kingdom in the 1960s and 1970s, by 2 years of

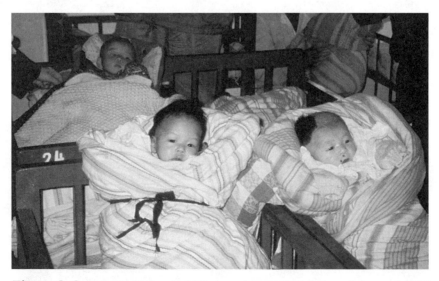

Figure 2–9 *Swaddled infants in a Chinese orphanage. Note the long sleeves on the child on the right. Children in orphanages often are dressed in ill-fitting clothing, as they have no personal possessions. Sleeves covering the hands interfere with fine motor activity. (Courtesy of N. Hendric, M.D.)*

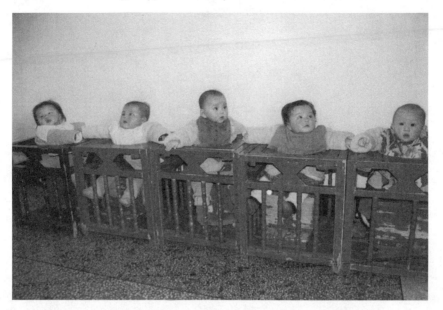

Figure 2–10 *Children are sometimes restrained in special "baby chairs" for many hours each day (some have built-in potty seats). Opportunity to practice gross motor activity is limited. (With permission.)*

age children had been cared for by 24 different adults, by 4 years by 40 different adults; and by 8 years of age by more than 80 different adults.[35,36] Of course, emotional neglect of a different type occurs in understaffed orphanages. Although it is hoped that this type of institution no longer exists, the 170 residents of the Romanian Babeni Orphanage for "unsalvageables" were cared for by one pediatrician and six attendants during the day, and three attendants at night.[37] Not surprisingly, 75% of children did not know their names or ages, 55% had failure to thrive, and 15% had obvious evidence of physical and sexual abuse. Multiple other severe diagnoses were present (Table 2–7). The situation at the Children's Institute in Leros, Greece, was described as "so gross that it almost defied belief."[38] Attachment disorders

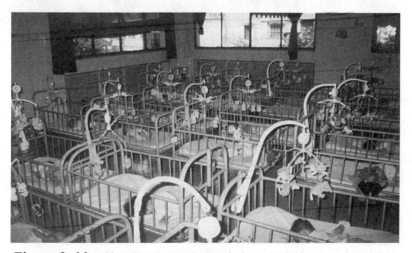

Figure 2–11 *This Vietnamese orphanage had over 30 children in each room. Although each crib had a mobile, children had few other toys during long hours in their cribs.*

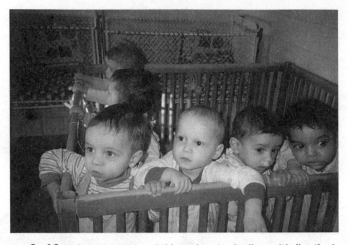

Figure 2–12 *These Romanian children sleep in the "cage-like" crib along the wall, then spend the entire day in a bare playpen. Nonetheless, they are bright, curious, and engaging children who actively seek stimulation and attention.*

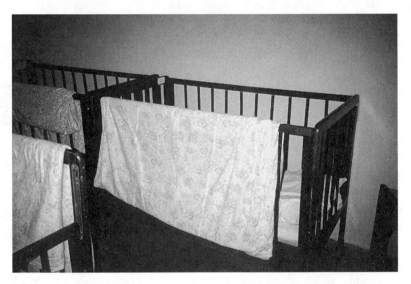

Figure 2–13 *This orphanage in Kazakhstan placed blankets on the edge of each crib for "infection control."*

and other emotional problems may thus occur after various types of institutional exposure (see Chapter 29).

Behavior Problems

Behavior problems are common among institutionalized children (Table 2–8) (see Chapter 30). For example, of 300 children age 12–21 years living in orphanages in Bangalore, India,[39] one-third had obvious behavior problems, and 10% of these required immediate psychiatric help. Problems were worse among those institutionalized before age 4 years. Similarly, Turkish boys living in orphanages had more mental symptoms than comparison children residing with their families.[40] In Iraqi Kurdistan, behavior problems worsened over time among orphans living in institutional care, but decreased among orphans assigned to foster care. The in-

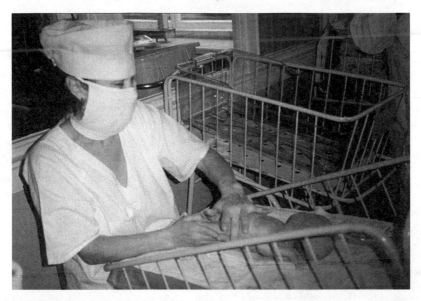

Figure 2–14 *Caregivers of young infants may all wear masks, depriving children of the view of human faces.*

Table 2–7 Neuropsychiatric diagnoses in a Romanian orphanage for "unsalvageables"

Diagnosis	%
Developmental language and speech disorder	94
Mental retardation	40
Reactive attachment disorder	24
Organic mental syndrome	16
Delirium	14
Pica	13
Autism	10
Depression	8
Attention deficit–hyperactivity disorder	8
Oppositional defiant disorder	4
Psychosis	4
Conduct disorder	3

Source: Data from Rosenberg et al.[37]

Table 2–8 Orphanage behaviors

Stereotypic behaviors such as rocking, head banging, head shaking, hand movements

Biting self and others

"Impossible" tantrums

Indiscriminate friendliness

Pain insensitivity or high pain threshold

Inappropriate behaviors (deliberately urinating in the living room, for example)

stitutionalized children also had a higher frequency of post-traumatic stress disorder.[41] Some of these behaviors can be considered "normal" responses to an abnormal environment. Russian investigators (among others) describe "orphan syndrome," characterized by "alteration in affective background" and "para-autistic appearance of deprivation character" as a consequence of maternal deprivation among institutionalized children.[42] "Autistic" or "quasi-autistic" behaviors were found in 12% of 111 children adopted from Romania by British families; some demonstrated gradual improvement over the early years after adoption.[43]

The time course of behavioral and emotional disturbances in institutionalized children was outlined in 1941 by Gesell and Amatruda.[44] (Table 2–9).

Sensory processing problems are seen in some institutionalized children. Compared with family-raised peers, 73 children adopted from Romania showed greater problems in 5/6 sensory processing domains: touch, movement-avoids, movement-seeks, vision, and audition, and 4/5 behavioral domains: activity level, feeding, organization, and social-emotional.[45] Eating

Table 2–9 Time course of emotional and behavioral disturbances after separation from family

Adverse Reaction	Time of Appearance
Diminished interest and reactivity	8–12 weeks
Reduced integration of total behavior	8–12 weeks
Excessive preoccupation with strange persons	12–16 weeks
General retardation	24–28 weeks
Blandness of facial expression	24–28 weeks
Impoverished initiative	24–28 weeks
Stereotypies of sensorimotor behavior	24–28 weeks
Ineptness in new social situations	44–48 weeks
Exaggerated resistance to new situations	48–52 weeks
Relative retardation in language behavior	12–15 months

problems, stereotypies, attachment disorders and indiscriminate friendliness are all more likely among post-institutionalized children.[46,47]

Abuse and Neglect

Sadly, even in institutions charged with protecting the welfare of children, physical and sexual abuse and dire neglect occur. In 1996, Human Rights Watch reported on the condition of children in some Chinese orphanages.[48] Of 55 children admitted to a particular orphanage

---

Juliana was adopted at age 5 from Bulgaria. She initially adjusted well to her new family. After several months, her father noticed that Juliana was behaving unusually when mom wasn't around. Juliana masturbated in front of him, tried to touch his genitals, and would seductively kiss him. She also began to have frequent nightmares and could only be comforted by her mother. By this time, she had learned English quite well. With the help of a child psychologist, the parents learned that Juliana had frequently been sexually abused by the night watchman at the orphanage.

---

in January and February 1992, 24 died within 9–10 months. The report implies that most of the children died of starvation. A report from Christian Solidarity International[49] describes a group of abandoned Russian children in government care, incorrectly confined to psychiatric facilities and subject to psychotropic medications and other treatments. Neglect and other horrific abuses have been delineated in some Russian orphanages in disturbing reports by Human Rights Watch.[50]

The Experience of Institutionalization

Surprisingly little is documented about the actual hour-by-hour experience of children living in institutional care. In one study, crying patterns among institutionalized Korean infants were compared with those of infants living with their families. The institutionalized children cried twice as much as the home infants (86 vs. 45 minutes/day), had half the contact period with caregivers (136 vs. 279 minutes/day), and were alone much longer 1089 vs. 1002 minutes/day).[51] In a time-use study comparison with family-reared children attending day care, orphanage children spent significantly less time with adults, engaged in significantly fewer activities, and spent less time in adult-led activities.[52] The children in the orphanage spent approximately 70% of waking time alone and only 30% with a caregiver; the children in day care showed the opposite pattern.

Orphanage Culture

Orphanages are part of the society in which they exist, and consequently reflect the beliefs and attitudes of that society. Abandoned children or handicapped individuals may be grouped with "unwanted and outcasts ... lepers ... convicts ... political prisoners and the mentally ill"[38] as people who must be isolated from society. Staff in such institutions may lack clinical skills, training, educational and financial resources.[38]

The psychological milieu of the orphanage is another factor that contributes to the outcome of the child. Orphanage staff views of the children reflect the attitudes of the culture and society, ranging from "all children are valuable" and "children are innocent" to "not even their parents want them, so why should we care" or "there must be some defect in these children or else they wouldn't be here." Torhild Andersen[53] described the mindset in Romanian orphanages where he worked: "A woman who abandons her child [is] a bad person regardless of her reason for this action . . . The way the parents are looked upon as persons is reflected in the way the child is treated . . . in institutions . . . the only thing one knows about the parents is that they abandoned the child. . . . this reflects badly on the child." To support his observations, he states that the treatment of children changes when the child is assigned for adoption: "The child will be taken special care of, given the best food, dressed better, hugged and given more attention". His interpretation is that the child then "starts to reflect the personality of the adoptive parents who are always thought of as rich and . . . civilised people."[53]

Thus, the experience of early deprivation in institutions may contribute to delayed growth, cognition, and socioemotional development. Children may demonstrate behavioral problems such as hyperactivity, indiscriminate demands for affection and attention, superficiality of relationships, and absence of normal anxiety to failure or rebuke.[17a] Psychiatric authorities state that "group rearing of abandoned children is inherently destructive and incompatible with normal psychological development."[54]

I was moving along the row of cribs. Babies were lying in the cribs, but seeing an adult they were getting livelier trying to attract attention. Suddenly my eyes came across a tiny creature staying quiet in his crib. I stopped. He looked like a child not older than 2 months. I asked, "Who is he?" "He is Zhenya, he is 5 months."

The baby huddled under my eyes. Unlike the others, he looked serious and strained. He was staring at me. He clenched his tiny fists and pressed them tightly to his chest. I softly called to him "Zhenechka." The baby winced and huddled even more, like a hedgehog. My heart sank out of pain and pity. I felt a lump in my throat. I held out my hands towards the baby, and I took him into my arms. I would like . . . I would like to do everything . . . But what can I do?

I brought the baby to the playroom. There was quiet music of Happy Baby Series. We settled down in an armchair. The boy still looked strained; he had a not childlike serious expression. "Eyes, Eyes, why are you staring at me like this?" The eyes winced. "I wish to get acquainted with you, Zhenechka! My name is Lyuda. I have two children, but they have grown up. I would like to take care of you and to become your friend. I will love you. May I? The eyes glittered and seemed to become quieter but the baby wasn't smiling yet. "Zhenechka, what a nice boy you are, you have large black eyes, black hair, a nose like a button. When you grow up and become a young boy, girls will like you." It was the first time the baby smiled. "What does this mean? Can he understand what I am saying or maybe it is just a coincidence?" I wanted the first to be true. I went telling him my dreams. I described his future life. He would have a loving family and they would gather together around a big family table in the evenings. Zhenechka was listening to my words very attentively and kept on smiling. Then I offered him a dance. Ave Maria was sounding. I raised him above my head and we began to spin around. The baby was flying through the air. And I was praying, "God, help him to live!" I felt the baby completely relax and put him on the table. Having bent over him I began to sing the tune "Ah-ah-ah . . ." Zhenya smiled wide and tried to imitate "Ah-ah" but choked and belched. Then he made another try and sang "Ah-ah-ah." May God bless you, Zhenya, and give you happiness![55]

Is There Such a Thing as a "Good Orphanage"?

Despite all the difficulties of caring for abandoned children in group settings, many orphanages make heroic efforts to provide good care under extremely difficult circumstances. Many orphanage workers dearly love and have deep compassion for the children in their care. At their best, orphanages provide physical safety and material needs, and promote health, developmental function, academic achievement, and psychological well-being. Various systems of care have evolved in different regions of the world, reflecting local cultural beliefs, financial constraints, and developmental awareness. For example, in Cambodia, most children share a single caregiver with two or three other children. The caregiver frequently holds or carries the children, and usually sleeps with them in a hammock. In many Russian orphanages, a multidisciplinary approach is taken. Orphanage staff often includes educators, speech therapists, physical therapists, and music therapists in addition to caregivers, medical staff, and support staff (Figs. 2–15 and 2–16). Children spend part of each day with the specialized therapists alone or in groups, and have the opportunity for individualized attention and to form an attachment to someone who will be consistent despite changes in group assignment. Many of the interventions that improve child welfare are low cost, and can be implemented even under difficult circumstances (Fig. 2–17). This was demonstrated in Eritrea, where restructuring of the Solumuna Orphanage resulted in remarkable reductions in neuropsychiatric symptoms among the children (Fig. 2–18).[54,56] The orphanage was restructured to mix the ages of the children, the staff lived with the children, children had personal possessions, spaces, and time, and orphanage policies were designed to promote the children's autonomy.[57] In contrast, another orphanage in the region had the same staff to child ratio, was segregated by age, policies were designed to promote security and predictability, and the staff functioned in a supervisory role. These children had more frequent behavioral symptoms, especially mood disorders.

In Ethiopia, orphanage children performed as well as family children on the Ravens Progressive Matrices and the Conservation Test, especially those who entered the orphanage early.[57] Superior social interactions with peers have been seen among orphans from Ethiopia and Romania.[31,58] Indeed, in many countries, orphanages may appear attractive to desperately poor families. Availability of food, clothing, shelter, education, and health care may persuade some impoverished families to place their children in institutional care. For example, children in Malawian orphanages for

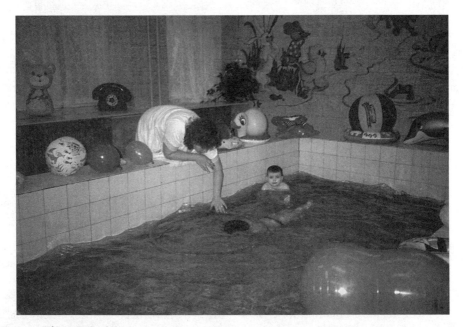

Figure 2–15 Swimming pools offer children in an orphanage in St. Petersburg, Russia the opportunity for some fun and physical activity.

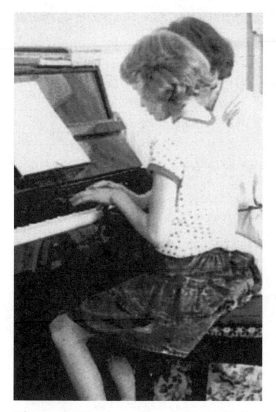

Figure 2–16 *Some orphanages for older children offer musical education. (With permission.)*

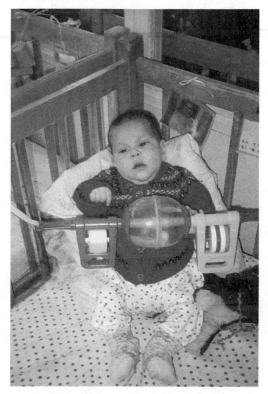

Figure 2–17 *Low-cost interventions can make a big difference in the baby's day. In this Romanian orphanage, a rolled blanket props the child in a seated posture, allowing her to view the activity in the room from a better vantage point. Age-appropriate toys are in reach. Her name is attached to the crib, encouraging caregivers to use it when interacting with her. A photo of her favorite caregiver is attached to the crib, perhaps as a reminder when she is not present.*

more than 1 year were less likely to be malnourished than village children.[22] In India, of 3822 children from 70 institutions, nearly all had signs of calorie, vitamin, and mineral deficiencies and of growth delays when compared to age-matched rural and urban poor, but the institutionalized children had better growth and better self-help, motor, socialization, and imagery skills. In an enriched setting in a Tehran orphanage, children "surpassed even American home-reared children from predominantly professional families" in achievement on developmental scales.[59]

Thus, under the best of circumstances, long-term permanent orphanage care may provide nurturing, stable, and consistent care[60] and be a realistic alternative for children in some circumstances where adoption and foster care are not options.[54]

Heterogeneity of the Orphanage Experience

Institutional life is extremely heterogeneous; thus, post-institutionalized internationally adopted children have come from widely variable backgrounds. Some factors that affect the quality of care in the institution are obvious, such as the staff/child ratio, staff training and awareness of basic child development needs, and the financial and other resources available. The philosophy of the institution is also vitally important. The most critical factor, however, is the

A 12-year-old boy wearing a sport hat ran into the room. "My little brother was just brought here. I want to see him. My brother's name is Pasha."

"You are right. He is here., but now you cannot see him. We have a quarantine. You may come later. Do you live far from here?"

"No, I don't, my orphanage is not far."

The doctor's heart sank. "What poor fellows they are!"

"Pasha's group is on the first floor. Come up to the window and I will show him to you."

It was winter, it got dark early outside, and to say the truth, the Polar Nights had already come to town. Bright light was coming through a large window. Within the light there was the familiar figure of the boy in a sport hat. Having seen his year-and-a-half-old brother behind the window, the boy began waving his hands and calling his brother.

"Pashka! It's me! Can you remember me?"

Pasha was staring but understood nothing.

Then the boy took off his hat and with tears in his eyes cried, "Pashka, what's up, you cannot recognize me? It's me! Why is it so? Pashka!"

The quarantine period ended and the elder brother began to visit Pasha every weekend. Each time he brought something tasty, an apple or a banana. He was likely to save that small treat in his orphanage for his brother.

"I will grow up and take Pashka home! If only he could remember me!"[55]

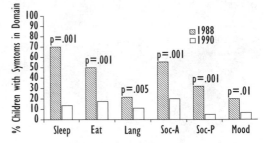

Figure 2–18 *Reduction in behavioral and emotional problems in children residing in Solumuna Orphanage, Eritrea, after restructuring of the orphanage. Interventions included assignment of children of different ages to mixed-age groups with stable caretakers and specialized staff training. When reassessed 2 years later, children's behavioral symptoms decreased significantly in all areas. Soc-A, social interactions with adults; Soc-P, social interactions with peers; Mood, mood disorders. (Reprinted from Wolff PH, Dawit Y, Zere B. The Solomuna Orphanage: a historical survey. Soc Sci Med 1995; 40:1136, with permission from Elsevier.)*

tention, compared to the child who is perceived as "difficult" or a "trouble maker." Thus, the effects of institutionalization—even in children of the same age, in the same room, in the same orphanage—are profoundly different.

Outcome of Children Raised in Orphanages

individual experience of the child. This overrides all other considerations. This experience is affected by the duration of institutionalization, the child's life experience prior to institutionalization (including genetic factors, prenatal exposures, family history, birth history), and the child's experience in the orphanage. The child in the crib that all adults must pass during the daily routine will likely have a different experience from that of the child whose crib is in the back corner of the room and whose needs are attended to last of the group. The social, engaging child likely will have these qualities reinforced, although a quieter, more timid child may be more readily ignored. The child who becomes a "favorite" may receive special privileges, foods, outings, and at-

Very few data exist on the long-term outcome of children raised in orphanages. Although some investigators believe that institutionalization in early childhood increases the likelihood of psychiatric impairments and joblessness as adults,[17a] this is not universally accepted, nor is the institutionalization always to blame. Deficits in language development, intellect, personality, and social skills among orphanage alumni are not necessarily caused by orphanage care.[61] Furthermore, although adverse childhood experiences result in increased frequency of acute and chronic psychosocial disorders in adult life, only a minority of exposed children are affected, and it is clear that variation in the severity, pervasiveness, individual differences in susceptibility, and interactions with later life stressors are all important.[62] Not surprisingly, institutional experience may affect later parenting style.[63]

One fascinating study[64] describes a survey of 1589 graduates of 9 orphanages (South and Midwest) who entered orphanage life between 1901 and 1961 (mean 1936) at ages 0–16 (mean 8 years). At the time of the survey, subjects were 45–101 years old. Fifty percent had spent greater than or equal to 9 years in orphanage. The survey compared these orphanage alumni to controls and found that in many aspects of life, the orphanage alumni had done well. For example, 88% had graduated from high school (compared with 75% of controls), 25% had received college degrees (compared with 16%), and 17% had received doctorates. More than twice the number of orphanage alumni had received master's degrees. Compared to the control group, the orphanage alumni had 10%–61% higher income, and 61% considered themselves to be happy (vs. 29%), 13% had sought psychiatric care (vs. 24%), only 1% were unemployed (vs. 4%), and only 2% had ever received any form of government assistance (vs. 21%). The only scale on which the orphanage alumni exceeded the control group was the frequency of divorce (44% vs. 32%). In further questions, 86% of alumni "never" or "rarely" wished for adoption, 72% preferred the orphanage to their own families, 89% preferred the orphanage to foster care (especially those who had experienced foster care), and 84% gave a "favorable" or "very favorable" rating to their orphanage experience. This surprisingly positive view of orphanage life may reflect the extreme difficulties these individuals faced prior to placement in the institution.

Such views are not universal, however. Among 32 adults raised in Quebec orphanages ($n = 32$), compared with income-, age-, and gender-matched controls, the orphanage graduates had less education (4 years vs. 8.4 years), fewer marriages (7% vs. 39%), lower scores on

Table 2–10 Risk pathways for internationally adopted children

Before Adoption
Genetics
Prenatal Exposures
Lack of prenatal care
Complications of labor and delivery
Abandonment
Institutionalization
Physical neglect
Malnutrition
Micronutrient deficiencies
Lack of stimulation and nurturing physical contact
Exposure to infections
Emotional neglect

After Adoption
Adjustment to new family, culture, country, language
Demands of new environment
Grief for loss of old environment and caregivers
Specific stressors of new environment
Parent and family stress
Educational demands
Adoption and identity issues

"well-being" scales, higher scores on "distress" scales, and more "stress-related" illnesses.[65] The outcome of children adopted from institutional care in other countries is at present unknown but is an area of active investigation. Although many children do well, some international adoptees have long-term cognitive, learning, or psychosocial problems.[1,43,45,46,61,66–68] Risk factors influencing outcome are summarized in Table 2–10.

The Rights of Institutionalized Children

The rights of institutionalized children are recognized by the UN Convention on the Rights of the Child. This international document includes the following provisions: all children have the right to education, the right to home, the right to family, the right to the highest standard of health and medical care available, and the right of protection from abuse and neglect.

Children without families are guaranteed "appropriate alternative family care or institutional placement," and disabled children are guaranteed the right to special care, education, and training "to help achieve the greatest degree of self-reliance and social integration possible." Finally, all institutionalized children are guaranteed the right to periodic review of placement. As of this writing it is embarrassing to report that this Convention has been ratified by all countries of the world except the United States and Somalia (2004). Nonetheless, this important document reflects a recognition by the international community of the inherent rights of children, and those specifically left without parental care. It is hoped that these rights will be recognized and protected for the hundreds of thousands of abandoned children throughout the world.

References

1. Chapin HD. A plan of dealing with atrophic infants and children. Arch Pediatr 1908; 25:491–496.

1a. Chapin HD. Are institutions for infants necessary? JAMA 1915; 64: 1–3.

2. Spitz RA. The First Year of Life: A Psychoanalytic Study of Normal and Deviant Development of Object Relations. New York: International Universities Press, 1965.

3. Bowlby J. Attachment and loss, Vol. 1. New York: Basic Books, 1969.

4. Shaginian N. The Influence of Psychological and Social Factors on Pregnancy and Abandoned Newborns. Joint Council of International Children's Services, Washington, DC: 2002.

5. Jellinek MS, Murphy JM, Bishop S, Poitrast F, Quinn D. Protecting severely abused and neglected children. An unkept promise. N Engl J Med 1990; 323:1628–30.

6. Abedin M, Young M, Beeram MR. Infant abandonment: prevalence, risk factors, and cost analysis. Am J Dis Child 1993; 147:714–6.

7. Fanshel D. The pediatrician and children in foster care. Pediatrics 1977; 60:255–7.

8. Wilson M. "Take this child": why women abandon their infants in Bangladesh. J Comp Fam Stud 1999; 30:687.

9. Cantwell N. Intercountry Adoption. Innocenti Digest, Vol. 4. Florence, Italy: UNICEF International Child Development Centre, 1998: 1–24.

10. Markel H. Orphanages revisited. Arch Pediatr Adolesc Med 1995; 149:609–10.

11. English PC. Pediatrics and the unwanted child in history: foundling homes, disease, and the origins of foster care in New York City, 1860 to 1920. Pediatrics 1984; 73:699–711.

12. Berkowitz CD. Children in orphanages: Newt Gingrich is not Daddy Warbucks. Pediatrics 1996; 97:288–89.

13. Thurston WF. In a Chinese orphanage. The Atlantic Monthly 1996; 277:28.

14. Gray C. Dr. Thomas Barnardo's orphans were shipped 500 km to save body and soul. CMAJ 1979; 121: 981–87.

15. Leslie LK, Hurlburt MS, Lanksverk J, Rolls JA, Wood PA, Kelleher KJ. Comprehensive assessments for children entering foster care: a national perspective. Pediatrics 2003; 112:134–142.

16. Simms MD, Dubowitz H, Szilagyi MA. Health care needs of children in the foster care system. Pediatrics 2000; 106:909–18.

17. Committee on Adoption and Dependent Care: the needs of foster children. Pediatrics 1975; 56:144–5.

17a. Frank DA, Klass PE, Earls F, Eisenberg L. Infants and young children in orphanages: one view from pediatrics and child psychiatry. Pediatrics 1996; 97:569–78.

18. American Academy of Pediatrics. Children in out of home child care. In: Pickering LK, ed. Red Book: Report of the Committee on Infectious Diseases, American Academy of Pediatrics, 2003: 123–37.

19. Hersh BS, Popovici F, Jezek Z, et al. Risk factors for HIV infection among abandoned Romanian children. AIDS 1993; 7:1617–24.

20. Hendrie NW. Survey of caregiver applicants in Cambodia, 2000 [unpublished].

21. Otieno PA, Nduati RW, Musoke RN, Wasunna AO. Growth and development of abandoned babies in institutional care in Nairobi. East Afr Med J 1999; 76:430–5.

22. Panpanich R, Brabin B, Gonani A, Graham S. Are orphans at increased risk of malnutrition in Malawi? Ann Trop Paediatr 1999; 19:279–85.

23. Chhabra P, Garg S, Sharma N, Bansal RD. Health and nutritional status of boys aged 6 to 12 years in a children observation home. Indian J Public Health 1996; 40:126–9.

24. Hostetter MK, Iverson S, Thomas W, McKenzie D, Dole K, Johnson DE. Medical evaluation of internationally adopted children. N Engl J Med 1991; 325:479–85.

25. Albers LH, Johnson DE, Hostetter MK, Iverson S, Miller LC. Health of children adopted from the former Soviet Union and Eastern Europe. Comparison with preadoptive medical records. JAMA 1997; 278:922–4.

26. Jenista JA, Chapman D. Medical problems of foreign-born adopted children. Am J Dis Child 1987; 141:298–302.

27. Johnson DE, Miller LC, Iverson S, et al. The health of children adopted from Romania. JAMA 1992; 268: 3446–51.

28. Miller LC, Hendrie NW. Health of children adopted from China. Pediatrics 2000; 105:E76.

29. Miller LC, Kiernan MT, Mathers MI, Klein-Gitelman M. Developmental and nutritional status of internationally adopted children. Arch of Pediatr Adolesc Med 1995; 149:40–4.

30. Kuhn CM, Schanberg SM. Responses to maternal separation: mechanisms and mediators. Int J Dev Neurosci 1998; 16:261–70.

31. Kaler SR, Freeman BJ. Analysis of environmental deprivation: cognitive and social development in Romanian orphans. J Child Psychol Psychiatry 1994; 35:769–81.

32. Sloutsky VM. Institutional care and developmental outcomes of 6- and 7-year old children. Int J Behav Dev 1997; 20:131–51.

33. Tabassam W, Hamayun S. Intelligence and personality differences among children from orphanages and intact families. J Indian Acad Appl Psychol 1993; 19:13–20.

34. Kalinina MA, Kozlovskaia GV, Koroleva TN. Depressive states at an early age. Zh Nevrol Psikhiatr Im S S Korsakova 1997; 97:8–12.

35. Tizard B, Hodges J. The effect of early institutional rearing on the development of eight-year-old children. J Child Psychol Psychiatry 1978; 19:99–118.

36. Tizard B, Rees J. The effect of early institutional rearing on the behaviour problems and affectional relationships of four-year-old children. J Child Psychol Psychiatry 1975; 16:61–73.

37. Rosenberg DR, Pajer K, Rancurello M. Neuropsychiatric assessment of orphans in one Romanian orphanage for 'unsalvageables'. JAMA 1992; 268:3489–90.

38. Kolvin I. Children in institutions. Br J Psychiatry 1995; 167:8–11.

39. Somen KS. Mental health problems of children in orphanages. Child Psychiatry Q1985; 18:62–70.

40. Kirpinar I. The distribution of mental symptoms of the adolescents living in Erzurum orphanage [in Turkish]. Tuerk Psikiyatri Dergisi 1992; 3:265–68.

41. Ahmad A, Mohamad K. The socioemotional development of orphans in orphanages and traditional foster care in Iraqi Kurdistan. Child Abuse Negl 1996; 20:1161–73.

42. Proselkova ME, Kozloskaia GV, Bashina VM. The characteristics of the mental development of young orphan children [in Russian]. Zh Nevropatol Psikhiatr Im S S Korsakova 1995; 95:52–6.

43. Rutter M, Andersen-Wood L, Beckett C, et al. Quasi-autistic patterns following severe early global privation. English and Romanian Adoptees (ERA) Study Team. J Child Psychol Psychiatry 1999; 40:537–49.

44. Gesell A, Amatruda C. Developmental diagnosis: normal and abnormal neuropsychologic development in infancy and early childhood (revised and enlarged, 1975). In: Knobloch H, Pasamanick B, eds. Developmental Diagnosis, 3rd Ed. Hagerstown, MD: Harper & Row, 1941: 1–506.

45. Cermak SA, Daunhauer LA. Sensory processing in the postinstitutionalized child. Am J Occup Ther 1997; 51:500–7.

46. Chisholm K. A three-year follow-up of attachment and indiscriminate friendliness in children adopted from Romanian orphanages. Child Dev 1998; 69:1092–106.

47. Fisher L, Ames EW, Chisholm K, Savoie L. Problems reported by parents of Romanian orphans adopted to British Columbia. Int J Behav Dev 1997; 20:67–82.

48. Watch HR. Death by Default: A Policy of Fatal Neglect in China's State Orphanages. New York: Human Rights Watch, 1996.

49. Cox C, et al. Trajectories of Despair: Misdiagnosis and Maltreatment of Soviet Orphans [synopsis]. Available at: http://www.adoption-research.org/despair.html.

50. Hunt K. Abandoned to the State: Cruelty and Neglect in Russian Orphanages. New York: Human Rights Watch, 1998.

51. Lee K. Crying patterns of Korean infants in institutions. Child Care Health Dev 2000; 26:217–28.

52. Daunhauer LA, Bolton A, Cermak SA. Time stands still: a comparison of time-use patterns between young children in an Eastern European orphanage and American children attending day care. In press, Am J Occup Ther, 2004.

53. Andersen TM. Social implications for institutionalized children. In: Rygvold A-L, Dalen M, Saeterdal B, eds. Mine–Yours–Ours and Theirs. Oslo: University of Oslo, 1999.

54. Wolff PH, Tesfai B, Egasso H, Aradom T. The orphans of Eritrea: a comparison study. J Child Psychol Psychiatry 1995; 36:633–44.

55. Levchuk L. Stories from a Russian Baby Home, 2002 [unpublished].

56. Wolff PH, Fesseha G. The orphans of Eritrea: a five-year follow-up study. J Child Psychol Psychiatry 1999; 40:1231–7.

57. Wolff PH, Dawit Y, Zere B. The Solomuna Orphanage: a historical survey. Soc Sci Med 1995; 40:1133–9.

58. Aboud F, Samuel M, Hadera A, Addus A. Intellectual, social and nutritional status of children in an Ethiopian orphanage. Soc Sci Med 1991; 33:1275–80.

59. Hunt JM, Mohandessi K, Ghodssi M, Akiyama M. The psychological development of orphanage-reared infants: interventions with outcomes (Tehran). Genet Psychol Monogr 1976; 94:177–226.

60. Wiener JM. Orphanages: an idea whose time has come again? Am J Psychiatry 1998; 155:1307–8.

61. McCall JN. Research on the psychological effects of orphanage care: a critical review. In: McKenzie RB, ed. Rethinking Orphanages for the 21st Century. Thousand Oaks, CA: Sage Publications, 1999: 127–150.

62. Maughan B, McCarthy G. Childhood adversities and psychosocial disorders. Br Med Bull 1997; 53:156–69.

63. Sigal JJ, Meislova J, Beltempo J, Silver D. Some determinants of individual differences in the behaviour of children of parentally deprived parents. Can J Psychiatry 1988; 33:51–6.

64. McKenzie RB. Orphanage alumni: how they have done and how they evaluate their experience. Child and Youth Care Forum 1997; 26:87–111.

65. Sigal JJ, Rossignol M, Perry JC. Some psychological and physical consequences in middle-aged adults of underfunded institutional care in childhood. J Nerv Ment Dis 1999; 187:57–9.

66. Benoit TC, Jocelyn LJ, Moddemann DM, Embree JE. Romanian adoption. The Manitoba experience. Arch Pediatr Adolesc Med 1996; 150:1278–82.

67. Carlson M, Earls F. Psychological and neuroendocrinological sequelae of early social deprivation in institutionalized children in Romania. Ann N Y Acad Sci 1997; 807:419–28.

68. Faber S. Behavioral sequelae of orphanage life. Pediatr Ann 2000; 29:242–8.

3

SPECIAL REGIONAL CONSIDERATIONS

Prospective parents often ask, "Which is the best country to choose for international adoption?" Overall, the individual experiences of the child (including genetics, prenatal exposures, nutrition, health, and environment) are more important determinants of the child's well-being than the colors of the flag flying over the orphanage. However, country-specific factors also influence the health of internationally adopted children. Financial resources, basic health indicators, and societal attitudes toward abandoned children[1] vary greatly among international adoption sending countries (see Chapter 2). The reasons why children are abandoned also differ between countries. Together, these factors shape the health, nutritional status, and development of children placed for international adoption.

Politics and economics determine which of the countless abandoned children in the world are adopted by foreigners (see Chapter 1). Adam Pertman writes, "Countries don't like to give up their children any more than parents do."[2] International adoption takes place only under particular social, economic, and political circumstances.[2–4] Many countries with large numbers of abandoned children prohibit international adoption, usually because of religious or political constraints. Countries that observe Shari'a (Islamic) law (e.g., Saudi Arabia and Afghanistan) do not permit adoption in a legal form that is recognized by the United States. Some countries alternately promote or ban foreign adoption. Some countries (e.g., Paraguay) have halted the practice until national adoption centers are established as mandated by the Hague Convention on Intercountry Adoption. Moratoria on international adoptions have been placed by Guatemala, Vietnam, Romania, Russia, and Cambodia in recent years; by 2004, only Russia and Guatemala have reopened for adoption (see below).

Personal and national economics also play a substantial role in international adoption. Sending countries and birth parents tend to be poor, while receiving countries and adoptive parents usually are well-off. The ethical concerns of this disparity are highlighted by Cheri Register's comments: "Wealth does not entitle us to the children of the poor. . . . International adoption is an undeserved benefit that has fallen to North Americans, West Europeans and Australians, largely because of the inequitable socioeconomic circumstances in which we live. In the long run, we ought to be changing those circumstances."[5]

Basic health, nutrition, education, and economic indicators vary enormously among international adoption sending countries (Tables 3–1 and 3–2).[6,7] These data provide a snapshot of the differences between some of the sending countries. The remainder of this chapter describes the "top five" sending countries for 2002 in detail (China, Russia, Guatemala, South Korea, and Ukraine), along with Romania, which played an important role in the history of international adoption in the United States. These countries and others are discussed in several other chapters (Chapters 4–7). For each country, the history of international adoption, logistics of adoption, general health of the population (focusing on tobacco, alcohol, and drug use), and special considerations for the children are reviewed. The story of international adoption in each country is intertwined with local politics, culture, and history.

servicemen after the Korean War. Told that there was no legal mechanism to accomplish this, they rallied enormous support and were able to persuade Congress just 2 months later to pass the 1955 Bill for Relief of Certain War Orphans. Eventually they adopted eight Amerasian children and founded the Holt agency, which continues to work actively in the region (and elsewhere). The Holt Agency Web site[8] states, "The Holts' adoption was revolutionary. Intercountry adoption had been done previously, but it was virtually unheard of at that time. The social work establishment of that time discouraged it. The common practice was to carefully match children by color and background which helped conceal the adoption." Korean adoptions thus paved the way for tens of thousands of international adoptions. The large influx of "obviously adopted" Korean children in the 1970–80s led to many changes in adoption practice, including more openness, recognition of the importance of maintaining cultural ties to the country of origin, and the acceptability of transracial adoption.[9]

South Korea was the major sending country of children to the United States until 1995 (except for 1991, when it was briefly displaced by Romania). Over 141,000 children have been adopted from South Korea by American families since 1955.[9] The number of children arriving each year from South Korea has been fairly consistent for about the past 10 years (see Table 3–3). Domestic adoption is limited in Korea because of the cultural importance of family "bloodlines."[10]

Korea (Republic of Korea, South Korea)

History of International Adoption

South Korea holds an important place in the history of international adoption in the United States (see Chapter 1). An Oregonian couple, Harry and Bertha Holt, decided to adopt some of the biracial children left behind by American

Logistics

Since the 1970s, intercountry adoption has been exceedingly well managed by the South Korean government. Four government-run and licensed Korean child welfare agencies (Eastern Social Welfare Society, Social Welfare Society, Holt Children Services, and Korea Social Services) handle all international adoptions. American adoption agencies are required to work

Table 3–1 Comparative indicators from top 15 sending countries

Country	U5 Mortality Rank[a,b]	Total Population 2001[b] (1000s)	GNI per Capita 2001[b] (U.S.$)	Life Expectancy at Birth[b] (years)	Total Adult Literacy Rate[b] (%)	Infants with Low Birth Weight[b] (%)	(% of) U5 with Moderate to Severe Underweight[b] (%)	Population with Access to Safe Water[b] (%)	Primary School Entrants Reaching Grade 5[b] (%)	Population Urbanized[b] (%)	Antenatal Care[b] (%)	Skilled Attendant at Delivery[b] (%)	Delivery in Health Facilities[c] (%)	Total Health Expenditure per Capita[c]	Adult HIV Prevalence Rate 15–49 years, 2001[b] (%)	Below Poverty Line[d] (%)	Unemployment[d] (%)
Belarus	125	10,147	1190	69	99	5	NA	100	96	70	100	NA	NA	430	0.27	22	2.1[e]
Bulgaria	138	7867	1560	71	99	9	NA	100	91	68	NA	NA	NA	198	<0.1	35	17.5
Cambodia	30	13,441	270	56	68	9	21	30	45	18	38	32	7	111	2.7	36	2.8
China	85	1,284,972	890	71	85	6	10	75	97	37	NA	89	51	205	0.11	10	10 (urban)[f]
Colombia	118	42,803	1910	71	92	7	7	91	69	76	91	86	77	616	0.40	55	17
Guatemala	72	11,687	1670	65	69	12	24	92	51	40	60	41	23	192	1.0	60	7.5
Haiti	38	8270	480	53	49	28	17	46	41	36	79	24	20	54	6.1	80	66
India	54	1,025,096	460	64	56	26	47	84	60	28	60	43	26	71	0.79	25	4.4
Kazakhstan	61	16,095	1360	65	98	6	4	61	92	56	91	99	95	211	0.07	26	10
Philippines	88	77,131	1040	70	95	18	28	86	69	59	86	56	28	167	<0.1	40	10
Romania	121	22,388	1710	70	98	9	6	58	96	55	NA	98	NA	190	<0.1	45	9.1
Russia	121	144,664	1750	66	99	7	3	99	NA	73	NA	NA	NA	405	0.9	40	8.7[e]
S. Korea	178	47,069	9400	75	98	NA	NA	92	99	82	96[c]	100	99	909	<0.1	4	3.9
Ukraine	125	49,112	720	68	99	6	3	98	98	68	NA	99	NA	152	NA	29	3.6[e]
Vietnam	88	79,175	410	69	93	9	33	77	83	25	68	68	70	129	0.3	37	25

GNI, gross national income; NA, not available; U5, under 5

[a] Rank of country out of all countries in the world. Lower numbers indicate higher mortality. Rate reflects the probability of dying between birth and age 5 years.

[b] Data from UNICEF.[6]

[c] Data from the World Health Organization.[7]

[d] Data from Central Intelligence Agency.[7a]

[e] Large number of unregistered unemployed or underemployed not included.

[f] "Substantial" in rural areas.

Table 3–2 An idiosyncratic, nonscientific view of international adoption from various countries

Country	Pre-adoptive Care	Post-adoption Snapshot	Comments
Kazakhstan	Orphanages—loving and attentive	Government requires ~2-week visitation prior to adoption; this eases adjustment.	Some kids may have been exposed to Kazakh and Russian languages; this may result in more language delays initially.
Vietnam	Orphanages—variable	Infants may be tiny; older kids are often small.	Parasites are common; growth recovers quickly.
Cambodia	Orphanages—variable; some have 1:2 live-in caregiver ratio	Infants may be tiny.	Infants who lived with their caregivers hate to sleep alone or be put down!
Philippines	Orphanages—variable; some extremely good	Older kids are well prepared for adoption.	Extensive medical records are often available and usually are very accurate.
India	Orphanages—variable; some very attentive	Infants may be tiny; older kids are often small.	Parasites are common. Medical records overall are quite accurate within limits of available testing.
Ethiopia	Orphanages—variable; some very attentive	Most in good health and nutritional state	Variable experiences prior to institutionalization
Colombia	Orphanages—variable; some extremely good	Most in good health and nutritional state; some may be small	Variable experiences prior to institutionalization
Bulgaria, Lithuania, Belarus	Orphanages—variable	Wide variation	Medical records are usually quite scanty.

See text for details about more frequent sending countries.

Table 3–3 South Korean children adopted by American families, 1989–2003

Year	n
1989	3544
1990	2620
1991	1818
1992	1840
1993	1775
1994	1795
1995	1666
1996	1516
1997	1654
1998	1829
1999	2008
2000	1794
2001	1870
2002	1779
2003	1790
Total	**29,298**

directly with these societies (see also adoptkorea.com[11]). Many professionals consider Korean adoptions a model for ethical practice.

Up-to-date information about the legal procedures for international adoption from Korea (and other countries) is available at the Web site for the U.S. State Department, Office of Children's Issues.[12] Children are usually escorted to the United States, although adoptive parents are permitted to travel to collect their children. Increasingly, parents are selecting this option.

General Health Issues in the Population

The prevalence of smoking (especially among women) and alcohol and drug use has recently increased. South Korea is considered one of the heaviest-smoking nations in Asia,[13] especially among men. Drinking is also common: about 65% of the population drinks. This proportion is much higher among students, >96% of whom drink regularly (males more than females). Beer and soju (25% alcohol) are the most popular alcoholic beverages.[14] Drug users prefer amphetamines, marijuana, opiates, inhalants, benzodi-

azepine, LSD, and cocaine.[15] In 1995, there were an estimated 2500 amphetamine injection drug users in the country.

Some infectious diseases that occur include dengue, filariasis, Japanese encephalitis, leishmaniasis, plague, and malaria. Three cases of severe acute respiratory syndrome (SARS) were confirmed as of September 2003.

Special Considerations for Children Adopted from South Korea

Before the adoption. Some birth mothers receive prenatal care through homes for unwed mothers if an adoption plan is made prior to delivery. Most Korean children live in loving, attentive foster care prior to adoptive placement. Children are carefully followed by well-trained physicians. If needed, specialty care is available (see Chapter 4).

After the adoption. Korean children are among the healthiest and most developmentally normal adoptees at arrival. Most arrive as infants ~5–9 months of age. The children are generally happy and well nourished (in some cases, overweight). Gross motor delays are common, possibly because the children are frequently carried by their foster mothers and floor time is restricted. Some children have markedly flattened occiputs (see Chapter 12). In the 1970s–80s, about 3%–5% of Korean adoptees had positive markers for hepatitis B surface antigen[16–20] (see Chapter 15). Through widespread implementation of vaccine programs and other public health measures, this number has been considerably reduced. Many early studies of internationally adopted children included large numbers of children from Korea.[17, 21–23] Conclusions about the health and well-being of international adoptees based on this cohort may not be applicable to children from more difficult backgrounds in other countries adopted in recent years.

Several specific studies of Korean adopted children are worthy of comment. Fundamental studies linking early malnutrition and cognitive achievement used Korean adoptees as research subjects[24, 25] (see Chapter 10). More recently, Korean adoptees were singled out for their excellent behavioral and cognitive outcomes. In one study, parents found no difference in adjustment and behavior between their birth children and their children adopted from Korea.[26] A 2000 study in The Netherlands of 159 7-year olds adopted as infants noted that 31% of the Korean adoptees in the group had intelligence scores >120.[27]

Questions have been raised regarding the validity of vaccines administered in many countries, however most experts agree that vaccine records of Korean children prior to adoption should be accepted.[28] Although lab work results from Korea are also likely to be reliable, it is sensible to obtain comprehensive testing of newly arrived Korean children, as for those from other countries.

The use of Korean growth charts is discussed in Chapter 4.

China

History of International Adoption

Very few children were adopted from China by Americans before 1994 (see Table 3–4). In 1995, suddenly the number entering the United States increased from ~200/year to 787. The following year, 2130 children arrived from China, the most from a single country. Since then, China has maintained its top position as a sending country (except for 1998–99, when Russia slightly surpassed it). China and Russia have each sent ~33,000 children to the United States since 1989.

Virtually all children adopted from China are girls. This peculiar lopsidedness reflects the strong Chinese preference for male children coupled with the government's mandated "one-child policy" (reviewed in Vonk et al.[29]). These social forces result in the selective abandon-

Table 3–4 Chinese children adopted by American families, 1989–2003

Year	n
1989	201
1990	28
1991	61
1992	206
1993	330
1994	787
1995	2130
1996	3333
1997	3597
1998	4206
1999	4101
2000	5053
2001	4681
2002	5053
2003	6859
Total	40,626

ment, abortion, infanticide, or failure to register births of female infants, and a skewed gender distribution of international adoptees and of children residing in institutional care. Population demographers estimate that over 1 million Chinese girls are "missing" each year.[30] Some regions report sex ratios as high as 145 males: 100 females[30]; overall there are about 116 boys for every 100 girls.[31]

The sociology of abandonment is complex and painful.[10,30] In one analysis, most of the 237 families who abandoned a child in the late 1980s–90s were married couples residing in rural villages (88%). The decision to abandon the child was usually made by the birth father or both parents together (40%). Gender, birth order, and gender composition of siblings determined who was to be abandoned; ~90% of the abandoned children were healthy girls. It was rare for the only or first girl born to be abandoned. Of the abandoned girls, 87% had no brothers, 40% were second daughters, and 36% were third daughters. Only 6% were first-borns. The few abandoned boys were usually disabled or ill or born to an unwed mother. Most children were abandoned within the first 6 months of life. Thus, the typical abandoned child was a healthy newborn girl with one or more older sisters and no brothers. Most abandonments took place at some distance from the family home, in a crowded location such as a market or bus station. Once the child was removed from the local jurisdiction, the incentive for local officials to investigate was reduced. Many of the girls were placed on doorsteps of families thought to be likely adoptive parents.

Only a small number of these abandoned girls are adopted, most by Americans (about 600/year go to other countries, usually Canada). In China, prosecution for abandonment is usually perfunctory, requiring fines similar to those for having an "over-quota" child. Occasionally, the birth mother is sterilized. However, abandonment is not regarded as criminal offense endangering the child.

Realistic estimates of the number of abandoned children are unavailable; as a rough estimate, only about 20% of abandoned children end up in government care. Some estimate that about 15 million baby girls have been abandoned since 1980.[32] From 1986 to 1990 in Hunan Province, over 16,000 abandoned children entered government care; 92% were girls and 25% were handicapped. In Hengyang City in Hunan Province, the number of abandoned children increased more than threefold within 3 years (1988, 233 children, 1989, 352, and 1990, 854) coincident with stricter enforcement of birth-planning policies. Between 1988 and 1993, as many as 16 children were abandoned each day in Shaoyang District.[30]

As many as 1 million Chinese children reside in orphanages.[33] Coincident with political enforcement of the "one child" policy, orphanage populations increased drastically in the late 1980s and early 1990s. During those years, mortality rates in orphanages exceeded 40%, and in some settings were as high as 80%. Most children died within the first few months after arrival. After sending 201 children to the United States in 1989, China virtually closed international adoption for the next 2 years. In the mid–1990s, an enormous controversy erupted after broadcast of a television documentary called

"The Dying Rooms" and the publication of *Death by Default,* a report by Human Rights Watch. These reports purported to show that the state-run orphanages practiced a "policy of fatal neglect" and that "most orphaned or abandoned children in China died within one year of their admittance to state-run orphanages.[34] The Human Rights Watch report accused the Shanghai Children's Welfare Institute of practicing "a deliberate policy of child murder in numerous cases," citing a mortality rate from the late 1980s to early 1990s that "was probably running as high as 90%."[34] After these accusations, an international furor arose. The charges were vigorously denied by the Chinese government.

Over the next few years, international adoptions increased and changes were made the care provided to abandoned children.[35] With revenue obtained from international adoptions, some of the larger orphanages improved their facilities and medical care. However, poorer welfare centers outside of major cities have not yet benefitted much from this.[10] Foster care programs have been initiated in some regions. Chinese adoptions are now overseen by the China Center for Adoption Affairs, a central authority, somewhat similar to the process in South Korea.[36] China now releases more detailed pre-adoptive medical information, permits healthy children to be adopted by foreigners, and has allowed considerably more transparency to enter the process.

Moreover, in 1999, Chinese couples were legally given the right to adopt abandoned children, something that had been banned or restricted. China does not have cultural traditions that preclude domestic adoption. Nonetheless, domestic adoption is uncommon: only about 8,000–10,000 per year are registered. Restrictions on adoption for Chinese citizens were recently liberalized, lowering the age from 35 to 30, but still require prospective adoptive parents to be childless (although this requirement may change soon).[10] Adoptive parents with children are punished and fined as if they themselves had violated birth planning by having an over-quota child. In a recent survey, only 11/392 of Chinese adoptive families received their child from a government welfare center. Most domestic adoptions are arranged informally.

Logistics

Adopting parents must travel to China and complete a legal adoption there. Many adoption agencies send families in large groups of 8–20. Such groups may be accompanied by a physician or nurse hired by the adoption agency. Some of the hotels that cater to Western tourists have (limited) medical facilities to evaluate and treat children during the adoption process.

General Health Issues in the Population

Tobacco, alcohol, and illicit drug use has expanded in China as in other Asian nations. Although men are the chief users, women are involved with these substances in increasing numbers. China is home to one-fifth of the world's population and one-third of the world's smokers.[37] Only about 4% of women smoke (compared with ~ 63% of men), but smoking is becoming more widespread among young people of both sexes. Alcohol use has increased substantially; in some studies nearly half of females use alcohol regularly (see Chapter 5), although, in general, alcohol use by women lags behind that of men.

Drug use is harder to quantify, and data about women are lacking. In 1995, there were ~100,000 drug users in Yunnan Province alone; in a single county (Kunming) there were an estimated 20,000 to 30,000 drug users, mostly injection drug users. Injection drug use varies in different regions (58% of drug users in Guangxi, 20%–30% in Guangdong and Sichuan, 5% in Guizhou in 1993; by 1996 rates increased to 75% in Xinjiang, 90% in Guangxi). The preferred drug is heroin; other favored choices include diazepam, opium, and cannabis. About 90% of drug users are below 30 years of age, and over 80% are male. In 1997, the estimated number of HIV infections was 200,000.[38]

Dengue, filariasis, Japanese encephalitis, leishmaniasis, plague, and malaria occur in China, as well as the recently identified SARS (over 5300 cases as of November 2003). In May 2003, foreign adoptions in China were temporarily halted in an attempt to reduce the transmission of SARS.[39]

Special Considerations for Children Adopted from China

Before the adoption.   Children reside in state-run orphanages prior to adoption. A small number of children are placed in foster care. Some children receive "modified institutional care," sometimes returning home at night with a caregiver but spending the day in the group setting. Some children are removed from foster care a month or two prior to adoption and returned to the orphanage "to prepare them for adoption." Sometimes parents do not know the living circumstances of their child prior to adoption. It remains unusual for adoptive parents to meet or be given contact information for foster parents, although in some regions this is changing.

Specific information about the arrival of the child into state care is sometimes given at the time of the adoption. Details about the location where the child was found may be provided (the market, the police station, etc.; see Chapter 4). Parents may be given notes found with the child, for example:

This healthy baby girl was born on—— 1992 at 5:30 am and is now 100 days old. . . . She is in good health and has never suffered any illness. Due to the current political pressures that are too difficult to explain, we, who were her parents for these first days, cannot continue taking care of her. We can only hope that in this world there is a kind-hearted person who will care for her. Thank you—In regret and shame, your father and mother.[30]

This female baby was born on March 15, 2002, in the morning at 9:30. Human beings in the world have as good hearts as biologic parents. We would like to express thanks to good-hearted people who will bring her up and keep her healthy, and we are quite sure that she will become a very good, active, lovely little girl when she grows up. We would like to express our heartfelt thanks again to whoever would bring her up.[40]

After the adoption. Are Chinese adoptees healthier and more developmentally intact than children from other countries? The young age of most children at the time of placement, better prenatal care, fewer adverse prenatal exposures, and superior institutional care have been cited as possible protective factors. No published studies have yet specifically compared the health of children adopted from China to that of adoptees from other countries. Most experts agree that the risks of fetal alcohol syndrome and fetal alcohol effect are considerably less than in children from Russia and other Eastern European countries. However, a survey of 452 children adopted from China reported prevalence of infectious diseases and growth and developmental delays similar to that of children from other countries.[41] Hepatitis B surface antigen was found in 6%, intestinal parasites in 9%, and latent tuberculosis infection in 3.5% of Chinese adoptees. Delayed growth was found in 39% of children for height, 18% for weight, and 24% for head circumference. Seventy-five percent of children had significant developmental delays in one or more domains; 44% had global delays. This report only evaluated children at entry into the United States; the prevalence of learning disabilities, language delays, persistent developmental delays, and behavioral and emotional problems was not assessed. Notably, 14% of the children had elevated lead levels,[41,42] a much higher prevalence than that for children from other countries. The long-term effects of lead intoxication may not be fully apparent until affected children reach school age.

Russia

History of International Adoption

The exponential rise in international adoptions from Russia (Table 3–5) parallels that for China over the past 12 years. Russia opened for international adoption as the Soviet Union disintegrated. The sudden availability of white children and the closure of Romania for international adoption rapidly accelerated interest in Russian adoptions. American parents were also enthusiastic about the provision of video tapes of the prospective child as part of the referral packet, first offered by a few agencies working in Russia in the early 1990s. Viewing video tapes of the prospective child made it easier for parents to connect with the child and also (often with professional assistance) to identify potential problems.

Italy, Canada, Israel, and New Zealand also receive children from Russia. Italy is second after the United States, receiving 197 Russian children in 1996 and 834 in 1999.[43]

The Ministry of Education is the central authority in Russia for international adoption, although officials and judges in each region have considerable autonomy to determine the actual legal process for adoption. As of 2000,

Table 3–5 Russian children adopted by American families, 1989–2003

Year	n
1989	0
1990	0
1991	12
1992	324
1993	746
1994	1530
1995	1896
1996	2454
1997	3816
1998	4491
1999	4348
2000	4269
2001	4279
2002	4939
2003	5209
Total	38,313

the government required accreditation of all foreign adoption agencies in Russia. Accreditation was offered only to those agencies with 5 or more years of experience in Russia. Accreditation obligates agencies to hire separate, salaried employees, to submit regular reports on their activities and income, and to pay taxes in full. About 50 American agencies are currently accredited. Agencies rely on local facilitators; previously some facilitators had simultaneous relationships with multiple adoption agencies and attorneys.[44] Some unscrupulous facilitators then offered children to multiple agencies, placing the child with the agency able to pay the highest fee. Shortly after taking office in 2000, Vladimir Putin signed a series of laws related to adoption practices. The laws were intended to halt corruption, child-selling, and other illegal activities related to international adoption.[43]

About 600,000–650,000 children reside in institutional care in Russia, with the number growing by ~100,000 each year.[45, 46] More than 90% are "social orphans"—children living in orphanages despite having parents.[46] Foster care is virtually nonexistent. Children are usually abandoned at birth, and enter residential care after a period (usually weeks to months) in the children's hospital or maternity home. Orphanages for young children, known as "baby homes," are usually under the jurisdiction of the regional health department. Older children reside in orphanages supervised by the regional education department. Children leave the "baby home" at about age 3; they are then assigned to a particular orphanage on the basis of results of a medical and developmental assessment. Some children enter state care after termination of parental rights (see Chapter 4). The type and quality of care vary enormously among different settings. Two exposés of conditions in Russian orphanages[47,48] attracted considerable media attention to the plight of institutionalized children in Russia. Some orphanages have far less than 50 U.S. cents per day to feed each child.[46] Other orphanages have plentiful food, multidisciplinary highly trained staff, and low caregiver-to-child ratios.

Logistics

In most regions, the process of international adoption now requires adoptive parents to make two trips before the adoption may be finalized. The purpose is first to identify the child and initiate legal proceedings and second to complete the adoption. A databank listing of available children (currently numbering 80,000) is maintained by government authorities. In theory, three Russian families must refuse the child before he or she is offered to foreigners. In practical terms, the child must remain on the databank for at least 6 months before a foreign adoption will be permitted. Both parents need not return for the second trip. Adoption proceedings must be completed before the immigrant visa is issued for travel to the United States.

General Health Issues in the Population

Russia has one of the highest smoking rates in the world[49]; smoking increased by 30% between 1995 and 1997. According to the Ministry of Health and Medical Industry in the mid-1990s, 67% of adult men and 25%–30% of adult women smoke. Smoking among adolescents has increased dramatically, especially among girls. A study in the early 1990s of over 36,000 students (age 15–17 years) revealed that smoking rates vary substantially, from around 25% in areas such as Kirov and Tver to around 46% in others areas, such as Moscow and Irkutsk. About 60% of 15-year-old boys and 44% of 15-year-old girls have tried smoking. Smoking prevalence in Moscow among 11 to 16 year-olds was estimated at ~42% (38% for girls). A high proportion of the cigarettes consumed (30%–40% of sales) are the traditional "papirosi," an unfiltered cigarette, consisting mainly of Oriental tobacco. Estimates of annual adult (age 15+) per capita consumption of cigarettes vary between 1156 and 2040 cigarettes.[50]

Alcohol use in Russia is staggering: the annual consumption is higher than anywhere else in the world. More than 30,000 Russians die each year of alcohol poisoning.[51] Annual consumption of alcohol is more than 10 liters per capita of pure alcohol—mostly in the form of vodka. This is a major factor in the decreased life expectancy for both men and women.[52] In 1993 the number of alcoholics in Russia rose by ~41%; alcoholism in women increased by 48%. In one survey, 80%–94% of girls between ages 15 and 17 drank "sometimes" and 17% drank "often."[53] More than 54,000 adolescents and 5500 children were referred to alcohol abuse treatment centers in 1998.[49] (see Erofeyev[51] for a readable description of the historical role of vodka in Russian society).

Illicit drug use has reached epidemic proportions in Russia. Cannabis, opium, and methamphetamine are the most popular drugs. Heroin is also increasingly popular. Six percent of 15 to 16 year-olds interviewed in Moscow in 1999 admitted to using heroin at least once. (Lifetime prevalence rate was <2% in all 21 other countries included in the same survey). A cross-road for the international drug trade, the Russian domestic market absorbs a growing and overwhelming portion of the illegal drugs that are produced, smuggled, and sold in the country.[54] Since 1990, the number of registered drug users has increased by almost 400%; in 1999, 359,067 drug users were registered in state drug-treatment centers. According to most experts, the true number of drug users is eight to ten times that figure. The Russian Ministry of the Interior, in a United Nations Office for Drug Control and Crime Prevention project, estimates that 2.5–3 million people regularly or occasionally use illegal drugs in Russia, representing >2% of the entire population.[55] The number of adolescent drug abusers increased 10-fold between 1988 and 1999; the incidence of substance abuse is 8.8 times greater among adolescents than the general population.[49]

The general health of the population has deteriorated in recent years. In a comprehensive series published in Newsday by prize-winning journalist Laurie Garrett, the Russian healthcare system was described as being "in a deadly state of shambles."[56] Diagnostic laboratories without electricity, running water, basic reagents, or apparatus; hospitals without supplies or equipment; and a moribund public health system are vividly described. Overall, Russia has the lowest life expectancy rates in Europe. The health of women is particularly poor.[57] Although 99% of births are attended, maternal mortality is more than six fold that of United States. Prenatal care is publicly funded, but refugees and immigrants are excluded. Sixteen percent of young women are susceptible to rubella, 30% of women are anemic during pregnancy (beyond physiologic anemia). Russian women have the highest abortion rate of any country in the world. The average Russian woman has between 3 to 8 abortions in her lifetime, 75% beyond 16 weeks gestation. Thirty-three percent of women smoke, and the prevalence of HIV/AIDS among young women is 0.3%. Domestic violence rates exceed those in the United States by four- to five-fold. Statistical estimates in Russia and other countries of the former Soviet Union do not always correspond to World Health Organization standards; underestimates of such indicators as infant mortality rate may result.[58]

Specific infectious risks in Russia include malaria (in very localized regions), tick-borne encephalitis, and diphtheria.

Special Considerations for Children Adopted from Russia

Before the adoption. Children reside in state-run orphanages. Foster care is virtually unknown. "Baby homes" provide care for children under 3 years of age. Children are then transferred to orphanages where they reside until age ~ 7 years. These homes are under the management of the Ministry of Health in each region (oblast). After age 7, children become the responsibility of the Ministry of Education, which supervises orphanage care until age ~17 years. At each transfer point, children are evaluated by a team of specialists to determine the appropriate placement (e.g., special needs facility, educational program, etc.).

Summer programs. A small number of "older" Russian children (5–12 years of age) follow an unusual pathway to adoption. These children participate in summer programs operated by adoption agencies and other humanitarian aid agencies. In Italy alone, over 60,000 children visited in the summer of 1997.[59] Although these programs are intended to provide only a summer holiday, sometimes the goal of the visit is adoptive placement. These children are considered good candidates for adoption by their orphanage caregivers, even though they are also viewed as "hard to match" because of their ages, the fact that they are part of sibling groups, or other factors. Generally a group of children from the same orphanage or region travel to the United States (or some other country) together. Each child or sibling group is assigned to a host family with whom they reside for several weeks. Occasionally, group activities are planned, and orphanage staff chaperones rotate among the host families for short periods during the visits. The children then return to their orphanages; families who agree to adopt their summer visitors proceed with the necessary legal procedures over the subsequent months. Such programs have the commendable goal of finding families for children, and indeed, many successful matches are made. Some adoption experts express concerns about these programs, particularly for those children not adopted by their host families. After experiencing family life in America, these children may have difficulties readjusting to orphanage life. Children not selected for adoption after participating in the summer program may become severely depressed. Programs that offer screening, training, and supervision for prospective parents likely make more successful placements.

After the adoption. Alcohol use is rampant in Russia. Parents unable to care for their children are more likely to use alcohol heavily than are other segments of the population. About 10%–15% of Russian adoptees have fetal alcohol syndrome (depending on criteria used for diagnosis).[60] This rate has not been formally compared with that of other countries, but most adoption medicine pediatricians find this condition more commonly in Russian children than among those adopted from Asia or Central or South America. In the absence of reliable markers of exposure (either phenotypic or biochemical), definitive determination is not possible. Learning disabilities and / or behavior problems during school years may reflect prenatal alcohol exposure. The prevalence of other medical problems is similar to that found in other countries. In a survey of children adopted from Eastern Europe (64% from Russia),[61] 2% had chronic hepatitis B, 5% had tuberculosis, and 51% had one or more intestinal pathogens. Growth delays (z scores < -1) were found in 44% of children for weight, 68% for height, and 43% for head circumference. Developmental delays in various domains were found in 53%–82% of the children.

Although most children have undergone assessment by several specialists as well as with ultrasound and laboratory testing, serious unrecognized diagnoses are sometimes found after arrival in the United States. In a review of 56 children adopted from Russia (and other countries of Eastern Europe),[61] chronic hepatitis B, optic nerve hypoplasia, orthopedic anomalies, severe unilateral hearing loss, renal calculi, mild spastic diplegia, and strabismus were identified after adoption. Impaired school performance, regulation of attention, and sensory integration are emerging in some Russian children as they progress through school.[62–65]

Romania

International Adoption History

During the 24 years of his regime, Romanian dictator Nicolae Ceausescu attempted to increase the population of Romania with draconian "pro-natalist" policies banning abortion and contraception. Social programs including nursing, social work, midwifery, psychology, and special education were dismantled.[66] Maternal deaths soared as illegal abortions were sought; thousands of unwanted children entered state institutions. After Ceausescu's execution in 1989, the world learned with horror of the more than 700 enormous state-run institutions housing 100,000 to 300,000 children, often in appalling conditions.[66–69] In Ungureni, for example, a home for 200 children, 40 children died every year from starvation and cold.[70] Many facilities provided bare subsistence levels of food, clothing, and shelter. Caregiver ratios were as high as 60:1. Conditions in institutions for "unsalvageables" were unspeakable.[71] (See Table 2–7) In less dire environments, children had severe delays in cognition, social function,[72] and motor skills.[73] Even neurologically normal children commonly exhibited self-stimulatory behaviors such as body rocking (35%–50%), wrist flapping (6%–10%), face guarding (10%–15%), and finger shadowing (18%–19%).[73]

Most adults today have vivid memories of the heart-wrenching photos released in the early 1990s of these confined children. Thousands of Americans, Europeans, and Canadians rushed to Romania to adopt children (See Table 3–6. Many children were placed with adoptive families in a process that was wildly unregulated and without government oversight (see Pertman,[2] pp 151–154 for an unimaginable story). Adoptions rose from <30 in 1989 to >10,000 in 1990.[59] In Canada, 1013 visas were issued to Romanian adopted children between January 1990 and April 1991.[68] Gradually, government regulations were enforced, and some semblance of order was imposed. Amidst concerns about corruption, however, international adoption from Romania has been off and on for the last 5 years. Presently (2004), a moratorium on international adoption remains in place, while government officials attempt to introduce and strengthen reforms. Concurrently, author-

Table 3–6 Romanian children adopted by American families, 1989–2003

Year	n
1989	138
1990	121
1991	2594
1992	121
1993	97
1994	199
1995	275
1996	555
1997	621
1998	406
1999	895
2000	1122
2001	782
2002	168
2003	200
Total	**8,294**

ity for the care of abandoned children has been transferred from national to local authorities and the child protection budget substantially increased. Efforts have been made in some localities to close large institutions and replace them with group homes or foster care.

Despite these reforms, more children reside in Romanian institutions today than 10 years ago:[74] 45,953 compared to 43,854. Including children in special residential schools, the total number of institutionalized children in Romania is nearly 100,000, even though 20,000 children have left the orphanages since 1989.

Logistics

International adoptions are currently banned in Romania. Some children who were matched to adoptive families prior to the ban are gradually being permitted to exit the country under special circumstances. The U.S. State Department's Office of Consular Affairs and the Romanian Embassy periodically post updates on their Web sites.[12,75]

General Health Issues
in the Population

Smoking is common: the annual adult (age 15+) per capita consumption of cigarettes in Romania averages around 1550–2100. Consumption is likely underestimated, as it has been reported that about 20% of cigarettes consumed in Romania are imported illegally. Smoking prevalence (daily and occasional) among adults age 20–29 is reported to be 55% of men and 20% of women.[49] Smoking is common in many social groups, including medical students (34%–54% smokers) and factory workers (69%–76% smokers).[76]

Alcohol use in Romania is estimated at 9.7 liters per capita, with 56% of adults reporting that they drink alcohol—74% of men and 40% of women. Drinking two to three times per week was reported by 17% of men and 2% of women. Romania's rate of cirrhosis remains among the highest in Europe.[49]

No reliable estimates of drug use in the population are available, as there are no drug treatment programs in either the public or private sector. Per capita income is low and most Romanians cannot afford to purchase illicit drugs.[77] However, some drug use occurs, and Romania is a major site for shipment of heroin and cocaine.[54] Inhalant use is widespread, especially among young people and street children.[49]

Tick-borne encephalitis is another local health risk.

Special Considerations for Children
Adopted from Romania

Before the adoption. Nearly all Romanian orphans live in institutions prior to adoption, although a small number reside in foster care. Just before the most recent international adoption moratorium, foster care was becoming more common, especially after children were matched to an adoptive family. As in the United States, the quality of this care varies greatly. Foster parents may lack the specialized training and resources to manage the problems of children institutionalized in deprived environments.

After the adoption. Romanian adoptees in Europe, Canada, and the United States constitute a special group. These children have been the focus of several extensive[62–64,67,68] and ongoing studies[78–84] that comprise most of what is known about adjustment and long-term outcome of post-institutionalized children after international adoption. Persistent developmental delays, frequent sensory dysfunction, and ongoing emotional and behavioral problems are unfortunately common in this group of children. It is not yet apparent how applicable these studies are to children adopted from less difficult early environments.

Romanian adoptees have been carefully scrutinized for health problems and developmental issues. In a survey of children adopted in the early 1990s, 53% had serologic evidence of past or present hepatitis B, 20% had positive tests for hepatitis B surface antigen, and 33% had intestinal parasites. Only 15% were judged to be physically healthy, and only 10% of children older than 12 months were developmentally normal.[67] In a comprehensive study of Romanian adoptees in Canada, 30% of those adopted at >8 months had several serious problems, even 3 years after adoption. Another one-third had a few serious problems but were progressing toward average levels of performance and behavior, while one-third of adoptees were doing well.[78] Adoption at young ages did not preclude persistent problems (Table 3–7).[68]

More recently, general health and development of newly arrived Romanian adoptees have improved. Rates for infectious diseases are similar to those found in children from other Eastern European countries. Many older children who arrived earlier demonstrate remarkable resilience and recovery from previous problems.

Table 3–7 Status of medical problems in Romanian adoptees (*n* = 130) in Canada at arrival and follow-up

Type of Problem	Children with Problems	
	Arrival (median age 6 months)	Follow-up (median age 3 years)
	(n)	(n)
Medical problems	80	41
Eating problems	62	28
Developmental delays	59	33
Stereotypical behaviors	39	27
Attachment problems	32	10
Tantrums	27	29

Source: Data from Marcovitch et al.[68]

Guatemala

History of International Adoption

The number of children adopted from Guatemala has risen steadily over the past 12 years, with a sharp increase in adoptions occurring most recently (Table 3–8). Guatemala has maintained its position among the "top five" sending countries since 1992. This increase results from the availability of infants and the increasing use of foster care prior to adoption. Suspensions and delays of adoptions from Cambodia and Romania have also coincided with this increase. Concerns about potential baby-selling and other scandals led to legal reforms to protect birth parents, children, and adoptive parents in the mid-1990s. Presently, Guatemala is the only country that provides a signed relinquishment document from the birth mother and results of DNA testing that verify the relationship of the mother and child (Fig. 3–1). The purpose of these documents is to ban adoption of children who have been obtained by illegal means (coercion, sold, stolen).[85] The U.S. Bureau of Citizenship and Immigration Services (BCIS) requires the DNA testing in all cases where the child is being released by an identifiable birth mother. Previously, unscrupulous women would pose as birth mothers to release the child. The blood samples are collected by an embassy-approved physician, then shipped to an authorized laboratory in the United States. The success of this effort has re-

Table 3–8 Guatemalan children adopted by American families, 1989–2003

Year	n
1989	208
1990	257
1991	329
1992	418
1993	512
1994	436
1995	449
1996	427
1997	788
1998	911
1999	1002
2000	1518
2001	1609
2002	2219
2003	2328
Total	13,411

> Conclusion
>
> The alleged mother, MARIA C., cannot be excluded as the biological mother of the child, MANUEL C., since they share genetic markers. Using the above systems, the probability of maternity is 99.99%, as compared to an untested, unrelated woman of the Guatemalan population.
>
> Combined Parentage Index: 126,400 to 1
> Probability of Maternity: 99.99%

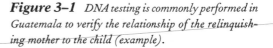

Figure 3–1 *DNA testing is commonly performed in Guatemala to verify the relationship of the relinquishing mother to the child (example).*

sulted in calls for similar programs in other countries.[86] The BCIS also requires that an HIV test be performed on the mother. Because of ongoing concerns in Guatemala about civil document fraud and corruption, occasionally the BCIS will interview and investigate the birth mother.

Presently, Guatemala does not have a central authority to oversee adoptions. Adoptions are arranged privately by local attorneys; final approval of the adoption is given by the Guatemalan Solicitor General's office. The legal process for a Guatemalan adoption, deemed "unique" by the United Nations Children's Fund (UNICEF), permits private adoptions with little state oversight.[87] Ongoing questions about legality remain; in 1999 UNICEF recommended that extrajudicial adoptions cease until Guatemala passed adoption laws consistent with The Hague Convention for International Adoptions and the International Convention on the Rights of the Child.[88] Nearly all adoptions in Guatemala are international; 62% of all adoptions go to U.S. families[87] and most of the remainder go to Canada. Although many reforms have been introduced into the legislature, the ~200 Guatemalan adoption lawyers represent a powerful lobby to maintain the status quo. Over 300 orphanages exist in the country, but few children from these orphanages are adopted because of the lengthy times it takes for an infant to be declared abandoned and eligible for adoption.

In an unusual case in 1998, an infant boy named Pablo was returned to his birth mother even though his adoption to a Spanish couple had been arranged. The birth mother stated that she had signed relinquishment documents under duress. The charitable organization Caza Alianza estimates that about 440 Guatemalan children were fraudulently adopted since 1996. Lawyers, in collusion with doctors, nurses, and social workers, pressure new mothers to relinquish their children. According to French adoption officials,[89] the children are placed in "clandestine orphanages" prior to adoptive placement.

Logistics

Numerous adoption agencies place children from Guatemala. The agencies contract with the private lawyers in Guatemala who oversee the adoption. Detailed procedures are available from the U.S. State Department, Office of Children's Issues[12] and are subject to frequent change.

General Health Issues in the Population

Smoking prevalence is approximately 38%–81% among men and 18%–34% among women.[90] Tobacco use increases with age: 8% of 12- to 14-year-olds, 25% of 15- to 19-year-olds, 34% of 20- to 24-year-olds, and 49% of 30- to 34-year-olds were smokers. The annual consumption of cigarettes per capita is estimated at 340. Alcohol use varies widely; between 20% and 48% of women use alcohol.[91] Various home brews are commonly consumed.

Drug abuse is prevalent in Guatemala. Use is increasing especially among mestizo, black, and Garifuna young people. Among teenagers, lifetime prevalence oscillates between 2% and 5% for cocaine consumption and between 4% and 7% for cannabis use. According the United Nations Office of Drug Control Programs, about 6% of the population abuses marijuana, 3% uses inhalants, and 3% uses tranquilizers.[92] Level of education determines drug of choice; marijuana is used by those with the lowest educational achievement and tranquilizers are used by those with the highest level. Guatemala is also a transit country for cocaine and heroin shipment and a minor producer of illicit opium poppy and cannabis (mostly for domestic consumption). Money laundering and corruption are also serious problems.[7a]

Other health risks include dengue, filariasis, leishmaniasis, onchocerciasis, American trypanosomiasis (Chagas disease), and malaria.

Special Considerations for Children Adopted from Guatemala

Before the adoption. Most Guatemalan children placed with American families reside in foster care prior to adoption. Adoptive parents usually travel to receive their child, but occasionally children may be escorted to the United States. Adoptive parents often meet their child's foster parents. This meeting can be extremely valuable, as it can ease the transition for the child and prepare the adoptive parents for future questions from their child ("who took care of me before I came home?"). Adoptive parents should be forewarned that foster care is not uniformly loving and attentive. As in the United States, foster parents vary in their motivation and ability to care for children. A few private orphanages place children for international adoption as well.

Information on birth families is limited. However, photographs are sometimes available. Birth mothers are commonly described as "domestico" (or maid) in legal documents; many are illiterate. Frequently, the relinquished child is the third or fourth in the family; the older children remain with the parent(s). Although referrals are usually offered within a few days or weeks of birth, legalities usually delay placement of the child for 7–9 months.

After the adoption. No particular medical problems have been identified in Guatemalan children after adoption. Physical condition and developmental skills reflect the type and quality of care received by the child prior to adoption. Medical problems (parasites, anemia, tuberculosis, etc.) occur in small numbers of children. Experts still disagree on the validity of vaccine records from Guatemala; efficacy of administered immunizations likely depends on their source, which may not be known with certainty (see Chapter 21). Although uncommon, serious unrecognized medical conditions have been found in Guatemalan adoptees, such as pervasive developmental delay, autism, hearing impairment, fetal alcohol syndrome, and cerebral palsy.[93]

Ukraine

History of international adoption

Adoptions from Ukraine are relatively recent. Ukraine first appeared on the list of "top 20" sending countries in 1998 (at #11, with 180 children). Since then, the number of Ukrainian children adopted in the United States has skyrocketed (Table 3–9). The reasons for this rise are complex. Closures in other countries prompted some families to investigate Ukraine. Some parents prefer the opportunity to "choose their own child," and some perceive the legal process as less cumbersome than in other countries. More than one child may be adopted at the same time. Because only a single trip is required, cost may be a factor. Ukraine has also been more receptive to nontraditional families than Russia: there are no firm age restrictions for adoptive parents.

Since the establishment of the National Adoption Center, about 10,000 children have been adopted by foreigners in the past 6 years. As Ukrainian adoption has become more pop-

Table 3–9 Children adopted from Ukraine, 1998–2003

Year	n
1998	180
1999	323
2000	659
2001	1246
2002	1106
2003	702
Total	4,216

ular, more concerns have arisen regarding corruption. In February 2003, Ukraine opened an investigation of foreign adoptions.[94] An initial inquiry revealed forged documents and other fraudulent material. The investigation is ongoing at present (June 2003). At least 36,000 homeless children remain in Ukraine. Adoptions in Ukraine will likely be subject to legal reform and political review in the near future.

Logistics

Ukraine has an unusual procedure for international adoptions. By law, prospective parents may not receive information about a specific child prior to arrival in Ukraine. Upon arrival, parents register with the National Adoption Center of Ukraine, which directs the parents to available children. Foreigners are permitted to consider only those children who have been on a national database for 1 year (this waiting requirement may be waived if the child suffers from certain medical conditions listed by the Ministry of Public Health Protection). This practice has proved extremely difficult for prospective adoptive parents, who must interpret complex medical information (usually without the benefit of medical consultation), assess the child's health and future potential, and make an adoption decision under extraordinary time and emotional pressures.

General Health Issues in the Population

Smoking starts at a very early age in Ukraine. In 1990, the prevalence of daily smoking was 10% among 12- to 13-year-olds and 40% among 16- to 17-year-olds. Smoking prevalence was 75% among students (principally 17- to 18-year-olds) at a technical college in Ukraine. Overall, smoking prevalence peaks in the age group 20–29 years (61% both sexes combined) and then declines to 50% in the age group 40–49

years and 33% in the age group 60–69 years. Smoking decreases with increasing levels of education and higher socioeconomic status. The annual per capita consumption of cigarettes is estimated at 1800.[95] The World Health Organization estimates smoking prevalence at 73% among men and 42% among women.[96]

Ukraine is one of the six European countries with the highest registered alcohol consumption.[97] According to the Ukrainian parliamentary committee on public health, more than 6.5 million citizens of working age have problems with alcohol. There are 670,000 chronic alcoholics registered in Ukraine.[98] Only 10% of Ukrainian men and 21% of women abstain from drinking. Ukraine's annual consumption of pure alcohol per capita is 11.5 liters, but including black market alcohol a better estimate is 13 liters.[97] Some 4% of the population consumes >50 grams of pure alcohol daily.[96]

Drug abuse is also widespread. The number of unregistered drug abusers is estimated at two to three times higher than 65,000, the number of officially registered addicts. Opium poppy straw extract continues to be the main drug of choice. Marijuana and synthetic drugs are growing in popularity among young people. Hard drugs such as cocaine and heroin are too expensive for the average Ukrainian citizen.[98] Most drug abusers are multidrug users of mostly marijuana and home-produced morphine derivatives.[96]

The effects of the Chernobyl disaster are discussed in Chapter 24. An excellent overview of health issues in Ukraine is available at the World Health Organization Web site,[96] and links from the Parent Network for Post-Institutionalized Children Web site.[99]

Special Considerations for Children Adopted from Ukraine

Before the adoption.   Children reside in government-run orphanages. These are set up similar to those in Russia (see above).

After the adoption. A recent review of the health of 76 children adopted from Ukraine[60] found frequent infections (giardia in 38%, tuberculosis in 25%, hepatitis B in 9%) and medical problems (middle ear disease in 20%, iodine deficiency in 10%). Strikingly, at least 15% had fetal alcohol syndrome (depending on criteria used for diagnosis).

Other Countries

Specific information about other countries may be found in Table 3–1, as well as in Chapters 5–7. Other helpful Web sites are the following:

http://www.euro.who.int/countryinformation
Country-specific overviews on health.

http://www.cdc.gov/tobacco/who/whofirst.htm
Country-specific information on tobacco use.

http://www.cia.gov/cia/publications/
factbook/
Country-specific information on illicit drugs.

http://www.cdc.gov/travel/
Travel information by country and disease

http://www.who.int/ith/
Travel information by country and disease

http://www.travel.state.gov/adopt.html
Country-specific information on international adoption regulations and logistics.

References

1. Andersen TM. Social implications for institutionalized children. In: Rygvold A-L, Dalen M, Saeterdal B, eds. Mine–Yours–Ours and Theirs. Oslo: University of Oslo, 1999: 118–24.

2. Pertman A. Adoption Nation: How the Adoption Revolution is Transforming America. New York: Basic Books, 2000.

3. Bartholet E. Family Bonds: Adoption, Infertility, and the New World of Child Production. Boston: Beacon Press, 1993.

4. Gailey CW. Race, class, and gender in U.S. international adoption. In: Rygvold A-L, Dalen M, Saetersdal B, eds. Mine–Yours–Ours and Theirs. Oslo: University of Oslo, 1999: 52–81.

5. Register C. Are Those Kids Yours? American Families with Children Adopted from Other Countries. New York: Free Press, 1991.

6. UNICEF. The State of the World's Children 2003. Available at: http://www.unicef.org/sowc03/tables.

7. World Health Organization. Countries. Available at: http://www.who.int/country.

7a. Central Intelligence Agency. http://www.cia.gov/cia/publications/factbook.

8. Holt International Children's Services. Available at: http://www.holtintl.org/.

9. Wetzstein C. Korean adoptees breached boundaries: wartime orphans celebrate making international adoptions acceptable. The Washington Times, Sept. 14 1999: 2.

10. Johnson K, Banghan H, Liyao W. Infant abandonment and adoption in China. Popul Dev Rev 1998; 24:469.

11. Adopting from Korea and afterwards. Available at: http://www.adoptkorea.com.

12. U.S. Department of State, Office of Children's Issues. International adoption. Available at: http://travel.state.gov/adopt.html.

13. Gluck C. South Koreans try to quit smoking. Available at: http://news.bbc.co.uk/1/hi/world/asia-pacific/1870627.stm.

14. Park, K. South Korea. Global Alcohol Policy Alliance, GAPA Bangkok Consultation, Alcohol in Asia. The Globe, Special Issue 4, 2001–2002. Available at: http://www.ias.org.uk/publications/theglobe/01issue3,4/globe01issue3_4.pdf.

15. The Asian Harm Reduction Network Country Assessment—South Korea. Available at: http://www.ahrn.net/regional/skorea.html.

16. Greenblatt M, Khoo EC. Incidence of hepatitis B carriers among adopted Korean children [letter]. N Engl J Med 1985; 312:1639.

17. Lange WR, Warnock-Eckhart E. Selected infectious disease risks in international adoptees. Pediatr Infect Dis J 1987; 6:447–50.

18. Nordenfelt E, Dahlquist E. HBsAg positive adopted children as a cause of intrafamilial spread of hepatitis B. Scand J Infect Dis 1978; 10:161–3.

19. Murray DL, Lynch M, Doughty A, Cho BK. Results of screening adopted Korean children for HBsAg [letter]. Am J Public Health 1988; 78:855–6.

20. Murray DL. International adoptees and hepatitis B virus infection [letter; comment]. Am J Dis Child 1990; 144:523–4.

21. Hostetter MK, Iverson S, Dole K, Johnson D. Unsuspected infectious diseases and other medical diagnoses in the evaluation of internationally adopted children [see comments]. Pediatrics 1989; 83:559–64.

22. Jenista JA, Chapman D. Medical problems of foreign-born adopted children. Am J Dis Child 1987; 141:298–302.

23. Hostetter MK, Iverson S, Thomas W, McKenzie D, Dole K, Johnson DE. Medical evaluation of internationally adopted children. N Engl J Med 1991; 325:479–85.

24. Lien NM, Meyer KK, Winick M. Early malnutrition and "late" adoption: a study of their effects on the development of Korean orphans adopted into American families. Am J Clin Nutr 1977; 30:1734–9.

25. Winick M, Meyer KK, Harris RC. Malnutrition and environmental enrichment by early adoption. Science 1975; 190:1173–5.

26. Kim WJ, Shin YJ, Carey MP. Comparison of Korean-American adoptees and biological children of their adoptive parents: a pilot study. Child Psychiatry Hum Dev 1999; 29:221–8.

27. Stams GJ, Juffer F, Rispens J, Hoksbergen RA. The development and adjustment of 7-year-old children adopted in infancy. J Child Psychol Psychiatry 2000; 41:1025–37.

28. American Academy of Pediatrics. Medical evaluation of internationally adopted children. In: Pickering LK, ed. Red Book: Report of the Committee on Infectious Diseases. Elk Grove Village, IL: American Academy of Pediatrics, 2003: 173–180.

29. Vonk ME, Simms PJ, Nackerud L. Political and personal aspects of inter-country adoption of Chinese children in the United States. Contemp Hum Serv 1999; 80:496.

30. Johnson K. The politics of the revival of infant abandonment in China, with special reference to Hunan. Pop Dev Rev 1996; 22:77.

31. Thurston WF. In a Chinese orphanage. The Atlantic Monthly 1996; 277:28.

32. Driedger SD. Bodies of evidence: China denies that its orphanages are death camps. Maclean's 1996; 109:52.

33. Duin J. Abandoned Chinese babies find homes. The Washington Times Nov 14, 2000: 2.

34. Human Rights Watch. Death by Default: A Policy of Fatal Neglect in China's State Orphanages. New York: Human Rights Watch, 1996.

35. Gillan A. Lost babies, found babies. London: European Intelligence Wire. Oct 12, 2002.

36. Cox SS-K. Adopted Asian children have entered the cultural mainstream in America. Asia Africa Intelligence Wire, Nov 9, 2002.

37. China plans smoking curbs in 2004. Asia African Intelligence Wire, Nov 17, 2003.

38. The Asian Harm Reduction Network Country Assessment—China. Available at: www.ahrn.net/regional/china.html.

39. Grauwels S. Taiwan's health chief quits over SARS crisis. The Boston Globe. May 16, 2003: A7.

40. Anonymous. Note found with my daughter. Personal communication to Miller LC, Boston, 2002.

41. Miller LC, Hendrie NW. Health of children adopted from China. Pediatrics 2000; 105:E76.

42. Aronson JE, Smith AM, Kothari V, et al. Elevated blood lead levels among internationally adopted children—United States, 1998. MMWR Morb Mortal Wkly Rep 2000; 49: 97–100.

43. Traynor I, Carroll R. Police raids uncover 'orphans for sale' racket: arrest of woman in Russia reveals web of bureaucratic corruption around adoption of 600 children by Italians. The Guardian (London), Guardian Foreign Pages, Feb 24 2001: 16.

44. Pertman A. Russia's reforms slow flow of US adoptions. The Boston Globe, National/Foreign, May 2 2000: A1.

45. Human Rights Watch. Available at: http://www.hrw.org/children/abandoned.htm.

46. Russia's Putin decries rise in orphan numbers. Reuters, March 2, 2000. Available at: http://www.cdi.org/russia/johnson/4146.html#12.

47. Cox C. Trajectories of Despair: Misdiagnosis and Maltreatment of Soviet Orphans. Zurich: Christian Solidarity International, 1991.

48. Hunt K. Abandoned to the State: Cruelty and Neglect in Russian Orphanages. New York: Human Rights Watch, 1998.

49. World Health Organization. Country information. Available at: http://www.euro.who.int/countryinformation.

50. Tobacco or health: a global status report. Russian Federation. Available at: http://www.cdc.gov/tobacco/who/russianf.htm.

51. Erofeyev V. The Russian God. The New Yorker, Dec. 16 2002: 56–63.

52. Vlassov V. The role of alcohol and social stress in Russia's mortality rate. JAMA 1999; 281:321–2.

53. Environmental and health atlas of Russia. Feshbach M, ed. Moscow and Chevy Chase, MD: "Paims" Publishing House, 1995.

54. Central Intelligence Agency. The World Factbook. Available at: http://www.cia.gov/cia/publications/factbook/geos/rs.html.

55. Paoli L, et al. Drug trafficking and related organized crime in Russia. Available at: http://www.iuscrim.mpg.de/forsch/krim/paoli2_en.html.

56. Garrett L. Crumbled empire, shattered health. Newsday, Oct 26–29, 1997.

57. Dymchenko LD, Callister LC. Challenges and opportunities: the health of women and newborns in the Russian Federation. J Perinat Neonat Nurs 2002; 16:11–22.

58. Wuhib T, McCarthy BJ, Chorba TL, Sinitsina TA, Ivasiv IV, McNabb SJN. Underestimate of infant mortality rates in one republic of the former Soviet Union. Pediatrics 2003; 111:e596–600.

59. Cantwell N. Intercountry Adoption. Innocenti Digest. Vol. 4. Florence, Italy: UNICEF International Child Development Centre, 1998: 1–24.

60. Johnson D. Adoption in Ukraine, Washington D.C.: Joint Council for International Children's Services, April 9, 2003.

61. Albers LH, Johnson DE, Hostetter MK, Iverson S, Miller LC. Health of children adopted from the former Soviet Union and Eastern Europe. Comparison with preadoptive medical records. JAMA 1997; 278:922–4.

62. Lin S. Sensory Integration in Post-institutionalized Eastern European Children. Occupational Therapy. Ph.D. Thesis. Boston: Boston University, 2002.

63. Cermak S, Groze V. Sensory processing problems in post-institutionalized children: implications for social workers. Child Adolesc Soc Work J 1998; 15:5–37.

64. Cermak SA, Daunhauer LA. Sensory processing in the post-institutionalized child. Am J Occup Ther 1997; 51:500–7.

65. Tirella LG, Miller LC. Educational achievements of 8- to12-year-old children adopted from Eastern Europe. Washington, DC: Joint Council for International Children's Services. April 10, 2002.

66. Children's Health Care Collaborative Study Group. Romanian health and social care system for children and families: future directions in health care reform. BMJ 1992; 304:556–9.

67. Johnson DE, Miller LC, Iverson S, et al. The health of children adopted from Romania JAMA 1992; 268:3446–51.

68. Marcovitch S, Cesaroni L, Roberts W, Swanson C. Romanian adoption: parents' dreams, nightmares, and realities. Child Welfare 1995; LXXIV:993–1017.

69. Johnson AK, Groze V. The orphaned and institutionalized children of Romania. J Emot Behav Prob 1993; 2:49–52.

70. Stojaspal J. Young folks at home: Ceausescu's monstrous orphanages begin to disappear as light and a little love get in. Time Int 2002; 160: 2002: 44–46.

71. Rosenberg DR, Pajer K, Rancurello M. Neuropsychiatric assessment of orphans in one Romanian orphanage for "unsalvageables." JAMA 1992; 268:3489–90.

72. Kaler SR, Freeman BJ. Analysis of environmental deprivation: cognitive and social development in Romanian orphans. J Child Psychol Psychiatry 1994; 35:769–81.

73. Sweeney JK, Bascom BB. Motor development and self-stimulatory movement in institutionalized Romanian children. Pediatr Phys Ther 1995; 7:124–32.

74. Mackie L. How to stop little children suffering: there are more orphans in Romania now than in 1989. New Statesman (1996); 128, 1999:30.

75. Embassy of Romania. Available at: http://www.roembus.org/english.communities/copii/link-copii.htm.

76. Centers for Disease Control and Prevention. Tobacco or Health: A Global Status Report–Romania. Available at: http://www.cdc.gov/tobacco/who/romania.htm.

77. U.S. Department of State. International Narcotics Control Strategy Report, March 1996: Romania. Available At:http://www.hri.org/docs/USSD-INCSR/95/Europe/Romania.html.

78. Ames EW. The development of Romanian orphanage children adopted to Canada. Burnaby, British Columbia, Canada: National Welfare Grants Program, Human Resources Development Canada, 1997.

79. Castle J, Groothues C, Bredenkamp D, Beckett C, O'Connor T, Rutter M. Effects of qualities of early institutional care on cognitive attainment. E.R.A. Study Team. English and Romanian Adoptees. Am J Orthopsychiatry 1999; 69:424–37.

80. Kreppner JM, O'Connor T, Rutter M. Can inattention/overactivity be an institutional deprivation syndrome? J Abnorm Child Psychol 2001; 29:513–28.

81. O'Connor TG, Rutter M, Beckett C, Keaveney L, Kreppner JM. The effects of global severe privation on cognitive competence: extension and longitudinal follow-up. English and Romanian Adoptees Study Team. Child Dev 2000; 71:376–90.

82. Rutter M, and English and Romanian Adoptees Study Team. Developmental catch-up, and delay, following adoption after severe global early privation. J Child Psychol Psychiatry 1998; 39:465–476.

83. Rutter M, Andersen-Wood L, Beckett C, et al. Quasi-autistic patterns following severe global privation. J Child Psychol Psychiatry 1999; 40:537–549.

84. Morison SJ, Ames EW, Chisholm K. The development of children adopted from Romanian orphanages. Merrill-Palmer Q 1995; 41:411–30.

85. Stefanova K. DNA testing used to ensure authenticity: Guatemalan babies, mothers screened. The Washington Times, World. July 5, 1999: 12.

86. Birchard K. Call for DNA testing for foreign adoptions. Lancet 1998; 352:633.

87. Adoption vs. trafficking in Guatemala. The Christian Science Monitor, October 17, 2000: 1.

88. UNICEF. Intercountry Adoption. Available at: http://www.unicef-icdc.org/publications/pdf/digest4e.pdf.

89. Jacot M. Adoption: for love or money? UNESCO Courier, February 1999:37.

90. Centers for Disease Control and Prevention. Tobacco or health: a global status report. Guatemala. Available at: http://www.cdc.gov/tobacco/who/guatemal.htm.

91. World Health Organization. Global Alcohol Database. Available at: http://www3.who.int/whosis/alcohol.

92. United Nation Office on Drugs and Crime. Guatamala country profile. Available at: http://www.odccp.org:80/mexico/country_profile_guatemala.html.

93. Miller LC, Comfort K, Tirella LG, Chan W. Health of children adopted from Guatemala, 2003, unpublished.

94. Ukraine opens criminal case over child adoption by foreigners. Asia Africa Intelligence Wire, Feb 6, 2003.

95. Centers for Disease Control and Prevention. Tobacco or health: a global status report. Ukraine. Available at: http://www.cdc.gov/tobacco/who/whofirst.htm.

96. World Health Organization. Highlights on Health in Ukraine. Available at: http://www.who.dk/document/e72372.pdf.

97. Knox K. Ukraine: the statistics sound good but don't toast sobriety yet. Available at: http://www.rferl.org/ca/features/2002/06/26062002163530.asp.

98. Ukraine reports statistics in drug and alcohol addiction. Asia Africa Intelligence Wire, Dec 1, 2003.

99. Ukraine: Environmental pollution, women and children's health, and birth defects. Available at: http://www.pnpic.org/ukraine.htm.

4

PRE-ADOPTION COUNSELING AND EVALUATION OF THE REFERRAL

The decision to adopt is often followed by a call to the pediatrician. Pediatric advice and suggestions are eagerly sought by most families interested in international adoption. Adoption-friendly practices offer pre-adoption visits as an opportunity for prospective parents to discuss concerns and questions. Once an individual child is offered to the family for consideration (known as the "referral" in adoption parlance), the pediatrician may become very involved in counseling the family about health risks. This chapter offers general guidelines for the pediatrician or family physician who offers pre-adoption counseling and reviews referrals for prospective adoptive families.

Pre-Adoption Counseling

Early Stages

Some prospective parents consult a pediatrician in the early stages of adoption (Table 4–1). Many of the subjects relevant to this process are ad-

dressed throughout this book. If a pediatrician does not feel qualified to address all of these topics; referral to social workers, adoption agencies, or mental health professionals may be necessary. Some of the more common questions, however, could be posed for biologic parenthood as well.

Pediatricians have special awareness of the difficulties for families of children with complex medical and developmental problems. Therefore, one of the most important functions

Table 4–1 Common pre-adoptive parent queries

Is adoption right for me?

How will adoption affect my other children?

Are healthy children available for international adoption? Which countries have the healthiest children?

What are the health risks for internationally adopted children?

How can I minimize these risks for myself and other family members?

How do "older children" adjust after adoption?

How do internationally adopted children fare long-term?

of a pediatrician may be to enlighten prospective adoptive families about subjects they may not have considered (Table 4–2). Adoptive parents sometimes express regrets that they were unaware of the potential problems of their adopted child. Although many adoption agencies carefully prepare parents and plentiful information is available on the Internet and elsewhere, some parents wish they had received more explicit information prior to the adoption about learning disabilities, hyperactivity, posttraumatic stress disorder, physical and sexual abuse, and attachment disorder.

A comprehensive, detailed description of the outcome of international adoption has not yet been published. Surveys published to date are limited by low numbers, selection biases, insufficient depth of analysis, and short periods of follow-up. Focus is usually limited to parent satisfaction, medical problems, growth, educational issues, or behavior. None of these alone gives a broad picture of international adoption. Furthermore, outcome may change as countries of origin and pre-adoptive experiences change over time. A large study of over 2000 international adoptees in Minnesota (the International Adoption Project) is currently being conducted,[1] with preliminary results indicating that the common medical problems among the children are chronic ear infections (17%), visual problems (17%), speech delays (10%), hearing impairment (8%), and behavioral disturbances (7%). The number of pre-adoption risk factors predicted the likelihood of later educational and behavioral problems (Table 4–3). In some

Table 4–2 Topics to discuss with prospective parents

Reasonable parental leave after adoption
Early intervention programs
School placement decisions
Insurance benefits for dental health services, if needed
Insurance benefits for mental health services, if needed
Insurance benefits for evaluation of school-related issues, if needed

Table 4–3 Pre-adoptive risk factors for later educational and behavioral problems

Prenatal exposure to alcohol (or other drugs of abuse)
Prenatal malnutrition
Prematurity
In an orphanage, baby home, or hospital for more than 6 months
Neglect of basic social needs such as food, clothing, or medical care (moderate or severe)
Physical abuse (moderate or severe)

Source: Minnesota International Adoption Project.[1]
See also Table 13–7.

cases, the presence of these risk factors may not be known with certainty. The number of risk factors varied with the country of origin of the child (nearly 2/3 of children from Russia and Eastern Europe had >4 risk factors) and age of the child at adoption (older children tended to have more risk factors). Emerging results from this important study are available at the project Web site.[1]

Parental leave is worth discussing at the beginning of adoption decisions. One parent should be prepared to stay home with the new child for 3 to 12 months. A minimum of 6 months is advisable in most circumstances. Single parents may need to plan carefully. If financial constraints dictate an earlier return to work, a nanny should be considered rather than group day care. Group day care, especially in large day care centers, may provide fragmented care similar to that found in orphanages. Focused, loving adult attention is the best means to help children recover from the effects of institutionalization (see Chapter 2) and to promote attachment to the family (see Chapter 29). Insurance benefits for the prospective adopted child should be maximized to allow comprehensive services if the need arises.

Some parents wish to adopt more than one child at a time. The desire for "instant family," cost considerations (reduction in travel expenses), the need to keep siblings together, or other factors may compel concurrent adoptions.

Siblings may provide support and security for each other through the adoption process, although some siblings may not be acquainted with each other. Parents considering concurrent adoptions should be counseled about the difficulties that may ensue with the simultaneous arrival of children with different and potentially challenging immediate needs. Reasonable parental leave is even more critical after concurrent adoptions.

Evaluating the Referral

Prospective parents usually consult a physician when they receive their "referral"—that is, the medical report of a child offered to them for consideration. Variable amounts of medical information are provided to prospective adoptive parents along with the referral. Legal considerations, cultural practices, medical facilities, and ethical concerns dictate the type and quality of the information provided. Most referrals include a medical report of variable length, photographs, and in some cases, especially Eastern Europe, videos. With the increasing availability of the Internet, more information is often available more quickly (see Chapter 1). However, practices in different countries change frequently as laws and adoption practices change. Specific pointers about referrals from the more common sending countries are described in Pre-adoptive Medical Reports by Country, below.

Although a great deal of information can be gleaned even from the most unpromising medical reports, it is important to educate parents about realistic goals of the consultation. Most parents are understandably anxious about the health of their prospective child, yet the value and scope of the consultation are constrained by the amount and quality of information provided. Reliability and completeness of information provided is never as meticulous or thorough as desired. Unscrupulous or careless preparation of documents in the sending country sometimes occurs; other difficulties include legal constraints, missing information, translation problems, lack of diagnostic testing capability, and cost restrictions. In most cases, physicians and orphanage staff in the sending countries attempt to be honest and straightforward advocates for the children. In other words, medical reports are not deliberately falsified to get the child out of the country, nor, except in unusual cases, is critical information withheld. More typically, problems arise from lack of awareness of potential problems, lack of tools to verify diagnoses, or assumptions that developmental delays and behavior problems are environmentally based. In addition to physician reports, much of the referral dossier provided to prospective parents derives from other sources. Translation problems can be significant for all documents.

Prospective international adoptive parents must recognize the limitations of the process of referral review (Table 4–4). Warnings and disclaimers are sometimes stamped on pages of the medical referral (Fig. 4–1). Perhaps

Table 4–4 Pre-adoptive assessments

What can we learn (if we're lucky)?
Maternal history
Birth information
Early life events
Growth patterns
Physical findings
Laboratory information
Developmental stage and play skills
"Obvious" problems
Personality

What can't we learn?
Language abilities
Behavior problems
Social skills and emotional status
Attachment disorder
Cognitive abilities
Risk of learning disabilities
Attention span
Likelihood of catch-up for growth and developmental delays
Exclusion of all medical and developmental problems

MEDICAL ACCURACY
NOT GUARANTEED
TRANSLATION NOT GUARANTEED

Figure 4–1 *Disclaimer found frequently on medical records given to prospective adoptive parents.*

it should be imagined that these are implied even if not explicitly stated. At best, such a review can exclude some obvious problems and yield some sketchy factual information that can contribute to the "image" of the child. It is *never* possible to provide guarantees about the physical, psychological, or emotional health of children. Furthermore, many concerns of pre-adoptive parents cannot be adequately addressed by the review process. Most prospective parents ask for an assessment of the child's future health, although their actual concern is for the child's cognitive, developmental, and behavioral function, which is much more difficult to predict. It is helpful to review this explicitly with prospective parents; as an example, a mentally retarded quadriplegic child can have excellent health, but extremely poor function.[2]

General Guidelines

Long before receiving their referrals, prospective parents are encouraged to discuss the type of medical information they will be given and the way in which questions arising from this material will be handled with their adoption agency or facilitator. Of the almost 10,000 medical reports reviewed in our International Adoption Clinic, few have been considered complete on the first review. Parents should discuss with their agency or facilitator in advance if they will have adequate time for medical consultation before a decision about the adoption is required. Because supplemental material is often needed to complete the pre-adoption consultation, prospective parents should discuss the expected time frame for decision making with their adoption agency in advance. Decision making under extreme pressure should be avoided.

When questions arise about the child's condition, or the medical report is unclear, it is helpful for counseling physicians to suggest questions which the prospective parents then convey to the adoption agency or facilitator. These are then translated and submitted to the child's caregivers and physicians in the child's birth country. It is critical to devise simple and direct questions, and to use the terminology that has been presented as a basis for the question. Sometimes, important questions should be phrased in alternative ways to lessen the chances for confusion as trained medical translators are only rarely involved. For example, asking "Is there any history of maternal alcohol use during pregnancy?" and "Does the child show any signs of problems from exposure to maternal alcohol use during pregnancy?" can both be helpful questions.

The medical dictionary can be helpful in demystifying some unusual medical terms, some of which turn out to be archaic but perfectly understandable. For example, *subnanism* means dwarfism (or failure to thrive); *couveuse* is an archaic term for incubator. Some of these confusions arise when nonmedical translators are involved in the process. Typographical errors, confusing terminology, and incomprehensible diagnoses are sometimes found in medical reports from all countries (Table 4–5).

Dates are common areas of confusion as well. In much of the rest of the world, 6/1 means January 6, not June 1 as in the United States. The adoption agency or facilitator should clarify any questions about these notations.

The most difficult area to assess is the child's language abilities. Because words like *babble* or *jabber* don't translate well, it's usually better to ask questions such as "Please describe the sounds the child makes" or, for older children, "Please give an example of something the child might say." Because this is rarely addressed on medical forms (and is nearly always impossible to assess in videos), it is reasonable to ask the local physicians to verify that the child can hear. Unrecognized hearing loss and

Table 4–5 Selected diagnoses quoted from medical referrals submitted for review

Free renal lumber

Began to mumble [This was the response to a query about language abilities]

Crush syndrome I

Paroxysmal alacrity as a residual from respiratory infection

Inkling for congenital syphilis

Xray of skull and cervical spine: occurrence of hypertension, block of C1, approach of arcs C2–3–4–5–6

Ear, nose, trout [Yes, it's a typo, but just a sample of what might appear]

The child worries periodically

Abstinent syndrome [drug withdrawal]

Ingenious jaundice

Dilution of the legs

Liquorodynamic dysfunction [This odd term refers to cerebrospinal fluid dynamics.]

He recovered and became cute

Hypertrophy of the fossils, first degree

Spasmophilia

All tests normal

Movement violation

Wavy course of perinatal lesson

Renal boxes painless

Presented fear zone

Astheno-neurotic syndrome

Lymphatic constitution

Compound genes

Dropsy (urogenital)

Oognyetyenie (oppression) syndrome

Increased speed in the flow in the spinal arteries (L>R)

Skin not snow white

EDS (express diagnosis of syphilis)

Cramps syndrome

Slow bottom paraparesis

Ulcus of the 12th appendage

Arouse onomatopoeia

Left site crooked jugulum

Hystedynemia [histidinemia, probably a transient metabolic disorder of no consequence]

Even reports of radiographs and ultrasounds can be difficult to understand, such as this neurosonogram report which nonmedical parents will expect to be interpreted for them: Non-homogeneous bilateral plexus choreiodus of side bellies, periventricularly high echodensity on VLP level.

---

deafness are surprisingly common among orphanage children.

Developmental information is also often hard to interpret. This may be provided by facilitators who are untrained in child development, who may see a happy, smiling child but not recognize that the child has significant developmental delays or behavioral disturbances. Again, communication with local medical personnel is the best way to ensure that accurate information is supplied.

Special Needs

Medical reports for children with identified special needs differ from those provided for healthy children. Most countries supply considerably more detailed medical and developmental information about children with special health care needs. For example, the medical report for a child from China with congenital heart disease may include reports and images of cardiac ultrasonographic examinations, as well as detailed physical examination findings. Actual radiographs (including computed tomography, ultrasounds, or magnetic resonance imaging studies), EEGs, EKGs, operative reports, and specialized laboratory test results are provided at times from China, South Korea, Guatemala, India, Philippines, or Colombia, allowing local review and interpretation. These supplemental materials are less often available from other frequent sending countries; in Russia, availability varies by region. Physicians and prospective adoptive parents should recognize that the special needs designation covers a wide range of problems, including many which may be readily remediable with resources available in the United States (i.e., supernumerary digit, mild club foot). Contrarily, other medical problems, for example strabismus (unless it is severe), may not qualify the child for special needs designation. In all sending countries, it is generally easier to engage physicians in the child's sending country in a dialogue about potential health issues when special needs are identified prior to referral.

Birth Information

Depending on the country and the age and individual circumstances of the child, variable amounts of information about the child's birth may be available. For nearly all children (except perhaps some from China whose mothers were hoping for boys), no prenatal care was received by the mother. Apgar scores are sometimes available, although occasionally only one number is provided without indication of whether it is the 1- or 5-minute score. The statement of the American Academy of Pediatrics on use and abuse of Apgar scores may be helpful for parents.[3] This elucidates the increased risk of cerebral palsy (from 0.3% to 1%) in term infants with extremely low Apgar scores (0–3). Although it is helpful to have Apgar scores, it is not critical, and most infants for evaluation are >6 months of age.

Of more concern is the lack of information about gestational age and the uncertainty of whether low–birth weight infants are truly premature, small for gestational age, or both. It is seldom possible to obtain gestational age information if it is not provided in the initial medical report. Birth mothers' reports of expected due dates may not be reliable. Furthermore, gestational age assessments may not have been done properly. Some small infants are assumed to be premature rather than growth retarded (or both). The circumstances of the child's birth are variably provided; most children are born in hospitals. Occasionally, children are born at home without medical attendants but then are admitted to hospitals, usually without detailed information about their condition at that time. For example, some children born at home may be left unattended, then later found (in hallways, streets, parks, etc) and taken emergently to a hospital. In these circumstances, it is reasonable to request details of the infant's condition when he or she entered care to assess the risks of hypoglycemia, hypothermia, and hypoxia. Very low-birth weight babies are sometimes born alive during attempted late-term abortions.

After birth, most infants remain in a maternity home or hospital for a period of weeks to months. Some children may be breast-fed during this time, either by their birth mothers or other mothers residing in the maternity home (acting as a wet-nurse). Occasionally this is due to medical problems, more frequently it is because the baby homes either do not wish to admit newborns or there is no space available for the child. Ideally, the different locations where the child has resided are clearly stated on the medical report, along with the reasons for and dates of transfer. No generalizations about the differences in quality of care between baby homes or children's hospitals are possible, although in specific circumstances such care may vary greatly.

An important part of this section of the medical report includes the reason this particular child is available for adoption. Most children are abandoned; however, in some, cases, parental rights have been terminated by court decree (see Chapter 2). Documents are sometimes available; following is an example, stating the reasons for termination of parental rights to Russian children.

The Plaintiff filed a petition for termination of parental rights due to parental neglect in regard to their minor children, daughter, M., son A., and son, I. It was stated that the parents neglect their children, abuse alcohol, the father wants to give up his children, the mother does not work, does not have a registered place of residence. The children do not attend school. They need to be bathed, are infested with lice, are hungry, walk unattended in the village. They were abandoned by their parents August 2, and the parents never inquired about them since. The parental neglect is very harmful for the children's well being and development. During the hearing, the representative of the Plaintiff supported the petition, and insisted on termination of parental rights of both Defendants in regard to their three minor children. Defendant O. did not appear in court, and V. appeared in court under the influence of alcohol.

Maternal gravidity and parity may also be stated, as well as the living circumstances and ages (and sometimes names) of older siblings. If these items are not included, parents should be encouraged to obtain this information, as their adopted child will certainly wish to know this information in the future.

Evaluation of young infants is extremely challenging. Usually, minimal maternal history is available, and birth information is incomplete. Parents must realize that it is difficult or impossible to (*1*) predict growth patterns from one or two time points, (*2*) differentiate "orphanage delays" from intrinsic problems, (*3*) assess most babies for fetal alcohol syndrome (see Chapter 5), and (*4*) predict future developmental concerns. Adoption of young infants with minimal exposure to institutional life is certainly desirable. However, evaluation of older children is in many ways more revealing. For example, it's easier to rule out cerebral palsy in a 3-year old than in a 6-month-old. However, the older child has experienced a longer period of institutionalization. The difference can be summed up as follows: the young ones are a mystery, the older ones have a history.

Growth Information

Ethnic growth charts. Ethnic growth charts are available for Korea, China, Vietnam, Thailand, Southeast Asia,[4] and India.[5-7] The source of the data used to generate these growth charts is in most cases unknown. Although ethnic differences in size do exist, the utility of these specific growth charts in assessing health risks before adoption is unclear. The growth charts published by the Centers for Disease Control and Prevention (CDC) in 2000[8] are based on the ethnically diverse population in the United States and now include measurements from the 3rd to 97th percentiles for height, weight, and head circumference in the normal range. These charts have been adopted as international standards by the World Health Organization, al-

lowing comparison of all children of the same age and gender without selection for economic or ethnic background.[9] Adequate information about relative size, growth velocity, and proportions can be readily assessed using these charts.

Growth data. Growth information, often the only objective information included in the referral, may be inaccurate, out of date, or incomplete. Most referrals include birth anthropometrics (except China, where occasionally measurements from the day the infant was found are available), and at least one other set of measurements. Sometimes series of measurements are provided. Dates of these measurements may not be apparent—occasionally designations such as "at present" are given. Clarifications should be requested. Current measurements should be provided. Referral measurements are often below the fifth percentiles for height, weight, and head circumference (Fig. 4–2). Medical information in the referral rarely suggests a specific diagnosis to account for the failure to thrive. Thus, parents must be informed that small size may be due to errors in measurement (although overmeasurement of height and weight is more typical), institutionalization-associated failure to thrive, or medical problems. Medical problems may range from "minor" conditions such as parasites, recurrent diarrhea, or recurrent respiratory problems to any pediatric condition that can impair growth. Most typically, the failure to thrive turns out to be due to a combination of factors and readily reverses after adoption (see Chapter 10). Nonetheless, parents must be educated about the long-term effects of malnutrition in early life on cognitive development and behavior (see Chapter 13).

Discussion of microcephaly with prospective adoptive parents is exceedingly more complex (see Chapter 12). Specific data do not yet exist to describe the outcome of microcephaly among international adoptees. Lessons from other pediatric populations suggest that chil-

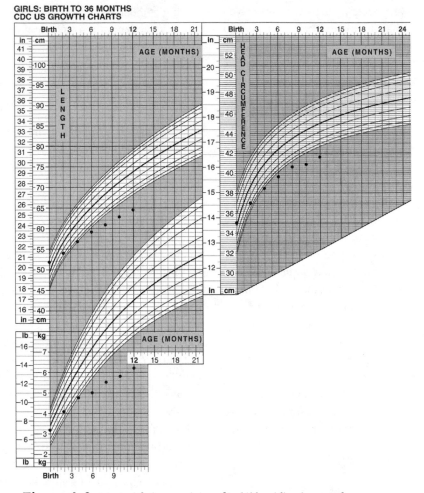

GIRLS: BIRTH TO 36 MONTHS
CDC US GROWTH CHARTS

Figure 4–2 *Typical failure-to-thrive of a child residing in an orphanage.*
Usually, only one or two points are provided for each growth parameter.

dren with microcephaly in early life have increased risk of cognitive delays, speech problems, arithmetic difficulties, and hyperactivity.[10–12] Unfortunately, incorrect or erratic head circumference measurements are common on the medical reports. Undermeasurements are more frequent than overmeasurements. Many children show remarkable improvement in head circumference measurement after adoption; however, early microcephaly may still represent a risk factor for later problems. The lack of certainty about gestational age makes interpretation of small head circumferences at birth even more problematic. However, differentia-

tion of acquired versus congenital microcephaly should be attempted. As with height and weight measurements, growth velocity is often more informative than one or two points in defining trends.

Medical Details

Most children have been examined by one or more physicians prior to adoption. This information is included in the medical report. Usually, reports are limited to "healthy," although sometimes specific diagnoses are given. Most reports contain a physical examination, which seldom includes comments about physical features suggestive of (or refuting) fetal alcohol syndrome. Obvious birth defects, skin lesions, and major physical findings are nearly always accurately described.

Hospitalizations (with reasons and duration) are sometimes included in the medical report. Laboratory testing is done on nearly all children, thus the report should have results for HIV enzyme-linked immunoadsorbent assay (ELISA), hepatitis B surface antigen, and syphilis serology (designated "RW" in Eastern Europe). These laboratory results are of great interest to prospective parents. However, (*1*) test results may be unreliable, (*2*) the tests must be repeated when the children return to the United States (and in the case of HIV, hepatitis B, hepatitis C, and Mantoux test they should be tested again 6 months later), and (*3*) the child may be infected even if the test is negative. Clinical laboratories may be unreliable, the child may become infected after the test was performed (or even by a contaminated needle used to draw blood for the test!), or the test may have been done during the incubation period of the infection. If the child was infected vertically with HIV, hepatitis B, or hepatitis C, early tests may not detect infection. Laboratory testing in the child's birth country thus provides a false sense of security at best, and at worst may actually expose the child unnecessarily to the very infections of concern. A helpful statement of these issues for families is available at the Web site for Families with Children from China.[13]

Occasionally, a child's medications are listed. These may usually be readily identified through various pharmacologic databases.[14,15]

Photographs and Videos

Most referrals include one or more photographs of the child. These can be extremely valuable, for medical and developmental assessment, especially when done well, and sometimes provide more information than videos. Photos of the child in several different positions can assist in determination of basic motor milestones. It is sometimes possible to observe and assess obvious anomalies and nutritional status (Fig. 4–3). If clear close-up views of the face are offered, determination of the risk of fetal alcohol syndrome can be made. Skull shape, ptosis, strabismus, and ear anomalies can offer clues about possible genetic diagnoses. Young infants are the most difficult to assess. Mongolian spots, or green or purple antiseptic applied to rashes, often alarm unsuspecting parents.

Videos are provided with most referrals from Russia, Kazakhstan, and Romania, and are sporadically available from other countries. At best, videos display the child's personality and abilities. However, videos show only a brief moment in time, during which the child may appear better or worse than he or she actually is. Children may be ill, sleepy, or frightened during the video. Often, the child is removed from the security of the group and

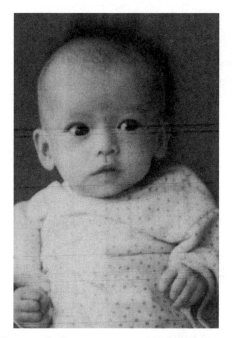

Figure 4–3 *Photographs often accompany the medical referral. This child weighed 9 pounds at 7 months of age. (With permission.)*

known caregivers, and taken to an unfamiliar office where strangers point cameras at the child and demand a "performance." Children do not realize that their video performance is actually an "audition" for a family, something no child should have to do. Videos must thus be viewed with great compassion for the child's circumstances. At times the child seems to be "frozen" in fear or uncertainty at placement in a completely unfamiliar environment without peers or familiar adults. Such children may quickly display rocking, head shaking, or other repetitive self-comfort behaviors. Some children appear to be in a trance, others smile vacantly at all the adults and then burst into tears. It is important to try to determine if the child is in a comfortable environment before making psychological or developmental assessments. Many wonderful children may not appear at their best in these unfamiliar, frightening situations. It is irresponsible to suggest to prospective parents that the child may have emotional difficulties, behavioral problems, or autism, based on a brief video possibly made under difficult circumstances.

Videos range from a 30-second view of the child in a caregiver's arms drinking from a bottle or sleeping to lengthy segments (1–2 hours) showing the child in a variety of settings (mealtimes, school, playground, dance performance, etc.). Most videos are under 10 minutes in duration. The most useful videos show the child's interactions with a familiar caregiver. Young infants are often shown unclothed. Ideally, the child is placed in various positions and several toys offered.

Motor function can be assessed qualitatively and quantitatively. Some infants have persistently fisted hands, which may be a sign of increased muscle tone, but more likely this is due to swaddling and lack of physical experience. Infants frequently resist weight bearing. Institutionalized infants lack the chance to be bounced on an adult lap and learn to extend their hips and knees. Some infants have tactile hypersensitivity on their soles; again this is due

to lack of experience with weight bearing. Infants frequently display considerable discomfort in prone lying; most spend their days supine, with little opportunity to practice trunk and neck extension.

Social and language skills are particularly difficult to demonstrate in a brief video. Eye contact, social and responsive smiles, and playful interactions are sometimes observed. However, more specific social milestones such as pointing, waving bye-bye, and imitation are rarely seen. Vocalizations of any kind by the child are rare (except for the school-age children who may answer questions, recite, or sing), emphasizing the delayed expressive language common among institutionalized children (see Chapter 31). Accurate assessment of the child's hearing based on the video is usually difficult. The ability of hearing-impaired or deaf children to follow instructions, engage with toys or people, and masquerade as a hearing child in a short video is quite astonishing.

If properly done, the video shows several close-up views of the child's face in repose to allow assessment of the risks of fetal alcohol syndrome. Camera angle, lighting, facial expression, close-ups, and focus must all be adequate to make an assessment. Videos are also useful to observe the presence of subtle anomalies that may not have been noted in the medical report. Ear symmetry, size, and placement can all be clues to genetic conditions. Ears may appear large if head circumference is small. Head circumference should be assessed subjectively and compared to measurements provided. Strabismus is also commonly observed or suspected.

Inspection of the environment in which the video was taken is also informative. The setting is often the orphanage director's office or a play room (large Oriental-style rugs are common in both; the director's office usually has couches and comfortable chairs). Some videos are filmed in the group day room or during a meal. It is useful to note if there is much crying in the background or, more frequently, utter silence. The activity and behavior of other children may give some clues about the environment. Sometimes a row of toddlers is observed rocking, swaying, or head banging, while the video "star" receives all the attention of the adults. If the video is taken during normal group activities, it is a challenge to keep track of the child in a roomful of active toddlers. In carefully done videos of adequate duration, a guess can be made about the child's activity level and attention span.

Changes in legal requirements (see below) mean that parents sometimes take their own videos of a prospective child. With advances in Internet technology, these are sent for review while the family is abroad. Children understandably may become frightened by the unfamiliar people who are so intently interested in them. Assessing the child's emotional well-being from these brief videos and extrapolating to a psychological diagnosis are impossible. By the same token, children who do well under these circumstances should be recognized for the excellent social skills that they possess. However, some may be displaying the "indiscriminate friendliness" that is common among this population (see Chapter 2).

"Two-Trip System"

Some countries, notably Russia and Vietnam, require adoptive families to make two trips to complete their adoptions. Variable amounts of information are provided before the first trip. Parents then meet the child, begin the adoption formalities, and return weeks to months later when a court date is set to finalize the adoption. Often they return from the first visit with more detailed medical information and a lengthy, self-made video. Prior to the first trip, it is helpful for the pediatrician to recommend what medical information should be obtained and to suggest the most useful activities to film (Appendix 4–1).

Pre-adoptive Medical Reports by Country

This section outlines the type of medical referral information provided by some of the more common sending countries. These comments are based on experience at the International Adoption Clinic at New England Medical Center since 1988 and, as such, are not comprehensive or complete. The exact content of medical reports from individual countries may vary enormously depending on the region, the local facilitators, and other factors. Quality and content also vary tremendously from year to year (see Chapter 3). Medical reports for children with identified special needs are addressed elsewhere in this chapter.

Eastern Europe and the Former Soviet Union

Medical reports from the former Soviet Union have been some of the most confusing and difficult to evaluate. Prospective adoptive families receive only an "extract," or summary, of the child's extensive medical record. These reports have sometimes created confusion, mistrust, and anxiety for adoptive parents. However, the reports are usually prepared in good faith, with an effort on the part of the local physicians to provide a complete and useful summary, given the information they have available.

Birth information is nearly always available. Gestational age assessments, especially for low-birth weight infants, are provided erratically. Sometimes "morphofunctional immaturity" is used as a synonym for prematurity, or prematurity is listed as a diagnosis without the number of weeks of gestation listed. Some referrals include the designation of a "degree" or "grade," with Roman numerals I–IV. These may reflect either gestational age, birth weight, or both (Table 4–6).[16]

Concerns about possible maternal drug or alcohol use or smoking are seldom addressed, even if the infant is low birth weight. Some-

Table 4–6 Stages of prematurity in Russia

Stage or Grade	Gestational Age (weeks)	Birth weight (g)
I	36–37	2001–2500
II	32–35	1501–2000
III	28–31	1000–1500
IV	<28	<1000

Source: Data from ref. 16.

Table 4–7 Syphilis terminology in Russian medical reports

Term	Translation
RW (or occasionally WR)	Wasserman test (non-treponemal tests)
RSK or RCK	Wasserman test
RIF	Immunofluorescence method with varying dilutions of the test serum. Sometimes this is listed as RIF 10 or RIF 200 (i.e., 1:10 or 1:200 dilutions)
RIBT	Treponemal immobilization test. Live treponemes are immobilized after exposure to the patient's serum (described in 1949 by Nelson and Mayer)[17]

Some of these tests are occasionally performed on spinal fluid (often translated into English as "liquor").

times the statement appears that the mother was "not on the Alcohol, Narcological or Venerealogical Registries"; this means simply that there is no record that the mother has sought care for those conditions. Supplemental information about maternal history may be available, especially in Eastern Europe, where many of the orphanages are in smaller towns and the mothers are known to the orphanage staff. "Assurances" about lack of alcohol or drug exposure are always welcome, although they may not be reliable.

Similarly, information about siblings may sometimes be obtained upon request. This may provide some clues about the mother's social situation (for example, six older siblings all living in orphanages present a different picture than three older children living with a married and employed mother and father whose fourth child could not be cared for because they lack financial resources). Sibling information will also be welcomed by the adopted child as he or she matures.

About 15% of the medical records reviewed from Russia and the former Soviet Union include a history of maternal syphilis (see Chapter 19). Generally, the local doctors do an excellent job diagnosing and treating syphilis. Even a remote history of syphilis in the birth mother usually provokes a course of treatment and careful monitoring of the infant. Long-bone radiographs and serial serologic testing results are often included in the medical report. Some of the serologic tests performed are shown in Table 4–7. Concerns related to syphilis include possible co-infection with other sexually transmitted diseases (HIV, hepatitis B, hepatitis C) and risk of exposure to one of these

blood-borne infections as a consequence of parenteral treatment. Penicillin is given by intramuscular injection in varying doses and regimens; details are rarely provided. Children may receive from 14 to more than 100 injections, depending on the schedule prescribed.

Perhaps the most problematic aspect of medical reports from Russia has been the confusing terminology related to neurologic diagnoses (Fig. 4–4). Virtually all medical reports

> DOB: August 15, 1994
> The child was born to a 17-year-old-mother. No father. Mother wrote a written relinquishment.
> Diagnosis: hypoxic-traumatic defect of the central nervous system
> hypertensive-hydrocephalic syndrome
> birth trauma of cervical section of the vertebrae
> rickets
> immaturity—III degree
> Birth: Weight: 2700 gr, height: 46 cm, head circumference: 32 cm, Apgar - 8/9.
> At present: Weight: 3800 gr, height: 56 cm, head circumference: 37 cm, chest circumference: 36 cm.

Figure 4–4 *Typical medical report provided from Russia. This child was neurologically normal, with minor developmental delays from which she quickly recovered.*

include multiple unfamiliar and frightening diagnoses (Table 4–8). The nearly universal presence of these diagnoses should be reassuring. Indeed, these diagnoses have not been confirmed among Russian children adopted by American families. Although many believe or suspect that these diagnoses have been placed on the child's medical report to make the child

Table 4–8 Neurologic diagnoses from 107 medical records from Eastern Europe[a]

Diagnosis	n	Diagnosis	n
Perinatal		Flexor tonus in limbs	1
Perinatal encephalopathy	43	Generalized muscular hypothony	1
Of hypoxical traumatic genesis	6	Generally weak	1
Of hypoxic genesis	3	Infantile cerebral paralysis	1
Of hypoxical etiology, late compensatory period	1	Lack of reflexes	1
Of mixed genesis	2	Mixed tetraparesis	1
Consequences of intrauterine hypoxia	1	Motive disorder	1
Early perinatal CNS pathology	1	Motor lesion syndrome	1
Early perinatal hypertension	1	Muscle hypotonus syndrome	5
Hypoxic perinatal CNS injury with hypertension syndrome	4	Neuromuscular disorder caused by hypoxia	1
Natal trauma of cervical spinal cord	3	Paraparesis of lower extremities	2
Neurotic syndrome of hypoxic genesis on background of morphofunctional immaturity	1	Spasm (or spastic) syndrome	3
		Spastic paresis of one foot	2
Organic defect of CNS (of hypoxical origin)	3	Spastic tetraparesis	3
Perinatal damage of CNS	6	Spastical	3
Perinatal hypoxia	3	Syndrome of motor disorders	2
Perinatal affection of the brain and spinal cord on the perinatal lesion of the brain	1	**Unknown Neurologic Disorders**	
		Cerebellar insufficiency	2
Anatomic		Cerebrostenic syndrome	4
(Intracranial) hypertension syndrome	8	CNS suppression syndrome	1
Congenital hydrocephalia	2	Hyperneuroreflectory activity	3
Congenital pathology of the skull	1	Hyperexcitability	10
Deformation of vascular plexuses, shades in gaps of ventricles, connected with vascular plexus (thrombus)	1	Hyperirritability	4
		Hypocorticism of the brain secondary to ECHO-EC	1
Hydrocephalic shape of head	2	Myotonic (or miotonical) syndrome	3
Hydrocephalic–hypertension syndrome	8	Neuroreflector syndrome	1
Hydrocephalus syndrome	5	Pyramidal insufficiency (or deficiency)	6
Injury of cervical spine and vertebral arteries	1	Residuals of organic damage of CNS	1
Intraventricular blood stroke	1	Slight cerebral dysfunction	2
Microcephaly	6	Syndrome of heightened neuroreflexical agitation	4
Spinal hernia	1		
Subarachnoid hemorrhage	1	**Unknown**	
		Continuous sluggish sepsis	1
Motor Disorders		Exudative diathesis	1
Adductor spasm	1	Hyperdynamic syndrome	1
Dyskinesia	1	Hypererethism	1
Dystonic syndrome	1	Left hemisyndrome	2
Equinovarus	2	Polycystosis	1
Flaccid tetraparesis	1	Secondary fermentopathy	1
		Subnanism (archaic name for dwarfism)	2
		Vegetative visceral syndrome	2

[a]See also ref. 18 for further explanations.

All children were examined in the International Adoption Clinic. Except for microcephaly, hypotonia, and developmental delay, no other conditions were confirmed.

eligible for foreign adoption, this is not true. For the most part, Russian physicians make these diagnoses in good faith; the diagnoses are consistent with their medical system and terminology. It is hard to understand how nearly 50% of infants can have "perinatal encephalopathy"; however, this term means something quite different to the Russian doctors than it does to those trained in the Western system of medicine. For example, the differences between increased neuroreflexive excitability and intracranial hypertension, adapted from the work of Y.A. Yakunin, are shown in Table 4–9. If only a few of the criteria are required for diagnosis, it's easy to see how these could be widely applied. Child neurology became an independent discipline in Russia in 1963.[18] A classification scheme of over 1000 nosologic forms was devised, and perinatal neurology emerged as a specialized area with the view that "many peculiarities and pathogenic mechanisms were revealed at different stages of development."[18] Overall, neurologic disease is considered to "represent the most common cause of disablement of children in Russia—almost 60%," with most morbidity related to central nervous system (CNS) prenatal and perinatal damage (36%) and residual neurologic deficits due to

this damage (24%).[18] It is believed that the most important stage of neurologic care is provided in the maternity home, when future problems can be prevented.[18] Extensive details about Russian medical terminology and neurology are found at the Russian Adoption Web site.[19]

The "flavor" of neonatal neurology can be seen in a recent survey[20] of the diagnoses given 41 abandoned infants in Moscow. Most children had multiple diagnoses; only seven were considered healthy. In the remaining 34, diagnoses included prematurity or hypotrophy (not differentiated) (12), intrauterine infection (28), disorder of the central nervous system (2), insufficiency of the cerebral circulation (26), excitability syndrome (26), and malformation (1). Intrauterine infection was a "social diagnosis" (e.g., no prenatal care increased the risk that the mother may have had undetected gonorrhea or syphilis). "Neurologic" diagnoses were seemingly applied in the absence of specific diagnostic criteria. In another study, 200/280 full-term newborns were considered to have moderate-to-severe perinatal hypoxic lesions by neurosonography.[21] A Russian explanation of perinatal encephalopathy is available at the Primavera Medica web site.[22]

Among the most useful features of Russian medical reports have been character or "pedagogical" statements (Fig. 4–5). These are usually offered for older children, and may describe the child's interests, academic performance, personality, behavior, and attitudes. Obviously prepared by those who know the child well, these statements offer a real sense of the child that bland medical data do not.

Table 4–9 Diagnostic criteria for "unusual" Russian medical conditions

Clinical Sign	Increased Neuroreflexive Excitability	Intracranial Hypertension
Tremor	+	+
Spontaneous Moro reflex	+	−
Horizontal nystagmus	+/−	+/−
Convergent strabismus	+/−	+/−
Agitation	+	+
Greffe symptom (sunset sign)	−	+/−
Eye protrusion	−	+/−
Fontanel bulging and skull sutures separation	−	+
Hyperesthesia	−	+
"Screaming out"	−	+

Source: Data from Yakunin.[23]

Romania

Medical reports from Romania vary widely. Typically, two- to three-page reports are provided, which list basic birth information (measurements and Apgar score: usually one score is given and frequently it is 9) and developmental milestones (all of which are checked off seemingly without regard for the actual devel-

```
┌─────────────────────────────────────────┐
│          CHARACTER STATEMENT             │
│              Nadezhda                     │
│          DOB: May 17, 1993                │
│                                           │
│              Nadya lives in the orphanage │
│  Mother:     Ludmila—died.                │
│  Father:     Igor—his parental rights were│
│              terminated.                  │
│                                           │
│  Nadya is a second grade student. She does│
│  well academically. She reads well and    │
│  retells short stories. She has a good     │
│  memory, easily changes types of           │
│  activities. She writes well, with few     │
│  spelling mistakes. She can solve simple   │
│  mathematical problems without help, loves │
│  learning. She can calculate within 10.    │
│                                           │
│  Nadya's speech is good. She is very       │
│  friendly with children. She loves drawing,│
│  painting, working with clay. She has good │
│  fine motor skills. Nadya has good         │
│  imagination, makes beautiful applique.    │
│  She is hard working, diligent, loves      │
│  sewing, knitting. Nadya participated in a │
│  performance contest and won a prize. She  │
│  loves singing and participating in        │
│  different contests.                       │
│                                           │
│  She has good hygiene skills.              │
│                                           │
│       Caregiver           signature        │
│       Orphanage director  signature        │
└─────────────────────────────────────────┘
```

Figure 4–5 *Pedagogical or character statements are sometimes provided for school age children. These offer descriptions of the child's interests, activity level, and achievements.*

opmental status of the child). Other referrals provide extensive medical information, including social background, family history, and standardized developmental assessments. Videos are sometimes available, especially for children in foster care. These typically show the child in the foster family's home, often interacting with family members. These videos can be quite lengthy (30–60 minutes) and may include the child playing various games indoors or out. Other times, the video content is less structured and captures random activity of the child while adults converse in the background. Little effort is usually made to engage the child in conversation, making language assessments difficult.

Ukraine

Laws in Ukraine are presently (2004) in flux. Currently, families are asked to travel before an individual child is identified to be assigned. On arrival in Ukraine, the family may be offered a "choice" of several children at once or serially. Information is provided only after a child is provisionally "selected"—at that time, the family may have a brief opportunity for medical consultation before the adoption decision is finalized. Families without medical background and knowledge of the risks common among institutionalized children need considerable support during this extraordinarily stressful process. Many seek emergency pre-adoptive counseling via the Internet, sending medical reports, photos, and video clips. Although helpful, opportunities to question, reflect, and assess are very limited.

Vietnam

Many children placed from Vietnam are young infants. The quality and quantity of information vary. Birth information is usually available. Health history, physical examinations, and basic laboratory tests may be provided; developmental information is minimal. Photographs are available sporadically (usually for older children). In some programs, adopting parents travel twice to Vietnam (see "the two-trip system" above). Children usually reside in state-run orphanages; some private orphanages also exist.

India and Phillipines

Reports from these countries are similar in quality and detail. Both provide extensive material for review. This may include information about the circumstances by which the child entered care, the child's physical condition, developmental information, intercurrent illnesses and hospitalizations, x-ray reports, laboratory tests, and, occasionally, ancillary information such as electroencephalograms (EEGs) or specialized scans. Results of testing for hepatitis B, HIV, and syphilis are usually included. The dossier usually includes considerable information collected over many months (or years), making it possible to monitor a child's progress. Reports from social workers describe the child's emotional state. Several photos are often included. On very rare occasions, videos are provided. Character descriptions of the child are often included as well. Questions addressed to the orphanages are usually answered directly. Both government and private orphanages exist.

South Korea

Pre-adoptive medical reports from South Korea comprise a very special category. Compared to other countries, a considerable amount of information is available about the birth mother and often the birth father as well. This may include not only physical information (height, weight, general appearance, medical problems) but also information about their educational and social backgrounds, interests, and occupations. Many pregnant mothers make adoption plans for their children prior to delivery and receive some prenatal care (although it may not be until late in the pregnancy). Virtually all the children are born in hospitals or maternity homes. Accurate birth information is available, although instead of Apgar scores the record usually indicates that "the baby cried immediately." Most (but not all) infants receive vaccination against hepatitis B within 48 hours of birth. Physical and developmental examinations are performed at least monthly, and results are sent to prospective adoptive parents (Fig. 4–6). Laboratory testing is generally reliable (although it should be repeated when children enter the United States). Nearly all the children live in foster care prior to adoption. Descriptions of the infant's daily routine, response to feeding and bathing, and sleep patterns are all provided to the adoptive family. The foster family is also described, along with their years of experience and family composition. Any

Development (I)

Gross Motor	prone lift head		(10°)
	chest up-arm support		( )
	bear weight on legs	some	(+)
		moderate	( )
		good	( )
	head lag on pull to sitting position		( )
	roll over		( )
	creep or crawl		( )
Fine Motor	follow to midline		( )
Adaptive	follow past midline		( )
	follow 180°		(+)
	hand sucking		(+)
	both hands together		( )
	reaches out for large object		( )
	grasp large object		( )
Personal-	regard face		(+)
Social	smile spontaneously		(+)
	smile responsively		(+)
	regard own hand		( )
Language	respond to bell		(+)
	coos		(+)
	laugh		( )
	turn to rattling sound		( )
	turn to voice		( )
	imitate speech sound		( )

Assessment of developmental age
  2-month-old level

Recommendation
  Adoptable

Figure 4–6 *Monthly updates of the prospective adoptee's developmental progress are often provided from Korea.*

medical issues appear to be thoroughly addressed by the local physicians, who have access to Western-style diagnostic equipment and tests. If anything, most local physicians appear to err on the side of caution (minor developmental delays or physical findings are extensively and carefully evaluated, beyond what would be standard practice in the United States). Questions raised by the medical reports are generally answered comprehensively. Full details are given about interim medical problems, hospitalizations, medications, and so on. Results of HIV testing and syphilis testing are provided inconsistently. Foster parents occasionally send pictures and letters with the child at the time of adoptive placement, which can be treasured forever. The following letter is an example:

Dear Parents: I am the foster mother of L.W. and my name is H.K. I took care of him for 1 year, and I fell in love with him. He is a very lovely baby boy. I would like to tell you about him beacase of worrying about him. He is a lovable and cute baby boy, and he grew up receiving abundant love from the foster family and neighbors. However, he is very shy with strangers. He took milk well, and smiled easily when he was with the family. He was playful with the family. However, when he was with unfamiliar people, he cried a lot, and did not get along with them. We think he will soon be one of your precious family members. It is my heartfelt wish that you will take good care of him, and your family will live happily with him forever. I wish that you stay healthy and happy always.

Guatemala

Children in Guatemala may live in orphanages or foster care prior to adoption. Both caregiving environments vary in quality. Medical reports of infants from Guatemala include results of DNA testing of the child and birth mother (see Chapter 3). Many of the birth mothers who make adoption plans for their newborns also provide blood samples, which are screened for hepatitis B and HIV. Young infants have scant medical records, with minimal birth information, a physical examination, and basic blood tests (CBC, syphilis, HIV). Referrals usually include three or four pictures of clothed infants. Occasionally more extensive reports are available. Follow-up growth information and photos are often available. Developmental information is sporadically supplied.

Cambodia

Most children adopted from Cambodia are young infants. Usually a brief medical report is available, with minimal developmental information. One or two photos, often miniature,

may accompany the medical report. Sometimes the age of the child is uncertain—in some cases because the child has been abandoned, in other cases because of confusion translating dates from the traditional Cambodian lunar calendar. Lab work may include screens for hepatitis B and HIV; occasionally polymerase chain reaction (PCR) results for HIV-DNA are obtained. American- or Western-trained pediatricians in Cambodia often supply superb information.

China

Referrals may include extremely minimal information. Birth information about Chinese children is virtually never available. For many years, families adopting from China received a standard two page report with a postage-stamp sized photograph of their prospective child's face. The report was often 6 or more months out of date, and listed a single set of measurements of height, weight, and head circumference. Weights were obtained clothed; many new arrivals in the United States weighed considerably less than expected (Fig. 4–7). The

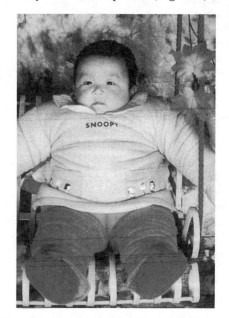

Figure 4–7 *Photos from China show fully clothed children. Many are weighed while dressed in heavy clothes. (With permission.)*

physical examination record, although complete in listing every organ system, was invariably filled in with the word "normal" after every designation (Fig. 4–8). Laboratory work

Health Examination Ruo Yang City #1	
Chen Xiao Xin	Sex: Female DOB: 11-22-2001
Placement Institute:	Ruo Yang Children's Center
Medical History:	No
Family History:	No
Hearing:	normal
Nose Sense of smell:	normal
Nose:	normal
Throat:	normal
Others:	normal
Teeth:	no
Oral cavity:	no
Palate:	normal
Others:	normal
Height:	68cm
Weight:	7.5kg (about 17lb)
Chest size:	40 cm
Head size:	39 cm
Skin:	normal
Lymph:	normal
thyroid gland:	normal
Spine:	normal
Limb:	normal
Flatfoot:	no
Joints:	normal
Anus:	normal
Uro-genital system:	normal
Hernia:	normal
Development:	normal
Nutrition:	normal
Nerve system:	normal
Heart:	normal
Lungs:	normal
Abdomen:	normal
Lab test:	normal (Nov. 9, 2002)
Liver function:	normal
Chest X-ray:	normal

Figure 4–8 *Typical medical report from China lists all physical findings as "normal."*

from China has typically included a CBC, hepatitis B serology (often surface antigen [sAg], surface antibody [sAb], coreAb, eAg, and eAb) liver function tests and occasionally also results of a chest x-ray and electrocardiogram. Several recent changes have enhanced the quality of information received from China. Developmental information is now usually included. This section of the medical referral lists a wide range of developmental milestones, usually with checkmarks to indicate those the baby has accomplished. Although somewhat helpful, these reports are of uncertain accuracy and may be incomplete or outdated. Specific descriptions of language abilities and verification of hearing are rarely satisfactory. For children living in foster care, more detailed information is usually offered. Nearly all referrals now include three or four photos of the infant at different ages and in different positions, allowing a better assessment of motor skills and physical appearance. However, photos always show the infant completely clothed. Laboratory test results for HIV and syphilis are now commonly included, although they may be out-of-date.

Key Points for Internationally Adopted Children (and Their Families)

- Pre-adoption counseling should cover many topics.
- Parent education and anticipatory guidance are critical.
- Adoption medicine consultants may provide useful information to parents and pediatricians throughout the process.
- Information provided in "referrals" must be carefully evaluated.
- Conversations prior to adoption about parental expectations and the child provide a sound basis for an ongoing and caring professional relationship between the pediatrician and the family.

Appendix 4–1 At the Orphanage

Parents usually have the opportunity to meet their child's caregivers and the orphanage director (usually a doctor) during the adoption process. The following list includes suggested topics to discuss during these meetings. This may be particularly helpful for parents who make two trips to complete the adoption (Russia and Vietnam) or who adopt from Ukraine (where no information is provided prior to travel).

Questions for Caregivers

1. Maternal history
   Medical history
   Obstetric history (previous pregnancies, outcome, where are children now? names available?)
   Known history of alcohol use? Drug use? Smoking?
   Maternal social history, occupation if known
2. Any paternal information, if available
3. Why is child in orphanage?
   Relinquishment at birth?
   Foundling? Circumstances when child was found? Condition of child when found?
   Termination of parental rights (are legal documents available?)
4. Previous placements (hospitals, other settings)
5. Date child entered orphanage
   Weight, height, head circumference
   Health issues
   Emotional and physical status
6. Health during time in orphanage
   Any hospitalizations? (Parents should be aware that children may be hospitalized for relatively minor illnesses.)
   Medical conditions?
   Medications?
   Blood tests? (hepatitis B, HIV, syphilis, hepatitis C)

Immunizations?
Growth measurements at different ages and currently
7. Developmental issues? Behavior problems? Emotional problems?
8. Language skills?
9. Any signs of fetal alcohol syndrome or fetal alcohol exposure (see Chapter 5)?
10. For older children
    Does the child have friends?
    School performance?
    Special interests, activities, or talents?
    Fits well into group?
    Wants to be adopted? Prepared?
11. Overall opinions about prognosis, recommendations for treatment

On-site Visits

1. Observe the child in a familiar environment with known caregivers, peers, and toys. Record behaviors, preferences, responses to environment and people. (Consider acute health issues, time of day, effect of disruption of routines, presence of strangers, etc.)
2. Listen carefully for vocalizations and speech. Your translator can be very helpful in assessing the child's language abilities. Look for the child's ability to understand (receptive language), use gestures, and use non-verbal communication.
3. Caregivers may be able to describe the child's personality and behaviors, the best techniques to soothe and comfort, and the child's special likes and dislikes. Do the caregivers seem to like the child?
4. Check out the daily routine schedule.
5. Visits over several days are better than a single visit to determine the child's abilities and function.
6. Caregivers may have specific information about the child's family, previous visitors, etc.
7. Observe the child's energy level and attention span

8. Observe self-stimulatory (rocking, head banging) or other unusual behaviors. See if other children in the group also have these behaviors.

9. Observe eye contact and whether the child has emotional interactions with others, and engages others in play.

Things to Bring (and Leave Behind) for Young Children

Simple cardboard books, ball, stacking cups or rings, cause/effect toy, music or squeak toy, unbreakable mirror, photos of you (wear the same clothes when you return), family members, house, and pets.

References

1. International Adoption Project. Available at: http://education.umn.edu/icd/iap/results4.25.htm.

2. Jenista JA. Medical issues in adoption. In: Marshner C, Pierce WL, eds. Adoption Factbook III. Waite Park, MN: National Council for Adoption, 1999: 417–422.

3. Committee on Fetus and Newborn, Committee on Obstetric Practice. Use and abuse of the Apgar score. Pediatrics 1996; 98:141–2.

4. Growth charts for children adopted internationally. Available at: http://www.comeunity.com/adoption/health/growth.html.

5. Agarwal DK, Agarwal KN, Upadhaya SK, Mittal R, Prakash R, Rai S. Physical and sexual growth patterns of affluent Indian children from 5 to 18 years of age. Indian Pediatr 1992; 29:1203–1268.

6. Agarwal DK, Agarwal KN. Physical growth of Indian affluent children (birth–6 years). Indian Pediatr 1994; 31:377–413.

7. Khadgawat R, Dabadghao P, Mehrotra RN, Bhatia V. Growth charts suitable for evaluation of Indian children. Available at: http://www.indianpediatrics.net/sept4.htm.

8. Centers for Disease Control and Prevention. Growth charts. Available at: http://www.cdc.gov./growthcharts.

9. http://www.fnri.dost.gov.ph/htm/2001updating.htm.

10. Desch LW, Anderson SK, Snow JH. Relationship of head circumference to measures of school performance. Clin Pediatr (Phila) 1990; 29:389–92.

11. Smith RD. Abnormal head circumference in learning-disabled children. Dev Med Child Neurol 1981; 23: 626–32.

12. Hack M, Breslau N, Weissman B, Aram D, Klein N, Borawski E. Effect of very low birth weight and subnormal head size on cognitive abilities at school age. N Engl J Med 1991; 325:231–7.

13. Jenista JA, Johnson DE, Miller LC, Murray DL. Hepatitis B: no guarantee. Available at: http://fwcc.org/hepatitisb.html.

14. Pharmaceutical agents commonly administered in Eastern European countries. Available at: http://www.peds.umn.edu.iac/for_families/before/pharmaceuticals.htm.

15. Medlineplus Drug Information. Available at: http://www.nlm.nih.gov/medlineplus/druginformation.htm.

16. Russian children and medical records. Adoption Medical News 1997; 3:1–7.

17. Nelson RA Jr, Mayer MM. Immobiliation of Treponema pallidum in vitro by antibody produced in syphilitic infection. J Exp Med 1949; 89: 369–93.

18. Petroukhin A. Child neurology in Russia: development of the traditions. Brain Dev 1998; 20:543–46.

19. Russian adoption medical report interpretation. Available at: http://www.russianadoption.org/adoptionfaq.htm.

20. Shaginian N. The influence of psychological and social factors on pregnancy and abandoned newborns. Washington, DC: Joint Council for International Children's Services, April, 2002.

21. Lobanova LV. Doppler study in the diagnosis and prediction of hypoxic lesions of the brain in mature newborn infants. Russ Bull Perinatol Pediatr 2001. Available at: www.mediasphera.aha.ru/pediatr/2001/4/e4-01ref.htm#3.

22. Semyonova KA. Perinatal encephalopathy. Available at: http://www.primavera.ru/english/enceph.htm#3.

23. Palchik AB, Shabalov NP. Hypoxic-ischemic encephalopathy of the newborn. St. Petersburg: Piter Publishing, 2000.

II

PRENATAL EXPOSURES

5

FETAL ALCOHOL SYNDROME

Alcohol is the most common teratogen on the planet and one of the most common identifiable causes of mental retardation.[1] Worldwide, between 1/1000 and 1/300 of infants are exposed prenatally to alcohol: some estimate the incidence as high as 1/100.[2] Fetal alcohol syndrome (FAS) is perhaps the leading cause of mental retardation in the United States;[3] precise statistics for other countries are not available. The prevalence of FAS in Russian orphanages is estimated at ~14%, based on physical criteria alone.[4]

Families adopting internationally have usually heard of FAS as a risk for their children. Few realize however, the spectrum of problems that occur after prenatal alcohol exposure, the lifelong disabilities these children experience, and the difficulty establishing this diagnosis in the absence of (reliable) maternal history. This section reviews the epidemiology of alcoholism in sending countries, the physical and neurobehavioral features of FAS, and the outcome of affected children. Because the outcome of children with FAS depends greatly on the prevention of "secondary disabilities,"[3,5] the long-term follow-up of children with FAS who have been adopted is highlighted.

History and Epidemiology

Alcohol has been recognized as a teratogen for decades.[6] The constellation of growth retardation, developmental delay, and unusual nail findings (onychodysplasia) was recognized in 1971.[7] The association of these findings with intrauterine alcohol exposure was described within a short time in both the United States and France.[8,9] Since then, an extensive literature on the effects of maternal alcohol ingestion during pregnancy has emerged.

Fetal alcohol syndrome has been identified among internationally adopted children from virtually *every* sending country. However, FAS is much more frequent in children from Russia, Ukraine, and other countries of the former Soviet Union. Adoptees from other Eastern European countries such as Romania have an intermediate incidence of FAS, whereas FAS is uncommon in children from Korea, Guatemala, and China. The incidence of FAS in international adoptees parallels the incidence of alcoholism in each sending country.

Accurate figures on alcohol consumption are difficult to ascertain. The World Health Organization Alcohol Database[10] provides com-

Gina's parents are both physicians. The medical report provided at the time she was referred to them raised concerns about the possibility of FAS, based on her facial characteristics and small size. However, they felt very drawn to her. They took advantage of the new laws in Russia to visit her twice prior to finalizing their adoption plans. "She does have some features of FAS," her mom said, "but we were amazed at her cognitive and language abilities when we visited her. She seemed to be developmentally head and shoulders above the other kids in her age group in the orphanage. We're not sure what lies ahead, but we just had to bring her home."

parable country-specific statistics compiled from reliable sources (Table 5–1). Data for other countries may be found at that Web site.

Definitions

Fetal alcohol syndrome is a constellation of physical and neurobehavioral abnormalities resulting from maternal ingestion of alcohol during pregnancy (Table 5–2).

Fetal alcohol syndrome results from high maternal blood alcohol concentrations after either regular or binge consumption. Maternal ingestion of 2 or more ounces per day of alcohol, especially early in gestation, promotes the development of the facial features of FAS. As little as 1.5 ounces of absolute alcohol (approximately

Nicholas was adopted from Russia at 2 years of age; his pre-adoption medical stated that he had "alcohol fetopathy." FAS was confirmed after arrival. He was tiny and developmentally delayed, but charming and sociable. Unlike his adopted sister, who did not have FAS, Nicholas did not display the typical catch-up in growth and development. After he'd been home for about 1 year, his parents requested that Nicholas's age be "reassigned" to reflect his actual size and functional abilities. Accordingly, this was done. However, 1 year later, Nicholas still lagged far behind his new peer group in both growth and developmental milestones.

three drinks) during pregnancy may significantly decrease cognitive scores, increase the frequency of minor neurological anomalies, reduce height, and promote facial dysmorphology.[11] The children of older mothers who engage in intermittent heavy drinking seem especially vulnerable to the effects of alcohol.[12] However, individual susceptibility clearly varies: dizygotic twins may differ in phenotypic expression of FAS.[13,14] Maternal alcohol dehydrogenase genotype contributes to susceptibility to prenatal alcohol exposure.[15] In a recent report, alcohol-induced damage to a specific neural cell adhesion molecule, L-1, was implicated in the pathogenesis of FAS.[15a] Further research in this area is eagerly awaited. No amount of alcohol ingestion during pregnancy is considered safe for the fetus.[16]

Fetal alcohol effect (FAE) is sometimes used to describe prenatally exposed children who lack the characteristic facial appearance of FAS; these children often have growth and developmental delays and neurobehavioral abnormalities. This term has become widely used, as it allowed some children to receive financial assistance, medical benefits, and educational interventions.[17] However, FAE lacks specific diagnostic criteria,[1] and is *not* a mild form of FAS. In 1996, the Institute of Medicine proposed the replacement of FAE with the terms *alcohol-related neurodevelopmental disorder* (ARND) and *alcohol-related birth defects* (ARBD).[18] Others suggest use of the term *fetal alcohol spectrum disorders.*"[19] These new terms reflect the reality of medical and developmental problems that occur after substantial regular intake or heavy episodic prenatal exposure to alcohol, *regardless* of the phenotypic appearance of the child (Fig. 5–1).[1]

The utility of these definitions for international adoptees is questionable. Many internationally adopted children have multiple, complex reasons for pre- or postnatal growth retardation (see Chapter 10). Likewise, neurobehavioral problems and cognitive delays may result from other exposures, including malnutrition, micronutrient deficiencies, institutionalization, stress, and prenatal drugs or tobacco (see Chapters 2, 6, 7, 8, 10, and 11).

Table 5–1: Epidemiology of alcohol use in top 15 sending countries[10]

Country	Per Capita Alcohol Consumption (liter/year)[a,b]				Drinking Habits (information from selected studies cited at Ref. 10)	Unrecorded Alcohol Use (illegal, home brew, etc.) not officially recorded in national statistics	Alcohol Content of Local Beverages
	Beer	Wine	Spirits				
Belarus	1.25	0.32	8.13		10% drink heavily	N/A	N/A
Bulgaria	1.79	3.58	2.85		*1993, students, age 14–18 years:* 66% drank alcohol, 20% drank regularly; 20% increased consumption recently; 1/3 disapproved of drinking. *1993, survey of 14- to 18-year-olds:* 77% were alcohol drinkers, 6–7% drank "often," 1% drank daily, 1.2% were dependent on alcohol. The average age of first use was 13–16 years old.	40%–70%	N/A
Cambodia	0.25	0.01	0.2		N/A	N/A	N/A
China	1.03	0.09	4.04		*University students:* males consumed significantly more alcohol than females, and had more problems from drinking. Beer was the preferred alcoholic beverage for both males and females. Of males, 10% indicated daily use; 19%, weekly use; 34%, monthly use; 8% were abstainers. Of females, 3% indicated daily use; 8%, weekly use; 24%, monthly use; 53% were abstainers. *445 high school seniors:* drinking was reported by 84% of males and 55% of females. Drinking one or two times in the previous 2 weeks was reported by 21 girls.	20%–30%	Alcohol content of yellow wine: 10%–15% Alcohol content of home brewed beverage: 10%
Colombia	3.75	0.08	2.54		*1987, alcohol consumed by both sexes:* 70% males, 42% females. Alcoholism in 8%, of the sample, alcoholism in 5% of females age 25–29 years and 20% of males age 38–49 years.	No clandestine production of alcoholic beverages has been reported.	N/A

(continues)

Table 5-1 (Continued)

Country	Per Capita Alcohol Consumption (liter/year)[a,b]	Beer	Wine	Spirits	Drinking Habits	Unrecorded Alcohol Use (illegal, home brew, etc.) not officially recorded in national statistics	Alcohol Content of Local Beverages
Guatemala	1.91	0.72	0.01	1.18	*Students in Guatemala City:* Lifetime prevalence of alcohol use, 26.5%. *Cross-sectional study:* 66% of males and 48% of females used alcohol, 27% currently used (20% of females). Highest rates were within the 35 to 39-year age group.	N/A	Aguardiente: 45 proof distilled Beverage (legal), Boj (Chicha, Guaro, Kuxa): indigenous, fermented product from sugarcane (10 proof)
Haiti	5.18	0.01	0.01	5.17	*Cross-sectional survey:* lifetime prevalence of alcohol use: 58% (60% for men, 56% percent for women); highest rate among 19 to 24-year-olds. About 1/3 initiated alcohol use before age 15; 7% of men, and 5% of females are current users.	N/A	N/A
India	1.01	0.03	0	0.98	*Alcohol use:* 25% of adults, 36% of males, 13% of females. Probable alcohol dependence in 6% of males, 0.5% of females. Varies among regions. *Rural Punjab:* 34% of males, 98% of females never used alcohol.	~50%	Country liquor (arrack), 65 proof, consumed in rural areas and by low-income groups in urban areas (especially South India)
Kazakhstan	2.76	0.32	0.14	2.28	*Women age 30–60 years:* 73% used alcohol at some time. Proportion of women involved in drunkenness is increasing, male/female ratio rose from 1:10 in 1990 to 1:8 in 1993	N/A	N/A
Korea (South)	6.78	1.78	0.02	2.01	N/A	2%	Soju, a local beverage, 44 proof. Also, sweet potato spirits (average 50 proof)
Russia	10.8	1.57	1.24	7.99	*Prevalence:* Only 1% of men and 16% of women abstain from alcohol. Alcohol-related disorders were reported by 73% of men and 10% of women.	Rural regions, ~80%–90% *1997 consumption:* ~1 billion bottles of perfume and 900,000 liters of window cleaning fluid were consumed for alcohol content,	Braga, a strong beer with alcohol content of 10%–15% ethanol

Country	Total	Beer	Wine	Spirits		Unrecorded consumption
Romania	9.65	2.93	4.91	1.78	*1992–1997:* self-reported mean alcohol consumption increased to 70.8 grams/week (men), 9.4 grams/week (women). *Cross-sectional survey:* 9% of men, 35% of women report "never drink alcohol"; 10% of men, 2% of women drink several times a week; 44% of men, 6% of women drink ~≥25 cl of vodka at a time; 31% of men, 3% of women do so at least once a month (25 cl of vodka contains 78.5 g of absolute alcohol). *1994 per capita consumption, liters per adult:* vodkas and vodka-based liquors: 13.7; Wines: 3.5; Brandies: 0.35; Champagnes: 1.02.	(~3.5–4 liters of pure alcohol per capita).
Phillipines	3.33	0.74	0.01	2.56	77% of males drink, 16% daily; 47% of women drink, 2% daily About 36% of high school and college students drink. When queried, 2%–3% had consumed alcohol that day, and 5%–10% that week. Rural students drink more than urban students. Male, female rates are similar (~35%).	N/A
Ukraine	3.9	0.75	0.26	2.86	*Teen rate:* 79% drank within last 12 months, 30% were drunk in last 12 months. Lifetime prevalence of alcohol use was 87% (equal for boys and girls). *Vocational-technical school students:* 66% drank alcohol *Rural secondary school students:* 16% drank alcohol.	Unrecorded consumption of pure alcohol estimated at 10.5 liters per capita (based on (*i*) production of Samogen, (*ii*) home production of wine, (*iii*) theft of alcohol intended for medical or industrial use, and (*iv*) illegally imported alcohol).	Samogen, potato or grain-based home brew of variable proof
Vietnam	1.32	0.45	0	0.88	N/A	N/A	N/A

[a]Estimated amount of pure ethanol in liters of total alcohol, and separately beer, wine and spirits consumed per adult (15 years and older). Numbers rounded in column 6.

[b]Estimates vary among different sources. See also Chapter 3.

Source: Data from World Health Organization.[10]

> Shortly after Elena was adopted from Russia, her pediatrician realized that she had FAS. He was reluctant to tell the family, thinking the diagnosis would break the newly forming bonds between parents and child, but finally did so. Their reaction surprised him: "Thank goodness we were able to bring her home where we can be sure she can get proper services and all the support she needs. Knowing the diagnosis helps us understand why her development and behavior are so different from our other children at this age."

> Alexander, age 7, has many features of FAS. His behavior seems to worsen every year, and he has difficulty playing with peers, making friends, and understanding the most basic principles of cause and effect. His parents are frantic with worry about his future, and consumed with anger and disappointment at the adoption agency who had promised them, "We don't place children with FAS." Both parents are in individual and marriage counseling, and are on antidepressant medication. "We'll do our best for Alex, and we love him dearly," say his parents, "but this is not the situation we expected for ourselves."

Table 5–2 Characteristics of fetal alcohol syndrome

- Pre- or postnatal growth retardation (below the 10th percentile)
- Facial dysmorphology (midline facial defects, micro-ophthalmia and/or short palpebral fissures, poorly developed philtrum, thin upper lip and absent cupid's bow, flattened maxillary area, and low-set ears)
- Central nervous system anomalies (developmental delay, intellectual impairment, behavioral disturbances, microcephaly [less than third percentile])

Furthermore, maternal history of alcohol ingestion is rarely available. Nonetheless, FAS and ARND/ARBD may be identified with certainty in some internationally adopted children. The preparation of adoptive families for the possibility that their child may have FAS varies greatly, as does their ability and willingness to grapple with the realities of parenting a child with this problem.

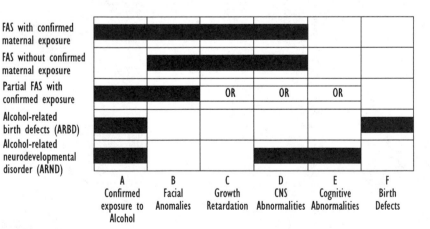

Figure 5–1 *Terminology related to prenatal alcohol exposure. FAS, fetal alcohol syndrome. Findings (A–F) are used to define specific diagnoses (left column). (Reproduced with permission from* Pediatrics, *Vol. 106, pp. 358–361, Figure 1, Copyright 2000.)*

Table 5–3 Physical features of fetal alcohol syndrome

Type	Feature
Skeletal	Clinodactyly, camptodactyly, radioulnar synostosis, flexion contractures, altered palmar creases, small distal phalanges, short fourth and fifth metacarpals, small fifth fingernails, short neck, cervical vertebral malformations, hemivertebrae, pectus excavatum or carinatum, rib anomalies, myelomeningocele, hydrocephalus, maxillary hypoplasia, and micrognathia
Cardiac	VSD, ASD, tetralogy of Fallot, coarctation of the aorta, aberrant great vessels
Craniofacial	Microcephaly, short palpebral fissures, epicanthal folds, ptosis (may be asymmetric), strabismus or myopia, micro-ophthalmia, increased retinal vessel tortuosity, optic nerve hypoplasia, strabismus, cleft lip ± palate, other orofacial clefts, maxillary hypoplasia, hypoplastic nasal bridge, short nose, anteverted nostrils, smooth philtrum with thin upper lip, absent cupid's bow, protruding auricles, low-set and posteriorly rotated ears
Renal	Aplastic, dysplastic, hypoplastic kidneys, horseshoe kidneys, hydronephrosis (although some authors[25] disagree)
Other	Hypoplastic labia majora, strawberry hemangiomata, accessory nipple, single umbilical artery

ASD, atrial septal defect; VSD, ventricular septal defect.

Source: Data from refs.[1,3,18,23,24]

Physical Features of Fetal Alcohol Syndrome and Alcohol-Related Birth Defects and Neurodevelopmental Disorders

Children with prenatal alcohol exposure have a variety of abnormal physical features (Table 5–3). The characteristic facial appearance is usually underrecognized in the newborn period, even among children of known alcoholics[20] (Fig. 5–2), but becomes more apparent during late infancy and early childhood (Fig. 5–3). In a large prospective longitudinal study,[21] only 50% of those children identified at age 4 with FAS had been identified at birth. Many of the facial features become less prominent as children enter adolescence[21,22] (Table 5–4). Recognition of characteristic facial appearance may be more difficult in Asian children with epicanthal folds. The face must be evaluated in repose; facial expressions interfere with determination of FAS (Fig. 5–4).

Growth delays are characteristic of FAS and ARBD. Nearly 80% of children have height, weight, and/or head circumference below the fifth percentile at birth, throughout infancy, and beyond.[26] The microcephaly results from poor brain growth. Alcohol impairs fetal brain synaptogenesis via blockade of *N*-methyl-*D*-aspartate (NMDA) glutamate receptors and activation of γ-aminobutyric acid (GABA) (A) receptors, leading to widespread neurodegeneration.[27] The fetal basal ganglia, corpus callosum, and cerebellum are especially

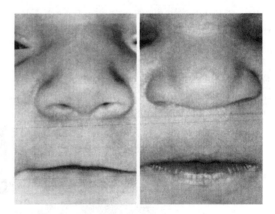

Figure 5–2 *Features of prenatal alcohol exposure may be more difficult to recognize in infants than in older children. Both infants shown have features of prenatal alcohol exposure (long and flat philtrums, thin vermillion, and depressed nasal bridges; infant on left also has anteverted nares). (From Stoler JM, Holmes LB. Under-recognition of prenatal alcohol effects in infants of known alcohol abusing women.* Journal of Pediatrics *1999; 135(4):434, with permission.)*

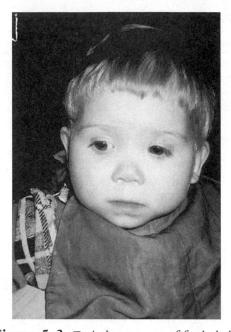

Table 5–4 Craniofacial dysmorphism in Fetal Alcohol Syndrome

Signs	Infants (%)	Adolescents (%)
Microcephaly	82	61
Short palpebral fissures	41	32
Epicanthal folds	62	16
Low nasal bridge, short nose	55	30
Micrognathia, flat midface	66	45
Thin upper lip	82	66
Indistinct philtrum	43	32
Hypoplastic/misaligned teeth	21	30
Strabismus	39	30
Minor ear anomalies (posterior rotation)	16	14
Increased growth of nose	0	80

Source: Adapted from Spohr et al.[22]

Figure 5–3 *Typical appearance of fetal alcohol syndrome. Characteristic features include thin upper lip, absent cupid's bow, flat, elongated philtrum, small palpebral fissures, and microcephaly.*

susceptible to alcohol exposure.[28] Postmortem studies of the brains of individuals with FAS show frequent neuroanatomic abnormalities, mostly affecting midline structures, such as micrencephaly (small brain), leptomeningeal heterotopias, holoprosencephaly, agenesis of the corpus callosum, dysgenesis of the cerebellum and brain stem, and neural tube.[28–31] For example, 6 of 10 children with FAS[32] evaluated by magnetic resonance imaging (MRI) had midline anomalies (agenesis or hypoplasia of the corpus callosum, cavum septi pellucidi, and cavum vergae). Seven had micrencephaly. Children with the most severe facial dysmorphology were more likely to have midline brain anomalies. Compared to other prenatal drug exposures, the congenital effects of alcohol are extensive (Table 5–5).[32a]

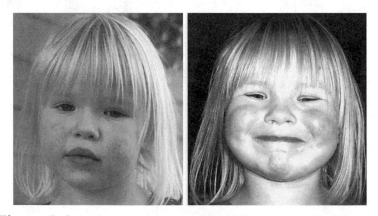

Figure 5–4 *Facial expression alters the appearance of features assessed for signs of fetal alcohol syndrome. Examination of the face in repose is essential. (With permission.)*

Table 5–5 Comparison of congenital effects from alcohol and other drugs

	Alcohol	*Cocaine*	*Heroin*	*Marijuana*
Decreased birth weight	+	+	+	+
Small for gestational age	+			
Mental retardation	+			
Newborn central nervous system problems	+	+	+	
Other central nervous system abnormalities	+	?		+
Withdrawal	+		+	
Physical anomalies	+			

Source: Weiner L, Morse BA, with permission.[32a]

Neurobehavioral Features of Fetal Alcohol Syndrome and Alcohol-Related Birth Defects and Neurodevelopmental Disorders

Impaired cognitive and psychosocial function are the most disabling features of FAS and ARBD.[33] Children with FAS have a broad range of IQs, but an average IQ of about 70. The severity of dysmorphic features relates to the degree of mental deficiency. Children with more severe manifestations have average IQs of 55, while those less severely affected have average IQs of 82.[34] However, cognitive deficits are common in children after heavy prenatal alcohol exposure with or without the physical features of FAS[35] (Fig. 5–5).

About 80% of children with FAS have obvious behavioral abnormalities by middle-school age[21] (Table 5–6). About 50% of affected children have some combination of poor coordination, hypotonia, or attention-deficit hyperactivity disorder (ADHD).[1] Children frequently have poor interpersonal skills (even when matched for IQ score to non-alcohol-exposed controls).[36] Some children have poor executive function, verbal learning, and memory deficits (especially spatial memory) even in the absence of mental retardation.[37–39] Abnormal ratings on the competence, problem, and summary scales of the Achenbach Child Behavior Check List are frequent among children with prenatal alcohol exposure, regardless

of physical findings and IQ.[40] While some children have intelligence in the normal range, many experience academic failure due to problems of activity and attention regulation (especially visual and auditory), severe learning disabilities, behavior disorders, delayed motor development, poor balance, and marked instability.[41–44] Children with FAS have abnormal cerebral metabolic rates (especially in the basal ganglia and thalamus)[45] and hypoperfusion of the left hemisphere (associated with arithmetic and logical–grammatical function and attentional problems) demonstrated by single photon emission computed tomography (SPECT) scan.[30]

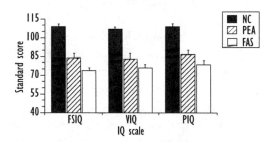

Figure 5–5 *The performance of children with fetal alcohol syndrome (FAS), prenatal exposure to alcohol (PEA), or matched normal controls (NC) on age-appropriate tests of IQ. Full-scale IQ (FSIQ), Verbal IQ (VIQ), performance IQ (PIQ). (From Mattson SN, Riley EP, Gramling L, Delis DC, Jones KL. Heavy prenatal alcohol exposure with or without physical features of fetal alcohol syndrome leads to IQ deficits. Journal of Pediatrics 1997; 131:718–21, with permission)*

Table 5–6 Neurobehavioral problems in 14-year-old children with prenatal alcohol exposure

Attentional regulation
Spatial memory and integration
Problem solving
Perceptual motor tasks
Arithmetic skills
Distractibility
Persistence
Organizational skills
Retaining information
Comprehension of words
Lack of tactfulness
Lower mean length of utterances
Decreased information processing
Restlessness
Reluctance to meet challenges

Source: Data from Streissguth et al.[21]

Many children also exhibit sleep disorders, abnormal habits, and stereotypy.[46,47] Auditory problems are also common, including (*1*) a developmental delay in auditory maturation, (*2*) sensorineural hearing loss, (*3*) intermittent conductive hearing loss due to recurrent serous otitis media, and (*4*) central hearing loss.[48–50]

Diagnosis

The diagnosis of FAS is based on clinical findings and maternal history. Because these lack precision and specificity, efforts have been made to establish standards for the phenotypic findings and to develop more accurate diagnostic measures. Computer-assisted analyses of facial photographs or craniofacial measurements of school-age children with FAS (most of them Caucasian) can identify affected individuals with nearly 100% accuracy, based on reduced palpebral length/inner canthal distance ratio, smooth philtrum, thin upper lip, (Fig. 5–6)[51,52] or head circumference and bigonial breadth.[53] These are helpful steps to improve case definition, but they must be expanded across the spectrum of ages (most children studied were

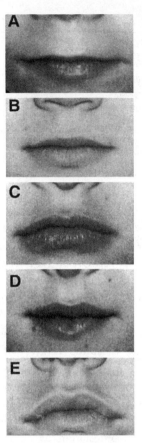

Figure 5–6 *The spectrum of dysmorphology of the lip and philtrum associated with prenatal alcohol exposure. Upper-lip thinness and philtrum smoothness are ranked from A (highest exposure) to E (lowest or no exposure). (From Astley SJ, Clarren SK. A case definition and photographic screening tool for the facial phenotype of fetal alcohol syndrome.* Journal of Pediatrics *1996; 129:36, with permission.)*

school-age) and different ethnic groups before used for practical diagnosis (Fig. 5–7).

Detection of markers of maternal alcohol use (whole blood-associated acetaldehyde, carbohydrate-deficient transferrin, γ-glutamyl transpeptidase, and mean red blood cell volume) in maternal blood during pregnancy or analysis of neonatal hair for fatty acid ethyl esters[54] may also be useful in the future to identify fetuses at risk for FAS.[55] However, such techniques are not presently applicable to international adoption.

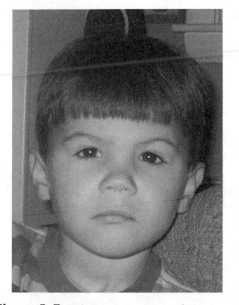

Figure 5–7 *Ethnic variation may make assessment of fetal alcohol syndrome difficult. This Russian boy has normal head circumference, superior cognitive skills, and excellent behavior. Ethnic heritage and prenatal exposure history are unknown. (With permission.)*

If diagnostic criteria are strictly applied, FAE or ARBD/ARND cannot be determined in the absence of maternal history. However, the combination of facial features, growth delays (especially microcephaly), and neurobehavioral abnormalities strongly suggest this diagnosis in international adoptees, especially in those from high-risk areas.

Differential Diagnosis

The clinical and physical characteristics of FAS are not specific. Other conditions to consider in differential diagnosis include Williams syndrome, maternal phenylketonuria, fetal hydantoin syndrome, prenatal toluene exposure, Cornelia de Lange syndrome, Noonan syndrome, velocardiofacial syndrome, and chromosomal abnormalities.[56] Consultation with a geneticist or dysmorphologist may be helpful to establish the diagnosis and exclude "look-alikes" (Table 5–7).

Outcome of Children with Fetal Alcohol Syndrome

The outcome of children with FAS is complicated by multiple pre- and postnatal factors.[57] Birth weight, microcephaly, gestational age, and prenatal exposure to drugs and tobacco may each independently influence outcome. Many children with FAS reside in homes of lower socioeconomic status, with lower parental educational level, exposure to violence, maternal depression, lead exposure, and ongoing parental drinking and drug use. With family dysfunction, children may experience frequent disruptive custody changes. Isolation of prenatal alcohol exposure as an independent variable in the assessment of outcome is difficult to achieve. Finally, referral and case ascertainment bias may select for children with more severe outcomes in some studies.

Outcome of growth deficits in children with FAS is relatively straightforward. The deficits in height, weight, and head circumference gradually improve during childhood.[58] Short stature and underweight persist in boys; girls generally achieve a normal weight by adolescence.[22] By 15 years of age, microcephaly persists in about 65% of children but improves in the remainder.[22,59] Persistent microcephaly is one of the major sequelae of severe intrauterine alcohol exposure.[60]

In a 10-year follow-up study of 60 German children diagnosed with FAS in infancy and childhood[22,60] (Table 5–4), craniofacial malformations diminished with time, as did skeletal abnormalities and some signs of neurologic dysfunction (hyperactivity, hypotonia, ptosis). Severely affected children were still easily recognizable in adolescence; in mildly affected children, physical signs of FAS were much less obvious. Overall, IQs were stable with time; in some children, IQ decreased or increased slightly. Only a "loose association" was found between microcephaly and mental retardation; microcephaly did not predict IQ at follow-up assessment. Overall, neurologic performance im-

Table 5–7 Differential diagnosis of fetal alcohol, Williams, Cornelia de Lange, and velocardiofacial syndromes

Factor	Fetal Alcohol Syndrome	Williams Syndrome	Cornelia de Lange Syndrome	Velocardiofacial Syndrome
Growth	Short stature, intrauterine growth retardation, microcephaly	Short stature, intrauterine growth retardation	Short stature, intrauterine growth retardation, microcephaly	Short stature, microcephaly
Eyes	Short palpebral fissures, epicanthal folds, ptosis (may be asymmetric), strabismus or myopia, micro-ophthalmia, increased retinal vessel tortuosity	Medial eyebrow flare, periorbital fullness, epicanthal folds, stellate pattern of iris, strabismus or myopia, increased retinal vessel tortuosity	Synophrys, myopia, long curly eyelashes	Narrow palpebral fissures, small optic discs, tortuous retinal vessels
Ears	Protruding auricles, low-set and posteriorly rotated ears		Low-set ears, hearing loss	Minor auricular anomalies
Nose	Depressed nasal bridge, anteverted nares, short nose	Depressed nasal bridge, anteverted nares	Depressed nasal bridge, anteverted nares	Square nasal root, decreased nasopharyngeal lymphoid tissue, prominent tubular nose, hypoplastic nasal alae, bulbous nasal tip
Mouth	Long, smooth philtrum with thin upper lip, absent cupid's bow, cleft lip/palate, other orofacial clefts	Long philtrum, thick lips, hypodontia, microdontia	Long philtrum, thin upper lip, downturned corners of the mouth, high arched palate, cleft lip/palate, widely spaced teeth, late-erupting teeth	Cleft palate, velopharyngeal insufficiency, small open mouth, pharyngeal hypotonia, Pierre Robin syndrome, retrognathia
General	Flat midface	Flat midface	Brachycephaly, short neck	Long face

Factor	Fetal Alcohol Syndrome	Williams Syndrome	Cornelia de Lange Syndrome	Velocardiofacial Syndrome
Cardiovascular	VSD, ASD, tetralogy of Fallot, coarctation of the aorta, aberrant great vessels	Supravalvular or valvular aortic stenosis, bicuspid aortic valve, mitral valve prolapse, mitral regurgitation, coronary artery stenosis, pulmonary valve stenosis, ASD, VSD, peripheral pulmonary artery stenosis, systemic hypertension	Sporadic	VSD, tetralogy of Fallot, right aortic arch, aberrant left subclavian, internal carotid artery abnormalities
Genitourinary	Aplastic, dysplastic, or hypoplastic kidneys, horseshoe kidneys, hydronephrosis	Small kidneys, solitary kidney, pelvic kidney, nephrocalcinosis, renal insufficiency, renal artery stenosis, vesicoureteral reflux, bladder diverticula, urethral stenosis, recurrent urinary tract infections		
Central nervous system	Mental retardation, myelomeningocele, hydrocephalus	Mental retardation (average IQ 56), relative sparing of language, poor visual–motor integration (range 41–80), hypersensitivity to sound, attention deficit disorder, cocktail party personality	Mental retardation, hypertonicity	Learning disability, mental retardation, behavioral/ psychiatric manifestations, blunt or inappropriate affect, psychotic illness

(continues)

Table 5–7 (*Continued*)

Factor	Fetal Alcohol Syndrome	Williams Syndrome	Cornelia de Lange Syndrome	Velocardiofacial Syndrome
Skeletal	Radioulnar synostosis, flexion contractures, altered palmar creases, small distal phalanges, short fourth and fifth metacarpals, small fifth fingernails, short neck, cervical vertebral malformations, hemivertebrae, pectus excavatum and carinatum, rib anomalies, micrognathia clinodactyly, camptodactyly	Radioulnar synostosis, hallux valgus, pectus excavatum, hypoplastic nails, kyphoscoliosis	Micrognathia, limited elbow extension, dislocation of the radial head, single transverse palmar crease, proximally placed thumbs, fifth finger clinodactyly, oligodactyly, syndactyly of toes 2 and 3	Slender hands and digits
Other	Hypoplastic labia majora, strawberry hemangiomata, accessory nipple, single umbilical artery	Vocal cord paralysis, inguinal hernia, chronic constipation, diverticulosis, hypercalcemia	Congenital diaphragmatic hernia, small nipples, gastroesophageal reflux, pyloric stenosis, cryptorchidism, hypoplastic male genitalia, cutis marmorata, hirsutism, low posterior hair line, low-pitched, growling cry in infancy	Nasal voice, inguinal hernia, umbilical hernia, neonatal hypocalcemia (rare)

proved, and EEGs became more normal. Individuals displayed improved psychiatric and cognitive function.[22] Nearly 70% of children were living with foster or adoptive families at the time of follow-up, but the effect of environment on outcome was not specifically addressed.

In a long-term study of 61 adolescents and adults with FAS,[3] the average IQ score was 68 but varied widely (Fig. 5–8). Patients achieved academic function at about the second- to fourth-grade levels, with special difficulties in arithmetic. Maladaptive behaviors such as poor judgment, distractibility, and difficulty perceiving social cues were common. Many individuals had poor concentration and attention, dependency, stubbornness or sullenness, social withdrawal, teasing or bullying, crying or laughing too easily, impulsivity, and periods of high anxiety. Many were noted to "lie, cheat, or steal, to show lack of consideration and to exhibit excessive unhappiness." None were receiving mental health services, and all had experienced "remarkably unstable family environments" with an average of five different homes placements each.

In a large longitudinal study from the same research group, ~500 children with prenatal alcohol exposure were followed prospectively until age 14 years.[21] These children were born to mothers considered representative of the general Seattle population of pregnant women receiving good prenatal care during 1974–75, a time before women knew it was inadvisable to drink during pregnancy. Socioeconomic status, home environment, and stability were not specifically addressed. Nonetheless, attentional problems, information processing, and learning problems were common among the subjects at age 14 (Table 5–5). As adults, impaired executive function was common and greater than that predicted from IQ scores.[19]

In another longitudinal study of 70 alcohol-exposed Finnish children followed until age 12 years, the duration and severity of intrauterine alcohol exposure correlated with the severity of neurobehavioral diagnoses and the likelihood of requiring special education or out-of-home placement.[61]

No studies to date specifically address the outcome of children with intrauterine alcohol exposure placed as newborns or infants in stable foster care or adoptive homes. In a large study that attempted to do so,[62] one or more adverse effects (alcoholism, anxiety, legal problems, depression, drug use, marital problems, psychological problems, divorce) were found in all of the adoptive homes of alcohol-exposed children. This precluded analysis of prenatal alcohol exposure as a single variable. Nonetheless, an adverse post-adoptive environment was more disruptive on the psychological development of children with prenatal alcohol exposure than those who had not been exposed. As adults, adoptees who had been prenatally exposed to alcohol and postnatally to adverse home circumstances had increased risk of substance abuse, various psychiatric symptoms, antisocial personality disorder, and depression. Many of the adoptees had psychiatric diagnoses, but 100% of those exposed to prenatal alcohol had multiple psychiatric diagnoses.

Several other studies report on the frequent placement of children with FAS in foster or institutional care. It is not clear if these placements are due to family problems or the child's

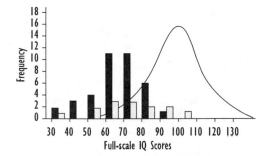

Figure 5–8 *Frequency distribution of IQ scores from the Wechsler Adult Intelligence Scale–Revised and the Wechsler Intelligence Scale for Children-Revised (as age appropriate). Mean chronological age was 18 years. The bell-shaped curve represents the normal distribution. Solid bars indicate fetal alcohol syndrome (n = 38, mean IQ = 66), open bars indicated fetal alcohol effects (N = 14, mean IQ = 73). (From Streissguth AP, Aase JM, Clarren SK, Randels SP, LaDue RA, Smith DF. Fetal alcohol syndrome in adolescents and adults. JAMA 1991; 265:1961–67. Copyright © 1991, American Medical Association. All rights reserved.)*

difficulties, and whether the child experienced neglect or deprivation prior to placement.[3,60,63,64] Early adoption would mitigate many of the confounding environmental effects known to be detrimental to these vulnerable children and would enhance "protective factors," such as early diagnosis, stable living environment, and provision of supportive services.[5]

Heritability of Alcoholism

Many adoptive and foster parents of children with FAS wonder if their child is at increased risk for development of alcoholism. While there is biochemical and molecular evidence that alcoholism may be inherited, environmental factors play a substantial role in determining the development and expression of this condition. Twin studies and adoption studies suggest that inheritance is complex and multifactorial and reflects biologic, psychologic, and environmental elements.[62,65-71] Conflict or psychopathology in the adoptive family increases the risk that their adopted children of alcoholic birth parents will themselves become alcoholic.[72] Early, concrete, and continuous education about alcohol use and decision making is recommended for children with FAS.[73]

Prevention of Secondary Disabilities

A child with fetal alcohol exposure presents many challenges. Parents may need support with many areas of child development (Table 5–8). Early Intervention (also known as "Birth to 3" programs in some regions) may provide ongoing physical, occupational, and speech therapy. Comprehensive educational support in the school should be instituted early, and changing needs should be addressed. As with all children with developmental concerns, assistance with adaptive skills, independent living, behav-

Table 5–8   Parenting concerns in raising a child with fetal alcohol syndrome[73]

Sleep disturbances (difficulty falling asleep, frequent wakening during night)

Poor appetite, difficulties coordinating sucking and swallowing

Developmental delays

Speech and language delays (expressive language usually better than receptive language)

Frequent ear infections, dental problems, upper respiratory infections

Sensory integration disorder (sensory defensiveness, gravitational and proprioceptive issues; see Chapter 33)

Hyperactivity, poor attention span

Learning disabilities, cognitive delays (often scattered)

Inappropriate social behaviors, unresponsiveness to social cues, poor judgment

Problems making or keeping friends

Parenting stress

ioral management, and employment can yield significant improvement in outcome.

Life History Interviews of 415 individuals (mean age 14.2 years, range 6–51 years) with FAS/FAE revealed the spectrum of secondary disabilities in this population.[74] Problems included mental health problems (90%), disrupted school experience (60%), trouble with the law (60%), confinement (in-patient mental health or substance abuse treatment or incarceration) (50%), inappropriate sexual behavior (50%), alcohol or drug problems (30%). Adults in the population had additional problems identified, including problems with employment (80%) and dependent living (80%). However, the study also identified numerous protective factors.[74] In order of strength, these include the following:

- Living in a stable and nurturant home for over 72% of life
- Being diagnosed before age of 6 years
- Never having experienced violence against oneself
- Staying in each living situation for an average of more than 2.8 years
- Experiencing a good-quality home from age 8 to 12 years

- Having applied for and been found eligible for developmental disabilities services
- Having a diagnosis of FAS rather than FAE (resulting in earlier diagnosis)
- Having basic needs met for at least 13% of life

Most adoptive homes supply these protective factors, and considerably more. The pediatrician should expect to be involved with a team of specialists to provide ongoing support to the child with FAS and ARBD and the family as different challenges emerge.

Finally, a number of positive characteristics have been identified in some children with FAS/FAE (Table 5–9).

Key Points for Internationally Adopted Children

- Alcohol exposure history is usually unknown for internationally adopted children
- Diagnosis is therefore based on characteristic facial appearance, growth delays, and neurobehavioral difficulties.
- Factors other than alcohol exposure can account for abnormal growth or neurobehavioral findings.

Table 5–9. Positive characteristics of some children with FAS/FAE.

Cuddly, cheerful, tactile
Friendly and happy
Caring, kind, loyal, nurturing, compassionate
Trusting and loving
Determined, committed, persistent
Curious, involved
Energetic, hard-working, athletic
Artistic, musical, creatively intelligent
Fair, cooperative
Highly verbal
Fair with younger children and animals
Able to have long-term visual memory
Able to participate in problem solving

Source: Data from Minnesota Dept. of Health.[75]

- Exposure is more likely in children adopted from Eastern Europe (especially Ukraine, Russia and other former Soviet Union countries).
- Adoption may ameliorate some of the long-term difficulties for children with FAS.
- Prevention of "secondary disabilities" is key to improving long-term outcome.

Resources

National Organization on Fetal Alcohol Syndrome. Available at: http://www.nofas.org/.

The ARC Fetal Alcohol Syndrome Resource Guide. Available at: http://thearc.org/misc/faslist.html.

Fetal Alcohol Syndrome Family Resource Institute. Available at: http://www.fetalalcoholsyndrome.org/.

University of Washington (Seattle) Fetal Alcohol and Drug Unit. Available at: http://depts.washington.edu/fadu/.

Dorris M. The Broken Cord. New York: Harper & Row, 1989. This is the true story of an American Indian child adopted from a reservation and his adoptive father's search to understand FAS.

Streissguth A, Kanter J. (ed) The Challenge of Fetal Alcohol Syndrome: Overcoming Secondary Disabilities. Seattle: University of Washington Press, 1997. This book contains proceedings from the International FAS Conference in Seattle, Washington.

Kleinfeld J, Wescott S. (ed). Fantastic Antone Succeeds! Experience in educating children with fetal alcohol syndrome. Fairbanks: University of Alaska Press, 1993, and the companion volume Fantastic Antone Grows Up. Kleinfeld J, Morse B, Wescott S (ed). Fairbanks: University of Alaska Press, 2000. These invaluable guides for parents and caregivers of children with FAS offer lots of practical advice, helpful strategies, and a positive outlook. The follow-up volume provides a guide to issues faced by adolescents and young adults with FAS.

FAQs

Q. Some prospective adoptive parents gave me a video and photograph to review of the child referred to them. I'm not sure I can tell from the facial features if FAS is present or not. What should I advise them?

A. Be honest. Some images are easy to categorize as definite FAS or definitely not FAS. However, most are indeterminate. Careful review of the medical history and growth measurements may help determine risk. Families must be aware that certain regions (Eastern Europe, Ukraine, Russia, and former Soviet Republics) are at higher risk, and that lack of characteristic facial findings is no guarantee that the birth mother did not ingest alcohol. When in doubt, request additional photographic or video material, verification of growth measurements (especially head circumference), and a direct query to the orphanage doctors about their assessment of the child's risk for FAS or related conditions.

Q. Can we "trust" the orphanage doctors to do this type of assessment?

A. The level of skills, training, and awareness varies enormously among physicians, even in regions of the world where alcohol use is extremely common. It's hard to be sure that the individual doctors recognize the signs of FAS, which may be subtle in infants and young children.

Q. Parents returned from Russia to my practice with a newly adopted child who has definite signs of FAS. What now?

A. You may wish to have a geneticist, dysmorphologist, or other specialist confirm the diagnosis. Additional medical work-up should be dictated by the child's medical findings (i.e., cardiac evaluation of heart murmurs, ophthalmologic intervention as necessary, etc.). There is an enormous amount of educational material available for families (see Resources). The family will clearly need your emotional and practical support. Early Intervention programs for young children, and programs through the public schools for older children should be contacted. Parent support groups (many of them specific for adoptive and foster parents of children with FAS) may also prove valuable. The key to management of children with FAS is prevention of secondary disabilities through provision of educational, developmental, and practical support services.

Q. One of my patients is a 7-year-old adopted from Lithuania. He has always been just below the fifth percentile for height, weight, and head circumfer-ence. He doesn't have the typical facial appearance of FAS, but some of his behaviors and cognitive problems make me think he could have been alcohol exposed in utero. How should I proceed?

A. This is tricky, as it is unlikely that you will ever to be able to confirm the diagnosis on maternal history. Mild growth retardation may reflect prenatal alcohol exposure, or other pre- and postnatal exposures. Regardless, he won't fit strict diagnostic criteria (Fig. 5–1): the only category without confirmed maternal exposure requires facial anomalies, growth retardation, and CNS abnormalities. A thorough neuropsychological evaluation might be helpful in pinpointing his neurobehavioral problems, which then can be addressed specifically with therapies and other interventions.

References

1. Committee on Substance Abuse and Committee on Children with Disabilities. Fetal alcohol syndrome and alcohol-related neurodevelopmental disorders. Pediatrics 2000; 106:358–61.

2. Sampson PD, Streissguth AP, Bookstein FL, et al. Incidence of fetal alcohol syndrome and prevalence of alcohol–related neurodevelopmental disorder. Teratology 1997; 56:317–26.

3. Streissguth AP, Aase JM, Clarren SK, Randels SP, LaDue RA, Smith DF. Fetal alcohol syndrome in adolescents and adults. JAMA 1991; 265:1961–67.

4. Warren KR, Calhoun FJ, May PA, et al. Fetal alcohol syndrome: an international perspective. Alcohol Clin Exp Res 2001; 25:202S–206S.

5. Streissguth AP. Fetal alcohol syndrome in older patients. Alcohol Alcohol Suppl 1993; 2:209–12.

6. Sullivan WC. A note on the influence of maternal inebriety on the offspring. J Ment Sci 1899; 45:489–503.

7. Senior B. Impaired growth and onychodysplasia. Short children with tiny toenails. Am J Dis Child 1971; 122:7–9.

8. Lemoine P, Harrousseau H, Borteyru JP, Menuet JC. Les enfants de parents alcooliques: anomalies observee: a propos de 127 cas. Ouest Med 1968; 8:476–82.

9. Jones KL, Smith DW, Ulleland CN, Streissguth AP. Pattern of malformation in offspring of chronic alcoholic mothers. Lancet 1973; 1:1267–71.

10. World Health Organization. Global Alcohol Database. Available at: http://www3.who.int/whosis/alcohol.

11. Larroque B, Kaminski M. Prenatal alcohol exposure and development at preschool age: main results of a French study. Alcohol Clin Exp Res 1998; 22:295–303.

12. Jacobson JL, Jacobson SW, Sokol RJ, Ager JW Jr. Relation of maternal age and pattern of pregnancy drinking to functionally significant cognitive deficit in infancy. Alcohol Clin Exp Res 1998; 22:345–51.

13. Christoffel KK, Salasky I. Fetal alcohol syndrome in dizygotic twins. J Pediatr 1975; 87:963–7.

14. Streissguth AP, Dehaene P. Fetal alcohol syndrome in twins of alcoholic mothers: concordance of diagnosis and IQ. Am J Med Genet 1993; 47:857–61.

15. Stoler JM, Ryan LM, Holmes LB. Alcohol dehydrogenase 2 genotypes, maternal alcohol use, and infant outcome. J Pediatr 2002; 141:780–5.

15a. Wilkemeyer MF, Chen S-Y, Menkari CE, et al. Differential effects of ethanol antagonism and neuroprotection in peptide fragment NAPVSIPQ prevention of ethanol-induced developmental toxicity. Proc Natl Acad Sci 2003; 100: 8543–48.

16. Savage DD, Becher M, de la Torre AJ, Sutherland RJ. Dose-dependent effects of prenatal ethanol exposure on synaptic plasticity and learning in mature offspring. Alcohol Clin Exp Res 2002; 26:1752–8.

17. Aase JM, Jones KL, Clarren SK. Do we need the term "FAE"? Pediatrics 1995; 95:428–30.

18. Stratton K et al. Fetal Alcohol Syndrome: Diagnosis, Epidemiology, Prevention, and Treatment. Institute of Medicine Committee to Study Fetal Alcohol Syndrome. Washington, DC: National Academy Press, 1996.

19. Connor PD, Sampson PD, Bookstein FL, Barr HM, Streissguth AP. Direct and indirect effects of prenatal alcohol damage on executive function. Dev Neuropsychol 2000; 18:331–54.

20. Stoler JM, Holmes LB. Under-recognition of prenatal alcohol effects in infants of known alcohol abusing women. J Pediatr 1999; 135:430–6.

21. Streissguth AP, Barr HM, Sampson PD, Bookstein FL. Prenatal alcohol and offspring development: the first fourteen years. Drug Alcohol Depend 1994; 36:89–99.

22. Spohr HL, Willms J, Steinhausen HC. The fetal alcohol syndrome in adolescence. Acta Paediatr. Suppl 1994; 404:19–26.

23. Hellstrom A. Optic nerve morphology may reveal adverse events during prenatal and perinatal life—digital image analysis. Surv Ophthalmol 1999; 44:S63–73.

24. Stromland K, Hellstrom A. Fetal alcohol syndrome—an ophthalmological and socioeducational prospective study. Pediatrics 1996; 97:845–50.

25. Taylor CL, Jones KL, Jones MC, Kaplan GW. Incidence of renal anomalies in children prenatally exposed to ethanol. Pediatrics 1994; 94:209–12.

26. Day NL, Leech SL, Richardson GA, Cornelius MD, Robles N, Larkby CA. Prenatal alcohol exposure predicts continued deficits in offspring size at 14 years of age. Alcohol Clin Exp Res 2002; 26:1584–91.

27. Ikonomidou C, Bittigau P, Ishimaru MJ, et al. Ethanol-induced apoptotic neurodegeneration and fetal alcohol syndrome. Science 2000; 287:1056–60.

28. Roebuck TM, Mattson SN, Riley EP. A review of the neuroanatomical findings in children with fetal alcohol syndrome or prenatal exposure to alcohol. Alcohol Clin Exp Res 1998; 22:339–44.

29. Johnson VP, Swayze VW II, Sato Y, Andreasen NC. Fetal alcohol syndrome: craniofacial and central nervous system manifestations. Am J Med Genet 1996; 61:329–39.

30. Riikonen R, Salonen I, Partanen K, Verho S. Brain perfusion SPECT and MRI in foetal alcohol syndrome. Dev Med Child Neurol 1999; 41:652–9.

31. Riley EP, Mattson SN, Sowell ER, Jernigan TL, Sobel DF, Jones KL. Abnormalities of the corpus callosum in children prenatally exposed to alcohol. Alcohol Clin Exp Res 1995; 19:1198–202.

32. Swayze VW 2nd, Johnson VP, Hanson JW, et al. Magnetic resonance imaging of brain anomalies in fetal alcohol syndrome. Pediatrics 1997; 99:232–40.

32a. Weiner L, Morse BA. Comparison of congenital effects from alcohol and other drugs. Alcohol, drugs and the fetus: a teaching package. ©1992. The Fetal Alcohol Education Program, Boston, MA.

33. Roebuck TM, Mattson SN, Riley EP. Behavioral and psychosocial profiles of alcohol-exposed children. Alcohol Clin Exp Res 1999; 23:1070–6.

34. Streissguth AP, Herman CS, Smith DW. Intelligence, behavior, and dysmorphogenesis in the fetal alcohol syndrome: a report on 20 patients. J Pediatr 1978; 92:363–7.

35. Mattson SN, Riley EP, Gramling L, Delis DC, Jones KL. Heavy prenatal alcohol exposure with or without physical features of fetal alcohol syndrome leads to IQ deficits. J Pediatr 1997; 131:718–21.

36. Thomas SE, Kelly SJ, Mattson SN, Riley EP. Comparison of social abilities of children with fetal alcohol syndrome to those of children with similar IQ scores and normal controls. Alcohol Clin Exp Res 1998; 22:528–33.

37. Uecker A, Nadel L. Spatial but not object memory impairments in children with fetal alcohol syndrome. Am J Ment Retard 1998; 103:12–8.

38. Mattson SN, Riley EP. Implicit and explicit memory functioning in children with heavy prenatal alcohol exposure. J Int Neuropsychol Soc 1999; 5:462–71.

39. Mattson SN, Goodman AM, Caine C, Delis DC, Riley EP. Executive functioning in children with heavy prenatal alcohol exposure. Alcohol Clin Exp Res 1999; 23:1808–15.

40. Mattson SN, Riley EP. Parent ratings of behavior in children with heavy prenatal alcohol exposure and

IQ-matched controls. Alcohol Clin Exp Res 2000; 24:226–31.

41. Connor PD, Streissguth AP, Sampson PD, Bookstein FL, Barr HM. Individual differences in auditory and visual attention among fetal alcohol-affected adults. Alcohol Clin Exp Res 1999; 23:1395–402.

42. Shaywitz SE, Cohen DJ, Shaywitz BA. Behavior and learning difficulties in children of normal intelligence born to alcoholic mothers. J Pediatr 1980; 96:978–82.

43. Lemoine P, Lemoine P. Outcome of children of alcoholic mothers. Ann Pediatr (Paris) 1992; 39:226–35.

44. Roebuck TM, Simmons RW, Richardson C, Mattson SN, Riley EP. Neuromuscular responses to disturbance of balance in children with prenatal exposure to alcohol. Alcohol Clin Exp Res 1998; 22:1992–7.

45. Clark CM, Li D, Conry J, Conry R, Loock C. Structural and functional brain integrity of fetal alcohol syndrome in nonretarded cases. Pediatrics 2000; 105:1096–9.

46. Steinhausen HC, Spohr HL. Long-term outcome of children with fetal alcohol syndrome: psychopathology, behavior, and intelligence. Alcohol Clin Exp Res 1998; 22:334–8.

47. Steinhausen HC, Willms J, Spohr HL. Long-term psychopathological and cognitive outcome of children with fetal alcohol syndrome. J Am Acad Child Adolesc Psychiatry 1993; 32:990–4.

48. Church MW, Abel EL. Fetal alcohol syndrome. Hearing, speech, language, and vestibular disorders. Obstet Gynecol Clin North Am 1998; 25:85–97.

49. Church MW, Eldis F, Blakley BW, Bawle EV. Hearing, language, speech, vestibular, and dentofacial disorders in fetal alcohol syndrome. Alcohol Clin Exp Res 1997; 21:227–37.

50. Church MW, Kaltenbach JA. Hearing, speech, language, and vestibular disorders in the fetal alcohol syndrome: a literature review. Alcohol Clin Exp Res 1997; 21:495–512.

51. Astley SJ, Clarren SK. A case definition and photographic screening tool for the facial phenotype of fetal alcohol syndrome. J Pediatr 1996; 129:33–41.

52. Stromland K, Chen Y, Norberg T, Wennerstrom K, Michael G. Reference values of facial features in Scandinavian children measured with a range-camera technique. Scand J Plast Reconstr Surg Hand Surg 1999; 33:59–65.

53. Moore ES, Ward RE, Jamison PL, Morris CA, Bader PI, Hall BD. The subtle facial signs of prenatal exposure to alcohol: an anthropometric approach. J Pediatr 2001; 139:215–9.

54. Klein J, Chan D, Koren G. Neonatal hair analysis as a biomarker for in utero alcohol exposure. N Engl J Med 2002; 347:2086.

55. Stoler JM, Huntington KS, Peterson CM, et al. The prenatal detection of significant alcohol exposure with maternal blood markers. J Pediatr 1998; 133:346–52.

56. Stoler JM. Reassessment of patients with the diagnosis of fetal alcohol syndrome [letter]. Pediatrics 1999; 103:1313–5.

57. Sood B, Delaney-Black V, Covington C, et al. Prenatal alcohol exposure and childhood behavior at age 6 to 7 years: I. Dose–response effect. Pediatrics 2001; 108:E34.

58. Day NL, Zuo Y, Richardson GA, Goldschmidt L, Larkby CA, Cornelius MD. Prenatal alcohol use and offspring size at 10 years of age. Alcohol Clin Exp Res 1999; 23:863–9.

59. Habbick BF, Blakley PM, Houston CS, Snyder RE, Senthilselvan A, Nanson JL. Bone age and growth in fetal alcohol syndrome. Alcohol Clin Exp Res 1998; 22:1312–6.

60. Spohr HL, Willms J, Steinhausen HC. Prenatal alcohol exposure and long-term developmental consequences. Lancet 1993; 341:907–10.

61. Autti-Ramo I. Twelve-year follow-up of children exposed to alcohol in utero. Dev Med Child Neurol 2000; 42:406–11.

62. Cadoret RJ, Riggins-Caspers K. Fetal alcohol exposure and adult psychopathology. In: Barth RP, Freundlich M, Brodzinsky D, eds. Adoption and Prenatal Alcohol and Drug Exposure. Washington, DC: Child Welfare League of America, 2000: 83–113.

63. Aronson M, Hagberg B. Neuropsychological disorders in children exposed to alcohol during pregnancy: a follow-up study of 24 children to alcoholic mothers in Goteborg, Sweden. Alcohol Clin Exp Res 1998; 22:321–4.

64. Steinhausen HC, Willms J, Spohr HL. Correlates of psychopathology and intelligence in children with fetal alcohol syndrome. J Child Psychol Psychiatry Allied Disc 1994; 35:323–31.

65. Ferguson RA, Goldberg DM. Genetic markers of alcohol abuse. Clin Chim Acta 1997; 257:199–250.

66. Koopmans JR, Boomsma DI. Familial resemblances in alcohol use: genetic or cultural transmission? J Stud Alcohol 1996; 57:19–28.

67. McGue M, Pickens RW, Svikis DS. Sex and age effects on the inheritance of alcohol problems: a twin study. J Abnorm Psychol 1992; 101:3–17.

68. Pickens RW, Svikis DS, McGue M, Lykken DT, Heston LL, Clayton PJ. Heterogeneity in the inheritance of alcoholism. A study of male and female twins. Arch Gen Psychiatry 1991; 48:19–28.

69. Johnson JL, Leff M. Children of substance abusers: overview of research findings. Pediatrics 1999; 103:1085–99.

70. Tishler PV, Henschel CE, Ngo TA, Walters EE, Worobec TG. Fetal alcohol effects in alcoholic veteran patients. Alcohol Clin Exp Res 1998; 22:1825–31.

71. Yates WR, Cadoret RJ, Troughton EP, Stewart M, Giunta TS. Effect of fetal alcohol exposure on adult symp-

toms of nicotine, alcohol, and drug dependence. Alcohol Clin Exp Res 1998; 22:914–20.

72. Cutrona CE, Cadoret RJ, Suhr JA, et al. Interpersonal variables in the prediction of alcoholism among adoptees: evidence for gene-environment interactions. Compr Psychiatry 1994; 35:171–9.

73. Morse BA, Weiner L. FAS: Parent and Child. Boston: Boston University School of Medicine, 1993.

74. Streissguth AP, Barr HM, Kogan J, Bookstein FL. Primary and secondary disabilities in fetal alcohol syndrome. In: The challenge of fetal alcohol syndrome: Overcoming secondary disabilities. Univ Washington Press, Seattle, 1997.

75. Guidelines for care of children with special health care needs: FAS and FAE. Available at: http://www.health.state.mn.us/divs/fh/mcshn/pdfdocs/fas.pdf.

6

PRENATAL DRUG
EXPOSURE

The prevalence of prenatal exposure to illicit drugs among international adoptees is unknown. Impoverished birth mothers who relinquish their children may lack the financial resources to purchase drugs. It is equally plausible to speculate that maternal drug abuse increases the likelihood of child relinquishment. In other circumstances, birth mothers hoping for a specific gender child (i.e., a male in China or India) may be unlikely to abuse drugs during the pregnancy. In the United States, it is estimated that about 11% of newborns are affected to some degree by prenatal substance exposure (including drugs and/or alcohol).[1] Among children residing in U.S. foster care, a group with sociologic and demographic similarities to abandoned children in other countries,[2] it is estimated that about 70% of those in the system for at least 17 months have substance-involved parents.[3]

Adoption referrals rarely contain information regarding maternal drug use during pregnancy. Lack of information should not be construed to indicate that drug use did not occur. Referrals from Eastern Europe occasionally include the term "narcomania," indicating narcotic addiction. Sometimes, there is a notation that the birth mother is listed on the "narcologic registry," indicating that at some time she was treated for drug abuse. Occasionally, the term "abstinent syndrome" is listed, indicating that the newborn experienced drug withdrawal. Court-ordered termination of parental rights or abandonment of previous children may suggest maternal drug abuse. Hepatitis C infection, prematurity, small size for gestational age, and/or congenital microcephaly all may result from prenatal drug exposure, although alternative explanations exist.

The possibility of prenatal drug exposure raises several questions for internationally adopted children. Most important are concerns about the effects of prenatal drug exposure on the child's growth, development, and behavior and whether adoption ameliorates these effects. In addition, adoptive parents often wonder if prenatal drug exposure increases the likelihood that the child will later become involved with drugs.

In this section, information about drug abuse in sending countries will be reviewed. Current knowledge of the effects of prenatal drug exposure on the child will be described, with a focus on adoption studies. Adoption studies that address the possibility of drug addiction in the offspring of drug-abusing mothers will be reviewed, along with recommendations for prospective pediatric monitoring of drug-exposed children.

Drug Abuse in Sending Countries

Accurate information about drug abuse in different countries is difficult to obtain. Many countries do not collect such information, nor do they wish it to be publicized. Underreporting is widespread, and outside verification of information is rarely available. Table 6–1 was prepared with information from United Nations Drug Control Program and Central Intelligence Agency Fact Book Web sites[4,5] and from Poshyachinda[6] (see Chapter 3).

Effects of Prenatal Drug Exposure

Over 2200 articles are listed in MEDLINE that describe the effects of prenatal drug exposure in children. In most, considerable difficulties confound interpretation of the results. The effects of prenatal drug exposure cannot be isolated from many other factors affecting developmental outcome[1] (Table 6–2). Furthermore, accurate history of all exposures during pregnancy is difficult if not impossible to ascertain. For example, in an anonymous prevalence study in an inner-city Maryland teaching hospital,[10] 18% of mothers admitted drug use, but 48% of infants had meconium analyses indicating recent drug exposures. Half had evidence of exposure to more than one drug. In a similar survey, 38% of women

Misha was 1800 grams at birth. No gestational age was recorded. No information about his birth mother was available, except that she had delivered four other children, all of whom were living in orphanages. Misha's test for hepatitis C antibodies was positive when he arrived home at 11 months of age. Follow-up tests were negative, suggesting that the initial results represented maternal antibody. He made fantastic progress in growth and development, and was a delight to his parents and older sister. When he entered school, however, he had difficulty sitting still and paying attention; receptive language scores were "borderline." Attentional regulation became more difficult; and by third grade, treatment with Ritalin was begun. "We know his medical history suggests that Misha may have been exposed to drugs before he was born," said his dad. "But we also know there were lots of other risk factors for his problems in his background, including 11 months of institutionalization and unknown genetics."

reported cocaine use during pregnancy, but 60% had positive results by hair sample analysis.[11] Multiple exposures are also common. For example, in a survey of 65 Swedish mothers evaluated for amphetamine use during pregnancy,[12] 30% also used heroin, 80% abused alcohol, and 80% smoked. Ninety-four percent of drug-abusing mothers in Holland[13] used multiple drugs (methadone, heroin, cocaine, amphetamines, tranquilizers), and all smoked. Regardless of the primary drug of choice, tobacco and alcohol are frequently combined (reviewed in Koren et al.[14]). Combinations of drugs may be more devastating than single agents for the developing fetus. Tobacco smoke and cocaine combine synergistically to increase the risks of prematurity and intrauterine growth retardation. Cocaine and alcohol together form cocaethylene, which is more neurotoxic than cocaine alone.[15,16] Thus studies that purport to show the effect of a single type of drug exposure on the fetus may be misleading. Accurate information on the type, potency, amount, frequency, and duration of drug use during pregnancy is essentially unavailable outside of laboratory animal settings.

Table 6–1 Drug use in sending countries

Country	Most Frequently Abused Drugs	Women and Drug Abuse	Other
Cambodia	Cannabis, amphetamines, inhalants (street children), ecstasy. Opium and heroin are limited	Increasing use among commercial sex workers	
China	Heroin, diazepam, opium, and cannabis	About 90% of drug users are below 30 years of age, and over 80% are male	~100,000 injection drug users in the Province of Yunnan alone
Guatemala	Cocaine, heroin, cannabis, inhalants, tranquilizers[8]	Increasing especially among young people	
India	Opium, cannabis, diazepam, antihistamines, codeine-containing cough syrup, buprenorphine	Many "drug widows" are infected with HBV, HCV, HIV	Polydrug and alcohol use are common. In Manipur, Nagaland, and Mizoram (states in NE India) IDU is especially widespread. HBV, HCV, HIV are common
Korea (South)	Amphetamines, marijuana, opiates, inhalants, benzodiazepine, LSD, cocaine[7]		
Romania	Heroin and cocaine		
Russia	Heroin, cocaine, amphetamines, methadone, phencyclidine, 3-methylfentanyl, codeine, buprenorphine	2.5–3 million people regularly or occasionally use illegal drugs	>450,000[a] people registered as drug addicts in 2000. IDU is increasing rapidly
Ukraine	Cannabis, opium[9]	Cocaine and heroin are too expensive for the average Ukrainian citizen	65,000[a] officially registered addicts
Vietnam	Heroin, amphetamines	Represent <6% of all addicts Increasing use among commercial sex workers	>100,000 registered addicts; drug use increasing among young

HBV, hepatitis B virus; HCV, hepatitis C virus; HIV, human immunodeficiency virus; IDU, injection drug use.
[a]Probably a grave underestimate of addicts.

Table 6–2 Confounding factors in prenatal drug exposure research

Lack of prenatal care
Prematurity
Intrauterine growth retardation
Microcephaly
Poor nutrition
Poverty
Multiple exposures including alcohol and tobacco
Unknown dose, potency, frequency, duration of exposure

Perinatal Effects of Maternal Drug Use

Regardless of the difficulties cited above, there are some consistent findings in infants after *in utero* drug exposure (Table 6–3). Prematurity, intrauterine growth retardation, microcephaly, and neurologic abnormalities have been reported after heroin, amphetamine, and cocaine exposure (even after controlling for tobacco use).[17] Withdrawal syndrome and less severe neurologic signs such as irritability, restlessness, and abnormalities in posture and tone occur after exposure to several types of drugs.

Table 6–3 Perinatal effects of maternal drug use

Drug	Generally Reported Findings	Other Effects

Cocaine	Preterm delivery
	Microcephaly
	Low birth weight,
	Lower Apgar scores
	"Disorganized behavioral state"
		Motor dysfunction
		Withdrawal symptoms
		Language and attentional problems
		Dose-dependent neurologic abnormalities
		  (global hypertonia)[11]
		Impaired visual orientation at 4 weeks[13]
		Vascular injury to CNS (subependymal
		  hemorrhage in caudothalamic groove)[20]
		Decreased autonomic stability[21,22]

Opiates	Preterm delivery Microcephaly Low birth weight Neonatal abstinence syndrome	Increased risk of sudden infant death syndrome Adjustment problems, psycholinguistic problems

Amphetamines and
  methamphetamines
	Inconclusive	Possibly increased aggression (or related to postnatal
		  environment?)

Marijuana	Low birth weight	Problems with verbal skills and memory

Source: Data from refs. 13, 17–19.

Internationally adopted children are seldom if ever placed as newborns, thus the immediate effects of prenatal drug exposure are unlikely to be observed by American parents or doctors. Toxicology screens are not helpful after the newborn period. Congenital effects of prenatal exposure to cocaine, heroin, or marijuana are compared to alcohol in Table 5–5.

Long-term Effects of Prenatal Drug Exposure

Evaluation of long-term consequences of prenatal drug exposure is confounded by multiple factors (Table 6–4); attribution of outcome to drug use alone is problematic. Inner city children are at risk for adverse developmental outcome regardless of in utero exposures.[23,24] Poor outcomes are strongly associated with poverty, unstable home conditions, violence in the home enviroment, and inadequate interaction with adult caregivers.[1]

Language, behavior, attention, and emotional regulation are particularly vulnerable to prenatal drug exposure (Table 6–5), perhaps in the context of other risk factors. A systematic analysis of 36 selected studies of the outcome of

children with prenatal cocaine exposure found no consistent negative associations with physical growth, developmental or language test scores, or behavior, but possible associations with decreased attentiveness, emotional expression, and "soft" neurophysiologic findings were found.[25] A meta-analysis of 101 studies of the effect on offspring of cocaine use during pregnancy[26] revealed a slight reduction in IQ and significantly lower scores for receptive and

Table 6–4 Confounding factors in evaluating late effects of prenatal drug exposure

Socioeconomic status	Alcohol use
Poverty	Ongoing drug use
Malnutrition	Parity
Anemia	Maternal depression
Maternal education	Chaotic home environment
Maternal age	Move more frequently
Psychiatric comorbidity	Spend less time with children
Single motherhood	Less adequate housing
Disruptive caretaking	Less contact with fathers
Reduced parenting skills	Fewer toys
Interruption of maternal bonding	Effect of peer group

Source: Data from refs. 14–16.

Table 6–5 Long-term effects of prenatal drug exposure (selected studies)

Drug	Effect
Cocaine[27]	Reduced language abilities at age 6 years
Cocaine[28]	At age 4, smaller head circumference and worse behavior (home environment was most predictive of cognitive level)
Cocaine[29]	More externalizing and delinquent behaviors for boys (but mostly related to environmental exposures)
Cocaine[23,24]	No neurologic findings at age 6 years but may not have detected problems in arousal, attention, recognition memory, impulse control
Cocaine[30,31]	Lower auditory comprehension and language
Heroin[17]	Reduced locomotor abilities, intellect, and Developmental Quotient at 1 year (controlled for nicotine exposure)
Heroin[18]	29% with muscle tone abnormalities, excess movements, poor coordination and balance; worse behavior and social competence
Amphetamine[12]	At age 10 years, normal intellectual capacity, but 12% were one grade behind; some aggression and peer problems
Polydrug[32]	Poor attachment (even after adoption) due to abnormal infant behaviors
Cocaine, heroin, methadone	Normal motor skills and EEGs, delayed language and cognition. At 18 months children were less active, less vocal, showed less initiative, made fewer demands. At age 5 they were more aggressive and more depressed, and had more social difficulties, "less ego resiliency"
Cocaine and/ or opiates	Prolonged auditory brain responses[33]

expressive language among cocaine-exposed children.

Protective Effects of Adoption on Drug-Exposed Children

Studies which evaluate drug-exposed children after adoption bypass many of the factors that contribute to poor outcome. However, such studies rarely account for the child's age at placement, circumstances of care prior to adoption, and new factors within the adoptive home.

In an "all adoption" study, 233 children were evaluated ~8 years after domestic adoption.[3] Compared to those without prenatal drug exposure, those with a history of prenatal drug exposure ($n = 121$, various combinations of cocaine, heroin, marijuana, PCP, as well as alcohol [85%] and tobacco [90%]) were twice as likely to be in enrolled in classes for the learning disabled. However, their parents reported similar closeness, quality of family relations, and satisfaction with the adoption to that of parents of non–drug-exposed children.

A series of Canadian studies compared 23 children adopted at birth after prenatal cocaine exposure to 23 non–cocaine-exposed, non-adopted children.[14–16] Adoptive mothers and control group mothers were matched for IQ and socio-economic status. The children were studied between 14 months and 6.5 years. Children with prenatal cocaine exposure had lower birth weights and younger gestational age than those without prenatal drug exposure. At birth and at followup, drug exposed children had smaller head circumferences. Although no differences between groups were found for global IQ, the cocaine-exposed group had poorer receptive and expressive language performance on the Reynell language test (Fig. 6–1), higher activity levels, less persistence and increased distractibility on temperament tests.[14–16]

Adopted 5- to 6-year-old Israeli children exposed prenatally to heroin performed as well developmentally as non-adopted, non-exposed controls, and outscored heroin-exposed children who remained with their birth mothers.[34] However, other studies have failed to show improvement after removal from the birth family.

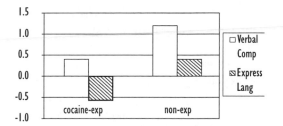

Figure 6–1 *Children exposed prenatally to cocaine had lower scores for verbal comprehension (open bars, p = .003) and expressive language (hatched bars, p = .001) compared to age-matched control children not exposed to cocaine. Adoptive families and control families were matched for maternal IQ and socioeconomic status. In this test, ʒero is the average score for age. For example, –0.4 is 4 months below the average score for age, and 0.6 is 6 months above the average age-appropriate score. (Data from Nulman I, Rovet J, Greenbaum R, et al. Neurodevelopment of adopted children exposed in utero to cocaine: the Toronto Adoption Study. Clin Invest Med 2001; 24:129–37.)*

One-year-olds living in adoptive or foster homes after prenatal exposure to cocaine[35] or opiates[17] scored similarly to exposed children living with their birth parents. Thus, research in this area is inconclusive, but adoption likely provides some benefits to drug-exposed children.

Prenatal Drug Exposure and Later Addiction

Adoptive parents may wonder if prenatally drug-exposed children are at increased risk of themselves becoming addicts as adolescents or adults. Few studies address this directly; much more is known about susceptibility to alcohol abuse among children of alcoholics. Predisposition to alcoholism is specific and separate from tendency toward other types of drug abuse[36] (see Chapter 5). However, biologic, psychologic, and environmental factors may predispose the child of a drug-abusing parent to become involved with drugs. Some evidence of a genetic predisposition to cocaine dependency has been suggested: specific alleles of the D2

dopamine receptor gene occur with higher prevalence among cocaine-abusing males.[37]

Adoption removes the child from the drug-abusing environment. Researchers in Iowa examined drug abuse among adults adopted at birth and characteristics of their birth parents.[38–41] Complex statistical analysis was used to isolate many factors, including variables within the adoptive family. Among 443 young adult adoptees, 15% of the men and 7% of the women were drug abusers. Drug abuse was highly correlated with an antisocial personality, which was predicted by an antisocial birth parent (information retrieved from adoption agency records).[38] Drug-abusing adoptees without antisocial personalities were likely to have had alcoholic birth parents. It is important to note that environmental factors in the adoptive family (divorce, psychiatric disturbances) were strongly associated with increased drug abuse among the adoptees (Table 6–6). It was

Table 6–6 Factors in adoptive family affecting drug use by adoptees (*n* = 443)

Factor	All Young Adult Adoptees (%)	Drug-Abusing Young Adult Adoptees (%)
Alcohol problem	19	20
Antisocial problem	9	12
Other psychiatric problem	22	27
Alcohol, antisocial, or psychiatric problem in adoptive parents or siblings	39	47
Physical problem in parent	39	40
Parent divorce or separation	5	18
Parent death (adoptee <19 years)	6	0
Home broken by parent death, divorce, or separation	11	17
Disturbed parent	20	40
Adoptee >5 months at placement	29	40

Source: Adapted from Cadoret et al.[38]

not determined if some of the problems in the adoptive families occurred as a result or cause of the drug-abusing child's behavior.

The same research group reported similar results in adult adoptees whose birth parents were alcoholics and/or had antisocial personalities (as determined from hospital and prison records).[39,41] The role of genetic factors or prenatal exposures shared by both birth parents and their relinquished children remains unknown.

Missing from these and other studies are any assessment of the effect of the peer group and social milieu. Undoubtably, these factors—and availability of drugs—greatly influence the susceptibility of adolescents and young adults to abuse drugs. These little-studied aspects of drug addiction may overshadow any putative genetic or "inborn" susceptibility. Overall, children prenatally exposed to drugs may have increased likelihood of behavioral, cognitive, and emotional disturbances that could contribute to an increased risk of drug dependency. However, it is also clear that many children from this background do well, and are indistinguishable from adopted children of non-drug-abusing birth parents.

Monitoring the Drug-Exposed Child After Adoption

The child with a definite or probable history of prenatal drug exposure should be monitored carefully after adoption. Like all children, growth and developmental milestones at entry to the United States should be documented. Hepatitis B, hepatitis C, and HIV serology should be obtained at entry and again 6 months later; viral PCR assays should be obtained in children <6 months of age, or those in whom initial screening tests indicate likely exposure. Language skills (including articulation), behavior, and attention span should be monitored at regular visits, and neurologic examination should be performed, including assessment of "soft signs" (finger-to-nose, rapid pronation-supination, heel-to-toe walking, balance on one foot, hop).[24] The pediatrician should assess the child's arousal, attention, recognition memory, and impulse control,[42] with the goal of providing supportive services if needed. Although prenatal drug exposure will usually not be known with certainty, anticipatory guidance will benefit many children.

Key Points for Internationally Adopted Children

• Prenatal drug exposures are usually not known prior to adoption.
• Behavioral, cognitive, and social development may be adversely affected by prenatal drug exposures.
• Adoption likely improves the outcome of prenatally drug-exposed children.

References

1. Freundlich M. The impact of prenatal substance exposure: research findings and their implications for adoption. In: Barth RP, Freundlich M, Brodzinsky D, eds. Adoption and Prenatal Alcohol and Drug Exposure. Washington, DC: Child Welfare League of America, 2000: 1–22.

2. Jenista JA. Medical issues in adoption. In: Marshner C, Pierce WL, eds. Adoption Factbook III. Waite Park, MN: National Council for Adoption, 1999:417–22.

3. Barth RP, Brooks D. Outcomes for drug-exposed children eight years post-adoption. In: Barth RP, Freundlich M, Brodzinsky D, eds. Adoption and Prenatal Alcohol and Drug Exposure. Washington, DC: Child Welfare League of America, 2000: 23–58.

4. United Nations Office on Drugs and Crime. http://www.undcp.org/unodc/en/global_illicit_drug_trends.html.

5. Central Intelligence Agency. The World Factbook. Ukraine. Available at: http://www.cia.gov/cia/publications/factbook/ geos/up.html.

6. Poshyachinda V. Drug injecting and HIV infection among the population of drug abusers in Asia. Bull Narc 1993; 45:77–90.

7. The Asian Harm Reduction Network. Country Assessment: Korea. Available at: http://www.ahrn.net/regional/skorea.html.

8. United Nations Office on Drugs and Crime. Guatemala country profile. Available at: http://www.odccp.org:80/mexico/country_profile_guatemala.html.

9. World Health Organization. Highlights on Health in Ukraine. Available at: http://www.who.dk/document/e72372.pdf.

10. Nair P, Rothblum S, Hebel R. Neonatal outcome in infants with evidence of fetal exposure to opiates, cocaine, and cannabinoids. Clin Pediatr (Phila) 1994; 33:280–5.

11. Chiriboga CA, Brust JC, Bateman D, Hauser WA. Dose–response effect of fetal cocaine exposure on newborn neurologic function. Pediatrics 1999; 103:79–85.

12. Eriksson M, Zetterstrom R. Amphetamine addiction during pregnancy: 10-year follow-up. Acta Paediatr Suppl 1994; 404:27–31.

13. van Baar AL, Soepatmi S, Gunning WB, Akkerhuis GW. Development after prenatal exposure to cocaine, heroin and methadone. Acta Paediatr Suppl 1994; 404:40–6.

14. Koren G, Nulman I, Rovet J, Greenbaum R, Loebstein M, Einarson T. Long-term neurodevelopmental risks in children exposed in utero to cocaine. The Toronto Adoption Study. Ann N Y Acad Sci 1998; 846:306–13.

15. Nulman I, Rovet J, Altmann D, Bradley C, Einarson T, Koren G. Neurodevelopment of adopted children exposed in utero to cocaine. CMAJ 1994; 151:1591–7.

16. Nulman I, Rovet J, Greenbaum R, et al. Neurodevelopment of adopted children exposed in utero to cocaine: the Toronto Adoption Study. Clin Invest Med 2001; 24:129–37.

17. Bunikowski R, Grimmer I, Heiser A, Metze B, Schafer A, Obladen M. Neurodevelopmental outcome after prenatal exposure to opiates. Eur J Pediatr 1998; 157:724–30.

18. Soepatmi S. Developmental outcomes of children of mothers dependent on heroin or heroin/methadone during pregnancy. Acta Paediatr Suppl 1994; 404:36–9.

19. Eyler FD, Behnke M, Conlon M, Woods NS, Wobie K. Birth outcome from a prospective, matched study of prenatal crack/cocaine use: I. Interactive and dose effects on health and growth. Pediatrics 1998; 101:229–37.

20. Frank DA, McCarten KM, Robson CD, et al. Level of in utero cocaine exposure and neonatal ultrasound findings. Pediatrics 1999; 104:1101–5.

21. Scafidi FA, Field TM, Wheeden A, et al. Cocaine-exposed preterm neonates show behavioral and hormonal differences. Pediatrics 1996; 97:851–55.

22. Delaney-Black V, Covington C, Ostrea E, et al. Prenatal cocaine and neonatal outcome: evaluation of dose–response relationship. Pediatrics 1996; 98:735–40.

23. Hurt H, Malmud E, Betancourt LM, Brodsky NL, Giannetta JM. A prospective comparison of developmental outcome of children with in utero cocaine exposure and controls using the Battelle Developmental Inventory. J Dev Behav Pediatr 2001; 22:27–34.

24. Hurt H, Giannetta J, Brodsky NL, Malmud E, Pelham T. Are there neurologic correlates of in utero cocaine exposure at age 6 years? J Pediatr 2001; 138:911–3.

25. Frank DA, Augustyn M, Knight WG, Pell T, Zuckerman B. Growth, development, and behavior in early childhood following prenatal cocaine exposure: a systematic review. JAMA 2001; 285:1613–25.

26. Lester BM, LaGasse LL, Seifer R. Cocaine exposure and children: the meaning of subtle effects. Science 1998; 282:633–4.

27. Delaney-Black V, Covington C, Templin T, et al. Expressive language development of children exposed to cocaine prenatally: literature review and report of a prospective cohort study. J Commun Disord 2000; 33:463–80.

28. Chasnoff IJ, Anson A, Hatcher R, Stenson H, Iaukea K, Randolph LA. Prenatal exposure to cocaine and other drugs. Outcome at four to six years. Ann N Y Acad Sci 1998; 846:314–28.

29. Delaney-Black V, Covington C, Templin T, et al. Teacher-assessed behavior of children prenatally exposed to cocaine. Pediatrics 2000; 106:782–91.

30. Singer LT, Arendt R, Minnes S, Salvator A, Siegel AC, Lewis BA. Developing language skills of cocaine-exposed infants. Pediatrics 2001; 107:1057–64.

31. Singer LT, Arendt RE. Prenatal cocaine exposure as a risk factor for later developmental outcomes. JAMA 2001; 286:45–6; discussion 46–7.

32. Dozier M, Albus KE. Attachment issues for adopted infants. In: Barth RP, Freundlich M, Brodzinsky D, eds. Adoption and Prenatal Alcohol and Drug Exposure. Washington, DC: Child Welfare League of America, 2000:171–198.

33. Lester BM, LaGasse LL, Seifer R, et al. The maternal lifestyle study (MLS): effects of prenatal cocaine and/or opiate exposure on auditory brain response at one month. J Pediatr 2003; 142:279–85.

34. Ornoy A, Michailevskaya V, Lukashov I, Bar-Hamburger R, Harel S. The developmental outcome of children born to heroin-dependent mothers, raised at home or adopted. Child Abuse Negl 1996; 20:385–96.

35. Thyssen Van Beveren T, Little BB, Spence MJ. Effects of prenatal cocaine exposure and postnatal environment on child development. Am J Hum Biol 2000; 12:417–428.

36. Johnson JL, Leff M. Children of substance abusers: overview of research findings. Pediatrics 1999; 103:1085–99.

37. Noble EP, Blum K, Khalsa E, et al. Allelic association of the D2 dopamine receptor gene with cocaine dependence. Drug Alcohol Depend 1993; 33:271–85.

38. Cadoret RJ, Troughton E, O'Gorman TW, Heywood E. An adoption study of genetic and environmental factors in drug abuse. Arch Gen Psychiatry 1986; 43: 1131–6.

39. Cadoret RJ, Yates WR, Troughton E, Woodworth G, Stewart MA. Adoption study demonstrating two genetic pathways to drug abuse. Arch Gen Psychiatry 1995; 52:42–52.

40. Cadoret RJ, Yates WR, Troughton E, Woodworth G, Stewart MA. Genetic–environmental interaction in the genesis of aggressivity and conduct disorders. Arch Gen Psychiatry 1995; 52:916–24.

41. Cadoret RJ, Yates WR, Troughton E, Woodworth G, Stewart MA. An adoption study of drug abuse/dependency in females. Compr Psychiatry 1996; 37:88–94.

42. Mayes LC. Developing brain and in utero cocaine exposure: effects on neural ontogeny. Dev Psychopathol 1999; 11:685–714.

7

PRENATAL EXPOSURE TO
MATERNAL SMOKING

Accurate information about birth mothers' tobacco use during pregnancy is rarely available for international adoptees. Like prenatal exposure to illicit drugs or alcohol, maternal smoking during pregnancy is linked to many problems in the fetus, infant, and child. Maternal smoking during pregnancy has long-term effects on the child's attention, behavior, and cognition in infancy, childhood, and adolescence. Some effects may persist to adulthood. Such problems are common among international adoptees, although the causes are multifactorial. This section surveys the epidemiology of smoking among women in sending countries. The long-term neurobehavioral effects on offspring after maternal smoking during pregnancy are reviewed. The effects of environmental tobacco smoke on other organ systems have been reviewed.[1]

Epidemiology of Tobacco Use

Tobacco use among women of child-bearing age varies considerably throughout the world (Table 7–1). Cultural, social, and economic factors determine the frequency of smoking among relinquishing birth mothers. In some countries, birth mothers are usually impoverished and unable to afford costly cigarettes. In other countries, cigarettes are relatively inexpensive and smoking is socially acceptable among women. Accurate statistics are difficult to obtain; few countries collect data about smoking among pregnant women. However, many nations report rapid increases in smoking among teenage girls. Worldwide there is very little awareness about the potential ill effects of maternal smoking on the developing fetus. Tobacco use sometimes occurs with other forms of substance abuse, such as illicit drugs and alcohol[1] (see Chapters 5 and 6).

Table 7–1 Smoking statistics for females in frequent sending countries

Country	Women Smokers (%)	Female Youth Smokers (%)[a]	Comments
Asia			
Cambodia	Rural women 10 Urban women 2–3	Rural children 20–30	
China	Most regions: 3–7	5	Some areas women smokers as high as 45% (Tibet, Tianjin)
India	7	1	About 33% of women smoke occasionally
Korea (S.)	8	16	
Nepal	15	7	Some areas women smokers as high as 72%
Philippines	18	19—age 10–14 years 38—age 15–19 years	
Thailand	2–6	0	Rate is higher in north
Vietnam	4		
Europe			
Belarus	5	4	
Kazakhstan	40[b]		
Lithuania	9	2	17% of women age 25–29 years smoke; 41% of 15-year-old girls have tried smoking
Moldova	3	<1	
Russia	14	6	In some regions about 25%–30% of women and 25%–40% of adolescent girls smoke
Romania	15	8	70% of women factory workers and 25% of women ages 25–44 years smoke
Ukraine	21	2	10% of 12–13 year olds, 40% of 16–17 year olds, 75% of students at technical college, and 61% of 20–29 year olds (M/F not differentiated)
Americas			
Bolivia	18–33	9[b]	
Brazil	29–42	2	
Colombia	19–21	<1	
Ecuador	17–28	4–15	
Guatemala	6–26	3	
Paraguay	6	N/A	
Peru	13–42	14[b]	
United States	10–28	6	

N/A, not available; M/F, male-to-female ratio

[a]Note: "Youth" defined differently in each study—could include any cluster from age 9 to 16 years

[b]Males and females combined

Source: Data from Centers for Disease Control and Prevention and World Health Organization.[2,3]

Long-term Neurobehavioral Effects of Prenatal Exposure to Maternal Smoking

Investigations of the long-term effects of prenatal exposure to maternal smoking have inherent difficulties. Animal studies demonstrate conclusively that prenatal smoke exposure alters brain chemistry. Neuronal cell proliferation and differentiation, nicotine receptor gene expression, and cholinergic, catecholaminergic, and peripheral autonomic pathways exhibit permanent changes after prenatal smoke exposure.[1,4–6] In human subjects, isolation of variables is problematic. As for studies of fetal alcohol or drug exposure, accurate ascertainment of dose, duration, and timing of maternal smoking exposure is difficult. Depending on the formulation of the cigarette, various compounds in addition to nicotine cross the placenta to enter the circulation of the fetus. Co-incident exposures, especially if covert, confound interpretation of outcomes. Unlike drugs or alcohol, postnatal exposures can continue via secondhand smoke. Potential confounding variables include socioeconomic disadvantage,[7,8] impaired child-rearing behaviors,[9] and emotional disturbances. In adults and adolescents, smoking is strongly associated with anxiety, depression, ADHD, and other psychiatric disorders.[1,4,10] It is not known if individuals with these problems are more likely to smoke, or if smoking contributes to these difficulties. These conditions are in part genetically mediated. Prenatal exposure to anxiety and depression may have long-lasting effects as well (see Chapter 8). Thus, smoking may indicate a cluster of risk factors for the infant. Some investigators have speculated that smoking during pregnancy is symptomatic of other maternal behaviors such as certain lifestyle and norm-breaking behavior, but does not directly contribute to adverse fetal outcomes.[11] Regardless, maternal smoking is a proxy for a disturbed prenatal milieu.

Attempts to isolate the effects of prenatal exposure to maternal smoking rely on special study designs and statistical methods. Because prenatal tobacco exposure often results in low birth weight and head circumference, some observed effects may be secondary to these growth disturbances[12–14] (see Chapters 10, 12). Maternal smoking may also induce fetal hypoxia, increase the likelihood of maternal complications, alter placental function, or act as a direct neuroteratogen. Few studies are able to differentiate prenatal from postnatal exposure to maternal smoking. Many adverse effects relate to the home environment of the child.[7,8,15]

Table 7–2 Long-term neurobehavioral effects of prenatal exposure to maternal smoking

Behavioral Problems

Attention deficit disorder, hyperactivity[1,17]

Externalizing (aggressive) behaviors[6,18] (almost double that of children of nonsmokers)

Various problem behaviors[16,19]

Criminal behavior (violent and nonviolent crimes)[20]

Conduct disorder[9,15,21,22,23]

Depression[21]

Substance abuse (drugs/alcohol)[12,21,22,24]

Impulsive behavior[24]

Cognitive and Learning Problems

Auditory processing deficits[17,25]

Reduced IQ[26,27] (although most investigators disagree with this[7,8,14,28])

Impaired cognitive function[24,29–32]

Language disabilities[30,31,33,34]

Decreased visuoperceptual function[35]

Impaired executive function[32]

Reading disabilities[34]

Disturbed memory function[24]

Hypertonicity, increased CNS excitation at 1 month of age[36]

Mental retardation[10]

Regardless of these study complications, numerous neurobehavioral problems are reported with increased frequency among children born after prenatal exposure to smoking (Table 7–2). Attentional problems, mild cognitive difficulties, and conduct disturbances occur more frequently in children born after exposure to maternal smoking. Children exposed to heavy smoking early in gestation fare worst.[16]

Key Points for Internationally Adopted Children

- Information about possible maternal smoking during pregnancy is rarely available
- Maternal smoking during pregnancy may adversely effect neurobehavioral outcome

- Problems with attentional regulation, behavior, mental function, and learning may occur in children exposed to maternal smoking during pregnancy

FAQs

Q. I was just asked to review two referrals for prospective adoptive parents; they want me to help them select the "lower-risk" child. Daria's medical history states that her birth mother smoked throughout the pregnancy—no amount is given. Anastasia's birth mother "drank a few times" during the pregnancy. Which is the lower risk situation?

A. Without knowing details of the amount, timing, and duration of exposure, it is hard to be precise. A volunteered smoking history is more likely to be accurate than a drinking history, the extent of which many women do not completely reveal. A careful look at other variables in the medical history (gestational age, birth measurements, subsequent growth, additional medical history, and assessment for risks in both girls of fetal alcohol syndrome) may help. Meanwhile, it is important to review potential concerns for both exposures to the prospective parents, and remember that either or both medical histories could be incomplete: perhaps both mothers drank and smoked!

References

1. American Academy of Pediatrics, Committee on Substance Abuse. American Academy of Pediatrics: Tobacco's toll: implications for the pediatrician. Pediatrics 2001; 107:794–8.

2. Centers for Disease Control and Prevention. National Tobacco Information Online System (NATIONS). Available at: http://apps.nccd.cdc.gov/nations.

3. World Health Organization Tobacco or Health Programme. Available at: http://www.cdc.gov/tobacco/who/.

4. Slotkin TA. Fetal nicotine or cocaine exposure: which one is worse? J Pharmacol Exp Ther 1998; 285:931–45.

5. Raine A. Annotation: the role of prefrontal deficits, low autonomic arousal, and early health factors in the de-velopment of antisocial and aggressive behavior in children. J Child Psychol Psychiatry 2002; 43:417–34.

6. Williams GM, O'Callaghan M, Najman JM, et al. Maternal cigarette smoking and child psychiatric morbidity: a longitudinal study. Pediatrics 1998; 102:e11.

7. Fergusson DM, Lloyd M. Smoking during pregnancy and its effects on child cognitive ability from the ages of 8 to 12 years. Paediatr Perinat Epidemiol 1991; 5: 189–200.

8. Baghurst PA, Tong SL, Woodward A, McMichael AJ. Effects of maternal smoking upon neuropsychological development in early childhood: importance of taking account of social and environmental factors. Paediatr Perinat Epidemiol 1992; 6:403–15.

9. Wakschlag LS, Lahey BB, Loeber R, Green SM, Gordon RA, Leventhal BL. Maternal smoking during pregnancy and the risk of conduct disorder in boys. Arch Gen Psychiatry 1997; 54:670–6.

10. Drews CD, Murphy CC, Yeargin-Allsopp M, Decoufle P. The relationship between idiopathic mental retardation and maternal smoking during pregnancy. Pediatrics 1996; 97:547–53.

11. Rantakallio P, Laara E, Isohanni M, Moilanen I. Maternal smoking during pregnancy and delinquency of the offspring: an association without causation? Int J Epidemiol 1992; 21:1106–13.

12. Ernst M, Moolchan ET, Robinson ML. Behavioral and neural consequences of prenatal exposure to nicotine. J Am Acad Child Adolesc Psychiatry 2001; 40:630–41.

13. Day N, Cornelius M, Goldschmidt L, Richardson G, Robles N, Taylor P. The effects of prenatal tobacco and marijuana use on offspring growth from birth through 3 years of age. Neurotoxicol Teratol 1992; 14:407–14.

14. Naeye RL, Peters EC. Mental development of children whose mothers smoked during pregnancy. Obstet Gynecol 1984; 64:601–7.

15. Wakschlag LS, Pickett KE, Cook E Jr, Benowitz NL, Leventhal BL. Maternal smoking during pregnancy and severe antisocial behavior in offspring: a review. Am J Public Health 2002; 92:966–74.

16. Fergusson DM, Horwood LJ, Lynskey MT. Maternal smoking before and after pregnancy: effects on behavioral outcomes in middle childhood. Pediatrics 1993; 92:815–22.

17. Kristjansson EA, Fried PA, Watkinson B. Maternal smoking during pregnancy affects children's vigilance performance. Drug Alcohol Depend 1989; 24:11–9.

18. Orlebeke JF, Knol DL, Verhulst FC. Child behavior problems increased by maternal smoking during pregnancy. Arch Environ Health 1999; 54:15–9.

19. Wasserman GA, Liu X, Pine DS, Graziano JH. Contribution of maternal smoking during pregnancy and lead exposure to early child behavior problems. Neurotoxicol Teratol 2001; 23:13–21.

20. Brennan PA, Grekin ER, Mednick SA. Maternal smoking during pregnancy and adult male criminal outcomes. Arch Gen Psychiatry 1999; 56:215–9.

21. Fergusson DM, Woodward LJ, Horwood LJ. Maternal smoking during pregnancy and psychiatric adjustment in late adolescence. Arch Gen Psychiatry 1998; 55: 721–7.

22. Weissman MM, Warner V, Wickramaratne PJ, Kandel DB. Maternal smoking during pregnancy and psychopathology in offspring followed to adulthood. J Am Acad Child Adolesc Psychiatry 1999; 38:892–9.

23. Maughan B, Taylor C, Taylor A, Butler N, Bynner J. Pregnancy smoking and childhood conduct problems: a causal association? J Child Psychol Psychiatry 2001; 42: 1021–8.

24. Fried PA, Watkinson B, Gray R. A follow-up study of attentional behavior in 6-year-old children exposed prenatally to marihuana, cigarettes, and alcohol. Neurotoxicol Teratol 1992; 14:299–311.

25. Fried PA, Watkinson B. 12- and 24-month neurobehavioural follow-up of children prenatally exposed to marihuana, cigarettes and alcohol. Neurotoxicol Teratol 1988; 10:305–13.

26. Milberger S, Biederman J, Faraone SV, Jones J. Further evidence of an association between maternal smoking during pregnancy and attention deficit hyperactivity disorder: findings from a high-risk sample of siblings. J Clin Child Psychol 1998; 27:352–8.

27. Weitzman M, Gortmaker S, Sobol A. Maternal smoking and behavior problems of children. Pediatrics 1992; 90:342–9.

28. Olds DL, Henderson CR Jr, Tatelbaum R. Intellectual impairment in children of women who smoke cigarettes during pregnancy. Pediatrics 1994; 93:221–7.

29. Richardson GA, Day NL, Goldschmidt L. Prenatal alcohol, marijuana, and tobacco use: infant mental and motor development. Neurotoxicol Teratol 1995; 17:479–87.

30. Fried PA, Watkinson B. 36- and 48-month neurobehavioral follow-up of children prenatally exposed to marijuana, cigarettes, and alcohol. J Dev Behav Pediatr 1990; 11:49–58.

31. Fried PA, O'Connell CM, Watkinson B. 60- and 72-month follow-up of children prenatally exposed to marijuana, cigarettes, and alcohol: cognitive and language assessment. J Dev Behav Pediatr 1992; 13:383–91.

32. Fried PA, Watkinson B, Gray R. Differential effects on cognitive functioning in 9- to 12-year olds prenatally exposed to cigarettes and marihuana. Neurotoxicol Teratol 1998; 20:293–306.

33. Tomblin JB, Smith E, Zhang X. Epidemiology of specific language impairment: prenatal and perinatal risk factors. J Commun Disord 1997; 30:325–43; quiz 343–4.

34. Fried PA, Watkinson B, Siegel LS. Reading and language in 9- to 12-year olds prenatally exposed to cigarettes and marijuana. Neurotoxicol Teratol 1997; 19:171–83.

35. Fried PA, Watkinson B. Visuoperceptual functioning differs in 9- to 12-year olds prenatally exposed to cigarettes and marihuana. Neurotoxicol Teratol 2000; 22:11–20.

36. Fried PA. Cigarettes and marijuana: are there measurable long-term neurobehavioral teratogenic effects? Neurotoxicology 1989; 10:577–83.

8

EFFECTS OF STRESS
IN EARLY LIFE

International adoptees encounter stress both prenatally and postnatally (Table 8–1). Most are products of unwanted pregnancies. After birth, many suffer from abandonment, institutionalization, malnutrition, recurrent illnesses, environmental deprivation, and/or emotional neglect. Some are physically or sexually abused, or witness distressing events. These stressful experiences in early life may permanently alter brain physiology and lead to long-lasting physiological, psychological, and behavioral changes.[1] Early stress may have life-long adverse effects on growth, development, health, behavior, learning, and memory. This section discusses how stress influences these areas, clinically and neurobiologically.

The Neurobiology of Stress

Stress is mediated via the hypothalamic–pituitary–adrenal axis. Stress induces excess or inappropriate production of corticotropin-releasing factor (CRF) or corticotropin (ACTH),

resulting in overproduction of cortisol. Stress also alters the regulation of glucocorticoid receptors in the brain, resulting in excessive binding of cortisol. Prolonged elevation of glucocorticoid levels adversely affects the brain (reviewed in Gunnar[2]). The hippocampus, involved in learning and memory, is especially vulnerable. Glucocorticoids inhibit glucose utilization in hippocampal neurons,[3] alter calcium metabolism, and stimulate glutamate release.[2] Glutamate inhibits proliferation of granule cell

Table 8–1 Sources of stress for institutionalized children

Prenatal exposure to maternal depression
Abandonment
Environmental deprivation
Malnutrition
Recurrent illnesses
Removal from familiar peer groups and caregivers
Physical neglect
Emotional neglect
Physical abuse
Sexual abuse

precursors in the hippocampal dentate gyrus;[4] these cells proliferate throughout life and thus are sensitive to environmental exposures and experience.[4] Elevated cortisol reduces the ability of hippocampal neurons to withstand insults such as seizures, ischemia, hypoglycemia, toxicity, and trauma.[3] Prolonged glucocorticoid exposure occurring with chronic stress is associated with structural changes in the hippocampus—and memory loss—in rats, primates, and humans.[5,6] Young rats given CRF have progressive loss of hippocampal CA3 neurons and reduced memory throughout life.[6] Centrally administered CRF induces many behavioral changes indicative of anxiety, such as lack of exploratory behavior and potentiation of acoustic startle response.[7]

The cingulate gyrus, amygdala (both parts of the limbic system), and frontal lobes are also involved in stress responses. These areas are rich in glucocorticoid receptors. The cingulate gyrus regulates effortful attention and self-control, the amygdala processes emotions, and cortical regions mediate behavioral response and cognitive appraisal of stressful situations.[7] The autonomic nervous system (via catecholamines), opioids, and serotonin also mediate response to stress.[8] However, less is known about these pathways.

Prenatal and Early Postnatal Stress

Even prenatal stress affects behavior and development of the offspring. Monkeys born to mothers stressed during pregnancy (e.g., exposed to unpredictable noises in a dark room) show decreased motor and exploratory behaviors, reduced cognitive ability, and delayed mastery of object permanence.[9] Similarly, children whose mothers were stressed during pregnancy have less optimal outcomes, including problems with emotional regulation, motor delays,[9] and intrauterine growth retardation.[10] Prenatal exposure to excess glucocorticoids may harm the developing brain.[9] Offspring of prenatally stressed rat or monkey mothers have increased basal levels

> Joshua, age 6 at adoption, arrived with his 3-year-old brother Jerald from Russia. Both had lived with their birth parents until 1 year before the adoption. Jerald was a happy-go-lucky little boy who adjusted well to his adoptive home, while Joshua seemed withdrawn, depressed, and usually near tears. He refused to sleep upstairs in his bedroom, but insisted on sleeping on the living room couch, and every night tried to prevent his brother from going upstairs to his bedroom. As his English skills developed, he was able to tell his adoptive parents that his birth father had thrown Jerald out of their fourth-floor apartment window one night when the baby wouldn't stop crying. Miraculously, Jerald survived with only a broken leg, which had long since healed prior to the adoption. Joshua was unable to forget his fright at witnessing this horrible event.

of plasma ACTH, increased ACTH in response to stressful situations, and decreased ability to adapt to ongoing stress. Human infants born to mothers with prenatal depression tend to be less active, less socially responsive, and fussier than unexposed peers, possibly via the same pathway. The possibility of "multigenerational effects" of stress has been suggested by animal studies. Infants prenatally exposed to stress have small heads; infants with small heads have abnormal stress responses.[9] Nonoptimal birth condition (microcephaly ± low Apgar scores) is associated with abnormal stress responses for at least the first 6 months of life.[11]

Maternal behaviors after birth also contribute to stress. Young animals and human infants have increased plasma cortisol levels and altered CRF levels and receptor number after maternal separation; these biochemical changes may persist until adulthood. Interestingly, the presence of a familiar social group and stable environment (as may occur in institutional care) reduces the endocrine effects of maternal separation.[9] The presence of younger animals ("peer therapists") also helped monkeys maintain normal psychosocial behaviors after maternal loss. The animals exhibit signs of despair, however, if removed from their peer group.

The infant experiences maternal depression as separation. Accordingly, infants of depressed mothers tend to be withdrawn, less active, and show altered sleep patterns, difficulty sustaining attention, poor mastery motivation, and limited responsivity to facial expressions. In addition, these infants have elevated norepinephrine and cortisol levels, EEG changes compatible with depression, and reduced vagal tone. Cognitive and language delays at 1, 4, and 12 years of age are more common in children born to depressed mothers than control children.[9,12] These children have more emotional or behavioral disorders, including problems in self-regulation, affect, peer relationships, sleep regulation, behavior, and academic achievement. Massage therapy improves weight gain, emotionality, sociability, soothability, and mental and motor scores and decreases stress hormones in infants of depressed mothers.[12]

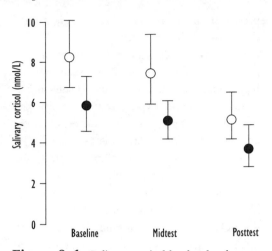

Figure 8–1 *Salivary cortisol levels related to nutritional status of children undergoing psychological tests (mental arithmetic, pegboard test, frustrating tasks, etc.). Results are shown at baseline, midtest, and posttest for stunted (open circles, n = 28) and nonstunted (closed circles, n = 23) children. (Reproduced with permission by the* American Journal of Clinical Nutrition. © *Am J Clin Nutr. American Society for Clinical Nutrition.)*

Growth and Stress

Growth and stress are interrelated. Poor nutrition is itself stressful. Children with acute marasmus or kwashiorkor have elevated free cortisol levels.[5] Stunted children have higher cortisol levels, higher heart rates, fewer vocalizations, more inhibitions, and less attentive behavior than their well-grown peers in response to physical and psychological stressors.[5] Their cortisol levels correlate with nutritional status (Fig. 8–1). Thus, prolonged cortisol exposure may mediate the heightened physiologic activation and poor cognitive performance common among poorly nourished children.[5]

Independent of malnutrition, stress itself directly affects growth. Prolonged exposure to stress inhibits secretion of growth hormone and other growth factors[5]; children with anxiety disorders tend to be shorter adults because of reduced growth hormone secretion.[13] The poor growth exhibited by many institutionalized children (see Chapter 10) likely reflects both

inadequate nutrition and other stressful environmental factors.

Stress and the Immune System

Stress also alters immune function. Stressed individuals tend to have leukocytosis (mostly neutrophils), reduced circulating T cells, altered immunoglobulin levels, and diminished mitogen proliferative responses and natural killer cell activity.[5,14–17] Chronic stress may also reduce antibody responses after immunization[18,19] (see Chapter 21) and have other long-term effects on health.

Stress and Attachment

Tactile contact is the strongest determinant of attachment among primates[3] (see Chapter 29); young individuals deprived of tactile contact may develop autistic-like behaviors. Early tactile deprivation reduces glucocorticoid binding sites in the hippocampus and frontal cortex. Thus, hypothalamic–pituitary–adrenal (HPA)-axis hormones mediate responses to tactile contact and subsequent attachment.[3] Newborn rats are hyporesponsive to HPA activation.[2] If removed from its mother, however, the young rat's HPA-axis becomes very reactive and may remain so throughout life. This hyperreactivity is tempered if some elements of maternal interaction are maintained (stroking, licking, feeding). Thus, maternal behaviors buffer HPA-axis reactivity.

In human children, diurnal patterns of cortisol production are established around 12 weeks of age. The ability to modulate stress reactivity emerges between 4 and 6 months of age.[3] Institutionalized children living in difficult circumstances in Romania lack diurnal variation in cortisol production (Fig. 8–2). Cortisol levels in institutionalized children in some settings correlate inversely to performance on the mental and motor scales of the Bayley test[3] and directly with length of institutionalization.[2] Among institutionalized children in France and Hungary, cortisol levels correlated with group size and ratio of children to caregivers.[2] Studies in noninstitutionalized children also support the notion that caregivers influence cortisol levels in young children. For example, stressful situations (such as immunization) induce higher levels of cortisol if the child is with an unfamiliar caregiver or is poorly attached[2] (Fig. 8–3). Similarly, cortisol levels in 9-month-olds left with an unfamiliar babysitter relate to the demeanor of the babysitter—children left with friendly, engaging sitters have lower levels than those left with withdrawn, unfriendly sitters.[2] Other studies suggest that attachment security and "fearfulness" relate to cortisol reactivity. For example, insecurely attached children have higher heart rates and cortisol concentrations, hyperactive HPA-axis and autonomic function, and increased limbic–hypothalamic arousal.[5] Somewhat counterintuitively, children placed in unfamiliar situations who become quiet, stop playing, do not

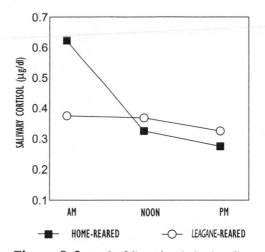

Figure 8–2 *Lack of diurnal variation in salivary cortisol levels in children reared in Romanian leagane (orphanages) compared with home-reared children. (From Carlson M, Earls F. Psychological and neuroendocrinological sequelae of early social deprivation in institutionalized children in Romania. Ann N Y Acad Sci 1997; 807:423, with permission.)*

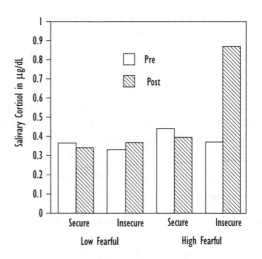

Figure 8–3 *Salivary cortisol levels in 18-month-old toddlers before and after novelty testing (approached by a clown who asked them to play). Low and high fear was based on a median split of approach–withdrawal to the novel stimuli.* Secure *and* Insecure *refer to parent–infant attachment quality as assessed using the Strange Situation. (Reprinted from Gunnar MR. Quality of early care and buffering of neuroendocrine stress reactions: potential effects on the developing human brain. Prev Med 1998; 27:210, with permission from Elsevier.)*

Jenny arrived at age 7 from Bulgaria. She adjusted well to her new mom and sisters but was cold and withdrawn to her new dad and brothers. She screamed and cried when her dad tried to cuddle or tickle her, and often refused to stay in a room alone with him. With the help of a bilingual therapist, the family learned of nearly nightly sexual abuse of Jenny (and many of the other girls in the orphanage) by the night watchman.

cry, and appear to sleep have the highest elevations of cortisol, while those who demand attention (climb into lap, bring toys, cry, fret, or tantrum) have lower levels. Sensitive, responsive, and secure caretaking thus buffers cortisol elevations in infants and young children. In contrast, depressed or withdrawn caregivers augment stress responses in young children, possibly increasing the later risk of emotional or behavioral disorders.

Stress and Mental Illness: Post-Traumatic Stress Disorder and Depression

Early childhood trauma, such as parental loss, physical or sexual abuse, or neglect, increases the risk of later mental disorders, including post-traumatic stress disorder (PTSD) and depression (Table 8–2). Post-traumatic stress disorder is mediated

Jessica's adoptive mother, Mrs. Q., was shocked when she arrived at her daughter's orphanage. The children spent most of the day confined to their cribs in darkened rooms. When picked up by their caregivers, the children would cry hysterically. After visiting for a few days, Mrs. Q. realized that the only times the children were physically touched was when they were bathed—rather roughly, and in ice-cold water. Jessica was apathetic, withdrawn, and "barely had any will to live," said Mrs. Q. "I'm sure she would have died from the next case of pneumonia or gastroenteritis that she had."

Table 8–2 Endocrine alterations in major depressive disorder and post-traumatic stress disorder

	MDD	*PTSD*
Cortisol	Increased	Decreased
Glucocorticoid receptor responsiveness	Decreased	Increased
Sensitivity of HPA-axis to negative feedback	Decreased	Increased
HPA-axis	Progressive desensitization	Progressive sensitization
Hippocampal volume	Decreased	Decreased

HPA, hypothalamic–pituitary–adrenal; MDD, major depressive disorder; PTSD, post-traumatic stress disorder.

Source: Adapted from Heim and Nemeroff[7] and Kendall-Tackett.[25]

in part via HPA-axis dysfunction.[8,20] It is characterized by "intrusive re-experiencing," autonomic hyperarousal, reduced responsiveness, intense emotional reactions, sleep problems, learning difficulties, memory disturbances, dissociation, aggression against self and others, and psychosomatic reactions.[21] Many of these symptoms are signs of an overactive amygdala. Acutely, patients feel as though the trauma were recurring. They experience sleep disturbances, hypervigilance, exaggerated startle response, and generalized anxiety or agitation. Chronically, children exhibit detachment, restricted range of affect, dissociative episodes, sadness, somatization, and feelings of hopelessness.[22] Many of these characteristics have been described in institutionalized and post-institutionalized children.[23] This condition is underrecognized post-adoption. Sometimes PTSD is complicated by the coexistence of mood, psychotic or other anxiety disorders, suicidal ideation, learning disabilities, or attentional difficulties.[20]

The age at which trauma occurs is critical. Traumatic experiences in infancy may permanently alter HPA-axis responsivity.[3] For example, rats removed from their mothers in infancy exhibit increased ACTH and corticosterone to a variety of stressors in adulthood.[7] Similarly, compared to nonabused controls, women with a history of physical or sexual abuse as children had elevated ACTH, cortisol, and heart rate when performing mental arithmetic in a laboratory setting (Fig. 8–4). Macaques raised in insecure conditions have elevated concentrations of CRF and reduced concentrations of cortisol in cerebrospinal fluid, the same findings as in humans with PTSD[7] (Fig. 8–5). One theory is that patients with PTSD develop hypothalamic and pituitary hypersensitivity to circulating levels of cortisol. As might be expected, patients with

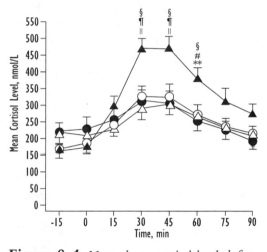

Figure 8–4 *Mean plasma cortisol levels before, during, and after psychosocial stress induction (public speaking and mental arithmetic) in women without a history of significant early-life stress and no psychiatric disorders (black circles), women with a history of childhood sexual or physical abuse without major depression (open circles), women with a history of childhood sexual or physical abuse and current major depression (black triangles), and women without a history of significant early life stress and a current major depression (open triangles). Symbols indicate significant differences in cortisol level of group with childhood abuse and depression compared with other groups. ***, p 0<.05 black vs. open triangles; #, p 0<.05 black triangle vs open circle; ||, p 0<.01. (From Heim C, Newport DJ, Heit S, et al. Pituitary-adrenal and autonomic responses to stress in women after sexual and physical abuse in childhood. JAMA 2000; 284(5):595, Copyright © [2000], American Medical Association. All rights reserved).*

Janice was just 3 months old when she was found nearly buried in a latrine in the Phillipines. Someone heard a faint crying, and realized that an infant had been dropped down the latrine. It took the villagers more than 12 hours to rescue her. For most of the time during the rescue, she cried hysterically, as if she couldn't understand why the people whose voices she heard weren't helping. She was nearly dead from hypothermia and dehydration when they reached her. She was taken to a hospital for several weeks, then transferred to a loving and attentive orphanage. Within 3 more months, she was adopted by an American family who were charmed by her robust good looks and engaging smiles. Knowing her history, they were not surprised after arrival home to realize that Janice was terrified to be alone in the dark. Going to sleep at night was extremely distressing. Her parents firmly believed that being alone in the dark must have triggered memories of her long ordeal of being "buried alive."

PTSD have marked hippocampal shrinkage (detectable by magnetic resonance imaging) and declarative memory deficits.[4,24] Furthermore, patients with PTSD have elevated catecholamines, independent of changes in cortisol.[25] In a recent study of 80 children adopted from Romania in the Netherlands, 20% fulfilled clinical criteria for PTSD 5 years after adoption.[26]

Major depression in adults is also linked to increased HPA-axis reactivity, elevated levels of cortisol, and relative insensitivity to cortisol feedback.[3] Thus, childhood trauma may result in neurobiological changes that extend into adulthood, including alterations in autonomic and catecholamine activity, dysregulation of HPA-axis function, increase in brain glucocorticoid receptor numbers, decrease in cortisol responsiveness, and reduction in volume of the hippocampus.[27]

Stress and Behavior

Stress in early life may have long-lasting effects on behavior. Concentration, distractibility, executive function, and emotional regulation may

An 8-year-old adopted from war-torn Sierra Leone was eating dinner in her Boston home. In the words of her mother, she "suddenly became catatonic, overcome with fear at the sound of bass vibrations from a stereo in a car out on the street, which she had mistaken for impending bombing. She was afraid to go to her room to bed, and clutched me inconsolably all night. 'I scared, Mama! Bad people!' is all she said." (Read the entire moving account of this family's adoption in Crosby.[32])

be adversely influenced by early exposure to stress.[28] Children who experience stress in early life in the absence of secure attachments may lose their ability to modulate impulsivity and the intensity of their feelings.[8] The manifestations may range from learning abilities to aggression against self or others. Children who have received inadequate early care may have higher rates of personality disorders, marital discord and disruptions, and difficulty with their own parenting abilities.[29] Previously abused or maltreated children have increased likelihood of depressive

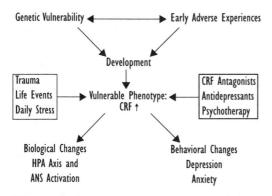

Figure 8–5 *Relationship between early life stress, sensitization of corticotropin-releasing factor (CRF) neuronal systems, and the development of depression and anxiety. ANS, autonomic nervous system; HPA, hypothalamic–pituitary-adrenal. (Reprinted from Heim C, Nemeroff CB. The impact of early adverse experiences on brain systems involved in the pathophysiology of anxiety and affective disorders. Biol Psychiatry 1999; 46:1518, with permission from Society of Biological Psychiatry.)*

and anxiety disorders, eating disorders, suicide attempts, substance abuse and addiction, criminal behavior, and other interpersonal difficulties.[29] The societal cost of neglect during critical periods of infant development is an increase in violence, crime, mental health disorders, unproductive adults, and unstable family situations.[2] Early exposure to stress may be ameliorated by a positive relationship with a competent adult, skill at learning and problem solving, engaging personality, competence and perceived efficacy by self or society, high IQ score, positive school experience, mastery of motivation, and previous successful coping experiences[27] and, later, marriage to a supportive, nondeviant partner.

Recently, a genetic basis for the variation in responses to stress has been identified. Work by Caspi and colleagues demonstrates that specific genetic polymorphisms relate to mental health after exposure to stress. For example, individuals with a short form of the serotonin transporter gene (5-HT T) are more likely to experience depression after emotional stress than those with the long form of this gene.[30] Similarly, a functional polymorphism in the gene encoding the neurotransmitter-metabolizing enzyme monoamine oxidase A (MAOA) influences the response to maltreatment in early childhood. Individuals with lower activity of the MAO gene are more likely to develop behavioral and mental disorders after stressful experiences in early childhood.[31]

Stress in early life thus has far-reaching effects on brain biochemistry and behavior, even into adult life. It should be assumed that internationally adopted children have experienced some degree of stress prior to placement with their adoptive families. Although a loving and supportive adoptive home may overcome some of the effects of stress in early life, some children may require specific treatment for prior stress. Vulnerable personality, genetic susceptibility, age at time of trauma, type and severity of trauma, and associated experiences all contribute to the outcome of children who have experienced stress in early life.

Key Points for Internationally Adopted Children

- Most international adoptees are exposed to stress pre- and postnatally.
- This exposure may have long-lasting effects on growth, the immune system, attachment, mental illness, and behavior.
- Genetic susceptibility and many other factors contribute to these responses.

Resources

Scheering MS, Gaensbauer TJ. Post-traumatic stress disorder. In: Zeanah CH (ed). Handbook of Infant Mental Health, 2nd ed. New York; The Guilford Press, 2000; 369–81.

References

1. Leutwyler K. Don't stress. Sci Am 1998; January: 28–30.

2. Gunnar MR. Quality of early care and buffering of neuroendocrine stress reactions: potential effects on the developing human brain. Prev Med 1998; 27:208–11.

3. Carlson M, Earls F. Psychological and neuroendocrinological sequelae of early social deprivation in institutionalized children in Romania. Ann N Y Acad Sci 1997; 807:419–28.

4. Gould E, Tanapat P. Stress and hippocampal neurogenesis. Biol·Psychiatry 1999; 46:1472–9.

5. Fernald LC, Grantham-McGregor SM. Stress response in school-age children who have been growth retarded since early childhood. Am J Clin Nutr 1998; 68:691–8.

6. Brunson KL, Eghbal-Ahmadi M, Bender R, Chen Y, Baram TZ. Long-term, progressive hippocampal cell loss and dysfunction induced by early-life administration of corticotropin-releasing hormone reproduce the effects of early-life stress. Proc Natl Acad Sci USA 2001; 98:8856–61.

7. Heim C, Nemeroff CB. The impact of early adverse experiences on brain systems involved in the pathophysiology of anxiety and affective disorders. Biol Psychiatry 1999; 46:1509–22.

8. van der Kolk BA, Fisler RE. Childhood abuse and neglect and loss of self-regulation. Bull Menninger Clin 1994; 58:145–68.

9. Dawson G, Ashman SB, Carver LJ. The role of early experience in shaping behavioral and brain development and its implications for social policy. Dev Psychopathol 2000; 12:695–712.

10. Durousseau S, Chavez GF. Associations of intrauterine growth restriction among term infants and maternal pregnancy intendedness, initial happiness about being pregnant, and sense of control. Pediatrics 2003; 111: 1171–5.

11. Ramsay DS, Lewis M. The effects of birth condition on infants' cortisol response to stress. Pediatrics 1995; 95:546–9.

12. Field T. Maternal depression effects on infants and early interventions. Prev Med 1998; 27:200–3.

13. Pine DS, Cohen P, Brook J. Emotional problems during youth as predictors of stature during early adulthood: results from a prospective epidemiologic study. Pediatrics 1996; 97:856–63.

14. Herbert TB, Cohen S. Stress and immunity in humans: a meta-analytic review. Psychosom Med 1993; 55: 364–79.

15. Pike JL, Smith TL, Hauger RL, et al. Chronic life stress alters sympathetic, neuroendocrine, and immune responsivity to an acute psychological stressor in humans. Psychosom Med 1997; 59:447–57.

16. Brosschot JF, Benschop RJ, Godaert GL, et al. Influence of life stress on immunological reactivity to mild psychological stress. Psychosom Med 1994; 56:216–24.

17. Irwin M. Immune correlates of depression. Adv Exp Med Biol 1999; 461:1–24.

18. Cohen S, Miller GE, Rabin BS. Psychological stress and antibody response to immunization: a critical review of the human literature. Psychosom Med 2001; 63:7–18.

19. Snyder BK, Roghmann KJ, Sigal LH. Effect of stress and other biopsychosocial factors on primary antibody response. J Adolesc Health Care 1990; 11:472–9.

20. van der Kolk BA, Pelcovitz D, Roth S, Mandel FS, McFarlane A, Herman JL. Dissociation, somatization, and affect dysregulation: the complexity of adaptation to trauma. Am J Psychiatry 1996; 153:83–93.

21. Famularo R, Kinscherff R, Fenton T. Symptom differences in acute and chronic presentation of childhood post-traumatic stress disorder. Child Abuse Negl 1990; 14:439–44.

22. Famularo R, Fenton T, Kinscherff R, Augustyn M. Psychiatric comorbidity in childhood post traumatic stress disorder. Child Abuse Negl 1996; 20:953–61.

23. Rutter M, Andersen-Wood L, Beckett C, et al. Quasi-autistic patterns following severe global privation. J Child Psychol Psychiatry 1999; 40:537–49.

24. Heim C, Newport DJ, Heit S, et al. Pituitary-adrenal and autonomic responses to stress in women after sexual and physical abuse in childhood. JAMA 2000; 284:592–7.

25. Kendall-Tackett KA. Physiological correlates of childhood abuse: chronic hyperarousal in PTSD, depres-

sion, and irritable bowel syndrome. Child Abuse Negl 2000; 24:799–810.

26. Hoksbergen RA, ter Laak J, van Dijkum C, Rijk S, Rijk K, Stoutjesdijk F. Posttraumatic stress disorder in adopted children from Romania. Am J Orthopsychiatry 2003; 73:255–65.

27. Pynoos RS, Steinberg AM, Piacentini JC. A developmental psychopathology model of childhood traumatic stress and intersection with anxiety disorders. Biol Psychiatry 1999; 46:1542–54.

28. Gunnar MR, Bruce J, Grotevant HD. International adoption of institutionally reared children: research and policy. Dev Psychopathol 2000; 12:677–93.

29. Maughan B, McCarthy G. Childhood adversities and psychosocial disorders. Br Med Bull 1997; 53:156–69.

30. Caspi A, Sugden K, Moffitt TE, et al. Influence of life stress on depression: moderation by a polymorphism in the 5-HTT gene. Science 2003; 301:386–9.

31. Caspi A, McClay J, Moffitt TE, et al. Role of genotype in the cycle of violence in maltreated children. Science 2002; 297:851–4.

32. Crosby SS. A mother's prayer. JAMA 2000; 283:1109–10.

III

TRAVEL AND TRANSITION

9

TRAVEL AND TRANSITION TO THE ADOPTIVE FAMILY

The moment the adopted child is placed with his or her new parents is an unforgettable emotional event for families. As in the delivery room, a scene familiar to pediatricians, the addition of a child to a family is one of the peak experiences of human life. An international adoption may follow months or years of waiting, often after the painful losses of infertility and the many anxieties and uncertainties related to bureaucratic hurdles. Parents have just arrived in a new and unfamiliar culture, and may be jet-lagged and exhausted. In some cases, parents will have already have met their child on a previous trip, as required in some countries (presently Russia and Vietnam). Usually, however, this is the first moment the parent beholds the child. Fantasies, expectations, and dreams suddenly confront the reality of the actual child.

The transition is a critical period in the creation of a new family unit. The experiences of parents and children vary dramatically during this time. The transition may be defined as the interval from meeting the child until settling into a routine at home (often weeks or several months after adoption). The pediatrician will be called upon to provide advice throughout this transition. In this section, several important aspects of the transition will be reviewed, including travel, transition behaviors, sleep, food, toileting, and institutional behaviors, with an emphasis on minimizing stressors for both the child and the parent(s).

Parent Health

In the excitement of planning an international adoption, many parents neglect their own health. Parents must prepare themselves for international travel well in advance of the trip. Parents with chronic medical conditions should consult their physicians about health precautions during travel. All parents should consult their physicians or travel medicine specialist about needed vaccines early in the adoption process. It is *essential* that prospective parents receive hepatitis B vaccination early in the adoption process. If necessary, the vaccine (Engerix-B™, 20 µg) can be administered on an accelerated schedule.[1,2] Hepatitis A vaccine should also be given, as well as updates of polio, tetanus, measles, varicella, and other vaccines as needed.

Inexperienced travelers need to be educated about basic travel hygiene (food, water, sanitation) and safety. Waterless hand cleansers (gels) are useful items to bring. Many travel clinics dispense prophylactic antibiotics to treat traveler's diarrhea. In some areas, malaria prophylaxis is needed. Adequate supplies of all prescription medicines should be taken in carry-on luggage. Parents may wish to consider purchasing emergency evacuation insurance if a prolonged trip is anticipated. (The child is not be eligible for such coverage until the adoption and U.S. immigration procedures are finalized). Guidance on health issues for traveling adults in different regions is available at the Centers for Disease Control and Prevention (CDC), World Health Organization (WHO), and other Web sites.[3–7] Accidents and injuries are the most common cause of serious problems among travelers.[8] Several books also provide useful travel advice.[9,10] Intrafamilial spread of infectious diseases after international adoption is reviewed in Chapters 14–18 and Chen et al.[11] Parents should recognize and try to compensate for the enormous emotional and physical stresses they experience from both the travel and the adoption.

Traveling with Other Children

Some families wish to travel with their older children to receive their adopted child. The pediatrician likely will be consulted about the advisability of including older siblings on such a trip. Several factors should be carefully considered. In addition to the usual concerns about international travel for young children, this type of trip presents special difficulties. In addition to helping the new child adjust to the radical life change, parents must also complete complex legal procedures. Time for play, relaxation, and sightseeing is limited. Parents are likely to be preoccupied with the details involved in completing the adoption. If there are legal or medical complications, the trip may be traumatic and difficult. Young children may not understand if something goes wrong and the child is unable to travel home with them ("But we can't leave my sister here"). It's often advisable for an additional adult to accompany the family. If someone becomes ill, an extra pair of hands is invaluable.

Children who have themselves been adopted may become anxious that they will be left behind or "replaced" by the new baby if they return to their birth country. Some children become frightened to hear their birth language again after adjusting to the adoptive family. Parents must balance these concerns with the difficulties of leaving young, insecurely attached children behind for several weeks. These concerns should be addressed early in the planning stages of a second adoption.

The health of traveling children should be ascertained carefully prior to departure. Schedules for accelerated immunization schedules are available if needed.[8,10] Traveling children should be up-to-date for age for diphtheria-tetanus-pertussis (DTaP), polio (IPV), *Haemophilus influenzae* (Hib), measles-mumps-rubella (MMR), pneumococcal, hepatitis B (HBV), and varicella vaccines. Early measles vaccine should be given to traveling children ages 6–11 months of age.[11a] Yellow fever vaccine may be given to children >9 months old if traveling to endemic areas in Africa or South America. Hepatitis A vaccine should be given to children >24 months old; although children rarely have severe disease, those infected efficiently transmit the infection to other children and to adults. In some regions, vaccination against meningococcal meningitis and Japanese encephalitis is needed (although the latter vaccine is controversial because of side effects[8]). Typhoid vaccine should be given to all children >2 years old[8] traveling to endemic regions.

Malaria prophylaxis should be discussed on an individual basis if traveling to endemic areas. Up-to-date recommendations for pediatric malaria prophylaxis are available on-line.[7] Traveler's diarrhea is more frequent and more severe in young children than in adults. Basic management of traveler's diarrhea in young children is described in Rose[9]. Parents should be prepared to manage traveler's diarrhea in their child with oral rehydration salts if necessary. Children accustomed to friendly neighborhood dogs must be cautioned about animal contacts, as rabies is a risk in some countries. Children should be tested for tuberculosis exposure before and after return from developing countries, especially if travel is prolonged and there is lengthy exposure to local citizens. Updated travel advice for young children is found at the Web site for the American Academy of Pediatrics.[12]

Traveling to Receive the Child

Most families travel to receive their child. The duration and timing of these trips vary depending on the legal requirements in the birth country. These requirements are subject to change, sometimes abruptly. The experience for prospective parents depends a great deal on the amount and quality of information available about the child prior to travel. The experience for the child relates to the child's age and preparation for adoption, as well as details of how the transition to the adoptive parents occurs. In most countries, families do not travel until a court date has been designated. The parents may arrive in the country only a day or two before the court date. Within several days, they receive the child and finalize the adoption, negotiating any necessary legal and bureaucratic hurdles. In some countries, an interval between meeting the child and the formal adoption is legally mandated, or a period of "residence" in the country is required, ranging from 1 to 12 weeks. Most regions in Russia require two trips for adoptive parents. Families receive minimal information about the child prior to the first trip. After meeting the child, they receive more detailed information if they indicate willingness to proceed with the adoption. A court date is set for 2–12 weeks in the future, at which time families return to complete the legal process. In Ukraine, families receive no information about a specific child prior to travel, but are offered a series of dossiers to review at the National Adoption Center until a "satisfactory candidate" is identified. Information about the child is then provided and the parents are taken to meet the child. If the parents accept the child, a court date follows quickly and the adoption is finalized. After a 1-month waiting period, the parent may assume custody of the child. In contrast, most Korean children are often escorted to the United States and first meet their families at the airport. The specific legal requirements of frequent sending countries is shown in Table 9–1. These requirements are subject to frequent change; updates are available at the Web site for the United States Department of State, Bureau of Consular Affairs.[13]

Table 9–1 Travel requirements for adoptive families

Country	Time in Sending Country to Complete Adoption (Approximate)
Cambodia (on hold)	4–7 days
China	2 weeks
Ecuador	Both parents travel; one may leave after 1 week, one stays 14–21 days
Guatemala	4–5 days; escort possible
India	7–10 days; escort possible
Kazakhstan	2–4 weeks, one parent may leave after court date
Nepal	Both parents, 2–3 weeks
Romania (on hold)	1 week
Russia	Two trips: the first 1 week, the second 2–3 weeks. Mandatory 10-day waiting period during second trip (as for all Russian civil court decisions)
Ukraine	1-month waiting period after adoption decree
Vietnam (on hold)	Two trips: the first 1 week, the second 2–3 weeks

Managing Health Problems During the Adoption

One of the greatest anxieties for traveling parents is the possibility that their new child will become ill. New parents worry especially about fevers, respiratory symptoms, and diarrhea. It is useful for the physician to meet with prospective parents well in advance of the travel date to review some basic precautions and to discuss management of possible illness. Parents should be instructed in how to take the temperature of the child so that this information is available if needed. Perhaps the most useful information to provide to traveling parents is how to reach the physician at home. Provision of e-mail, fax numbers, and on-call phone numbers is reassuring and will promote good management of any intercurrent illnesses. Parents should be assured that in most cases, the orphanage physicians are available to care for the child or to refer the child appropriately for more serious conditions. In capital and large cities, the U.S. embassy or consulate will recommend physicians, hospitals, and laboratories in the case of emergency and provide other assistance (see also ref. 13 or Web site for specific embassy) for parents or for the child. In addition, the American Academy of Pediatrics Directory lists foreign members by city and country; occasionally these physicians may serve as local resources for traveling parents.

What to Bring

Many families worry that needed medications may not be available, or if injections are necessary that sterile needles and syringes may not be used. Several medical kits specifically designed for children are available commercially (Table 9–2). These usually include basic medical supplies, such as antipyretics, thermometer, ointments, and explanatory reading material (for example, see Web site for Families with Children from China).[14] Many parents ask the pedi-

Table 9–2   Basic supplies for traveling parents (adjust as appropriate for child's age)

Alcohol wipes
Amoxicillin
Antibacterial wipes
Antibiotic ointment
Antihistamine
Antipyretic (acetaminophen, ibuprofen)
Azithromycin (or cefixime)
Band-aids
Cold or cough preparation
Diaper rash cream
Dosage syringe
Insect repellent
Nasal aspirator
Pedialyte, oral rehydration salts
Permethrin (Elimite)
Sunscreen
Sodium sulfacetamide optic drops (Sulamyd)
Thermometer
Vaseline
Waterless soap gel

Source: Adapted from Borchers.[15]

atrician to prescribe broad-spectrum antibiotic(s) and appropriate-sized needles and syringes as well. (A letter on office stationery stating the purpose of these latter items may prevent unnecessary questions at border crossings.) Families should be encouraged to donate unused material to the orphanage when they depart. Large cities in most sending countries have reasonably well-stocked pharmacies; sterile needles and syringes are available for purchase without prescriptions. Smaller cities may have fewer supplies available; however, most orphanages have basic medications on hand. Nevertheless, most families will feel more secure when traveling with some basic supplies.

Meeting the Child

Most families carefully evaluate the referral information about their child prior to travel. They have some general idea of the child's health, as well as specific questions for the caregivers. The degree of growth delay may also be anticipated, especially if updated measurements are provided close to the time of travel. If a video has been reviewed, the parents may have some sense of the degree of developmental delay to expect, as well as some preconceptions about the child's personality and behavior ("she's smiley and sociable," or "he's a serious child"). Because the videos are brief snippets of a child's day and may be months out of date by the time the family travels, these expectations may be incorrect. Furthermore, the stress of the transition may alter the child's demeanor and behavior. Major questions about the child's health, development, and behavior should be addressed prior to travel if possible, as analysis and interpretation of this sensitive and important information is difficult at the last minute.

The quality of the initial encounters of the parent and child depends on various factors. Parents have usually been well prepared by their adoption agencies about what to expect when they travel to receive their child; they must remember that the child often has had no preparation. Although little may be done to prepare young infants, older children have surprising ability to understand some of what happens with an adoption. In orphanages where children are frequently adopted, children may recognize that the appearance of strangers is followed by disappearance of one of their group. This may create a great deal of anxiety. If the transition is gradual, children may see that the child being adopted gets special attention as she comes and goes from the group. When the child returns from outings with her parents, she may have new clothes and toys. Jealousy, anxiety, and fear may create misbehaviors and emotional upset in the entire group of children.

Some children are understandably terrified of the adopting parents (Fig. 9–1). Although the parents have had months to study their child's photograph (and possibly video), the child abruptly experiences a removal from all famil-

Kristo and Alla, ages 4 and 6 years, were sleeping soundly in their orphanage. Although they were brother and sister, they were in different groups and rarely saw each other, and certainly had no special relationship. One night, both were awoken, hurriedly changed from pajamas to clothes, and handed over to a strange man who carried them to a car. Except for the night watchman and the occasional workman, the children rarely saw men during their daily lives. As he drove them away, both children cried with fear—neither had ever been in a car before and the sensation of movement was terrifying. After 2 hours, tear stained and exhausted, they were carried into a brightly lit hotel. They felt more terror as they were carried into an elevator, another new experience. With a knock on the door, two jet-lagged Americans were roused from their sleep. "Here are your children," said the man. "I'll be back at 9 AM so we can go to court." He handed the children over, and departed.

iar sights, sounds, smells, tastes, and people. In extreme cases this is emotionally comparable to kidnapping. Many orphanages are sensitive to these issues for the children and are willing to help prepare children for adoption. Parents sometimes prepare a family book with photos of family members, pets, the house, neighborhood, and other appropriate things (Table 9–3). If labeled in English and the local language, caregivers may review the photo album with the child in advance of the adoption. Even for infants, a photo of the parents to place by the bedside may ease the transition. Some parents send audio tapes of their voices singing or reading stories (and electronically compatible tape-players). A special toy sent in advance, joined by a matching one at adoption, may help children make the transition to their new family more comfortably.

After receiving the new child, most parents undress the child and anxiously inspect the child's body. Families should be prepared prior to travel for likely physical findings, including a Bacille Camille-Guérin (BCG) vaccination scar (see Chapter 14), Mongolian spots (Fig. 9–2),

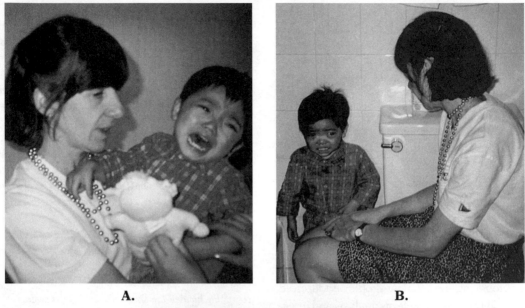

A.   B.

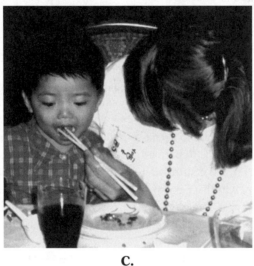

C.

Figure 9–1 *The first few hours of transition to the new family may be difficult. A. N. is handed by her nanny to her new mother. Too young to understand, she is old enough to realize that something serious is happening in her life and that she is being separated from familiar people. B. Thirty minutes later, N. is still terrified. Who is this woman who keeps following me around? What are all these strange things in this room? Where is everyone I know and love? Why can't this person understand me when I talk? C. One hour later, N. contentedly accepts food from her new mother. Note that N.'s mother wisely did not change her daughter's clothing during this difficult time. At the moment that N. lost her beloved caregivers, her home, her language, and her culture, all that remained was her familiar clothing. Retaining this remnant of her identity may have helped N. with this difficult transition. (With permission.)*

buttock fat atrophy from multiple injections (Fig. 9–3), and dental caries (Fig. 9–4). Any scars or unusual findings should be noted. Some children have circumferential scars around the wrists or ankles (Fig. 9–5). This can be alarming to parents who assume these result from ties or restraints. Although this is a possible explanation, such marks may also result from elastic bands

Diana, age 3 years, had lived in an orphanage in Kazakhstan her entire life. One day, her beloved nanny scooped her up on her lap and said "I have something wonderful to show you." She then sat with Diana and showed her a book of photos from America. The photos showed people, houses, toys, and even a dog. The photos were labeled in Russian, so the nanny was able to tell Diana "This is your new Mama, this is your new Papa, this is your house, your toys. . . . They will come to get you soon, and take you on a big trip to your new home!" The nanny read the book to Diana every night for 4 weeks at bedtime. One day, the orphanage director said to Diana, "Today is a wonderful day, Diana! Your Mama and Papa have come to meet you!" Diana was dressed by the nanny in her best clothes, and a big bow placed in her hair. Her nanny walked with her down to the director's office, and when they opened the door, there was Mama and Papa! Diana clung to her nanny for a few minutes, then her Mama showed Diana that she had a book. It was the same as the book her nanny had read to her! Diana looked at the book, and looked at Mama and Papa. After a few minutes, she was content to sit on Mama's lap, and look at the familiar pictures with her, marveling that the people in the photos were now here. Mama and Papa hugged her and gave her a special dolly, and said they'd be back tomorrow to play and visit some more. Over the next 3 weeks, they gradually spent more time together, and started to take her out of the orphanage, first for walks on the grounds, then gradually for short car rides, to restaurants, to shops, and to their hotel. At first, Diana was frightened to leave, and cried a bit, but after a week or so, she started to feel sad when she returned to the orphanage. One day, her Mama said that Diana could stay overnight at the hotel with them. Her nanny made sure she understood, and gave Diana her special pillow from the orphanage to take. A few days later, Mama and Papa told Diana they would go on a long trip together. Diana trustingly gave Mama her hand, and walked out to the taxi to go the airport.

Scene: Twenty adopting parents anxiously wait in the hotel conference room in China. The clock ticks slowly; where are the babies? Suddenly, the door opens, and the room fills with nannies; crying, sleeping, or wary infants; officials; translators; and facilitators. Every parent strains to see their child—often they've only had a postage stamp–sized photo to hold on to for the months between the referral and the actual adoption. As each parent finds their child, tears, laughter, crying babies, crying nannies all swirl together in a kaleidoscope of emotion.

Scene: An orphanage in Russia. The parents sit nervously in the director's office. After an interminable wait, a nanny comes in, leading a 14-month-old by the hand. The child is wide-eyed with fright. As the strange people on the couch rise to greet him, he bursts into tears and buries his face in his nanny's shoulder. "Stop that, Sergei! Here's your Mama and Papa come to get you!" says the director sharply. She peels him away from the nanny and hands him to the bewildered parents who try ineffectually to comfort him.

Scene: The airport. The whole family is waiting, grandma, grandpa, brothers, sisters, parents, aunts and uncles. Finally the plane is announced. Down the long hall come three Korean women, each carrying two infants. The women are exhausted. After careful checking, the babies are handed to their parents; the whole family crowds around to get a good look, and everyone takes a turn holding the new arrival.

on clothes that were too small for the child, unfortunately a common occurrence in orphanages. Other unexplained scars are sometimes found.

Traveling with the New Child

Depending on the country, parents may suddenly receive custody of their new child. Childproofing the hotel room is essential—children from institutions may have no sense of safety and

Table 9–3 Aiding the transition of the newly adopted child: advice for prospective parents

Send a family book; make several copies.

Label photos in local language and English.

Send a special toy; bring a matching one when you arrive.

Make a tape of your voices—greetings, songs, nursery rhymes, etc. Send along with a tape recorder with lots of batteries or appropriate plug adapter.

When visiting young babies, wear the same perfume or scented lotion everyday. Leave a pillow scented with the same fragrance, and wear the same scent when you return.

Prepare a laminated photo of yourself to tie to the baby's crib.

Wear the same clothes as in the photo when you meet the child for the first time.

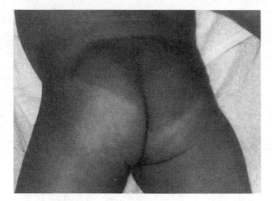

Figure 9–2 *Adoptive parents may not be prepared for the appearance of extensive Mongolian spots. Children from Asia, the Near East, Central and South America, and Africa commonly have Mongolian spots. Typically, these occur in the sacrogluteal area or lumbar region, but may also occur on the extremities. This normal blue-purple pigment usually fades by 5 years of age.*

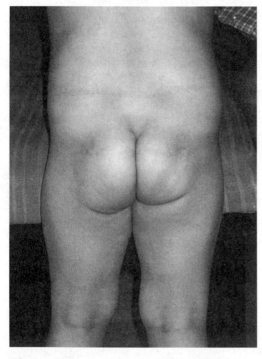

Figure 9–3 *Fat atrophy of the upper outer quadrant of the buttocks occurs after multiple intramuscular injections in this site. This is found most commonly in children adopted from Russia or Eastern Europe. In children without fat atrophy, careful inspection of this site often reveals multiple blue-gray puncture marks left by injections. (With permission.)*

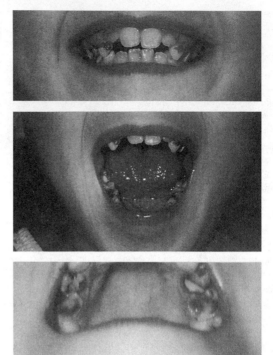

Figure 9–4 *Dental caries are common in children adopted from orphanages. Tooth-brushing and dental care are frequently lacking. Severe caries may cause painful mastication, reducing food intake. (With permission.)*

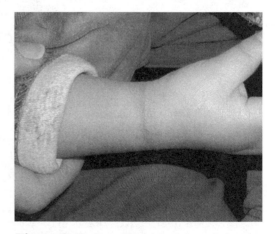

Figure 9–5 *Circumferential marks on the extremities may result from restraints or from tight elastic bands on ill-fitting clothing.*

no familiarity with common objects. At the same time, the child usually has a strong drive to explore. New parents may not recognize potential hazards and should be instructed to observe their environment carefully to prevent problems.

Many newly adopted children have never traveled in motor vehicles. Motion-sickness is a common complaint; parents should be prepared for this possibility. Lengthy air travel is another challenge for the new family; common-sense advice is available at the Web site Flying with Kids.[16]

Child Behavior During the Transition

For first-time parents, a review of expectations for normal behavior, sleeping, eating, and elimination, including the wide range of normal and common alterations seen in children from orphanages, will be reassuring. Behaviors such as hyperactivity, passivity, clinginess, and temper tantrums may be prominent in the first few weeks after adoption but quickly abate afterwards. Children may become distressed when confronted with unfamiliar routines, for example, with food, bathing, and toileting. Whatever techniques parents use are different from what is familiar to the child: from the child's point of view, everything the parents do is "wrong." Parents must understand the immensity of the transition their child is experiencing and be empathetic about the adjustments the child is making to new styles of care and parenting.

Sleep

Sleep schedules. Many parents are given their child's daily schedule from the orphanage and wonder how strictly to adhere to this after adoption. Most orphanage schedules include lengthy nap times and early bed times. In Romania, one orphanage for healthy 4- to 7-year-old children enforced a 3-hour nap for the children every afternoon. Children may be accustomed to such schedules, but quickly adapt to change. Jet lag may interfere with sleep schedules for a time after arrival home.

Sleep quality. Sleep disturbances are extremely common among international adoptees, especially in the first few months after adoption. Children often display anxiety at bed or nap times. Nightmares, "daymares" (during naps), and night terrors are common among this group of children, but these usually subside over the first few weeks after adoption. Most children have never been alone in a bed and definitely not alone in a room. The American custom of placing children in their own rooms to sleep may be frightening. Some children (notably those from Korea and Cambodia) have become accustomed to sleeping with caregivers and are inconsolable when expected to sleep alone. Some children awake crying and become alarmed when their parents arrive to comfort them—some parents have felt the children were expecting someone else (a previous caregiver, for example)—and are disoriented to find someone else responding to them. For some children, sleep states seem to be associated with grieving for lost caregivers; some children cry sadly and deeply when going to sleep or awakening.

Psychological processing of the immense changes in the child's life may manifest as sleep disturbances, although this is difficult to prove. Parents must recognize that insecurity and anxiety underlie most of these "early-onset" sleep disturbances among internationally adopted children. This is in contrast to manipulative behaviors related to sleep and bedtime that sometimes develop in young children. Management of these sleep problems requires specific attention to the underlying psychological issues. Many parents find that co-sleeping for the first few weeks or months after adoption greatly reduces the child's anxiety. Transition to more conventional sleep arrangements is easily accomplished when bonding to the family is more firmly established. Repeated expressions of love and provision of needed attention and security are key methods to manage sleep problems in newly adopted children.

Food

Amount. Unusual behaviors related to food are common among post-institutionalized children. Parents frequently report that their children are ravenous, consuming "unbelievable amounts" of food, and still wanting more. Most children with these behaviors have suffered significant hunger and should be offered food freely. Older children may be more confident about the food supply if given a small box to store a personal supply of food to consume as wished. Other children inspect the refrigerator and cupboards frequently to be sure that food is available; others hoard or hide food or stuff it in their mouths ("chipmunk cheeks"). Parents should be encouraged to offer food freely; usually the voracity diminishes within a few days or weeks when the child becomes confident that the food supply is reliable. Some parents find it useful to calmly offer more food to the child after he is done eating, even if he has eaten an enormous amount of food.

Sensory issues related to food. A surprising number of children have sensory issues related to food. The most common is an inability to tolerate textures. Many children have subsisted on soups, liquids, and purees, and have missed

Beth was adopted at age 14 months from China. She was bright and beautiful, and a joy to her new parents. However, they were concerned that she refused all solid foods and was content to remain on the bottle. Their pediatrician told them not to worry, and that she would "grow out of it." The parents frequently offered solid foods but were always rebuffed. At her 4-year check-up, their pediatrician was shocked to learn that Beth was still being fed infant formula in a "sippy cup," occasional juice, and yogurt, and had never taken a bite of solid food.

Kenny, age 3 years, was adopted from Lithuania. His mom reported a "typical lunch" for him, 1 month after adoption: 7 ounces of vegetable soup, two peanut butter and jelly sandwiches cut in quarters, eight celery sticks, four baby carrots, 8 ounces of milk, a banana, half an apple, and five chocolate chip cookies. Three hours later, he was ready for snack.

some of the oral-motor milestones related to chewing solids. Nipples used for bottle feeding in many orphanages have large openings, probably to speed feeding. Children fed in this manner develop oral-motor reflexes to prevent choking, but have reduced oral-motor tone. These children may be "open mouthed" in appearance and may drool excessively. When offered conventional nipples, the children have difficulty producing an adequate suck to withdraw the formula. These children may have considerable difficulty tolerating a spoon because of overactive tongue thrust and may become distressed when presented with foods containing any texture (lumps). Some of these children also have "chipmunk cheeks"; one speculation has been that overstretching of baroreceptors in the oropharynx is needed for the child to sense where the food is in the mouth. Usually these difficulties abate within a few weeks, but some children have exceptional difficulties and may benefit from the assistance of a feeding team. In some children, esophageal reflux contributes to food aversions.

Introducing a new diet. Parents often wonder if the orphanage diet should be maintained during the transition, and especially whether formula must be gradually switched from a local brand to an American brand. Although some children appear sensitive to changes in diet, the vast majority of children do well, and graded switching is not necessary. Misplaced concerns about lactose intolerance in Asian infants often need to be allayed (see Chapter 28).

Some children display a pronounced unwillingness to try new foods. Whether this relates to taste or texture can be difficult to determine. Orphanage diets tend to be bland and predictable. For children in this category, slow introduction of new foods may be better tolerated than presentation of a wide array of tastes and textures.

Indifference to food. Surprisingly, some children, even if malnourished, are indifferent to food. These children usually have significant failure to thrive, but normal or near-normal cognitive development. These children often seem oblivious of hunger and never request snacks and meals. Their dismayed parents are at a loss to understand why a malnourished child refuses food or is indifferent to food; psychological problems between parent and child often ensue. These children must be carefully evaluated for medical reasons for failure to thrive (see Chapter 10). Occasionally, supplemental nighttime feeds are needed, and may eventually trigger normal hunger responses. The etiology of this syndrome is not clear. Delayed gastric emptying, inadequate food in the orphanage, and the extra attention from caregivers for the child refusing food may interact to alter the biochemical signals of hunger and satiety. Careful interventions may allow these children to eventually learn to eat properly; many never seem to particularly enjoy eating.

Toileting

Toilet training expectations and methods differ among cultures and are managed differently in institutional care than in families. Many parents are told in advance that their child is "potty-trained," only to discover to their chagrin (especially if they have come without diaper supplies) that this is not true. Most orphanages regularly schedule "potty-time" after each meal or snack. Infants even as young as 6 months may be placed on a potty—often tied on to the potty seat if too young to maintain balance—for lengthy periods after eating. This routine minimizes the number of soiled or wet diapers over the course of the day. Adoptive parents inevitably abandon this schedule because of the irregular events during the transition period (court appearances, travel, etc.), with the result that the "potty-training" vanishes. Parents adopting children less than age 3 or even 4 years of age should prepare for diapers, at least until they return home and establish some routine in the course of the day.

Many children are remarkably apprehensive about diaper changes. Prior painful experiences during diaper changes, the proprioceptive stimulus of being placed supine, fear of clothing removal, or simply a change in the technique of the diapering could contribute to the child's anxiety. Regardless of the cause, this fear usually abates within a short time.

Bathing

Attempts to bathe the child may be met with crying and distress. In orphanages, bathing may not be a pleasant experience (cold water, rough wash cloths and towels, etc.). Understandably, orphanage workers must bathe many children quickly. Bathing usually does not include pleasant, soothing waterplay. Children take some time to realize that bath-time means warm water, enjoyable sensations, and a chance for interesting play.

Clothes and Toys

One of the tangible expressions of the adoptive parents' love for the new child is the desire to provide material items such as clothing and toys. Usually one of the strongest urges of a new parent is to undress and inspect the child, then to bathe her and dress in her in all new clothing. Parents should be cautioned to restrain these impulses during the early hours of the transition. Under most circumstances, the child has abruptly lost all that is familiar—language, culture, people, places, and things. All that remains is her clothes, which smell and feel familiar. These should be removed and replaced only after the child has had a period of time with her new family. Stiff, new clothes may feel uncomfortable and unfamiliar; new clothes are a rarity in the orphanage. Most items should be washed prior to use and tags removed to prevent irritation.

Similarly, encounters with multiple new toys may be unfamiliar and frightening for children who have never had personal possessions. A child living in institutional care may never have had someone show him how to play with (as opposed to fling or bang) toys. Assisting the child's interaction with toys is a valuable activity for parents in the early days of the transition.

Institutional Behaviors

Institutional behaviors often are noted in the early hours and days after adoption. These behaviors may be upsetting to unprepared parents. Occasionally institutional behaviors are captured on videos supplied to parents prior to adoption; however, this is uncommon. More frequently, these behaviors are observed after the child is placed with the family. These behaviors provide self-comfort, sensory stimulation, or attract adult attention (Table 9–4). For children lacking physical comfort, toys, social interactions, and other experiences, these behaviors are adaptive and promote neurologic

development in an abnormal environment. Some of these behaviors may be considered survival skills.

The list of self-stimulating or self-soothing behaviors is lengthy (see Chapter 2). Children who have been physically deprived of proprioceptive, visual, and auditory stimulation often develop behaviors that stimulate these senses. The most common is rocking, which can be either on hands and knees, or in a sitting position flexing forward at the waist. Other behaviors include swaying from side to side, head banging, finger flicking, hair or ear twisting, and head butting. Some children hold or move their fingers and hands in unusual positions and stare fixedly at them (Fig. 9–6). Others are mesmerized by fans, lights, or corners, seemingly attracted by shadows, textures, and other subtleties. Curiously, thumb sucking is rare, probably because it is physically strongly discouraged in most orphanages. Other sensory behaviors commonly seen are altered responses to pain, usually manifest as an extremely high

Table 9–4 Institutional behaviors

Rocking
Swaying or "bobbing"
Head banging
Head shaking
Head bopping
Hand staring or flapping
Spacing out (dissociating)
Staring at lights, fans, shadows
Biting, hitting, or scratching self or others
Smelling objects
Hair twirling or ear pulling
Bruxism (teeth grinding)
Looking at objects very closely

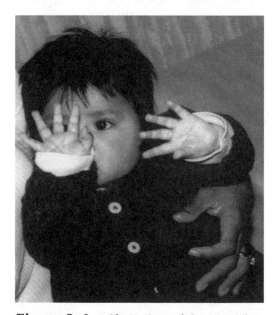

Figure 9–6 *Self-stimulatory behavior, such as hand gazing, may increase in frequency and intensity during the stressful early phases of the transition. For this child, this behavior disappeared within a few days after the adoption. (With permission.)*

pain threshold, and "daredevil" behaviors, or lack of sense of safety. Some investigators have speculated that dysregulation of neurotransmitters or cortisol underlie the physiologic reasons for these behaviors[17–20] (see Chapter 8).

Some of these behaviors can be so pronounced as to raise the question of autism. Indeed, some children have such persistent behaviors that the diagnosis of "acquired institutional autism" seems appropriate[21,22] (see Chapter 13).

A wide variety of attention-getting behaviors may be observed in internationally adopted children. These include biting, spitting, scratching, and various tantrums and inappropriate behaviors. These unpleasant and difficult behaviors may have earned the child some extra attention in an environment where even negative attention (discipline) was preferable to no attention. New parents must direct their attention to the good behaviors the child exhibits, while ignoring or correcting these negative behaviors. With time, children realize that the route to adult attention has changed.

Survival skills include some of the eating behaviors discussed above. Also important are the social skills children develop to survive emotionally in an orphanage environment with multiple caregivers. Some of these behaviors may also be seen in the spectrum of reactive attachment disorder. The most common of these behaviors is overfriendliness. This behavior—superficial charm and sociability with strangers—is an adaptive response to inconsistent caregivers. Although these children are pleasant to encounter, they must be monitored closely for appropriate attachment to their parents (see Chapter 29).

Although some of these behaviors may occur in children raised in a family, institutionalized children often display them repetitively or obsessively. For most children, these behaviors resolve over a few weeks as the environment is enriched. For some, however, the behaviors are deeply ingrained and persist for years. Most common are self-rocking or head-shaking behaviors prior to sleep or during times of frustration.

The Post-Arrival Visit

At long last, the new family is home. Many families are instructed by their adoption agency to be seen "immediately" by the child's physician after arrival in the United States. Unless the child is ill, this is usually unnecessary and may add undue stress. Certainly a visit to the physician within the first 4–5 days is useful. At this time it is important to obtain accurate anthropometric data and perform a physical examination to detect major problems and get a general sense of the developmental status of the child. Vaccinations and blood tests are not warranted at the first visit, except under unusual circumstances. Illness in other family members after international travel must be carefully assessed.[23] Fever, diarrhea, and dermatologic conditions are the most common complaints.

A more complete evaluation should be performed 2–4 weeks after the child arrives home. At this time, the child should be thoroughly examined, remeasured to assess early signs of catch-up growth, and have screening blood tests performed (Table 9–5). Vaccinations can be administered and a plan for completing needed vaccines made. Parents should be thoroughly questioned about the child's health and well-being, appetite and dietary preferences, sleep behaviors at night and at nap-time, defecation and urination patterns, and the presence of orphanage or other unusual behaviors. Questions about attachment and bonding are also appropriate at this visit and should be repeated at subsequent visits. Open-ended questions such as "Is she what you expected?" or "How does it feel to be a parent?" or "Tell me what kind of boy he is" may pave the way for useful discussions.

It is useful to have a somewhat standardized format for the post-arrival visit. During this visit, the pediatrician may observe the interactions between the parents and child,

Table 9–5 Screening tests for new arrivals

CBC
Lead level
RPR or VDRL test
Hepatitis B sAg, sAb, core Ab[a]
Hepatitis C antibody[a]
HIV-1 and HIV-2 ELISA (consider DNA-PCR for infants <6 months)[a]
Liver function tests
Thyroid function tests
Stool for ova and parasites, *Giardia* antigen
If diarrhea: stool for *Salmonella, Shigella, Campylobacter*
Tuberculin skin test (PPD)
Urinalysis

Consider

- Newborn screen to State Board of Health (This includes a hemoglobin electrophoresis in most states. Although it also includes a TSH/T4, these assays are optimized for newborns and may not be accurate for older children.)
- Varicella titer: if immune, varicella vaccination can be deferred
- *Helicobacter pylori* antibody ELISA (see Chapter 20)
- Hearing screen: mandatory in any child with significant language delay, strongly suggested in any child with history of multiple episodes of otitis media prior to adoption

Ab, antibody; Ag, antigen; CBC, complete blood (cell) count; ELISA, enzyme-linked immunosorbent assay; PCR, polymerase chain reaction; PPD, purified protein derivative; RPR, rapid plasma reagent; VDRL, Venereal Disease Research Laboratory.

[a]Repeat 6 months after arrival.

generally observe the child's activity level and attention span, and perform a developmental screening assessment (see Chapter 13). In addition, the following focused questions may reveal some areas of concern and suggest avenues for further investigation. These questions are suggested as a supplement to routine pediatric age-appropriate inquiries.

Questions on Child's History

What information was available to you prior to adoption?

Did you receive additional information when you received your child?

Do you have a vaccine record?

Where did your child reside?

Did you get to visit the facility?

Did you meet any of your child's caregivers?

Did your child seem to have a special caregiver?

Do you have any way of maintaining contact with that caregiver?

For children who have been in foster care

Did you meet the foster family? How did their relationship to the child seem?

Do you have any way of maintaining contact with the foster family?

Questions on Transition

How did she do with the transition to you?

Was there a lot of crying, grieving, withdrawal?

Were there problems with feeding, sleeping, or behavior? Have these improved?

For older children

How was she prepared for the transition? Was this helpful?

For families who make two trips to complete the adoption

What was the time interval between the trips?

How much time did you spend with her during each visit?

Do you think she remembered you from the first visit?

Did she leave the orphanage willingly with you?

Questions on Health

Were there any health issues during the time in the birth country or since arrival home?

Was the child receiving any medications when you received him?

Have you noticed anything about him physically that you especially wish me to check?

Questions on Attachment

Is she showing some early signs of attachment?

Does she make good eye contact with you?

Does she turn to you for approval? Turn to you for reassurance and comfort?

Is she "overfriendly" to outsiders?

How does she behave with unfamiliar people or situations?

Are you feeling connected to her?

For two-parent families
Are you both feeling connected to her?

Is there a difference in how she relates to each of you?

Questions on Sleep

Are there any sleep issues?

What are the sleeping arrangements?

Is there any trouble separating from you for sleep?

Are there any nightmares? Night terrors?

For children in cribs
Does he call for you in the morning to come get him?

Questions on Diet

What types of food does she eat? What amounts?

How is her appetite?

Does she hoard food? Hide food? Stuff her cheeks (chipmunk cheeks)?

Can she chew?

How does she handle different textures?

Are there any significant food refusals? Food cravings?

Are there any anxieties or unusual behaviors related to food?

Questions on Elimination

How frequently does he have bowel movements?

What is the consistency?

Is there any distress when defecating?

Were you told he was potty trained? Is he?

For boys
Have you observed the urine stream?

Questions on Hearing

Can your child hear? How have you determined this?

Questions on Language

How much of your child's birth language did she understand?

How much could she say? (ask for concrete examples)

Has she been exposed to speakers of her birth language since arriving home? How did she react?

Questions on Behavior

Has your child exhibited any "orphanage behaviors" such as rocking, head banging, head shaking, trances, staring spells, or staring at hands, lights, or fans? Tell me more about these. When do these episodes occur? How long do they last?

Have you tried to interrupt these behaviors?

Has your child exhibited any other behaviors that have concerned you?

How would you describe this child?

Questions on Family Situation

Who lives in the household?

Who will be caring for the child?

How will you juggle work and child care?

For families with other children
How are the other kids reacting to the new sibling?

Did the other kids travel with you, or did they stay home? How did that go for them?

Questions on Parent Stress

Are you feeling comfortable about how things are going?

Is parenthood what you expected?

Is the child what you expected?

How is the extended family responding to the new child?

Physical Examination

A very thorough physical examination is mandatory at arrival. Special points to note include the following:

General appearance and demeanor (alert, curious, engaging, withdrawn, frightened, eye contact, attention span, response to commands)

Relationship to parent (clinging, secure, disengaged)

Head: shape (asymmetry, occipital flattening), careful measurement of head circumference

Eyes: strabismus is common.

Ears: verify bilateral hearing; if there is any concern, conduct an audiologic evaluation. You may need to disimpact cerumen.

Throat: verify intact palate. Count teeth, assess condition (caries common), differentiate primary and secondary dentition.

Hair: texture, thickness, any bald spots, color if unusual

Nails: unusual appearance may indicate iron deficiency, vitamin deficiency, prenatal alcohol exposure (fifth digits).

Lymph nodes: lymphadenopathy that could be consistent with tuberculosis

Skin: Mongolian spots, BCG scar (usually left deltoid), scars, any notable findings (injection marks are often seen in upper outer quadrant of buttocks, sometimes with associated fat atrophy; see Fig. 9–3)

Perineum: careful inspection for obvious signs of sexual abuse

Musculoskeletal: muscle tone (usually hypotonic)

If possible, measure mid-arm circumference/triceps skin fold thickness as measurements of body fat.

References

1. Bock HL, Loscher T, Scheiermann N, et al. Accelerated schedule for hepatitis B immunization. J Travel Med 1995; 2:213–7.

2. Marsano LS, Greenberg RN, Kirkpatrick RB, et al. Comparison of a rapid hepatitis B immunization schedule to the standard schedule for adults. Am J Gastroenterol 1996; 91:111–5.

3. The American Society of Tropical Medicine and Hygiene. Travel Clinic Directory. Available at: http://www.astmh.org.

4. The International Society of Travel Medicine. Travel Clinic Directory. Available at: http://www.istm.org.

5. Pan American Health Organization. EID weekly updates. Available at: http://www.paho.org.

6. World Health Organization. International travel and health. Available at: http://www.who.int/ith.

7. National Center for Infectious Diseases. Traveler's Health. Available at: http://www.cdc.gov/travel.

8. Hostetter MK. Epidemiology of travel-related morbidity and mortality in children. Pediatr Rev 1999; 20:228–33.

9. Rose SR. International Travel Health Guide. Northampton, MA: Travel Medicine, Inc., 2001.

10. Centers for Disease Control and Prevention. Health Information for the International Traveler, 2001–2002. Atlanta: U.S. Department of Health and Human Services, Public Health Service, 2001.

11. Chen LH, Barnett EA, Wilson ME. Preventing infectious diseases during and after international adoption. Ann Intern Med 2003; 139:371–8.

11a. American Academy of Pediatrics. Immunization in special clinical circumstances. In: Pickering, L., ed. 2003 Red Book. Report of the Committee on Infectious Diseases. Elk Grove Village, IL: American Academy of Pediatrics, 2003, 93–98.

12. American Academy of Pediatrics. Available at: http://www.aap.org.

13. U.S. Department of State. Medical information for Americans traveling abroad. Available at: http://www.travel.state.gov/medical.html.

14. Families with Children from China. Travel Medical Kit. Health and medical information. Available at: http://www.fwcc.org/healthinfo.htm.

15. Borchers DA. Helpful medical items to take to China for your child. Available at: http://www.fwcc.org/medicalitems.html.

16. Fly with Kids. Available at: http://www.flyingwithkids.com/.

17. Carlson M, Earls F. Psychological and neuroendocrinological sequelae of early social deprivation in institutionalized children in Romania. Ann N Y Acad Sci 1997; 807:419–28.

18. Cermak SA, Daunhauer LA. Sensory processing in the post-institutionalized child. Am J Occup Ther 1997; 51:500–7.

19. Cermak S, Groza V. Sensory processing problems in post-institutionalized children: implications for social workers. Child Adolesc Soc Work J 1998; 15:5–37.

20. Gunnar MR. Quality of early care and buffering of neuroendocrine stress reactions: potential effects on the developing human brain. Prev Med 1998; 27:208–11.

21. Rutter M, Andersen-Wood L, Beckett C, et al. Quasi-autistic patterns following severe global privation. J Child Psychol Psychiatry 1999; 40:537–49.

22. Rutter M. Developmental catch-up and delay, following adoption after severe global early privation. J Child Psychol Psychiatry 1998; 39:465–76.

23. Ryan ET, Wilson ME, Kain KC. Illness after international travel. N Engl J Med 2002; 347:505–16.

IV

GROWTH AND DEVELOPMENT

10

MALNUTRITION

Malnutrition afflicts more than 200 million children throughout the world and is responsible for 50% of deaths that occur before age 5. Malnutrition robs young children of good health, growth, and development. Many internationally adopted children are malnourished prior to adoption (see Chapter 2). Prenatal malnutrition is common: more than 25% of international adoptees are low birth weight.[1–3] Because of uncertainty about gestational age in most children, determination of intrauterine growth retardation is difficult. Postnatal malnutrition befalls children who reside with impoverished or neglectful birth families, in institutions, or in indifferent foster care. Some children suffer from prolonged, severe, and/or recurrent episodes of malnutrition. Others endure a single episode of malnutrition due to illness, food shortages, or loss of a beloved caregiver. Poor appetite, impaired oral-motor function, and improper feeding techniques (bottle-propping) all reduce food intake. Chronic undernutrition is much more common than malnutrition, and has long-lasting effects as well.

Although most international adoptees display remarkable growth recovery after adoption, the consequences of early malnutrition or undernutrition may still be observed in some children years later. Genetic factors, prenatal exposures, and neglect all amplify the effects of early malnutrition. This chapter describes the interactions of malnutrition and neglect, and the effects of malnutrition on growth, cognition, behavior, and immunity. The effects of recovery from malnutrition on growth, cognition, and behavior are reviewed, along with practical considerations for internationally adopted children.

Malnutrition and Neglect

Malnutrition often occurs in conjunction with neglect. The combination is far more devastating than malnutrition alone. Experimental animals exposed to both malnutrition and environmental isolation have more severe and persistent behavioral problems than after exposure to either one separately.[4] Both malnutrition and neglect commonly result in behavioral withdrawal. These factors thus act synergistically to isolate the infant from the stimulation necessary for normal development.[4-6] Malnutrition in the absence of neglect is less harmful. For example, among equally malnourished infants in Chile,[7] developmental abilities were better among those who were the product of "wished-for pregnancies," "separated less from their mother's side," and received more stimulation from their mothers. Similarly, many Dutch children born during World War II suffered from pre- and postnatal malnutrition[6] but had normal development and behavior (see exceptions below).

Definitions

Children with malnutrition by definition are *underweight* (<–2 standard deviation [SD] from median weight for reference population). They may also be *wasted* (weight for height <–2 SD for reference population) or *stunted* (height <–2 SD from median height for reference population). Among 1445 children evaluated on arrival in our International Adoption Clinic, 30% were stunted, 18% were underweight, and 13% were both. The most severe forms of malnutrition are marasmus and kwashiorkor. *Marasmus* results from inadequate caloric intake, manifest first by poor weight gain, then by weight loss. Skin turgor diminishes as subcutaneous fat disappears, the abdomen may become distended, and muscles become atrophic. The child may be irritable, then becomes progressively more apathetic. Appetite decreases, and infrequent or "starvation" stools appear due to changes in intestinal mucosa, decrease in digestive enzymes, and inadequate intake of essential amino acids, folic acid, and other water-soluble vitamins. *Kwashiorkor* results from severe deficiency of protein intake, or, more precisely, an abnormal ratio of dietary calories to essential amino acids.

Biochemically, lipid peroxidation is increased and antioxidative capacity reduced.[8,9] Children have poor growth, loss of muscular tissue, edema or ascites, hepatomegaly, and increased susceptibility to infections. There may be evidence of collateral circulation on the abdominal wall. Generalized dermatitis is common (especially in children with hypophosphatemia[10]): usually there is erythema and hyperpigmentation of the skin, which may be cracked, peeling, and secondarily infected. Children may also have sparse, straight, easily uprooted hair. Reddish tint of the hair may be related to specific amino acid deficiencies. Children may be lethargic, apathetic, or irritable. The combination of marasmus and kwashiorkor, sometimes called protein-calorie or *protein-energy malnutrition*, is the most common form of malnutrition. Malnutrition rarely occurs in the absence of iron, vitamin, zinc, and/or other micronutrient deficiencies (see Chapter 11). Many international adoptees have mild to moderate malnutrition; severe malnutrition and kwashiorkor are rare. Many more have chronic undernutrition (impaired growth that does not fulfill the criteria for underweight, wasting, or stunting). This often becomes obvious after adoption when growth improves (e.g., from 5th to 50th percentile).

Effects of Malnutrition

Malnutrition has broad effects on growth, development, cognition, behavior, and immune function. All of these areas are linked and are subject to multiple other influences. Isolating the effects of malnutrition is impossible outside of experimental settings. Early malnutrition has effects throughout the lifespan. Adults malnourished as children are more likely to develop coronary artery disease, type 2 diabetes, and hypertension.[11,12] Prenatal malnutrition also affects health in adult life. Dutch children born after the "Hunger Winter" imposed by the Nazi blockade were more than twice as likely to develop schizophrenia if their mothers were malnourished during the first trimester of pregnancy.[13] Impaired glucose tolerance developed more frequently in those children whose mothers were malnourished during the last trimester of pregnancy.[11,14] Infants born small for gestational age are more likely to develop insulin resistance, dyslipidemia, and "syndrome X" (hypertension, type 2 diabetes, and obesity).[15,16] Nutritional deprivation in early life may also impair cognitive function in old age.[17]

Malnutrition and Growth

The most obvious effect of malnutrition is on growth. The severity, timing, and duration of caloric deprivation determine the degree of growth inhibition. In growing children, height best reflects overall nutritional condition: body weight and amount of subcutaneous fat depend on recent intake rather than on the duration of undernutrition. In severe cases of malnutrition, growth ceases. In less extreme conditions, growth velocity is reduced. Young infants are more vulnerable to the effects of malnutrition on growth than older children. Children with chronic caloric undernutrition are short, have retarded bone ages, and normal dental ages. Although weight is below normal for age, weight for height is often normal (due to the reduction in height).

Like height and weight, head circumference may be reduced by malnutrition (see Chapter 12). Although height tends to catch up with time, head circumference in children who suffer early malnutrition becomes progressively more abnormal.[18] Indeed, "suboptimal head circumference may be the most sensitive physical index of prolonged undernutrition during infancy."[18,19] Sometimes, however, head circumference is relatively preserved (Fig. 10–1).

In some children, the combination of neglect and malnutrition results in psychosocial dwarfism. Biochemical tests in these children are indistinguishable from those seen in idiopathic hypopituitarism, including abnormalities of growth hormone, ACTH, and thyroid function. The children are short, appear younger

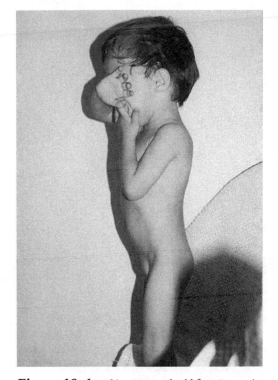

Figure 10–1 *Thin, 30-month-old from Romania. Weight was 7.6 kg (weight for age 7 months), height was 79 cm (height for age 17 months), and head circumference was 47 cm (head circumference for age 20 months). (With permission.)*

than their chronological age (immature facial features and body structure), and have delayed dental and bone ages[20] (Fig. 10–2). Some children have widened cranial sutures.[21] In extreme cases, children exhibit bizarre eating and drinking behavior (polydipsia), sleep disturbances with nighttime roaming, and foraging (beyond the usual post-adoption arrival behaviors; see Chapter 9). Poor sleep relates to growth delays: in one study, children who slept well grew 1.04 cm/month, while those who slept poorly grew 0.34 cm/month.[22,23] Some children with psychosocial dwarfism also have pain agnosia.[22,24]

Growth Delays and International Adoptees

Growth delays are common among international adoptees. Many have low birth weights,

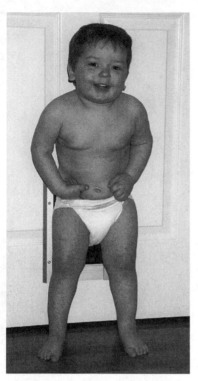

Figure 10–2   *This 32-month-old boy from Russia had normal weight and head circumference (25th percentile) but short stature (<3rd percentile; height for age 18 months) on arrival. Bone age was delayed nearly 12 months. (With permission.)*

Multiple factors contribute to malnutrition among institutionalized children (see Chapter 2). Duration of orphanage confinement is an important variable. In three distinct populations of adoptees (Romanian, Chinese, Russian),[3,27,30] length of institutionalization related directly to linear growth lags. For every 2.86–5 months orphanage life, children lost 1 month of linear growth (see Fig. 2–2).

Malnutrition and Cognition

In addition to reducing growth, malnutrition also impairs cognitive ability. Malnutrition during the period of most rapid brain growth (last trimester of pregnancy through the first 9–12 months of postnatal life) diminishes brain size, brain DNA content, myelinization, cortical dendritic growth, and neurotransmitter content.[6,32] Some of these changes may be ameliorated by environmental enrichment.

A linear correlation between growth and developmental delays has been identified in children with protein-energy malnutrition.[33] Similarly, malnourished international adoptees are more likely to be developmentally delayed than are better-nourished children (Fig. 10–3).[26]

Numerous studies[18,34–46] (but not all[47,48]) find permanent reductions in cognitive ability after significant malnutrition in early childhood. Studies in Jamaica and South Africa show reduced IQ as long as 20 years after recovery from malnutrition.[18,44,46] The elegant longitudinal studies of Galler and Ramsey in Barbados demonstrate that children sustain a loss of ~12.5 IQ points as long as 10 years after a single episode of malnutrition[34–40] (Fig. 10–4).

Malnutrition also alters subtle neurocognitive function. Memory and attention appear to be particularly vulnerable to early malnutrition. Visuomotor and perceptual abilities were impaired in South Africans diagnosed with malnutrition 20 years previously, unrelated to their IQ scores. Some children had changes in the temporoparietal brain regions, made visible by computed tomography.[46] Fine motor delays are

although these are difficult to interpret in the absence of (reliable) information about gestational age. Mean birth weights of 135 children adopted from India were 1.82 kg for males and 1.79 kg for girls.[25] Of 114 Indian children adopted in Sweden, most had birth weights <2.5 kg; 27% were <2.0 kg.[1,2] Mean birth weight of 42 Russian adoptees was 2.73 kg (range 1.14–4.10 kg).[3] Malnutrition may develop or worsen during institutional life. Small size at birth, intercurrent medical problems (recurrent infections, for example), insufficient calories, and lack of nurturing physical contact all contribute to ongoing malnutrition (see Chapter 2). Many international adoptees are malnourished at arrival, as assessed using z scores (Table 10–1) or proportion of children with measurements less than the third or fifth percentiles (Table 10–2).

Table 10–1 Nutritional status of newly arrived international adoptees (mean z scores)

Country of Origin (N)	Receiving Country	Weight z Scores	Height z Scores	Head Circumference z Scores	Comments
Mixed, most from Romania or China (129)[26]	United States	−0.76	−1.36	−1.03	Nutritional status correlates with gross and fine motor development. Those with severe cognitive and language delays have lower z scores for all measurements. Delays correlate with z scores for height, weight, and head circumference.
Russia (56)[3]	United States	−1.05	−1.41	−1.25	One month of linear growth delay for every 5 months in the orphanage
China (192)[27]	United States	−1.17	−1.51	−1.43	Weight z scores correlate with height and head circumference z scores; 1 month of linear growth delay for every 2.86 months in the orphanage
India (114) [1,2]	Sweden	−2.30	−2.20 (−3.00 for those >24 months)	−2.00	

Table 10–2 Nutritional status of newly arrived international adoptees

Country of Origin (N)	Receiving Country	Less than Third Percentile Weight	Less than Third Percentile Height	Less than Third Percentile Head Circumference
Most from Korea and India (100)[28]	Australia	30%	30%	—
Most from Africa/Indian Ocean (68)[29]	France	31% [a]	—	—
India (200)[25]	United States	86%	80%	—
Romania (65)[30]	United States[b]	15%	31%	26%
Age at arrival (months)		<15 >15	<15 >15	<15 >15
Less than third percentile (%)[c]		18 13	24 39	15 39
Romania (22)[31, d]	Canada	36%	32%	45%
Age at arrival (months)		<6 7–12 13–24 >24	<6 7–12 13–24 >24	<6 7–12 13–24 >24
Less than fifth percentile (%)		0 60 50 33	0 20 50 67	17 60 62 33

[a]Many required hospitalization for nutritional rehabilitation.

[b]Percentage <−2 z score.

[c]Calculated from data in 31.

[d]Percentage of children with measurements less than fifth percentile (%)

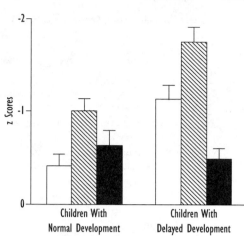

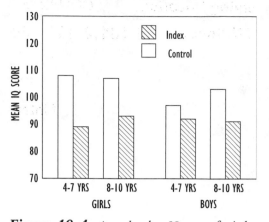

Figure 10–3 *Z scores for weight (open bars), height (shaded bars), and head circumference (solid bars) were lower in internationally adopted children with developmental delay (*n = 64*) compared with those with normal development (*n = 65*) when evaluated at arrival to the United States. Note y-axis orientation. (Adapted from Developmental and nutritional status of internationally adopted children. Arch Pediatr & Adolesc Med 149:40–4, 1995. Copyright © 1995, American Medical Association. All rights reserved.)*

Figure 10–4 *Age related to IQ scores for index (hatched bars) or control (open bars) children. Children were 5- to 11-year-olds in Barbados. Index children had histories of moderate to severe protein-energy malnutrition in the first year of life. Mean IQ of the index children was 12 points lower than the mean IQ of the comparison children. There was a disproportionate number of cases at the lower end of the distribution curve for the index group: 17% of the 127 control children had IQs <90; 50% of the 119 index cases had IQs <90. Socioeconomic conditions did not differ between the two groups of children. (From Galler JR, Ramsey F, Solimano G, Lowell WE, Mason E. The influence of early malnutrition on subsequent behavioral development. I. Degree of impairment in intellectual performance. J Am Acad Child Psychiatry 1983; 22:13, with permission.)*

found in some children at least through 18 years of age,[36] years after malnutrition has resolved. Even children with temporary malnutrition due to pyloric stenosis in infancy have impaired auditory and visual memory at age 5–14 years, especially if their weight deficit reached 11% or more.[32] These children also have lower scores on the Parental Estimate of Development Scale. Other studies show sensory integration disorder, learning disabilities, abnormal auditory evoked responses, and impaired school performance long after a single episode of malnutrition.[39] Researchers in South Africa[18] state that the "association of a small head and impaired visuo-motor functioning may be the most reliable indicator of children at a cognitive disadvantage after undernutrition in infancy" (Fig. 10–5).

Maternal or other environmental factors that frequently coexist with malnutrition are also important and contribute to outcome.

Mothers of malnourished children have higher maternal depression scores; maternal depression correlated with the behavioral and cognitive functioning of the child during the school years, regardless of the child's IQ. Thus maternal depression, or conditions leading to it—hospitalization, lack of bonding—may be an independent factor contributing to behavioral and cognitive deficits in children with an early history of malnutrition.[37,48] Malnourished infants are more likely to be described by their mothers as "difficult." It is not known if these findings can be extrapolated to foster mothers or orphanage caregivers. In all settings, malnutrition is usually complicated by concurrent exposures to social and economic disadvantage, poor housing, ill health, and family disruption

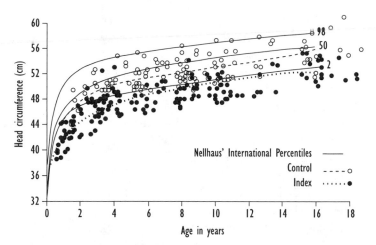

Figure 10–5 *Mean head circumference measurements for control (open circles) and index (black circles) children compared with percentiles 2, 50, and 98 (Nellhaus). Forty South African children were followed longitudinally for 20 years; the 20 index children had malnutrition in early infancy. (From Stoch MB, Smythe PM, Moodie AD, Bradshaw D. Psychosocial outcome and CT findings after gross undernourishment during infancy: a 20-year developmental study. Dev Med Child Neurol 1982; 24:422, with permission.)*

or disorganization, all factors capable of influencing intellectual development.[44]

The timing of malnutrition markedly influences its effects on neurocognitive outcome. The risks are greatest when the malnutrition coincides with periods of rapid brain growth.[44] Production of brain DNA is two-thirds complete by birth then ceases at 1 year of age[32]; brain growth is largely complete by 3 years of age.[18] Low–birth weight infants generally have inferior cognitive outcomes.[49–58] When evaluated in early childhood and during school-age and teenage years, these children tend to have difficulties in coordination, lateralization, spatial and graphomotor skills, attention, and cognition. Smaller head circumferences (see Chapter 12) and adverse sociodemographic factors are both strongly linked to worse outcome.

In children without prenatal growth retardation, malnutrition anytime within the first 3 years of life is more likely to result in impaired intellectual development than if it occurs later during childhood.[18] Cognitive outcome may be worse in children who experience malnutrition within the first 6 months of life,[59–62] although other studies demonstrate no difference

in outcome after malnutrition at any time within the first 2 years.[44] Cognitive recovery may only be possible during the period of rapid brain growth, although some[63] believe it may occur at any time. Varied outcomes likely result from the testing measures used and characteristics of the study population.

Even in adequately nourished children, specific dietary deficiencies (protein, cholesterol, polyunsaturated fatty acids) may reduce speech and language, gross motor function, and perception and visual motor skills.[64] Neuroanatomic abnormalities found in infants with severe protein-calorie malnutrition suggest a possible basis for their neuropsychological deficits.[65]

Malnutrition and Behavior

In addition to its effects on growth and cognition, malnutrition also affects behavior. Malnutrition rarely occurs in isolation; it is usually accompanied by deprivation of social, sensory, and environmental stimulation.[6] Thus it is difficult to ascribe behavioral problems seen after malnutrition to that factor alone.[43] Malnourished individuals are apathetic and tend to avoid new experiences, show overly emotional responses to aversive or stressful stimuli, and exhibit less locomotor activity.[6] Malnourished infants are lethargic and suck poorly, which further contributes to poor nutrition.[66] These children are classified as "ineffectual, immature, and dependent" when assessed in nursery school.[66] Animal studies suggest that malnutrition "functionally isolates" the individual, limiting enriched experiences needed for optimal cognitive development.[4] Malnutrition reduces curiosity, the major impetus for learning in young infants.[6]

Even a single episode of malnutrition in early life can result in long-lasting behavioral changes. Jamaican boys with a period of malnutrition before age 2 years had poor attention span, poor memories, more distractibility, less cooperation with teachers, more isolation from peers, fewer positive peer relationships, and more frequent behavior or conduct problems at ages 5–10 years than their well-nourished siblings and classmates.[45] There was no relation to the timing of the malnutrition within the first 2 years of life and behavioral outcome. Children with pyloric stenosis in infancy have significantly more problems related to social immaturity, overactivity, and conduct when studied at school age. Those children in whom onset of starvation was between 21 and 30 days of life have more difficulties than children with later onset of starvation. The authors of this study concluded that "even a brief period of severe starvation in early infancy, uncontaminated by socioeconomic conditions, has a long-lasting effect on learning abilities and general adjustment as measured at 5–14 years of age."[32] Similarly, Barbadian children with a single episode of malnutrition in infancy had short attention spans, poor memories, distractibility, restlessness, poorer social interaction with teachers and peers, low self-esteem, and more emotional lability years later.[34–39] These behavioral problems were unrelated to IQ. There was a fourfold increase in the frequency of attention-

deficit hyperactivity disorder at age 15 years (60% of previously malnourished children vs. 15% of control children).[40] The attention-deficit behaviors persisted to at least age 9 to 15 years.[39] Finally, although previously malnourished South African children were well integrated into their communities 20 years later, many individuals showed lack of drive, initiative, enterprise, and social maturity.[46]

Malnutrition and Immune Function

Malnutrition is the most common cause of immunodeficiency in the world. Malnutrition and undernutrition clearly increase susceptibility to infection. Pneumonia and measles are among the most common acute infections in malnourished children and contribute to the deaths of many. Other infections are also more common among malnourished children. In one study, hepatitis B surface antigenemia was more common among Thai children with malnutrition than in well-nourished children (29% vs. 7.4%).[67]

Many components of the immune system are affected by malnutrition (Table 10–3). One of the most striking findings in malnutrition is a generalized increase in serum immunoglobulins, likely a response to increased antigen exposure (via chronic dermatitis, increased intestinal permeability, which enhances systemic absorption of food antigens and microbial toxins, and more frequent intestinal parasites).[68] C3 levels may be diminished because of reduced hepatic production or increased catabolism. Undernutrition or malnutrition may impair responses to vaccines (see Chapter 21). Children with severe malnutrition may harbor severe infections (bronchopneumonia, pyelonephritis, septicemia) without the usual clinical signs of infection.

Many of these changes in the immune system reverse with improved nutrition. However, improvement in immune function lags considerably behind nutritional rehabilitation.[70,71] Recovery of some immune functions,

Table 10–3 Effects of malnutrition on the immune system

Defects of neutrophils
  Decreased bactericidal and candidicidal activity
  Impaired myeloperoxidase killing (possible)
  Decreased migration to bacterial chemotactic factors
  Decreased adherence
Decreased complement components (except C4)
Compromised integrity of skin and mucosal surfaces
Abnormalities of immunoglobulins
  Normal or increased (may be low in young infants
    with severe marasmus)
  Reduced secretory IgA
  Impaired antibody responses to some vaccines
    (typhoid, diptheria, influenza, yellow fever)
      (responses to tetanus, pneumococcus, polio,
      measles vaccines usually normal)
  High levels of IgE (but allergy is rare)
Cellular immunity
  Thymic atrophy
  Lymphopenia
  Reduced T cell numbers
  Impaired delayed type hypersensitivity
  Altered lymphocyte proliferation
  Decreased serum leptin

Source: Adapted from Stiehm[68] and Chandra.[69]

especially cell-mediated immunity, may be incomplete.[71] Ongoing micronutrient deficiency, chronic exposure to infectious diseases, or other environmental factors may impede complete restitution of the immune system. Thus, the malnourished international adoptee may be more susceptible to infection for some time even after nutritional rehabilitation is complete.

Recovery from Malnutrition

Physical Effects

Supplemental calories and a nurturing environment are both needed for optimal physical recovery from malnutrition. When both components are provided, most children demonstrate remarkable growth catch-up after malnutrition. Adequate dietary amino acids, phosphorus, and sulfur are particularly important to promote growth recovery.[72] The velocity and amount of catch-up vary depending on many factors: the age of the child, the severity, duration, and cause of the malnutrition, and concurrent health problems. Children who suffer substantial malnutrition in early childhood likely end up shorter and lighter (and with smaller head circumferences) than their genetic potential indicates[47] (similar to most studies of intrauterine growth–retarded infants[51,53]). In some circumstances, children may achieve their full growth potential or nearly so.[18,46,73] If the height deficit is <5%–8%, chances for a complete recovery are good. If the height deficit is ≥15%, the possibility of achieving normal height is less. Weight usually recovers prior to height.[74]

After adoption, most malnourished children demonstrate remarkable growth recovery. Indian children adopted in Sweden improved their height and weight measurements from about −2.2 SD to −0.7 SD within about 2 years[1,2] (Fig. 10–6A). Children with less linear catch-up growth had lower birth weights. Those with lower height for age at adoption had the most marked catch-up but ultimately remained smaller (Fig. 10–6B). Likewise, malnourished Korean children adopted by American families eventually surpassed typical height and weight measurements for Korean children, but remained shorter and lighter than American controls.[5,75]

Onset of puberty may be affected by malnutrition. Girls with a history of marasmus (but not kwashirokor) often have significant delays in onset of menarche,[38] although precocious puberty may occur in children after recovery from malnutrition (see Chapter 27). Twelve-year-old children born small for gestational age have increased adrenocortical and adrenomedullary hormones; some have elevated cortisol and cholesterol levels.[76]

Serum aminotransferase levels are sometimes transiently elevated during early recovery from malnutrition.[61] Ingestion of a high-calorie, high-carbohydrate diet (especially sucrose) or increased physical activity (that accompanies

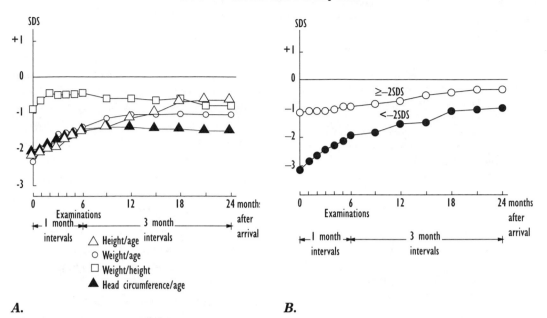

A.   **B.**

Figure 10–6 *A. Growth recovery after adoption. Height, weight, head circum-ference, and weight-for-height were measured serially in 114 Indian children adopted in Sweden for the first 2 years after arrival. B. Height recovery during the first 2 years after adoption. Stunted children (closed circles) showed faster catch-up growth than non-stunted children (open circles). (With permission from Taylor & Francis, Stockholm, Sweden.)*

improved stamina)[77] have been suggested as possible causes.[78,79]

Cognition and Behavior

Environmental stimulation can remediate the behavioral and cognitive effects of malnutrition and is probably more effective than achieving optimal nutrition.[48,60] Environmental stimulation long after an acute period of malnutrition may modify or diminish some behavioral changes.[6] Home visitors and other low-cost enrichment programs improve the developmental scores of children after malnutrition, although the sustainability of these benefits is controversial.[41–43] Although low–birth weight children are more likely to experience learning difficulties and attentional problems as adolescents,[16,80] recent work demonstrates that cognitive function improves over time (years) in very low–birth weight infants; this may provide a model

for other high-risk conditions in early life.[81] Adequacy of catch-up growth determines neurodevelopmental outcome in very low–birth weight infants[82]; similar studies have not yet been reported after early malnutrition.

Adoption is the most dramatic intervention after malnutrition. Adoption provides "a total and permanent improvement of the environment,"[5] optimizing both nutrition and surroundings. Studies of Indian, Korean, and Chilean adoptees all address this question. Indian children adopted in Sweden achieved normal psychomotor scores within 2 years, although milestones were initially delayed in ~30% of the children, especially those who were stunted or underweight.[1,2] Average age at follow-up was 39 months. In another study, Korean children in the United States were evaluated 6 or more years after adoption; all were in grades 1–8.[5,75] The nutritional status of the children at the time of entry into pre-adoptive (foster) care (<2 years of age) predicted IQ scores (see Chapter 3). All 138 children adopted before age 3 years had above-average IQ scores. However, mean IQs increased with better nutritional status (malnourished = 102, moderately nourished = 106, well-nourished = 112)[5] (Fig. 10–7). Nutritional status of Korean children adopted at older ages (between age 2 and 5 years) also predicted IQ. Those with severe malnutrition at entry did not achieve average IQ scores, but moderately malnourished and well-nourished children scored *above* average.[75] Finally, Chilean children with malnutrition in infancy achieved higher IQ scores after adoption than those consigned to institutions or those who returned to their biologic families.[83] These studies are all testaments to the "special stimulatory character of the adoptive home."[75]

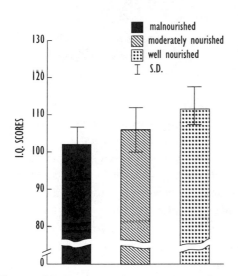

Figure 10–7 *IQs of 138 Korean children adopted to the United States before age 2 years and now in grades 1–8. Nutritional condition on entry to foster care in Korea was classified as malnourished (<3rd percentile for both height and weight), moderately nourished (3rd to 24th percentile for both height and weight), and well-nourished (>25th percentile for both height and weight). (Reprinted with permission from Winick M, Meyer KK, Harris RC. Malnutrition and environmental enrichment by early adoption. Science 1975; 190:1173. Copyright ©1975, American Association for the Advancement of Science.)*

Malnutrition and International Adoption: Practical Considerations

When caring for the malnourished or undernourished new arrival, the pediatrician should explicitly discuss feeding practices with the family (see Chapter 9). Voracious or ravenous children should be allowed to eat freely. Rapid weight gain allows a quicker return to normal body composition in malnourished children, and free access to food is important psychologically for the hungry child. Vitamin and mineral supplements (especially zinc) should be considered for significant malnutrition (less than third percentile for weight). Occasionally, elevations of alkaline phosphatase and/or aminotransferases are seen during growth recovery; these usually return to normal within weeks. Temporary widening of the cranial sutures occasionally occurs during growth recovery in infants.

Rapid growth recovery is the rule in malnourished children after adoption (Figs. 10–8 and 10–9). If substantial physical catch-up does not occur within the first 6 months, medical or behavioral causes preventing recovery should be sought (Table 10–4). The list of possibilities is substantial, and a comprehensive approach must be taken (Table 10–5). Curiously, some children with growth retardation from malnutrition and neglect become accustomed to low-caloric intakes, and do not appear to be hungry even if presented with adequate amounts of food. This may reflect disordered regulation of the complex pathways that determine appetite and satiety.[84] However, until these pathways are more clearly elucidated, a behavioral approach to nutritional rehabilitation is necessary for these children.

In conclusion, many international adoptees are malnourished to some degree at arrival to the United States. Others have endured unrecorded episodes of malnutrition prior to adoption. Even children with measurements greater than the fifth percentile may be undernourished, as demon-

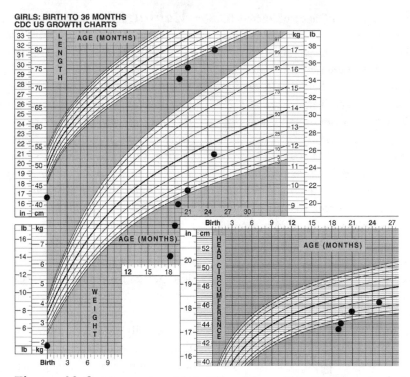

Figure 10–8 *Many malnourished children have rapid catch-up growth after adoption. Exceptions to this pattern should be investigated. (Growth charts from Centers for Disease Control and Prevention [CDC]).*

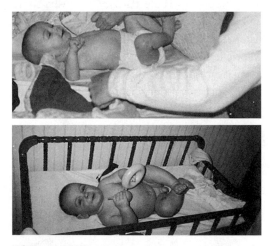

Figure 10–9 *Within 3 months of adoption, this child's physical appearance is transformed. (With permission.)*

strated by the rapid catch-up growth to an appropriate percentile curve. Most children quickly recover weight; height, and head circumference growth recovery usually follow. Micronutrient deficiencies and immune function impairments may outlast growth deficits. Long-term, many factors influence whether previously malnourished international adoptees reach their full potential for growth and cognitive development. Those without rapid physical recovery should be evaluated more fully. Some children likely have permanent behavioral or neurocognitive effects from early episodes of malnutrition.

Key Points for Internationally Adopted Children

- Malnutrition is common in new arrivals.
- Most children exhibit rapid catch-up in growth measurements.

Table 10–4 Medical reasons for poor catch-up growth in internationally adopted children

Gastrointestinal (see Chapters 15, 16, 20, and 28)
Reflux
Milk protein intolerance
Lactose intolerance
Hepatitis
Celiac disease
Malabsorption
Helicobacter pylori infection

Renal
Urinary tract infection
Renal tubular acidosis

Pulmonary
Cystic fibrosis

Endocrine
Growth hormone deficiency
Hypothyroidism
Iodine deficiency (see Chapter 11)
Hypopituitarism

Infectious (see Chapters 14, 17, and 18)
Intestinal parasites (including "occult" parasites)
Bacterial infection of intestinal tract
Tuberculosis
HIV infection
Dental problems
Bacterial overgrowth

Behavioral (see Chapters 13, 31, and 33)
Oral-motor immaturity
Emotional conflict
Oral hypersensitivity
Delayed gastric emptying
Abnormal hunger/satiety axis

Miscellaneous (see Chapters 11 and 24)
Lead poisoning
Zinc deficiency
Psychosocial growth delay

Table 10–5 Suggested initial evaluation for poor growth recovery after adoption[a]

History and physical examination
Calorie counts
Laboratory tests (CBC, albumin, BUN, creatinine, liver
    function tests, thyroid function tests, urinalysis,
    electrolytes, calcium, phosphorus, random growth
    hormone, anti-endomysial/anti-gliadin antibodies,
    IgA, tissue transglutaminase)
Evaluation for *H. pylori*
Stool ova and parasites, culture
Bone age radiograph
Sweat chloride
Chest radiograph
Renal ultrasound

[a]These tests should be considered supplements to the
    recommended screening tests for new arrivals.

- Early malnutrition may have long-term effects on growth, cognition, behavior, immunity, and health.
- Malnourished children who do not have rapid growth recovery after arrival should be carefully evaluated.

References

1. Proos LA, Hofvander Y, Wennqvist K, Tuvemo T. A longitudinal study on anthropometric and clinical development of Indian children adopted in Sweden. II. Growth, morbidity and development during two years after arrival in Sweden. Ups J Med Sci 1992; 97: 93–106.

2. Proos LA, Hofvander Y, Wennqvist K, Tuvemo T. A longitudinal study on anthropometric and clinical development of Indian children adopted in Sweden. I. Clinical and anthropometric condition at arrival. Ups J Med Sci 1992; 97:79–92.

3. Albers LH, Johnson DE, Hostetter MK, Iverson S, Miller LC. Health of children adopted from the former Soviet Union and Eastern Europe. Comparison with preadoptive medical records. JAMA 1997; 278:922–4.

4. Levitsky DA, Barnes RH. Nutritional and environmental interactions in the behavioral development of the rat: long-term effects. Science 1972; 176:68–71.

5. Winick M, Meyer KK, Harris RC. Malnutrition and environmental enrichment by early adoption. Science 1975; 190:1173–5.

6. Barnes RH. Dual role of environmental deprivation and malnutrition in retarding intellectual development. A. G. Hogan Memorial Lecture. Am J Clin Nutr 1976; 29:912–7.

7. Alvarez ML, Concha X, Elordi M, Lamilla C, Ramos C, Perez P. Infant malnutrition, development rate and its relation to the environment: a pilot study. Rev Saude Publica 1991; 25:282–8.

8. Lenhartz H, Ndasi R, Anninos A, et al. The clinical manifestation of the kwashiorkor syndrome is related to increased lipid peroxidation. J Pediatr 1998; 132:879–81.

9. Manary MJ, Leeuwenburgh C, Heinecke JW. Increased oxidative stress in kwashiorkor. J Pediatr 2000; 137:421–4.

10. Manary MJ, Hart CA, Whyte MP. Severe hypophosphatemia in children with kwashiorkor is associated with increased mortality. J Pediatr 1998; 133:789–91.

11. Rosenbloom AL. Fetal nutrition and insulin sensitivity: the genetic and environmental aspects of "thrift". J Pediatr 2002; 141:459–61.

12. Godfrey KM, Barker DJ. Fetal nutrition and adult disease. Am J Clin Nutr 2000; 71:1344S–52S.

13. Goldberg C. What happens in the womb can follow you to the tomb. The Boston Globe, Dec 3, 2002: C14.

14. Ravelli A, van der Meulen JH, Michels RP, Osmond C, Barker DJ. Glucose tolerance in adults after prenatal exposure to famine. Lancet 1998; 351:173–7.

15. Lee PA, Kendig JW, Kerrigan J. Persistent short stature, other potential outcomes, and the effect of growth hormone treatment in children who are born small for gestational age. Pediatrics 2003; 112:150–62.

16. Pomerance JJ. Management of short children born small for gestational age. Pediatrics 2003; 111:180–2.

17. Abbott RD, White LR, Ross GW, et al. Height as a marker of childhood development and late-life cognitive function: the Honolulu-Asia aging study. Pediatrics 1998; 102:602–9.

18. Stoch MB, Smythe PM. 15-year developmental study on effects of severe undernutrition during infancy on subsequent physical growth and intellectual functioning. Arch Dis Child 1976; 51:327–36.

19. Skull SA, Ruben AR, Walker AC. Malnutrition and microcephaly in Australian aboriginal children. Med J Aust 1997; 166:412–4.

20. Barnett WS. Long-term cognitive and academic effects of early childhood education on children in poverty. Prev Med 1998; 27:204–7.

21. Gloebl HJ, Capitanio MA, Kirkpatrick JA. Radiographic findings in children with psychosocial dwarfism. Pediatr Radiol 1976; 4:83–6.

22. Money J. The Kaspar Hauser Syndrome of "Psychosocial Dwarfism". Buffalo, NY: Prometheus Books, 1992.

23. Honda Y, Takahashi K, Takahashi S, et al. Growth hormone secretion during nocturnal sleep in normal subjects. J Clin Endocrinol Metab 1969; 29:20–9.

24. Money J, Wolff G, Annecillo C. Pain agnosia and self-injury in the syndrome of reversible somatotropin deficiency (psychosocial dwarfism). J Autism Child Schizophr 1972; 2:127–39.

25. Smith-Garcia T, Brown JS. The health of children adopted from India. J Community Health 1989; 14:227–41.

26. Miller LC, Kiernan MT, Mathers MI, Klein-Gitelman M. Developmental and nutritional status of internationally adopted children. Arch Pediatr Adolesc Med 1995; 149:40–4.

27. Miller LC, Hendrie NW. Health of children adopted from China. Pediatrics 2000; 105:E76.

28. Nicholson AJ, Francis BM, Mulholland EK, Moulden AL, Oberklaid F. Health screening of international adoptees. Evaluation of a hospital-based clinic. Med J Aust 1992; 156:377–9.

29. Bureau JJ, Maurage C, Bremond M, Despert F, Rolland JC. Children of foreign origin adopted in France. Analysis of 68 cases during 12 years at the University Hospital Center of Tours [in French]. Arch Pediatr 1999; 6:1053–8.

30. Johnson DE, Miller LC, Iverson S, et al. The health of children adopted from Romania. JAMA 1992; 268:3446–51.

31. Benoit TC, Jocelyn LJ, Moddemann DM, Embree JE. Romanian adoption. The Manitoba experience. Arch Pediatr Adolesc Med 1996; 150:1278–82.

32. Klein PS, Forbes GB, Nader PR. Effects of starvation in infancy (pyloric stenosis) on subsequent learning abilities. J Pediatr 1975; 87:8–15.

33. Sathy N, Elizabeth KE, Nair MK, Bai NS. Growth faltering and developmental delay in children with PEM. Indian Pediatr 1991; 28:255–8.

34. Galler JR, Ramsey F, Solimano G, Lowell WE. The influence of early malnutrition on subsequent behavioral development. II. Classroom behavior. J Am Acad Child Psychiatry 1983; 22:16–22.

35. Galler JR, Ramsey F, Solimano G, Lowell WE, Mason E. The influence of early malnutrition on subsequent behavioral development. I. Degree of impairment in intellectual performance. J Am Acad Child Psychiatry 1983; 22:8–15.

36. Galler JR, Ramsey F, Solimano G, Kucharski LT, Harrison R. The influence of early malnutrition on subsequent behavioral development. IV. Soft neurologic signs. Pediatr Res 1984; 18:826–32.

37. Galler JR, Ramsey F, Solimano G. Influence of early malnutrition on subsequent behavioral development. V. Child's behavior at home. J Am Acad Child Psychiatry 1985; 24:58–64.

38. Galler JR, Ramsey F. A follow-up study of the influence of early malnutrition on development: V. Delayed development of conservation (Piaget). J Am Acad Child Adolesc Psychiatry 1987; 26:23–7.

39. Galler JR, Ramsey F. A follow-up study of the influence of early malnutrition on development: behavior at home and at school. J Am Acad Child Adolesc Psychiatry 1989; 28:254–61.

40. Galler JR, Barnett LR. Children and famine: long-term effects on behavioral development. Ambulat Child Health 2001; 7:85–95.

41. Grantham-McGregor S, Schofield W, Harris L. Effect of psychosocial stimulation on mental development of severely malnourished children: an interim report. Pediatrics 1983; 72:239–43.

42. Grantham-McGregor S, Schofield W, Powell C. Development of severely malnourished children who received psychosocial stimulation: six-year follow-up. Pediatrics 1987; 79:247–54.

43. Grantham-McGregor SM. Assessments of the effects of nutrition on mental development and behavior in Jamaican studies. Am J Clin Nutr 1993; 57: 303S–309S.

44. Hertzig ME, Birch HG, Richardson SA, Tizard J. Intellectual levels of school children severely malnourished during the first two years of life. Pediatrics 1972; 49:814–24.

45. Richardson SA, Birch HG, Grabie E, Yoder K. The behavior of children in school who were severely malnourished in the first two years of life. J Health Soc Behav 1972; 13:276–84.

46. Stoch MB, Smythe PM, Moodie AD, Bradshaw D. Psychosocial outcome and CT findings after gross undernourishment during infancy: a 20-year developmental study. Dev Med Child Neurol 1982; 24:419–36.

47. Drewett RF, Corbett SS, Wright CM. Cognitive and educational attainments at school age of children who failed to thrive in infancy: a population-based study. J Child Psychol Psychiatry 1999; 40:551–61.

48. Lloyd-Still JD, Hurwitz I, Wolff PH, Shwachman H. Intellectual development after severe malnutrition in infancy. Pediatrics 1974; 54:306–11.

49. Volpe JJ. Cognitive deficits in premature infants. N Engl J Med 1991; 325:276–8.

50. Hack M, Breslau N, Weissman B, Aram D, Klein N, Borawski E. Effect of very low birth weight and subnormal head size on cognitive abilities at school age. N Engl J Med 1991; 325:231–7.

51. Teplin SW, Burchinal M, Johnson-Martin N, Humphry RA, Kraybill EN. Neurodevelopmental, health, and growth status at age 6 years of children with birth weights less than 1001 grams. J Pediatr 1991; 118: 768–77.

52. Paz I, Laor A, Gale R, Harlap S, Stevenson DK, Seidman DS. Term infants with fetal growth restriction are not at increased risk for low intelligence scores at age 17 years. J Pediatr 2001; 138:87–91.

53. Leitner Y, Fattal-Valevski A, Geva R, et al. Six-year follow-up of children with intrauterine growth retardation: long-term, prospective study. J Child Neurol 2000; 15:781–6.

54. Harvey D, Prince J, Bunton J, Parkinson C, Campbell S. Abilities of children who were small-for-gestational-age babies. Pediatrics 1982; 69:296–300.

55. Hack M, Klein NK, Taylor HG. Long-term developmental outcomes of low birth weight infants. Future Child 1995; 5:176–96.

56. Barker DJ. The long-term outcome of retarded fetal growth. Schweiz Med Wochenschr 1999; 129:189–96.

57. Villar J, Smeriglio V, Martorell R, Brown CH, Klein RE. Heterogeneous growth and mental development of intrauterine growth-retarded infants during the first 3 years of life. Pediatrics 1984; 74:783–91.

58. Sommerfelt K, Markestad T, Ellertsen B. Neuropsychological performance in low birth weight preschoolers: a population-based, controlled study. Eur J Pediatr 1998; 157:53–8.

59. Cravioto J, Delicardie ER. Mental performance in school age children. Findings after recovery from early severe malnutrition. Am J Dis Child 1970; 120:404–10.

60. Cravioto J, Delicardie ER. The relation of size at birth and preschool clinical severe malnutrition. Acta Paediatr Scand 1974; 63:577–80.

61. Zenel JA. Failure to thrive: a general pediatrician's perspective. Pediatr Rev 1997; 18:371–8.

62. Skuse D, Pickles A, Wolke D, Reilly S. Post-natal growth and mental development: evidence for a "sensitive" period. J Child Psychol Psychiatry 1994; 35:521–45.

63. Evans DE, Moodie AD, Hansen JDL. Kwashiorkor and intellectual development. South Afr Med J 1971; 45:1413–26.

64. Rask-Nissila L, Jokinen E, Terho P, et al. Effects of diet on the neurologic development of children at 5 years of age: the STRIP project. J Pediatr 2002; 140:328–33.

65. Benitez-Bribesca L, Rosa-Alvarez I, Mansilla-Olivares A. Dendritic spine pathology in infants with severe protein-calorie malnutrition. Pediatrics 1999; 104:e21.

66. Pollitt E. Behavior of infant in causation of nutritional marasmus. Am J Clin Nutr 1973; 26:264–70.

67. Suskind RM, Olson LC, Olson RE. Protein calorie malnutrition and infection with hepatitis-associated antigen. Pediatrics 1973; 51:525–30.

68. Stiehm ER. Humoral immunity in malnutrition. Fed Proc 1980; 39:3093–7.

69. Chandra RK. Nutrition and the immune system from birth to old age. Eur J Clin Nutr 2002; 56:S73–6.

70. Chevalier P, Sevilla R, Sejas E, Zalles L, Belmonte G, Parent G. Immune recovery of malnourished children takes longer than nutritional recovery: implications for treatment and discharge. J Trop Pediatr 1998; 44:304–7.

71. McMurray DN, Watson RR, Reyes MA. Effect of renutrition on humoral and cell-mediated immunity in severely malnourished children. Am J Clin Nutr 1981; 34:2117–26.

72. Golden MHN. Is complete catch-up possible for stunted malnourished children? Eur J Clin Nutrit 1994; 48:S58–71.

73. Galler JR, Ross RN. Malnutrition and Mental Development. The Post (Parent Network for the Post-Institutionalized Child), 1998; 20:1–7. Meadowlands, PA.

74. Walker SP, Golden MH. Growth in length of children recovering from severe malnutrition. Eur J Clin Nutr 1988; 42:395–404.

75. Lien NM, Meyer KK, Winick M. Early malnutrition and "late" adoption: a study of their effects on the development of Korean orphans adopted into American families. Am J Clin Nutr 1977; 30:1734–9.

76. Tenhola S, Martikainen A, Rahiala E, Parviainen M, Halonen P, Voutilainen R. Increased adrenocortical and adrenomedullary hormonal activity in 12-year-old children born small for gestational age. J Pediatr 2002; 141:477–82.

77. Meeks Gardner J, Grantham-McGregor SM, Chang SM, Himes JH, Powell CA. Activity and behavioral development in stunted and nonstunted children and response to nutritional supplementation. Child Dev 1995; 66:1785–97.

78. Porikos KP, Van Itallie TB. Diet-induced changes in serum transaminase and triglyceride levels in healthy adult men. Role of sucrose and excess calories. Am J Med 1983; 75:624–30.

79. Sibille M, Durieu I, Durand DV. Elevated liver enzymes in asymptomatic patients. N Engl J Med 2000; 343:662, discussion 663.

80. O'Keeffe MJ, O'Callaghan M, Williams GM, Najman JM, Bor W. Learning, cognitive, and attentional problems in adolescents born small for gestational age. Pediatrics 2003; 112:301–7.

81. Ment LR, Vohr B, Allan W, et al. Change in cognitive function over time in very low-birth-weight infants. JAMA 2003; 289:705–11.

82. Latal-Hajnal B, von Siebenthal K, Kovari H, Bucher HU, Largo RH. Postnatal growth in VLBW infants: significant association with neurodevelopmental outcome. J Pediatr 2003; 143:163–70.

83. Colombo M, de la Parra A, Lopez I. Intellectual and physical outcome of children undernourished in early life is influenced by later environmental conditions. Dev Med Child Neurol 1992; 34:611–22.

84. Korner J, Leibel RL. To eat of not to eat—how the gut talks to the brain. N Engl J Med 2003; 349:926–30.

11

MICRONUTRIENT
DEFICIENCIES

Micronutrients are essential for the healthy development of young children. Micronutrient deficiencies, common throughout the world, impair growth, development, behavior, and health. Because most micronutrient deficiencies accompany protein-energy malnutrition and environmental deprivation, it is difficult to isolate the effects of single-nutrient deficiencies. Some occur in the absence of malnutrition and may be overlooked.

Internationally adopted children have many risk factors for micronutrient deficiencies (Table 11–1). However, precise diagnosis may be difficult or impossible after their arrival in the United States. By then most children have already enjoyed several weeks of improved nutrition in the care of their adoptive parents while awaiting completion of legal proceedings in their birth country. Nonetheless, some micronutrient deficiencies have long-lasting effects on growth, behavior, or cognition. Many

international adoptees have problems in these areas, possibly a result of micronutrient deficiencies suffered in early life. This chapter reviews the initial and long-term effects of deficiencies of iron, iodine, zinc, vitamin A, and several other micronutrients.

Iron Deficiency

Iron deficiency is perhaps the most common disease on earth, afflicting more than 2 billion people. The World Health Organization estimates that about 25% of the world's children have iron deficiency anemia; many more are iron deficient. In deprived populations, as many as 45% of children have iron deficiency anemia.[5] An even larger percentage of children under age 5 years may be affected. Iron is essential for normal brain growth, cell differentiation, protein synthesis, hormone production, and cellular energy metabolism. Brain cells require iron for cellular

Table 11–1 Risk factors for micronutrient deficiencies in internationally adopted children

Risk Factor	Resulting Micronutrient Deficiency
Poor prenatal care	Iron, folate, iodine
Toxic exposures in utero	
Alcohol	Zinc[1]
Radiation	Iodine
Low birth weight	Vitamin A, vitamin E, iron, folate[2]
Lack of breast feeding	Water-soluble vitamins[3]
Deficient diet	
Hypocaloric	Protein-energy malnutrition
Deficient micronutrients	Specific deficiencies
Early introduction or overreliance on cow's milk	Iron
Medications	Vitamin K, niacin, vitamin B_6, folate
Intestinal parasites	Iron
Recurrent diarrhea	Zinc, vitamin A, folate, vitamin B_{12}, copper
Chronic infections (e.g., tuberculosis)	Iron, zinc, vitamin A[4]
Lack of sun exposure	Vitamin D

oxidative and synthetic processes, and production and catabolism of neurotransmitters.[6] Thus it is not surprising that children with iron deficiency anemia have developmental delays.

Iron Deficiency and Internationally Adopted Children

Internationally adopted children are particularly susceptible to iron deficiency. Many are low birth weight. Few birth mothers have adequate prenatal care; many likely have iron deficiency anemia. Prolonged bottle feeding is common in institutions, with late introduction of weaning foods (see Chapter 2). Infant foods and formulas available in orphanage diets often lack iron fortification; meat or other iron-rich foods may not be provided. Tea (often given to children in orphanages), cereals, and legumes contain phytates and phenols, which may inhibit iron absorption. Some children have con-

current lead poisoning (see Chapter 24), although iron deficiency is an independent risk factor for reduced Mental Development Index scores, and on a global basis probably has more severe developmental consequences.[7] Some children have pathologic blood loss due to intestinal parasites (especially the hookworms *Necator americanus* and *Ancylostoma duodenale*), *Helicobacter pylori*–induced gastritis, or urinary schistosomiasis[8,9] (see Chapters 17 and 20). Infection and low body weight greatly increase the risk of anemia (by 51% and 21%, respectively, in Honduran children).[10] The prevalence of anemia varies considerably among different reports of international adoptees, depending on definition, ages, and countries of origin of the children studied (Table 11–2; see Chapter 23).

Developmental Delays

Iron deficiency anemia in newborns and infants is linked to reduced cognitive performance,[18–20] which persists to later childhood.[21–23] For example, iron-deficient infants 19–24 months old are delayed in language, vocalization, social contact, active vocabulary, and eye–hand coordination.[24] Six- to 12-year-old Mexican children with iron deficiency (but not anemia) scored significantly lower on the Wechsler Intelligence Scales for Children for information, comprehension, verbal performance, and full-scale IQ,

Table 11–2 Anemia in international adoptees

Country of Origin (N)	Adoptees with Anemia (%)
Mixed, mostly Korea (293)[11]	2.3[a]
Mixed, mostly Korea (128)[12]	3.4[a]
Mostly Africa and Indian Ocean countries (68)[13]	8.8[a]
Mostly Korea and India (100)[14]	12
India (200)[15]	18.5[a]
Mixed (129)[16]	31[a]
China (452)[17]	35

[a]Differentiation of iron deficiency from other causes of anemia not indicated. Definitions of anemia varied among studies.

and had slower EEG activity.[25] Iron-deficient American adolescents, with or without anemia, have poorer math achievement scores[26] than their iron-replete classmates.

Alterations in mood, affect, and motivation have also been attributed to iron deficiency: iron-deficient infants appear unhappy, tense, fearful, or withdrawn, and older children seem less attentive (reviewed in Pollitt[27]). Although other nutritional or social factors contribute to these findings,[28] iron deficiency is undoubtably a key element.

The reversibility of these problems is uncertain. In a 1978 study of 24 infants with iron deficiency anemia, Bayley Scale of Infant Mental Development scores improved ~13.6 points 1 week after treatment with parenteral iron. The children had improved alertness, responsiveness, and gross and fine motor coordination.[29] Older children studied in Indonesia improved their cognitive processes, visual attention,[30] mental, and motor scores[31] after iron repletion. However, other studies demonstrate persistent developmental problems even after correction of iron deficiency. For example, Guatemalan 5-year-olds who had been briefly iron deficient as infants (hemoglobin ≤100 grams/liter) had lower mental and motor scores even after their growth and hematologic status normalized.[23] Similarly, Israeli second-graders who had been anemic in infancy had lower learning achievement scores than those of matched peers without history of anemia.[21] Likewise, well-nourished Costa Rican 11- to 14-year-olds who had been severely iron deficient in infancy had lower mental and motor scores, specifically in arithmetic, written expression, motor function, spatial memory, and selective recall. More of the previously anemic children had repeated a grade or were referred for special services. Parents and teachers rated their behavior as more problematic in several areas, including increased anxiety and depression, diminished social skills, and poor attention spans.[22] Similarly, former WIC participants (Women, Infants, Children—a dietary supplementation program for low-income women and their children in the United States) were more likely to have mild or moderate mental retardation at 10 years of age if they had been anemic in early life.[32] This finding was independent of other risk factors.[32] Finally, first-graders who had been anemic at 6–18 months had lower IQ scores and more "soft" neurologic signs.[33]

Thus, iron deficiency during infancy has long-lasting effects on cognitive function.[21] This may be mediated by the reduction in noradrenaline, serotonin, and dopamine levels in iron deficiency, and ensuing decreases in attention and arousal.[34] In animal models, early iron deficiency irreversibly alters brain iron content and distribution, resulting in changes in neurotransmitters, behavior,[18] and responses to stress.[35] Iron deficiency also prolongs auditory brain stem conduction time, suggesting that myelin synthesis is to some extent iron dependent.[36] Thus iron deficiency is detrimental to brain development in ways similar to more global malnutrition.[36]

Clinical Findings in Iron Deficiency

Anemia is a late manifestation of iron deficiency. Earlier findings include reduction in serum ferritin, followed by reduction in serum iron levels, increased iron binding capacity, and reduced transferrin saturation. Reduced mean cell volume, hemoglobin, and hematocrit appear only after tissue iron stores are markedly depleted. Spoon nail deformities, glossitis, and congestive heart failure signal severe iron deficiency.

Treatment

Newly adopted children benefit from iron-fortified cereals and formulas. Intake of iron-rich foods (meat, spinach, beans, peas) should be encouraged. Cow's milk should be limited to 16 ounces daily in the second year of life, and indeed should be given only to children with adequate growth (see Chapter 10) who are lactose tolerant (see Chapter 28). Iron-enriched formulas are preferred for underweight children <36 months. Additional iron supplements should be prescribed for anemic children. Poor response to iron supplementation may reflect concurrent deficiencies of vitamins A, E, or B$_{12}$,[37] or a hemoglobinopathy (see Chapter 23).

Zinc Deficiency

Clinical zinc deficiency was first recognized more than 40 years ago among children with short stature and pubertal delay. Since then, zinc deficiency has been implicated in growth and developmental delays, cognitive deficits,[38] attention-deficit hyperactivity disorder (ADHD), and immune dysfunction. Even marginal zinc deficiency may cause problems. The prevalence of zinc deficiency in developing countries is unknown, but is estimated to affect anywhere from 5% to 60% of children worldwide.[39,40] Children at risk include those whose diets lack meat, shellfish, or poultry, or those who consume foods high in phytates or fiber (such as legumes or cereals) which inhibit zinc absorption. Such diets are typical in orphanages throughout the world. Reduced dietary intake of zinc-containing foods is rapidly followed by zinc deficiency.[41] Zinc deficiency has not been specifically identified in internationally adopted children, but likely is present in some.

Measurement of plasma or serum zinc is widely used to detect zinc deficiency, although this method may not accurately assess total body zinc stores. Circulating levels of zinc, like iron, are reduced during the acute-phase response.[42] Thus interpretation of zinc levels during infection is problematic. Some investigators instead measure hair zinc levels, or use indirect methods such as tests of taste acuity, mental concentration, short-term memory, and cell-mediated immunity, and estimates of dietary consumption.[43] The clinical response to supplemental zinc is sometimes used to diagnose zinc deficiency.

The clinical signs of severe zinc deficiency are nonspecific,[44] such as hepatosplenomegaly, irritability, and diarrhea.[45] Cutaneous manifestations include erythematous, scaly, vesiculobullous rashes around the eyes, nose, mouth, and perineum, angular stomatitis, alopecia, and poor wound healing.[45]

Growth Delays

Zinc is an important cofactor for DNA, RNA, and protein synthesis. Zinc is also involved in regulation of gene expression and hormone synthesis (including growth hormone, androgens, and thyroid hormone[39,41,46]). Thus it is not surprising that zinc deficiency is associated with growth delays. Some of the evidence for this connection is indirect. For example, zinc supplements improved weight gain in infants with nutritional failure to thrive.[47] Furthermore, French children with marginal zinc status had low weight for height[48] and delayed somatic growth and pubertal development, without other obvious explanations.[49] More recently, moderate zinc deficiency was found in a group of short Japanese boys without endocrine abnormalities. After supplementation with oral zinc, the boys improved their caloric intake and growth velocity, as well as a number of biochemical measures (serum zinc, calcium, and phosphorus concentrations, alkaline phosphatase activity, tubular reabsorption of phosphorus, serum osteocalcin, and plasma insulin-like growth factor-1). Urinary excretion of growth hormone did not change during the study, which suggests that the effects of zinc supplementation were not mediated via this pathway.[50]

Among severely malnourished children, zinc deficiency may specifically limit growth. Supplemental zinc improved weight gain by ~75% in malnourished children during nutritional rehabilitation in Bangladesh,[51] Ethiopia,[52] and Guatemala.[43] However, deficient stores of zinc are not universally found in malnourished populations,[53] and zinc supplementation does not always improve growth.[54]

Susceptibility to Infection

In the developing world, zinc deficiency is strongly associated with increased susceptibility to infections and prolonged recovery time from infections. Children residing in institutional settings frequently suffer from recurrent infections; the possible contribution of zinc deficiency has not been investigated. Zinc is necessary for the development and function of neutrophils, natural killer cells, B cells, and macrophages. Repeated infections undoubtably contribute to poor growth; some of the favorable effects of zinc supplementation on growth may result from reduced frequency or severity of infections. Intestinal parasites are better able to survive in zinc-deficient hosts, as shown in a mouse model.[55] In children, zinc deficiency is associated with increased risk of serious infectious diseases such as diarrhea, pneumonia, and malaria.[56] Even 3 months after recovery from acute diarrhea, plasma zinc levels in Indian children correlated with morbidity from diarrheal and respiratory disease.[57] Stool losses of zinc during diarrhea further exacerbate zinc deficiency and contribute to poor growth.[58] Dietary supplementation with zinc reduces the severity and duration of diarrheal episodes[56] and other infections,[54] especially in children with stunted growth.[59] Zinc supplementation may also reduce the incidence of dysentery, pneumonia, and mortality.[60–63] Zinc supplements improved the linear growth of stunted Ethiopian infants, possibly via reduction of anorexia and decreased morbidity from intercurrent illnesses (cough, diarrhea, fever, vomiting).[52]

Cognitive Delays

The effects of zinc deficiency on cognition vary depending on the severity and age at which it occurs. In animal models, severe zinc deficiency during pregnancy is associated with structural brain abnormalities in offspring, such as anencephaly, microcephaly, or hydrocephaly. Less severe zinc deficiency during pregnancy results in impaired learning, reduced attention, and poor memory in offspring in mice, rats, or monkeys.[64] Other animal models of zinc deficiency demonstrate behavioral problems, impaired responses to stress, reduced activity, deficits in short-term memory and spatial learning, and difficulty in re-

taining previously learned visual discrimination problems and learning new problems.[65] Children appear particularly vulnerable to the cognitive effects of zinc deficiency during periods of rapid growth. Guatemalan infants given zinc supplements were more physically active than those given placebo, and less likely to cry or whine.[66] Likewise, healthy Chinese first-graders given supplemental zinc performed better on neuropsychological tests (continuous performance, perception, and visual memory) than those given other micronutrients alone.[67] Children given zinc plus other micronutrients outperformed those given either supplement alone.[68]

Zinc is a cofactor for the metabolism of neurotransmitters, fatty acids, prostaglandins, and melatonin. Therefore, some investigators speculate that zinc may play a role in the pathophysiology and treatment of ADHD. Indirect evidence for this relationship includes the hyperactivity and behavior abnormalities seen in animal models of zinc deficiency.[69] Furthermore, several reports indicate that children with ADHD have lower serum zinc levels than those of controls.[69,70] Response to pharmacologic treatment of ADHD is also influenced by zinc status.[71] A role for zinc in learning disabilities was indirectly suggested by the finding that dyslexic British children had lower zinc concentrations in their sweat than healthy controls.[72] Curiously, children with fetal alcohol syndrome (FAS) have relative zinc deficiency due to increased urinary zinc clearance.[1] The relationship of this to the dysmorphic features and other clinical manifestations of FAS is unknown (see Chapter 5).

Iodine

Iodine deficiency is the most common cause of preventable mental retardation[73] worldwide; more than 1 billion people are at risk.[74] Many internationally adopted children come from regions with reduced consumption of iodized salt and endemic iodine deficiency (Fig. 11–1). 10% of children adopted from China have mildly abnormal thyroid function on arrival to the

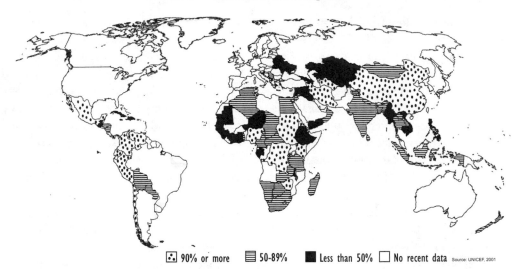

Figure 11–1 *Iodine deficiency is endemic throughout the world. Map shows percentage of households consuming iodized salt. (From UNICEF, 2001. This map does not reflect a position by UNICEF on the legal status of any country or territory or the delimitation of any frontiers.)*

United States.[17] Among affected populations, iodine deficiency reduces the mean IQ by 10–15 points. Iodine deficiency disorders include goiter, endemic cretinism, psychomotor delay, and increased perinatal mortality. The link between maternal hypothyroidism caused by iodine deficiency during pregnancy and mental retardation in the child is well established: both maternal and fetal thyroid function are affected. Borderline maternal thyroid function during pregnancy (even in the absence of iodine deficiency) results in permanent neuropsychologic dysfunction in the child.[75] Even transient hypothyroidism in infancy may have devastating long-term effects on neurologic outcome.[76] A Russian survey reported that 5.3% of neonates in Saratov region of Russia (452 miles southeast of Moscow) had transient hypothyroidism.[77]

The thyroid status of birth mothers of internationally adopted children is unknown. Obvious signs of iodine deficiency are found in ~24% of pregnant women in Indian slums[78] (15% had iron deficiency anemia as well). In several European countries that lack national standards for iodination of salt, as many as 18%

of teenage girls have goiter.[79,80] Country-specific information about iodine deficiency is readily available.[81]

Clinical Iodine Deficiency

Children born and raised in iodine-deficient areas generally have reduced intellectual capacity compared to children residing in iodine-sufficient areas, as reported from China,[82] Iran,[83] Sikkim,[84] India,[85] and Tuscany.[86] Specific deficits include reduced motivation and achievement,[85] delayed reaction time,[86] poor visuomotor coordination, and reduced IQ (IQ <70 in 21%–72%).[82,84] In one study, impaired language, memory, conceptual thinking, numerical reasoning, and motor skills were found in >80% of children with iodine deficiency.[84] Some children also have nerve deafness, spasticity, and pyramidal signs.[82] However, intellectual deficits do not occur in all iodine-deficient areas, as reported from Nigeria[87] and Malaysia.[88] In these regions, the effects of iodine deficiency may be masked by other problems that also affect IQ.

Intervention studies conducted in iodine-deficient regions where iodine supplements are given to pregnant women or directly to children generally show improved intellectual capacity among treated subjects (Benin[89] and Ecuador[90]). However, some studies fail to demonstrate improvement after supplementation, suggesting that other factors contribute to performance or that intervention treatments were insufficient or offered too late[74,82,91] to benefit the subjects.

Although iodine deficiency is a serious concern, in some regions iodine excess is more problematic. Chinese children from high-iodine areas have lower IQs than children from control areas.[92] These areas also have high fluorine; 73% of children also had dental fluorosis.

Iodine and Radiation

Some internationally adopted children come from regions where pre- or postnatal exposure to radiation is possible (see Chapter 24). Although radiation exposure in utero or during young childhood increases the risk of later thyroid disorders, the effects cannot be separated from concurrent iodine deficiency, as shown in Lithuania,[93] Chernobyl,[94] and the Marshall Islands.[95] Prenatal exposure to radiation may have other effects as well. Children exposed prenatally to radiation in Chernobyl had relative psychological impairment, more speech–language disorders and emotional problems, lower mean IQ scores, and more cases of borderline IQ than a "non-contaminated control group" at age 6–7 or 10–11 years. However, the effects of radiation exposure could not be separated from the coincident social disruption[96] and possible exposure to other contaminants. Radiation exposure of mothers in Chernobyl correlates with vitamin A and E deficiencies in their children[97] (management of children with possible radiation exposure prior to adoption is discussed in Chapter 24).

Iodine and Selenium Deficiency

Iodine deficiency sometimes occurs in combination with selenium deficiency.[98] Both elements are involved in thyroid hormone production, the structural integrity of glutathione peroxidase,[99] and other metabolic pathways. Deficiencies of selenium and iodine coexist in the same geographic regions, most notably China, Siberia, Korea, and Central Africa, and, to a lesser extent, South America.[100] Many international adoptees arrive from these areas. Selenium deficiency has been implicated in the pathogenesis of two diseases, Keshan disease (cardiomyopathy)[101] and Kashin-Beck disease (osteonecrosis of long-bone epiphyses, short stature),[102–104] although other factors contribute to disease expression. The onset of bony changes of Kashin-Beck disease can be as young as 4 years.[105] These diseases are endemic in some areas of China and Russia, the major sending countries for international adoption. Selenium deficiency also causes anemia,[106] and has variable effects on the neurologic complications of iodine deficiency.[73]

Vitamin Deficiencies

Vitamin A

Vitamin A is another vital micronutrient. It is essential to the function of retinal photoreceptors necessary for vision. Xerophthalmia due to vitamin A deficiency is the major cause of blindness in children worldwide.[107] Vitamin A is also necessary for the growth and differentiation of epithelial cells and hematopoietic cells, especially CD4 cells in lymph nodes, thymus, and spleen. Vitamin A deficiency impairs the mucosal immune responses in respiratory and gastrointestinal tracts, especially in undernourished children.[108] Children with vitamin A deficiency have poorer immunoglobulin G (IgG) responses to tetanus toxoid, lower CD4/CD8 ratios, and abnormal distribution of circulating T cells.[109] Vitamin A deficiency markedly increases the mortality of measles infection[110] and increases susceptibility to diarrhea and respiratory diseases.[109]

Vitamin A status relates to undernutrition,[111] as well as history of diarrhea, measles, and acute respiratory infections.[112] Fat malabsorption or prolonged poor dietary intake contributes to vitamin A deficiency. Infection increases the risk of subclinical vitamin A deficiency (serum retinol level <20 μg/dl) more than threefold.[10] All of these factors may affect children residing in orphanages. Not surprisingly, vitamin A deficiency often coexists with iron deficiency,[8,9] zinc deficiency, and malnutrition. Caregiver behaviors may contribute to vitamin A and other dietary deficiencies. In one study, vitamin A–deficient Nepali children were treated more harshly or neglected and were given less encouragement to eat and fewer offers of food by their caregivers than their vitamin A–sufficient siblings.[113] These caregiver behaviors may be applicable to children living in institutional care as well.

Newborns have limited stores of vitamin A; premies have almost none. Vitamin A deficiency usually becomes apparent between 36 and 72 months of age.[114] The incidence of subclinical vitamin A deficiency ranges from 6% to 46% in Panama,[115] El Salvador,[115] Honduras,[10] India,[112,116] Vietnam,[5] and Bangladesh.[8] Many more children have borderline levels.

Night blindness, xerophthalmia (xerosis of conjunctivae and cornea, Bitot's spots [superficial foamy gray triangular spots on conjuctiva, consisting of keratinized epithelium; Fig. 11–2], and corneal ulcerations), follicular hyperkeratosis, corkscrew hairs, and poor growth are signs of vitamin A deficiency.[45] In vulnerable populations, such as certain regions of Ethiopia, xerophthalmia can affect as many as 53% of individuals.[114]

Vitamin A supplements improve growth and sometimes anemia[117] in stunted children,[5]

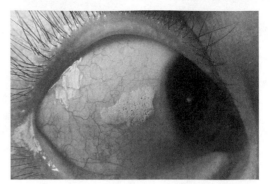

Figure 11–2 *Ophthalmologic findings in xero-ophthalmia associated with vitamin A deficiency include xerosis of conjunctivae and cornea, Bitot's spots (superficial foamy gray triangular spots on conjuctiva, consisting of keratinized epithelium), and corneal ulcerations. (From Sight and Life, TALC, with permission.)*

especially those with lower serum retinol levels at baseline.[111] Stunted children given multiple micronutrient supplements in addition to vitamin A had the most improved growth.[5,117] A recent meta-analysis of vitamin A supplementation suggests that this treatment offers no protective effect on the incidence of diarrhea and slightly increases the incidence of respiratory tract infection.[118] However, some studies in the meta-analysis included healthy children without signs of vitamin A deficiency.

Vitamin E

Vitamin E deficiency is rare, but can occur with protein energy malnutrition. In this situation, vitamin E is critical for normal neurologic structure and function. Serious neurologic signs such as fine motor incoordination, ataxia, weakness, hyporeflexia, impaired vision, pigment retinopathy, delayed somatosensory conduction, and reduced amplitude of electroretinograms are more common in malnourished children with concurrent vitamin E deficiency.[119,120] Premature infants or children with fat malabsorption are particularly susceptible to vitamin E deficiency.[45]

Vitamin D

Vitamin D deficiency is discussed in Chapter 25.

Vitamin C

Vitamin C deficiency, or scurvy, is rare in international adoptees. Unusual dietary intake can occur in some institutionalized children because of behavioral problems, presumed "allergies," or unavailability of particular nutrients. Children with scurvy present with malaise, nausea, and hemorrhagic rash on the extremities (which may be subtle). Long-bone radiographs show subperiosteal hemorrhages (Fig. 11–3).

Franny, born at 1700 grams, was adopted at age 18 months from Sochi, Russia (on the Black Sea). Her mom reported that the orphanage diet seemed to consist totally of fish, with no dairy products, fruits, or vegetables offered. Franny had prominent radial heads, 15° genu valgus, rachitic rosary, and frontal bossing. She was unable to stand independently. Three weeks after arrival in the United States, laboratory test results included alkaline phosphatase 2355, with normal calcium, phosphorus, and parathyroid hormone. Skeletal survey for vitamin deficiency showed evidence of scurvy in addition to rickets (Fig. 11–3).

Vitamin B$_{12}$

Vitamin B$_{12}$ deficiency is a rare cause of failure to thrive and developmental delay. Strict vegetarian diet, intestinal bacterial overgrowth, or parasitic infection (among other causes) may result in vitamin B$_{12}$ deficiency, especially in children whose mothers were deficient during pregnancy. Children present with irritability, weakness, vomiting, lethargy, and hypotonia. Some have tremors, twitches, chorea, or myoclonus.

Multiple Micronutrient Deficiencies

In the real world, micronutrient deficiencies rarely occur in isolation. Micronutrients interact in various biochemical pathways; their absorption, regulation, and metabolism are linked. For example, zinc levels are lower in patients with iron deficiency anemia.[121] Furthermore, most micronutrient deficiencies occur in the context of generalized malnutrition or undernutrition. Deficiency of multiple micronutrients may interfere with responses to supplementation with a single micronutrient.[68] Short children given both zinc and iron supplements improve their growth velocity.[122] Furthermore, vitamin A levels improve in children given supplemental iron, zinc, or both.[123] Vitamin A and iron deficiency often coexist. Vitamin A supplementation may improve iron absorption and mobilization of iron from tissue stores.

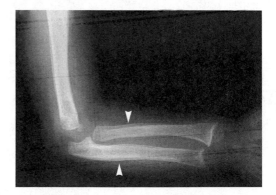

Figure 11–3 *Radiograph of long bones of child with scurvy. Subperiosteal hemorrhages (arrow) result in periosteal elevation. Epiphyseal spurs are common.*

Key Points for Internationally Adopted Children

- Internationally adopted children are at risk for multiple micronutrient deficiencies.
- Micronutrient deficiencies contribute to growth and developmental delays, behavioral problems, and increased susceptibility to infection.
- Deficiencies of iron, zinc, and iodine are most common among international adoptees.
- Iron and iodine deficiencies require careful treatment and monitoring.
- Most other micronutrient deficiencies respond to normal diet; however, some adverse effects of these deficiencies may persist even after treatment.

FAQs

Q. When children first arrive from the orphanage, so many of them have thin, fine hair. Is this a sign of a specific micronutrient deficiency? And what should I do about it?

A. The typical "orphanage hair" is sign of poor nutritional status, but rarely is a single micronutrient at fault. A multivitamin and mineral preparation is reasonable to offer. Younger children taking adequate volumes of vitamin and trace mineral–fortified formula probably don't need supplements.

Q. What guidelines should be used to treat iron deficiency?

A. Iron stores should be replaced quickly. Supplemental iron (3–4 mg/kg per day in two divided doses) is well tolerated and well absorbed. The dose should reflect the degree of anemia (lower dose for hemoglobin >9). Multivitamins with iron have little role in managing the anemic child; the amount of iron is inadequate to correct iron deficiency.[124] With compliance, hemoglobin should be normal within 4–6 weeks. Don't forget to check carefully for intestinal parasites and other causes of iron (blood) loss, as well as for lead poisoning.

Q. My patient has intractable diarrhea but otherwise seems healthy. Could he have zinc deficiency?

A. The long list of causes of diarrhea includes zinc deficiency. Antecedent malnutrition, vitamin A deficiency, intestinal infection with bacterial or other pathogens (including cryptosporidium), and bovine milk sensitivity[125] can all lead to persistent diarrhea in the international adoptee and should be considered. If all else is excluded, it may be worth a brief trial of zinc supplementation.

Q. A 15-month-old in our practice just arrived from China and broke out with measles! Should I prescribe vitamin A?

A. Supplements should certainly be considered if the child is young and severely ill. Current recommendations are 200,000 IU orally for children 1 year of age and older, and 100,000 IU orally for children 6–12 months of age. Children with ophthalmologic evidence of vitamin A deficiency should be retreated the next day and again 4 weeks later.[126,127]

Q. It seems very common to find odd thyroid test results in my newly arrived patients. Some have elevations of both T4 and TSH. What does it all mean?

A. It's not always clear how to interpret these results. As many children come from areas with endemic iodine deficiency, it is possible that these abnormal thyroid function tests reflect recovery from iodine deficiency and adaptation to an iodine-replete diet. In other cases, recovery from protein-energy malnutrition has affected the thyroid-binding globulin level, resulting in odd test results. It's very important to follow up abnormal test results; occasionally you will identify a child who is developing thyroid insufficiency.

Resources

International Council for the Control of Iodine Deficiency Disorders. Communication Focal Point. Available at: http://www.tulane.edu/~icec/iddcomm.htm.

U.S. Agency for International Development. MOST—The USAID Micronutrient Program. Available at: http://www.mostproject.org/index.htm.

Opportunities for Micronutrient Interventions (OMNI). Available at: http://www.jsi.com/intl/omni/home#language.

Australian Iron Status Advisory Panel. Australian medical group with interest in iron disorders; good flow charts for diagnosis and treatment. Available at: http://www.ironpanel.org.au/AIS/AISdocs/index.html.

References

1. Assadi FK, Ziai M. Zinc status of infants with fetal alcohol syndrome. Pediatr Res 1986; 20:551–4.

2. Rondo PH, Abbott R, Rodrigues LC, Tomkins AM. Vitamin A, folate, and iron concentrations in cord and maternal blood of intra-uterine growth retarded and appropriate birth weight babies. Eur J Clin Nutr 1995; 49:391–9.

3. Allen LH. Maternal micronutrient malnutrition: effects on breast milk and infant nutrition, and priorities for intervention. SCN News 1994; 11:21–4.

4. Karyadi E, Schultink W, Nelwan RH, et al. Poor micronutrient status of active pulmonary tuberculosis patients in Indonesia. J Nutr 2000; 130:2953–8.

5. Thu BD, Schultink W, Dillon D, Gross R, Leswara ND, Khoi HH. Effect of daily and weekly micronutrient supplementation on micronutrient deficiencies and growth in young Vietnamese children. Am J Clin Nutr 1999; 69:80–6.

6. Beard J. One person's view of iron deficiency, development, and cognitive function. Am J Clin Nutr 1995; 62:709–10.

7. Wasserman G, Graziano JH, Factor-Litvak P, et al. Independent effects of lead exposure and iron deficiency anemia on developmental outcome at age 2 years. J Pediatr 1992; 121:695–703.

8. Persson V, Ahmed F, Gebre-Medhin M, Greiner T. Relationships between vitamin A, iron status and helminthiasis in Bangladeshi school children. Public Health Nutr 2000; 3:83–9.

9. Olivares M, Walter T, Hertrampf E, Pizarro F. Anaemia and iron deficiency in children. Br Med Bull 1999; 55:534–43.

10. Nestel P, Melara A, Rosado J, Mora JO. Vitamin A deficiency and anemia among children 12–71 months old in Honduras. Rev Panam Salud Publica 1999; 6:34–43.

11. Hostetter MK, Iverson S, Thomas W, McKenzie D, Dole K, Johnson DE. Medical evaluation of internationally adopted children. N Engl J Med 1991; 325:479–85.

12. Jenista JA, Chapman D. Medical problems of foreign-born adopted children. Am J Dis Child 1987; 141:298–302.

13. Bureau JJ, Maurage C, Bremond M, Despert F, Rolland JC. Children of foreign origin adopted in France. Analysis of 68 cases during 12 years at the University Hospital Center of Tours [in French]. Arch Pediatr 1999; 6:1053–8.

14. Nicholson AJ, Francis BM, Mulholland EK, Moulden AL, Oberklaid F. Health screening of international adoptees. Evaluation of a hospital based clinic. Med J Aust 1992; 156:377–9.

15. Smith-Garcia T, Brown JS. The health of children adopted from India. J Community Health 1989; 14:227–41.

16. Miller LC, Kiernan MT, Mathers MI, Klein-Gitelman M. Developmental and nutritional status of internationally adopted children. Arch Pediatr Adolesc Med 1995; 149:40–4.

17. Miller LC, Hendrie NW. Health of children adopted from China. Pediatrics 2000; 105:E76.

18. Walter T. Effect of iron-deficiency anaemia on cognitive skills in infancy and childhood. Baillieres Clin Haematol 1994; 7:815–27.

19. Lozoff B, Brittenham GM, Viteri FE, Wolf AW, Urrutia JJ. The effects of short-term oral iron therapy on developmental deficits in iron-deficient anemic infants. J Pediatr 1982; 100:351–7.

20. Tasunenobu T, Goldenberg RL, Hou J, et al. Cord serum ferritin concentrations and mental and psychomotor development of children at five years of age. J Pediatr 2002; 140:165–70.

21. Palti H, Meijer A, Adler B. Learning achievement and behavior at school of anemic and non-anemic infants. Early Hum Dev 1985; 10:217–23.

22. Lozoff B, Jimenez E, Hagen J, Mollen E, Wolf AW. Poorer behavioral and developmental outcome more than 10 years after treatment for iron deficiency in infancy. Pediatrics 2000; 105:E51.

23. Lozoff B, Jimenez E, Wolf AW. Long-term developmental outcome of infants with iron deficiency. N Engl J Med 1991; 325:687–94.

24. Lozoff B, Brittenham GM, Viteri FE, Wolf AW, Urrutia JJ. Developmental deficits in iron-deficient infants: effects of age and severity of iron lack. J Pediatr 1982; 101:948–52.

25. Otero GA, Aguirre DM, Porcayo R, Fernandez T. Psychological and electroencephalographic study in school children with iron deficiency. Int J Neurosci 1999; 99:113–21.

26. Halterman JS, Kaczorowski JM, Aligne CA, Auinger P, Szilagyi PG. Iron deficiency and cognitive achievement among school-aged children and adolescents in the United States. Pediatrics 2001; 107:1381–6.

27. Pollitt E. Iron deficiency and cognitive function. Annu Rev Nutr 1993; 13:521–37.

28. Evans DI. Cerebral function in iron deficiency: a review. Child Care Health Dev 1985; 11:105–12.

29. Oski FA, Honig AS. The effects of therapy on the developmental scores of iron-deficient infants. J Pediatr 1978; 92:21–5.

30. Soewondo S. The effect of iron deficiency and mental stimulation on Indonesian children's cognitive performance and development. Kobe J Med Sci 1995; 41:1–17.

31. Idjradinata P, Pollitt E. Reversal of developmental delays in iron-deficient anaemic infants treated with iron. Lancet 1993; 341:1–4.

32. Hurtado EK, Claussen AH, Scott KG. Early childhood anemia and mild or moderate mental retardation. Am J Clin Nutr 1999; 69:115–9.

33. Cantwell RJ. The long-term neurological sequelae of anemia in infancy [abstract]. Pediatr Res 1978; 8:342.

34. Parks YA, Wharton BA. Iron deficiency and the brain. Acta Paediatr Scand Suppl 1989; 361:71–7.

35. Beard J, Connor JR, Jones BC. Iron in the brain. Nutr Rev 1993; 51:157–66.

36. Roncagliolo M, Garrido M, Walter T, Peirano P, Lozoff B. Evidence of altered central nervous system development in infants with iron deficiency anemia at 6 mo: delayed maturation of auditory brainstem responses. Am J Clin Nutr 1998; 68:683–90.

37. Allen LH, Rosado JL, Casterline JE, et al. Lack of hemoglobin response to iron supplementation in anemic Mexican preschoolers with multiple micronutrient deficiencies. Am J Clin Nutr 2000; 71:1485–94.

38. Castillo-Duran C, Cassorla F. Trace minerals in human growth and development. J Pediatr Endocrinol Metab 1999; 12:589–601.

39. Favier AE. Hormonal effects of zinc on growth in children. Biol Trace Elem Res 1992; 32:383–98.

40. Allen LH. Zinc and micronutrient supplements for children. Am J Clin Nutr 1998; 68 (Suppl):495S–8.

41. Ploysangam A, Falciglia GA, Brehm BJ. Effect of marginal zinc deficiency on human growth and development. J Trop Pediatr 1997; 43:192–8.

42. Brown KH. Effect of infections on plasma zinc concentration and implications for zinc status assessment in low-income countries. Am J Clin Nutr 1998; 68:425S–429S.

43. Prentice A. Does mild zinc deficiency contribute to poor growth performance? Nutr Rev 1993; 51:268–70.

44. Goskowicz M, Eichenfield LF. Cutaneous findings of nutritional deficiencies in children. Curr Opin Pediatr 1993; 5:441–5.

45. Balint JP. Physical findings in nutritional deficiencies. Pediatr Clin North Am 1998; 45:245–60.

46. Nishi Y. Zinc and growth. J Am Coll Nutr 1996; 15:340–4.

47. Walravens PA, Hambidge KM, Koepfer DM. Zinc supplementation in infants with a nutritional pattern of failure to thrive: a double-blind, controlled study. Pediatrics 1989; 83:532–8.

48. Chakar A, Mokni R, Walravens PA, et al. Plasma zinc and copper in Paris area preschool children with growth impairment. Biol Trace Elem Res 1993; 38:97–106.

49. Fons C, Brun JF, Fussellier M, Cassanas G, Bardet L, Orsetti A. Serum zinc and somatic growth in children with growth retardation. Biol Trace Elem Res 1992; 32:399–404.

50. Nakamura T, Nishiyama S, Futagoishi-Suginohara Y, Matsuda I, Higashi A. Mild to moderate zinc deficiency in short children: effect of zinc supplementation on linear growth velocity. J Pediatr 1993; 123:65–9.

51. Simmer K, Khanum S, Carlsson L, Thompson RP. Nutritional rehabilitation in Bangladesh—the importance of zinc. Am J Clin Nutr 1988; 47:1036–40.

52. Umeta M, West CE, Haidar J, Deurenberg P, Hautvast JG. Zinc supplementation and stunted infants in Ethiopia: a randomised controlled trial. Lancet 2000; 355:2021–6.

53. Takyi EE, Asibey-Berko E. Zinc nutritional status in preschool children in different communities in southern Ghana. East Afr Med J 1999; 76:13–8.

54. Rosado J, Lopez P, Munoz E, Martinez H, Allen LH. Zinc supplementation reduced morbidity, but neither zinc nor iron supplementation affected growth or body composition of Mexican preschoolers. Am J Clin Nutr 1997; 65:13–9.

55. Scott ME, Koski KG. Zinc deficiency impairs immune responses against parasitic nematode infections at intestinal and systemic sites. J Nutr 2000; 130: 1412S–20S.

56. Black RE. Therapeutic and preventive effects of zinc on serious childhood infectious diseases in developing countries. Am J Clin Nutr 1998; 68:476S–479S.

57. Bhandari N, Bahl R, Hambidge KM, Bhan MK. Increased diarrhoeal and respiratory morbidity in association with zinc deficiency—a preliminary report. Acta Paediatr 1996; 85:148–50.

58. Hambidge KM. Zinc and diarrhea. Acta Paediatr Suppl 1992; 381:82–6.

59. Sazawal S, Black RE, Bhan MK, Bhandari N, Sinha A, Jalla S. Zinc supplementation in young children with acute diarrhea in India. N Engl J Med 1995; 333:839–44.

60. Sazawal S, Black RE, Bhan MK, et al. Zinc supplementation reduces the incidence of persistent diarrhea and dysentery among low socioeconomic children in India. J Nutr 1996; 126:443–50.

61. Sazawal S, Black RE, Menon VP. Zinc supplementation in infants born small for gestational age reduces mortality: a prospective randomized, controlled trial. Pediatrics 2001; 108:1280–86.

62. Penny ME, Peerson JM, Marin M, et al. Randomized, community-based trial of the effect of zinc supplementation, with and without other micronutrients, on the duration of persistent childhood diarrhea in Lima, Peru. J Pediatr 1999; 135:208–17.

63. Zinc Investigators Collaborative Group. Prevention of diarrhea and pneumonia by zinc supplementation

in children in developing countries: pooled analysis of randomized controlled trials. J Pediatr 1999; 135:689–97.

64. Wasantwisut E. Nutrition and development: other micronutrients' effect on growth and cognition. Southeast Asian J Trop Med Public Health 1997; 28:78–82.

65. Black MM. Zinc deficiency and child development. Am J Clin Nutr 1998; 68:464S–469S.

66. Bentley ME, Caulfield LE, Ram M, et al. Zinc supplementation affects the activity patterns of rural Guatemalan infants. J Nutr 1997; 127:1333–8.

67. Penland JC, Sandstead HH, Alcock NW, et al. A preliminary report: effects of zinc and micronutrient repletion on growth and neuropsychological function of urban Chinese children. J Am Coll Nutr 1997; 16:268–72.

68. Sandstead HH, Penland JC, Alcock NW, et al. Effects of repletion with zinc and other micronutrients on neuropsychological performance and growth of Chinese children. Am J Clin Nutr 1998; 68(Suppl):470S–5.

69. Toren P, Eldar S, Sela BA, et al. Zinc deficiency in attention-deficit hyperactivity disorder. Biol Psychiatry 1996; 40:1308–10.

70. Bekaroglu M, Aslan Y, Gedik Y, et al. Relationships between serum-free fatty acids and zinc, and attention deficit hyperactivity disorder: a research note. J Child Psychol Psychiatry 1996; 37:225–7.

71. Arnold LE, Pinkham SM, Votolato N. Does zinc moderate essential fatty acid and amphetamine treatment of attention-deficit/hyperactivity disorder? J Child Adolesc Psychopharmacol 2000; 10:111–7.

72. Grant EC, Howard JM, Davies S, Chasty H, Hornsby B, Galbraith J. Zinc deficiency in children with dyslexia: concentrations of zinc and other minerals in sweat and hair. BMJ (Clin Res Ed) 1988; 296:607–9.

73. Delange F. The role of iodine in brain development. Proc Nutr Soc 2000; 59:75–9.

74. Maberly GF. Iodine deficiency disorders: contemporary scientific issues. J Nutr 1994; 124:1473S–78S.

75. Haddow JE, Palomaki GE, Allan WC, et al. Maternal thyroid deficiency during pregnancy and subsequent neuropsychological development of the child. N Engl J Med 1999; 341:549–55.

76. Rapaport R. Congenital hypothyroidism: expanding the spectrum. J Pediatr 2000; 136:10–2.

77. Svinarerv MY, Kolyadenko VF, Kurmacheva NA, Yevstifeyeva LP, Stepanishchenko IN. Epidemiology of iodine deficiency in the Saratov region: results of congenital hypothyroidism screening. Russ J Pediatr 2000; 4:http://www.medlit/ru/medeng/ped00e0421.htm.

78. Kapil U, Pathak P, Tandon M, Singh C, Pradhan R, Dwivedi SN. Micronutrient deficiency disorders amongst pregnant women in three urban slum communities of Delhi. Indian Pediatr 1999; 36:983–9.

79. Delange F, Van Onderbergen A, Shabana W, et al. Silent iodine prophylaxis in Western Europe only partly corrects iodine deficiency; the case of Belgium. Eur J Endocrinol 2000; 143:189–96.

80. Manz F, van't Hof MA, Haschke F. Iodine supply in children from different European areas: the Eurogrowth study. Committee for the Study of Iodine Supply in European Children. J Pediatr Gastroenterol Nutr 2000; 31 (Suppl 1):S72–5.

81. WHO global database on iodine deficiency disorders. Available at: http://www3.who.int/whosis/mn/mn_iodine/mn_iodine.cfm.

82. Boyages SC, Collins JK, Maberly GF, Jupp JJ, Morris J, Eastman CJ. Iodine deficiency impairs intellectual and neuromotor development in apparently normal persons. A study of rural inhabitants of north-central China. Med J Aust 1989; 150:676–82.

83. Azizi F, Sarshar A, Nafarabadi M, et al. Impairment of neuromotor and cognitive development in iodine-deficient schoolchildren with normal physical growth. Acta Endocrinol (Copenh) 1993; 129:501–4.

84. Sankar R, Rai B, Pulger T, et al. Intellectual and motor functions in school children from severely iodine deficient region in Sikkim. Indian J Pediatr 1994; 61: 231–6.

85. Tiwari BD, Godbole MM, Chattopadhyay N, Mandal A, Mithal A. Learning disabilities and poor motivation to achieve due to prolonged iodine deficiency. Am J Clin Nutr 1996; 63:782–6.

86. Aghini Lombardi FA, Pinchera A, Antonangeli L, et al. Mild iodine deficiency during fetal/neonatal life and neuropsychological impairment in Tuscany. J Endocrinol Invest 1995; 18:57–62.

87. Ojule AC, Osotimehin BO. The influence of iodine deficiency on the cognitive performance of school children in Saki, south-west Nigeria. Afr J Med Med Sci 1998; 27:95–9.

88. Osman A, Zaleha MI, Iskandar ZA, et al. Levels of thyroxine, TSH, thyroid volume and mental performance among Orang Asli in selected settlements in Malaysia. East Afr Med J 1996; 73:259–63.

89. van den Briel T, West CE, Bleichrodt N, van de Vijver FJ, Ategbo EA, Hautvast JG. Improved iodine status is associated with improved mental performance of schoolchildren in Benin. Am J Clin Nutr 2000; 72:1179–85.

90. Fierro-Benitez R, Cazar R, Stanbury JB, et al. Effects on school children of prophylaxis of mothers with iodized oil in an area of iodine deficiency. J Endocrinol Invest 1988; 11:327–35.

91. Fu LX, Chen ZH, Deng LQ. Effects of iodine nutritional status of fetuses, infants and young children on their intelligence development in the areas with iodine-deficiency disorders [in Chinese]. Zhonghua Yu Fang Yi Xue Za Zhi 1994; 28:330–2.

92. Yang Y, Wang X, Guo X. Effects of high iodine and high fluorine on children's intelligence and the

metabolism of iodine and fluorine [in Chinese]. Zhonghua Liu Xing Bing Xue Za Zhi 1994; 15:296–8.

93. Nedveckaite T, Motiejunas S, Kucinskas V, et al. Environmental releases of radioactivity and the incidence of thyroid disease at the Ignalina Nuclear Power Plant. Health Phys 2000; 79:666–74.

94. Vermiglio F, Castagna MG, Volnova E, et al. Post-Chernobyl increased prevalence of humoral thyroid autoimmunity in children and adolescents from a moderately iodine-deficient area in Russia. Thyroid 1999; 9:781–6.

95. Takahashi T, Fujimori K, Simon SL, Bechtner G, Edwards R, Trott KR. Thyroid nodules, thyroid function and dietary iodine in the Marshall islands. Int J Epidemiol 1999; 28:742–9.

96. Kolominsky Y, Igumnov S, Drozdovitch V. The psychological development of children from Belarus exposed in the prenatal period to radiation from the Chernobyl atomic power plant. J Child Psychol Psychiatry 1999; 40:299–305.

97. Neyfakh EA, Alimbekova AI, Ivanenko GF. Vitamin E and E deficiencies in children correlate with Chernobyl radiation loads of their mothers. Biochemistry (Mosc) 1998; 63:1138–43.

98. Untoro J, Ruz M, Gross R. Low environmental selenium availability as an additional determinant for goiter in East Java, Indonesia? Biol Trace Elem Res 1999; 70:127–36.

99. Neve J, Vertongen F, Molle L. Selenium deficiency. Clin Endocrinol Metab 1985; 14:629–56.

100. Vanderpas JB, Contempre B, Duale NL, et al. Iodine and selenium deficiency associated with cretinism in northern Zaire. Am J Clin Nutr 1990; 52:1087–93.

101. Aro A, Kumpulainen J, Alfthan G, Voshchenko AV, Ivanov VN. Factors affecting the selenium intake of people in Transbaikalian Russia. Biol Trace Elem Res 1994; 40:277–85.

102. Peng A, Yang C, Rui H, Li H. Study on the pathogenic factors of Kashin-Beck disease. J Toxicol Environ Health 1992; 35:79–90.

103. Allander E. Kashin-Beck disease. An analysis of research and public health activities based on a bibliography 1849–1992. Scand J Rheumatol Suppl 1994; 99:1–36.

104. Moreno-Reyes R, Suetens C, Mathieu F, et al. Kashin-Beck osteoarthropathy in rural Tibet in relation to selenium and iodine status. N Engl J Med 1998; 339:1112–20.

105. Zhai SS, Kimbrough RD, Meng B, et al. Kashin-Beck disease: a cross-sectional study in seven villages in the People's Republic of China. J Toxicol Environ Health 1990; 30:239–59.

106. Fondu P, Hariga-Muller C, Mozes N, Neve J, Van Steirteghem A, Mandelbaum IM. Protein-energy malnutrition and anemia in Kivu. Am J Clin Nutr 1978; 31:46–56.

107. McLaren DS. Vitamin A deficiency disorders. J Indian Med Assoc 1999; 97:320–3.

108. Molina EL, Patel JA. A to Z: vitamin A and zinc, the miracle duo. Indian J Pediatr 1996; 63:427–31.

109. Semba RD, Muhilal, Ward BJ, et al. Abnormal T-cell subset proportions in vitamin-A deficient children. Lancet 1993; 341:5–8.

110. Villamor E, Fawzi WW. Vitamin A supplementation: implications for morbidity and mortality in children. J Infect Dis 2000; 182 (Suppl 1):S122–33.

111. Hadi H, Stoltzfus RJ, Dibley MJ, et al. Vitamin A supplementation selectively improves the linear growth of Indonesian preschool children: results from a randomized controlled trial. Am J Clin Nutr 2000; 71:507–13.

112. Khandait DW, Vasudeo ND, Zodpey SP, Kumbhalkar DT. Risk factors for subclinical vitamin A deficiency in children under the age of 6 years. J Trop Pediatr 2000; 46:239–41.

113. Gittelsohn J, Shankar AV, West KP, Faruque F, Gnywali T, Pradhan EK. Child feeding and care behaviors are associated with xerophthalmia in rural Nepalese households. Soc Sci Med 1998; 47:477–86.

114. Haidar J, Demissie T. Malnutrition and xerophthalmia in rural communities of Ethiopia. East Afr Med J 1999; 76:590–3.

115. Mora JO, Gueri M, Mora OL. Vitamin A deficiency in Latin America and the Caribbean: an overview. Rev Panam Salud Publica 1998; 4:178–86.

116. Aspatwar AP, Bapat MM. Vitamin A status of socio-economically backward children. Indian J Pediatr 1995; 62:427–32.

117. Mwanri L, Worsley A, Ryan P, Masika J. Supplemental vitamin A improves anemia and growth in anemic school children in Tanzania. J Nutr 2000; 130:2691–6.

118. Grotto I, Mimouni M, Gdalevich M, Mimouni D. Vitamin A supplementation and childhood morbidity from diarrhea and respiratory infections: a meta-analysis. J Pediatr 2003; 142:297–304.

119. Kalra V, Grover J, Ahuja GK, Rathi S, Khurana DS. Vitamin E deficiency and associated neurological deficits in children with protein-energy malnutrition. J Trop Pediatr 1998; 44:291–5.

120. Satya-Murti S, Howard L, Krohel G, Wolf B. The spectrum of neurologic disorder from vitamin E deficiency. Neurology 1986; 36:917–21.

121. Ece A, Uyanik BS, Iscan A, Ertan P, Yigitoglu MR. Increased serum copper and decreased serum zinc levels in children with iron deficiency anemia. Biol Trace Elem Res 1997; 59:31–9.

122. Perrone L, Salerno M, Gialanella G, et al. Long-term zinc and iron supplementation in children of short stature: effect of growth and on trace element content in tissues. J Trace Elem Med Biol 1999; 13:51–6.

123. Munoz EC, Rosado JL, Lopez P, Furr HC, Allen LH. Iron and zinc supplementation improves indicators of vitamin A status of Mexican preschoolers. Am J Clin Nutr 2000; 71:789–94.

124. Buchanan GR. The tragedy of iron deficiency during infancy and early childhood. J Pediatr 1999; 135:413–5.

125. Bhan MK, Bhandari N, Bhatnagar S, Bahl R. Epidemiology and management of persistent diarrhoea in children of developing countries. Indian J Med Res 1996; 104:103–14.

126. D'Souza RM, D'Souza R. Vitamin A for the treatment of children with measles—a systematic review. J Trop Pediatr 2002; 48:323–7.

127. American Academy of Pediatrics. Measles. In: Pickering LK, ed. Red Book: 2003 Report of the Committee on Infectious Diseases. Elk Grove Village, IL: American Academy of Pediatrics, 2003:419–29.

12

MICROCEPHALY AND EARLY
BRAIN INJURY

Their heads sometimes so little that there is no room for wit;
sometimes so long that there is no wit for such room.

Thomas Fuller, *Of Natural Fools*, 1642[1]

Growth delays are common in international adoptees at arrival to the United States (see Chapter 10). However, short stature and underweight are not as worrisome as microcephaly, a reflection of impaired brain growth. Microcephaly is common in newly arrived international adoptees (Table 12–1). Prenatal exposures, intrauterine growth retardation, birth injuries, environmental deprivation, malnutrition, micronutrient deficiencies, and other factors all contribute to the prevalence of microcephaly in this population of children (see Chapters 2, 5–8, 10, and 11). These exposures affect brain size as well as function. Although microcephaly is a surrogate marker for early brain injury, not all normocephalic children escape exposures that adversely affect brain function. Conversely, some children with microcephaly appear to be functionally and cognitively intact.

Head circumference measurement is one of the few objective items provided in preadoption medical referrals (although it may be inaccurate; see Chapter 4). About 40% of preadoptive referrals indicate that the child has microcephaly. The pediatrician must understand the relationship of head size and outcome to advise prospective adoptive parents of these children (see also Johnson[2] for an excellent parent-friendly review of this topic). This knowledge also helps provide suitable anticipatory guidance for microcephalic children after adoption. This chapter reviews the intriguing relationship of brain size and early-onset brain injury to cognitive and behavioral outcomes.

Definition of Microcephaly

Microcephaly is usually defined as head circumference <−2 standard deviations (SD) for age

Table 12–1 Prevalence of microcephaly in newly arrived international adoptees, z scores

Country of Origin (N)	Receiving Country	Adoptees with Microcephaly (%)
Romania (65)[3]	United States	7% of infants <10 months old had z scores <–2, 41% of children >10 months had z scores <–2; HC decreased with duration of orphanage confinement
Romania (22)[4]	Canada	45% less than fifth percentile
Various (129)[5]	United States	Mean z score –1.03 (range –5.31 to 1.37); lower scores corresponded to more severe GM, FM, language, and cognitive delays
Eastern Europe (56)[6]	United States	43% with z score <–1; mean z score –1.25 (range –3.7 to 0.62)
China (192)[7]	United States	24% with z score <–2; mean z score –1.43 (range –5.2 to 1.37)
India (114)[8]	Sweden	Mean z score at arrival –2.1; 2 years after adoption ~–1.6

FM, fine motor; GM, gross motor; HC, head circumference.

(comprising the lowest 2.3% of the population).[9] Some investigators use a limit of <–3 SD (the lowest 0.1% of the population); others define microcephaly as head circumference less than the fifth to tenth percentile or use z scores (child's measurement minus mean measurement for age divided by SD for age) $\leq$ –2. Regardless of definition, head circumference relates to brain size, brain protein and DNA content, and number of neurons.[10] The rare exceptions are conditions that affect skull morphology or soft tissue structure, such as craniofacial malformations (craniosynostosis, Crouzon or Apert syndromes), intracranial pathology (hydrocephaly, anencephaly, and variants), and scalp edema or overriding sutures (in newborns). Rickets, a relatively common problem among international adoptees, occasionally causes significant frontal bossing that can falsely inflate head circumference measurement (see Chapter 25).

Microcephaly may be congenital or acquired. Congenital microcephaly is usually genetic (autosomal dominant, autosomal recessive, and X-linked) or due to prenatal exposures (maternal phenylketonuria [PKU], maternal malnutrition, radiation, viruses, or teratogens such as drugs or alcohol).[11] Brain growth during the second trimester is especially vulnerable to such insults.[1,12] Acquired microcephaly usually results from birth trauma, head injury, postnatal infection, or malnutrition. Malnourished children have reduced head circumferences; their brains have diminished cell number, DNA and protein content, and weight.[10]

Some studies suggest that children with primary microcephaly fare better than those with secondary microcephaly,[13] but effects on intelligence depend on the extent and type of underlying pathology. Abnormal brain imaging (cerebral atrophy, cortical dysplasia, myelination delay, white matter hypoplasia) more accurately predict developmental performance than the degree of microcephaly.[14]

Early Brain Injury and Development

Early brain injury often results in microcephaly. This is not always true, however—some children have normal head growth after focal or global brain injuries. Thus a normal head circumference should not be assumed to indicate a normally functioning brain. After prefrontal or more diffuse brain injuries in early life, some children exhibit significant cognitive and behavioral impairments. Such injuries may follow prenatal exposures to alcohol or drugs, trauma, neglect, or other insults. Disorders of personality, social behavior, and executive functions

Table 12–2 Executive function deficits after brain injury

Area	Types of Problems
Organization	Attention, decision making, planning, sequencing
Regulation	Initiation, repetition, temper control
Awareness	Denial of "deficits," unintentional noncompliance
Motor planning	"Unconscious" tasks require concentration
Verbal fluency	Impaired fluency
Focus	Unable to shift mental sets, perseverative tendencies

Source: Data from Tepper.[18]

(planning and decision making) are some of the devastating consequences of such damage[15–17] (Table 12–2). Some children compensate for early-onset brain injuries and, indeed, this seems to be true to a large extent for speech and motor function. The development of personality, social cognition, moral reasoning, and executive function, however, seem particularly vulnerable to brain injury in early life. In ways that are not yet completely understood, brain injury and dysfunction, especially in prefrontal regions, impede the acquisition of social knowledge. Children who experience such injuries display difficulties in planning, judgment, and decision making, which may adversely affect their ability to live independently, work, and develop social relationships. Such difficulties are not usually fully manifest until adolescence or young adulthood. Early brain injuries may also contribute to the development of nonverbal learning disability, attention-deficit hyperactivity disorder, autism spectrum disorders, and conduct disorders, although these pathways have yet to be defined.[15]

Microcephaly and Development

The link between small head size and impaired mental development has been recognized for centuries. In more modern times, the association of microcephaly and mental retardation was noted by Kind in 1876 in a study of 500 "mentally defective" individuals and by Tarbell in 1883 in a study of Boston school children.[1,12,19] These observations were confirmed in descriptions of children in institutions for the mentally retarded or in specialty clinics.[11,20–23] For example, a 1965 Mayo Clinic review of 134 children with microcephaly, dwarfism, or mental or developmental retardation found that all whose head circumferences were <-2 SD were "mentally sub-normal." Those with lower IQs had lower head circumferences.[23] The investigators concluded that all microcephalic children, with rare exceptions, were mentally retarded. (They also noted that these children frequently had short stature.) In this population, only a single child with microcephaly and normal mental ability was found (although five additional children with microcephaly and normal IQ were later reported[24]). However, several other studies of children in specialty clinics revealed that not all microcephalic children were retarded. For example, Pryor and Thelander[20] identified 4.2% of microcephalic children in a birth defects clinic with normal intelligence. Moreover, 60% of 31 microcephalic children exposed to atomic radiation as fetuses in utero had normal intelligence, including 14 of 17 children with head circumferences of <-2 to -3 SD.[25]

Some children with small head circumferences due to congenital heart disease, malabsorption, or hypopituitarism have normal intelligence.[24,26] However, other neurobehavioral problems may be present. For example, in a referral population of children with neurologic or cognitive problems, 27 of the 202 with microcephaly (13.3%) had normal IQ scores but more than half had minimal cerebral dysfunction.[27] Similarly, another group of microcephalic children with normal IQ scores had many other problems, including deafness, cerebral palsy, attention-deficit disorder, perceptual dysfunction, and learning disabilities.[28] Another survey recognized abnormal head circumferences in 15/73 children with learning disabilities: 8 with macrocephaly and 7 with microcephaly.[29]

What is the relationship of microcephaly to mental ability in children outside of specialized settings? Several studies address the question of whether some microcephalic individuals have normal intelligence and function. One such study compared anthropometric measurements to IQ, reading ability, and social class among 334 grade-school boys.[30] Socioeconomic status best predicted psychometric test scores, but head circumference was the second best predictor (and related closely to IQ) (Fig. 12–1). In a similar study, 1.9% of 1006 children in regular school classes in Seattle were microcephalic.[31] Although the mean IQ of the microcephalic children did not differ from that of their classmates, they had significantly lower academic achievement scores. Using a different approach, head circumference and standardized test results were compared in 360 school children. Full-scale IQ results correlated directly with head circumference, but learning disabilities were less frequent in microcephalic children compared with macrocephalic or normocephalic children (23%, 54%, and 39%, respectively).[21] Finally, in a long-term study of monozygotic twins, the lighter/smaller of each pair had both smaller head circumference and lower global and performance IQ at 13 years of age.[32]

Several studies using data derived from patients entered into the National Perinatal Collaborative Project address the effects of microcephaly on intellectual outcome. Head size at 1 year of age was analyzed as a predictor of IQ at 4 years of age among 9379 children[33] (Fig. 12–2). Head circumference at age 1 year correlated directly with IQ at age 4 years; however, there was no head size that gave more than a 50% probability of IQ <80 at 4 years of age. Even among children with the smallest 0.67% of head circumference measurements, half had IQs within the normal range (but none achieved IQ of 120 or greater). Outcome at 4 years of age was also influenced by the educational achievements of the mother and the child's height (although these relations were less pronounced than head circumference). In this population,

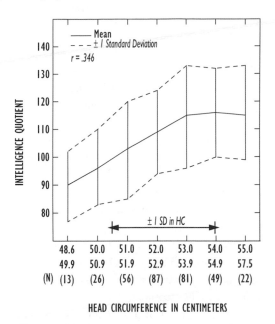

Figure 12–1 *IQ related to head circumference (cm) in 334 grade school–age boys in St. Louis. Mean IQ increased approximately 6 points with each increment of 1 cm in head circumference up to 54 cm. (From Weinberg WA, Dietz SG, Penick EC, McAlister WH. Intelligence, reading achievement, physical size and social class. A study of St. Louis Caucasian boys aged 8-0 to 9-6 years, attending regular schools. J Pediatr 1974; 85:484, with permission.)*

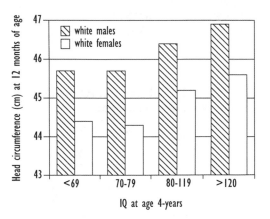

Figure 12–2 *Head circumference at age 12 months predicts IQ at age 4 years. (Data from Nelson and Deutschberger.)[33]*

the authors concluded that 1-year-old children with head circumference measurements <43 cm (boys) or <42 cm (girls) have approximately a 50% chance of an IQ <80 at 4 years of age and very little chance of superior intelligence.

Another study used this database to assess IQ at age 7 years in children with persistent microcephaly (at birth, 1 year, and 7 years of age) (Table 12–3).[9] Of the 28,820 children studied, 25 had isolated microcephaly; of these, only 25% of these were mentally retarded. Thus head size of <–2 SD had "very low predictive value" for mental retardation for an individual child. However, two-thirds of children with head circumferences <–3 SD had IQs <80. As in other studies, short stature was also associated with worse mental outcome.

A third study of 31,173 infants from the Collaborative Perinatal Project evaluated the developmental outcome of children with "low normal" head circumferences at birth.[22] Developmental outcome at 8 months, 4 years, and 7 years of age did not differ between those with "low normal" head circumference at birth and those whose measurements were in the mid-normal range. Thus, although microcephaly is strongly associated with reduced intelligence, a few children with small head size have normal intelligence. It is likely, however, that microcephalic children with normal IQs have more learning disabilities and functional difficulties with school performance.

Table 12–3 Distribution of IQ in children with persistent microcephaly

	(N)	children with IQ in each range (%)			
		<70	71–80	81–100	>100
Normal	28,665	2.6	7.4	40.9	36.4
–2 SD	114	10.5	28.1	43	14
–3 SD	41	51.2	17.1	29.3	0

IQ not known for some children.

Source: Data from Dolk.[9]

Patterns of Microcephaly

Internationally adopted children may have congenital (primary) or acquired (secondary) microcephaly. Congenital microcephaly means decreased head circumference at birth, after correction for gestational age.[34] Acquired microcephaly occurs after normal prenatal growth (and normal measurement at birth): brain growth decelerates following infection, trauma, toxic exposures, metabolic disease, environmental deprivation, or brain degeneration. At any age, head circumference may be absolute or relative (a small head on a small child). Some children have temporary periods of microcephaly, preceded or followed by more normal brain growth patterns. Although the accuracy of measurements may be questioned, it is likely that episodes of illness, malnutrition, or perhaps even emotional deprivation (loss of a beloved caregiver, transfer to a new room, etc.) may temporarily impede brain growth.

Proportionality

In some children, small head circumference is proportional to other anthropometric measurements. Children with global growth delays due to hypothalamic or pituitary dysfunction or other chronic medical problems usually have proportional microcephaly.[9,24,35] Some researchers suggest that such children have better IQ scores, academic achievement, and intellectual prognosis than those whose head circumference is disproportionately smaller than other measurements.[31,34] Others disagree, however, pointing out that children with global growth delays are more likely to be mentally subnormal.[23] Some teratogens—alcohol, for example—cause both microcephaly and growth retardation.[9] Height has been linked to cognitive ability in several large studies,[9,33] although this relationship is less well established than head circumference and cognitive ability. However, for any given head circumference, IQ generally rises as length or height increases.[33] Thus the short child with a small head is likely to be less intelligent than a taller child with the same head size.

Congenital Microcephaly

Full-term or premature newborns may have microcephaly alone or in conjunction with intrauterine growth retardation, which also reduces height and weight. Congenital microcephaly is associated with abnormalities in fetal neurogenesis, neuronal migration, and cell differentiation.[36] Children with microcephaly beginning early in gestation have worse school performance and ability to concentrate than those with later-onset microcephaly.[37] An extensive literature describes the neurodevelopmental outcome of low–birth weight (for example, see Botting et al.[38]) or intrauterine growth retarded infants.[37,39–42] Many studies refer to the extra risk conferred by congenital microcephaly, with many children demonstrating lower scores on intelligence testing (Table 12–4),[43–45] poorer academic achievement,[46] and worse visuospatial and other perceptual abilities.[46,47] In a review of 249 very low–birth weight children followed until age 8 years,[48] subnormal head size at 8 months of age was an independent risk factor for diminished verbal and performance IQ scores, receptive language, speech, reading, and mathematic and spelling abilities, and a higher incidence of hyperactivity. Nonetheless, study infants with normal head circumferences comprised 77% of those with IQ scores <85. In another study of children with very low birth weight who were small for gestational age, those with normalization of head growth by 12 months had significantly higher energy-nutrient intake than those without improvement in microcephaly.[49]

Environmental factors, such as maternal education and socioeconomic status, play an important part in the ultimate achievement of children with congenital microcephaly. Nonetheless, early microcephaly affects verbal recognition, spatial working memory, recognition memory, or other subtle neuropsychological functions, even if IQ is preserved.[50] An association of congenital microcephaly with schizophrenia has also been noted.[51,52]

Acquired Microcephaly

Two-thirds of total head growth occurs in the period from birth to 24 months.[53] Acquired microcephaly results from birth trauma, head injury, infection, environmental deprivation, or malnutrition. These insults all impede neuronal growth, arborization, synaptogenesis, and cellular differentiation during the first years of life.[54] Acquired microcephaly most often results from malnutrition and associated sociocultural deprivation (see Chapter 10). Children who suffer from these problems are at increased risk of neurocognitive deficits in later life.[36,55–61] In addition to reduced IQ, children with acquired microcephaly due to malnutrition may exhibit behavioral disturbances (apathy), learning disabilities, attentional problems, impaired sensory integration, and lowered self-esteem.[57] Other studies show no alteration in neurocognitive abilities in children age 7–9 years with previous failure to thrive and microcephaly in infancy.[62]

Acquired microcephaly is frequent among institutionalized children[2] (Fig. 12–3), probably from the combined effects of malnutrition and lack of environmental stimulation. No studies have yet reported the neurocognitive outcome of adopted children with acquired microcephaly. Two reports suggest that head circum-

Table 12–4 Mean IQ at age 4 years, in relation to head circumference at birth, in 118 low–birth weight infants

Head circumference percentile at birth	<10	10–25	26–50	>50
IQ at age 4 years	82.8	91.9	91.7	100.6

Source: Data from Gross et al.[43]

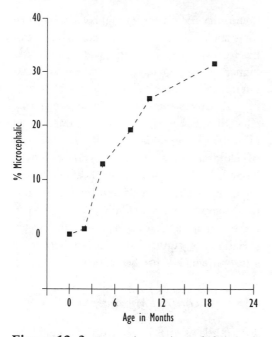

Figure 12–3 *Progression to microcephaly in institutionalized Russian children normocephalic at birth. (Courtesy of Dana E. Johnson, M.D.)*

ference measurements improve after adoption[4,8] (birth measurements were not available for the children in either study) (Table 12–5).

Ethnic Variation in Head Circumference

Does head size vary with ethnicity? Unlike measurements of height and weight, head cir-

Table 12–5 Children with head circumference less than fifth percentile (*n* = 22)

	Age at Adoption (months)			
	<6	7–12	13–24	>24
% at arrival	17	60	62	33
% at follow-up (mean, 12 months after adoption)	0	40	25	33

Source: Data from Benoit et al.[4]

cumference standards have not been published by the World Health Organization. Although racial differences in head circumference have been reported,[53] the etiology of these differences has not been established, nor have the relative contributions of genetics and environment been distinguished. Some ethnic-specific head circumference growth standards are available (for example, Chinese, Korean), but the specific populations used to develop these charts (and their nutritional status) are not always clearly defined (see Chapter 4). About 50% of normal head size variation is familial.[63]

American pediatricians favor the head circumference chart developed by Nellhaus, especially for children older than 3 years. This chart, published in 1968, combined 14 reports of head circumference standards from the world literature.[53] The included reports were derived from measurements of 125 to 1670 children of different ages who had been full-term infants and were "physically and mentally well." The composite graphs include results of studies of African-American, Japanese, Alaskan Eskimo, and Caucasian children (from Scotland, United States, Belgium, Switzerland, England, Sweden, Finland, and Czechoslovakia). Notably absent are South Asian, African, and Hispanic children. Nonetheless, Nellhaus subtitled the paper "Practical Composite International and Interracial Graphs" and concluded that "race causes no appreciable difference in head circumference in either sex."

In a follow-up report, Nellhaus added information on 150 Hispanic children. Their head circumference measurements fell within his previously established normal ranges. In contrast, Chinese children living in Hong Kong had head sizes 1–1.3 cm smaller than these ranges after the first year of life (although their measurements were normal at birth[26]). In contrast to the accelerated body growth observed among American children after World War II (due to improved child nutrition and other sanitary measures), Nellhaus did not observe a similar effect on head growth.

The Nellhaus charts are still widely used, especially for children over 3 years of age. The newly revised growth charts for American children, published by the National Center for Health Statistics[64] include forms for head circumference of children less than 36 months of age. The charts, developed between 1992 and 1997, are based on survey data collected between 1963 and 1994, including longitudinal studies conducted by the National Center for Health Statistics and the National Health and Nutrition Examination Surveys (NHANES) I, II, and III. These surveys evaluated an ethnically and racially diverse sample of American children and should therefore suffice for any young child. These charts replace the 1977 version which were criticized for their bias towards Caucasian individuals (published by the National Center for Health Statistics, the charts from birth to age 3 years were developed at the Fels Research Institute.)

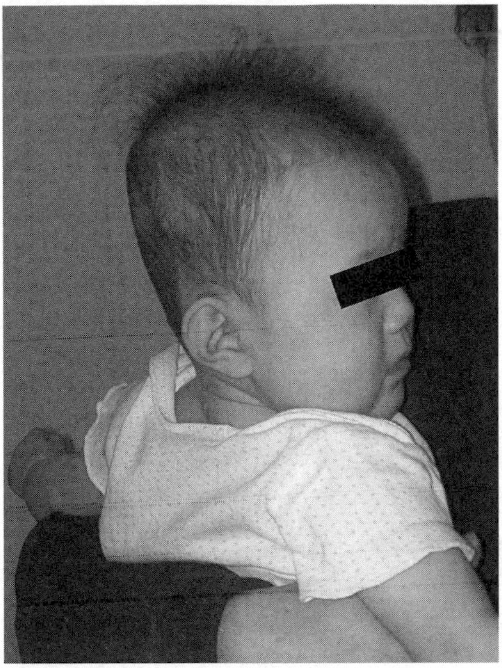

Figure 12–4 *Some children have markedly flattened occiputs after prolonged positioning in supine posture. (With permission.)*

Variation in Head Shape

Head shape varies with gestational and chronological age, ethnicity, and genetics. Environmental factors, especially sleeping position, also contribute to head shape. Many young children residing in orphanages spend their days swaddled and virtually immobilized in their cribs. Children always placed in the same position often develop molding deformities of the skull (Fig. 12–4). Occipital flattening is the most common deformity. Some children have associated torticollis, ear flattening, or other facial asymmetries. If extreme, occipitofrontal circumference is reduced, although cranial volume is normal. This positional plagiocephaly responds well to conservative treatments such as alteration in position, physical therapy for associated torticollis, and, if needed, a cranial orthosis (molding helmet).[65–67] Even without specific intervention, this cosmetic deformity (partially) corrects over time. Deformational plagiocephaly and scaphocephaly are associ-

ated with increased likelihood of requiring special services in school[68] and auditory processing disorders.[69,70] True craniosynostosis must be differentiated from deformational plagiocephaly (Table 12–6); occasionally radiographs or computed tomography may be necessary.

Head Circumference Assessment in Pre-Adoptive Medical Records

Head circumference and other measurements are sometimes the only objective information offered in pre-adoptive medical records (see Chapter 4). Birth measurements may be the only information available from the neonatal period; specifics about maternal history, prenatal course, labor and delivery, and neonatal course are usually lacking. Gestational age assignments are infrequently listed in preadoptive

Table 12–6 Differentiation of deformational plagiocephaly and lambdoid craniosynostosis

Deformational Plagiocephaly	Lambdoid Craniosynostosis
Flat occiput on one side of head with prominence on contralateral side	Same
Frontal prominence ipsilateral to occipital flattening	Same but generally less severe
Ear ipsilateral to flattened occiput is typically displaced anteriorly	Ear ipsilateral to flattened occiput is typically displaced posteriorly and inferiorly
Not observed	Posterior basal skull tilted with prominent mastoid
Ipsilateral cheekbone and forehead are prominent	Minimal if any facial deformity

Source: Adapted from Persing et al.[67]

medical reports, making interpretation of head size problematic. Under more ordinary circumstances, birth head circumference can serve as a "proxy" for gestational age: among 1535 prematurely born infants, head circumference correlated closely with gestational age.[53]

Serial measurements of head circumference may be provided in the pre-adoptive medical report. The accuracy of such measurements is sometimes questionable. Measurement techniques may not be standardized, and measurements may not be repeated to ensure accuracy, especially in squirmy children. As with other growth parameters, serial measurements are far more useful than a single data point. Although Nellhaus[53] gloomily states, "Even a single head circumference measurement of two standard deviations below the mean for age and sex justifies the suspicion of mental retardation," this generalization does not seem applicable for international adoptees.

Many of these children do surprisingly well, despite a period of microcephaly in early infancy. Some exhibit remarkable recovery of head growth after adoption (Fig. 12–5). The long-term outcome of children with micro-

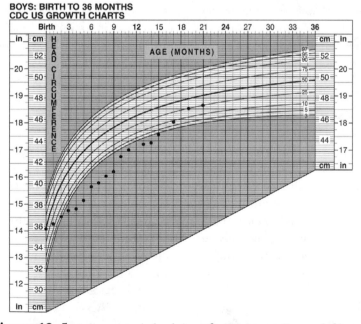

Figure 12–5 *Improvement in head circumference occurs to a remarkable extent in some children after adoption (Growth charts from Centers for Disease Control and Prevention [CDC]).*

cephaly at arrival to the United States is not yet defined. Although it is suspected that children with early microcephaly are at increased risk for later learning or behavioral problems, this has not been demonstrated with certainty. The combination of improved nutrition and nurture in the adoptive home may considerably improve outlook.

Key Points for Internationally Adopted Children

- Microcephaly is commonly noted on pre-adoptive medical referrals.
- Many new arrivals have microcephaly (z scores <-2).
- In this population, microcephaly usually reflects early brain injury (possibly from toxic exposures and/or environmental deprivation).
- Microcephaly may reduce IQ and increase the likelihood of neuropsychological dysfunction (learning disabilities, academic performance, behavior, executive function).
- The long-term outcome of international adoptees with microcephaly on arrival to the United States has not been completely defined.

References

1. Hecht F, Kelly JV. Little heads: inheritance and early detection. J Pediatr 1979; 95:731–2.

2. Johnson DE. Does size matter, or is bigger better? The use of head circumference in preadoption medical evaluation and its predictive value for cognitive outcome in institutionalized children. Available at: http://www.peds.umn.edu/iac/sizematter.pdf.

3. Johnson DE, Miller LC, Iverson S, et al. The health of children adopted from Romania. JAMA 1992; 268:3446–51.

4. Benoit TC, Jocelyn LJ, Moddemann DM, Embree JE. Romanian adoption. The Manitoba experience. Arch Pediatr Adolesc Med 1996; 150:1278–82.

5. Miller LC, Kiernan MT, Mathers MI, Klein-Gitelman M. Developmental and nutritional status of internationally adopted children. Arch Pediatr Adolesc Med 1995; 149:40–4.

6. Albers LH, Johnson DE, Hostetter MK, Iverson S, Miller LC. Health of children adopted from the former Soviet Union and Eastern Europe. Comparison with preadoptive medical records. JAMA 1997; 278:922–4.

7. Miller LC, Hendrie NW. Health of children adopted from China. Pediatrics 2000; 105:E76.

8. Proos LA, Hofvander Y, Wennqvist K, Tuvemo T. A longitudinal study on anthropometric and clinical development of Indian children adopted in Sweden. II. Growth, morbidity and development during two years after arrival in Sweden. Ups J Med Sci 1992; 97:93–106.

9. Dolk H. The predictive value of microcephaly during the first year of life for mental retardation at seven years. Dev Med Child Neurol 1991; 33:974–83.

10. Winick M, Rosso P. Head circumference and cellular growth of the brain in normal and marasmic children. J Pediatr 1969; 74:774–8.

11. Dorman C. Microcephaly and intelligence. Dev Med Child Neurol 1991; 33:267–9.

12. Haslam RH, Smith DW. Autosomal dominant microcephaly. J Pediatr 1979; 95:701–5.

13. Qazi QH, Reed TE. A problem in diagnosis of primary versus secondary microcephaly. Clin Genet 1973; 4:46–52.

14. Custer DA, Vezina LG, Vaught DR, et al. Neurodevelopmental and neuroimaging correlates in nonsyndromal microcephalic children. J Dev Behav Pediatr 2000; 21:12–8.

15. Tranel D, Eslinger PJ. Effects of early onset brain injury on the development of cognition and behavior: introduction to the special issue. Dev Neuropsychol 2000; 18:273–80.

16. Anderson SW, Damasio H, Tranel D, Damasio AR. Long-term sequelae of prefrontal cortex damage acquired in early childhood. Dev Neuropsychol 2000; 18:281–96.

17. Connor PD, Sampson PD, Bookstein FL, Barr HM, Streissguth AP. Direct and indirect effects of prenatal alcohol damage on executive function. Dev Neuropsychol 2000; 18:331–54.

18. Tepper T, for Parents Network for the Post-Institutionalized Child. Executive function. Available at: http://www.pnpic.org/exec_fun.htm.

19. Mosier HD Jr, Grossman HJ, Dingman HF. Physical growth in mental defectives. A study in an institutionalized population. Pediatrics 1965; 36:(Suppl):465–519.

20. Pryor HB, Thelander H. Abnormally small head size and intellect in children. J Pediatr 1968; 73:593–8.

21. Desch LW, Anderson SK, Snow JH. Relationship of head circumference to measures of school performance. Clin Pediatr (Phila) 1990; 29:389–92.

22. Brennan TL, Funk SG, Frothingham TE. Disproportionate intra-uterine head growth and developmental outcome. Dev Med Child Neurol 1985; 27:746–50.

23. O'Connell EJ, Feldt RH, Stickler GB. Head circumference, mental retardation, and growth failure. Pediatrics 1965; 36:62–6.

24. Cloutier MD, Stickler GB. Head circumference in children with idiopathic hypopituitarism. Pediatrics 1968; 42:209–10.

25. Wood JW, Johnson KG, Omori Y. In utero exposure to the Hiroshima atomic bomb. An evaluation of head size and mental retardation: twenty years later. Pediatrics 1967; 39:385–92.

26. Nellhaus G. Head circumference in children with idiopathic hypopituitarism. Pediatrics 1968; 42:210–1.

27. Martin HP. Microcephaly and mental retardation. Am J Dis Child 1970; 119:128–31.

28. Przytycki A, Burgin R. Microcephalic children without mental retardation. Harefuah 1992; 122:566–8.

29. Smith RD. Abnormal head circumference in learning-disabled children. Dev Med Child Neurol 1981; 23:626–32.

30. Weinberg WA, Dietz SG, Penick EC, McAlister WH. Intelligence, reading achievement, physical size and social class. A study of St. Louis Caucasian boys aged 8-0 to 9-6 years, attending regular schools. J Pediatr 1974; 85:482–9.

31. Sells CJ. Microcephaly in a normal school population. Pediatrics 1977; 59:262–265.

32. Henrichsen L, Skinhoj K, Andersen GE. Delayed growth and reduced intelligence in 9–17 year old intrauterine growth retarded children compared with their monozygous co-twins. Acta Paediatr Scand 1986; 75: 31–5.

33. Nelson KB, Deutschberger J. Head size at one year as a predictor of four-year IQ. Dev Med Child Neurol 1970; 12:487–95.

34. Opitz JM, Holt MC. Microcephaly: general considerations and aids to nosology. J Craniofac Genet Dev Biol 1990; 10:175–204.

35. Dacou-Voutetakis C, Karpathios T, Logothetis N, Constantinidis M, Matsaniotis N, Michalopoulou E. Defective growth hormone secretion in primary microcephaly. J Pediatr 1974; 85:498–502.

36. Morgane PJ, Austin-LaFrance R, Bronzino J, et al. Prenatal malnutrition and development of the brain. Neurosci Biobehav Rev 1993; 17:91–128.

37. Parkinson CE, Wallis S, Harvey D. School achievement and behaviour of children who were small-for-dates at birth. Dev Med Child Neurol 1981; 23:41–50.

38. Botting N, Powls A, Cooke RW, Marlow N. Cognitive and educational outcome of very-low-birthweight children in early adolescence. Dev Med Child Neurol 1998; 40:652–60.

39. Westwood M, Kramer MS, Munz D, Lovett JM, Watters GV. Growth and development of full-term nonasphyxiated small-for-gestational-age newborns: follow-up through adolescence. Pediatrics 1983; 71:376–82.

40. Pryor J, Silva PA, Brooke M. Growth, development and behaviour in adolescents born small-for-gestational-age. J Paediatr Child Health 1995; 31:403–7.

41. Markestad T, Vik T, Ahlsten G, et al. Small-for-gestational-age (SGA) infants born at term: growth and development during the first year of life. Acta Obstet Gynecol Scand Suppl 1997; 165:93–101.

42. Fattal-Valevski A, Leitner Y, Kutai M, et al. Neurodevelopmental outcome in children with intrauterine growth retardation: a 3-year follow-up. J Child Neurol 1999; 14:724–7.

43. Gross SJ, Kosmetatos N, Grimes CT, Williams ML. Newborn head size and neurological status. Predictors of growth and development of low birth weight infants. Am J Dis Child 1978; 132:753–6.

44. Strauss RS, Dietz WH. Growth and development of term children born with low birth weight: effects of genetic and environmental factors. J Pediatr 1998; 133:67–72.

45. Teplin SW, Burchinal M, Johnson-Martin N, Humphry RA, Kraybill EN. Neurodevelopmental, health, and growth status at age 6 years of children with birth weights less than 1001 grams. J Pediatr 1991; 118:768–77.

46. Hack M, Breslau N. Very low birth weight infants: effects of brain growth during infancy on intelligence quotient at 3 years of age. Pediatrics 1986; 77:196–202.

47. Sommerfelt K, Markestad T, Ellertsen B. Neuropsychological performance in low birth weight preschoolers: a population-based, controlled study. Eur J Pediatr 1998; 157:53–8.

48. Hack M, Breslau N, Weissman B, Aram D, Klein N, Borawski E. Effect of very low birth weight and subnormal head size on cognitive abilities at school age. N Engl J Med 1991; 325:231–7.

49. Brandt I, Sticker EJ, Lentze MJ. Catch-up growth of head circumference of very low birth weight, small for gestational age preterm infants and mental development to adulthood. J Pediatr 2003; 142:463–8.

50. Georgieff MK. Intrauterine growth retardation and subsequent somatic growth and neurodevelopment. J Pediatr 1998; 133:3–5.

51. Cantor-Graae E, Ismail B, McNeil TF. Neonatal head circumference and related indices of disturbed fetal development in schizophrenic patients. Schizophr Res 1998; 32:191–9.

52. Kunugi H, Takei N, Murray RM, Saito K, Nanko S. Small head circumference at birth in schizophrenia. Schizophr Res 1996; 20:165–70.

53. Nellhaus G. Head circumference from birth to eighteen years. Practical composite international and interracial graphs. Pediatrics 1968; 41:106–14.

54. Volpe JJ. Cognitive deficits in premature infants. N Engl J Med 1991; 325:276–8.

55. Barnes RH. Dual role of environmental deprivation and malnutrition in retarding intellectual development. A. G. Hogan Memorial Lecture. Am J Clin Nutr 1976; 29:912–7.

56. Colombo M, de la Parra A, Lopez I. Intellectual and physical outcome of children undernourished in early life is influenced by later environmental conditions. Dev Med Child Neurol 1992; 34:611–22.

57. Galler JR. Malnutrition and mental development. The Post (Parent Network for the Post-Institutionalized Child), 1998:20 1–7. P.O. Box 613, Meadowlands, PA.

58. Grantham-McGregor S, Schofield W, Powell C. Development of severely malnourished children who received psychosocial stimulation: six-year follow-up. Pediatrics 1987; 79:247–54.

59. Handler LC, Stoch MB, Smythe PM. CT brain scans: part of a 20-year development study following gross undernutrition during infancy. Br J Radiol 1981; 54:953–4.

60. Sathy N, Elizabeth KE, Nair MK, Bai NS. Growth faltering and developmental delay in children with PEM. Indian Pediatr 1991; 28:255–8.

61. Stoch MB, Smythe PM, Moodie AD, Bradshaw D. Psychosocial outcome and CT findings after gross undernourishment during infancy: a 20-year developmental study. Dev Med Child Neurol 1982; 24:419–36.

62. Drewett RF, Corbett SS, Wright CM. Cognitive and educational attainments at school age of children who failed to thrive in infancy: a population-based study. J Child Psychol Psychiatry 1999; 40:551–61.

63. Weaver DD, Christian JC. Familial variation of head size and adjustment for parental head circumference. J Pediatr 1980; 96:990–4.

64. National Center for Health Statistics. 2000 CDC Growth Charts: United States. Available at: http://www.cdc.gov/growthcharts/.

65. Moss SD. Nonsurgical, nonorthotic treatment of occipital plagiocephaly: what is the natural history of the misshapen head? J Neurosurg 1997; 87:667–70.

66. Maughans TA. The misshapen head. Pediatrics 2002; 110:166–7.

67. Persing J, James H, Swanson J, Kattwinkel J. Prevention and management of positional skull deformities in infants. Pediatrics 2003; 112:199–202.

68. Miller RI, Clarren SK. Long-term developmental outcomes in patients with deformational plagiocephaly. Pediatrics 2000; 105:E26.

69. Balan P, Kushnerenko E, Sahlin P, Huotilainen M, Naatanen R, Hukki J. Auditory ERPs reveal brain dysfunction in infants with plagiocephaly. J Craniofac Surg 2002; 13:520–5; discussion 526.

70. Virtanen R, Korhonen T, Fagerholm J, Viljanto J. Neurocognitive sequelae of scaphocephaly. Pediatrics 1999; 103:791–5.

13

DEVELOPMENTAL DELAY

Developmental delays may be broadly categorized as "disorders that interfere with the child's ability to communicate, relate and think creatively and logically" in an age-appropriate manner, or as "disorders in the regulation of activity and attention."[1] Using this definition, nearly all internationally adopted children are developmentally delayed at arrival (Table 13–1). Less is known about the long-term developmental outcome of this group and the incidence of learning disabilities and cognitive delays (see Chapters 31–33). Many factors contribute to the prevalence of these problems in international adoptees (Table 13–2). This chapter reviews the components that influence developmental delay, learning disabilities, and cognition among international adoptees. The results of interventions to treat developmental delay, suggested screening techniques for this special population, and current knowledge of the developmental and cognitive outcome of internationally adopted children are also discussed.

Developmental Delay in Internationally Adopted Children

The prevalence of developmental delay among internationally adopted children at arrival varies from 10% to 90%,[2,3] depending on the methods used to identify delay (mail survey, screening assessment, detailed assessment), the definition of delay, the ages of the children studied, and the time after adoptive placement (Table 13–1). When examined as a separate variable, duration of institutionalization correlates with the prevalence of developmental delays in adopted infants[3,4] (Fig. 13–1). Moreover, growth retardation and concurrent medical problems are linked to the frequency and severity of delay.[4,5] The applicability of these findings to children adopted after ~3 years of age is complicated by the heterogeneous nature of this population (placed in care after initial residence with birth family, selection bias for adoptive placement of developmentally normal children, etc.).

Table 13–1 Prevalence of developmental delay among newly arrived international adoptees

Country of Origin (N)	Receiving Country	Comments
China (192)[4]	United States	75% had developmental delay; including GM 55%, FM 49%, cognition 32%, language 43%, S/E 28%, ADL 30%, global 44%
		Delays correlated with growth z scores and duration in orphanage (for ADL and language)
India (114)[6]	Sweden	29% with developmental delays
Eastern Europe (56)[7]	United States	Types of delay: GM 70%, FM 82%, language 59%, S/E 53%
India (200)[8]	United States	18% with developmental delays
22 countries (129)[5]	United States	50% had developmental delays; including GM 33%, FM 40%, language 18%, cognition 16%, global 14%.
		Delays correlated with growth and medical problems
Romania (22)[9]	Canada	Global developmental delays at arrival (DQ ~ 80)
		Improvement to normal range (DQ ~ 90) at follow-up ~12 months later[a]
Romania (65)[3]	United States	65% of infants at ≤6 months were normal; only 30% of infants 7–12 months old were normal, only 10% of children 12–24 months old were normal, and only 10% of those >24 months old were normal
Southeast Asia (28)[10]	Belgium	When assessed 4–12 years after adoption, IQ scores surpassed those of Belgian general population[a]
Asia/Latin America (128)[2]	United States	36% had visual impairment, 36% had hearing problems, 9% had developmental delay, 1% had mental retardation
Asia, Pacific or Caribbean countries, or South America (100)[11]	Australia	2% had hearing problems, 6% had visual problems
Africa, Indian Ocean countries, Southeast Asia (68)[12]	France	22% had psychomotor delays (variable definition)
Romania (44)[13,14]	Canada	Delays in all areas of development at arrival
		Improved ~2 DQ points per month in adoptive homes[a]
Romania (111) (all adopted before age 2 years)[15]	United Kingdom	About half of children were below the third DQ percentile
		Cognitive recovery was nearly complete in most about 2–3 years later[a]

ADL, activities of daily living; DQ, developmental quotient; FM, fine motor; GM, gross motor; S/E, social emotional.

[a]Follow-up information. Definitions of delay differed among studies.

Table 13–2 Possible causes of developmental delay

Genetic/metabolic

Anatomic

Prenatal exposures (drugs, alcohol, toxins) (see Chapters 5–7)

Perinatal events (including prematurity, intrauterine growth retardation, perinatal complications)

Malnutrition (see Chapter 10)

Micronutrient deficiencies (see Chapter 11)

Toxic exposures (lead, mercury, radiation, others) (see Chapter 24)

Illness

Deprived environment (swaddling, lack of nurturing physical contact, auditory and visual deprivation, rote care, long naps, lack of experience, neglect, abuse, trauma) (see Chapter 2)

Unknown

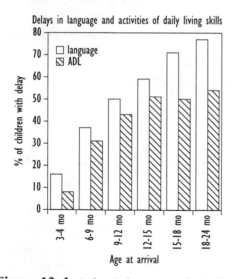

Figure 13–1 *Delays in language and activities of daily living skills tend to increase with duration of orphanage confinement in children adopted from China. (Reproduced by permission of Pediatrics, Vol. 105, p e76. Copyright 2000.)*

Risk Factors for Developmental Delay in Internationally Adopted Children

Environmental Deprivation

Numerous factors may contribute to developmental delay among internationally adopted children (Table 13–2); many may affect the same individual. Environmental deprivation is one of the chief causes of developmental delay. In experimental animals, environmental deprivation alters the actual structure of the brain. Animals raised in complex, enriched environments have more brain synapses, brain weight, cortical thickness, dendritic arborization, and new blood vessels, and better learning abilities and memory than animals raised in non-enriched environments.[16,17] Critical periods occur during which specific types of experience are needed for the brain to develop normally.[17] During these critical periods, the organism is biologically prepared for specific sensory inputs or experiences—if these are not encountered, then structural development of the brain may be impaired. Development of language[18] and visual pathways[19] is clearly dependent on appropriate input during critical periods. Children adopted from Romania who experienced severe environmental deprivation have altered brain metabolic activity[20] demonstrable by positron emission tomography (PET) scanning.

Children residing in orphanages throughout the world have decreased developmental abilities, compared with family-raised children.[21–28] Reduction in IQ score of as much as 30 points has been found in 3- to 4-year-old children of similar backgrounds residing in orphanages rather than foster homes.[29] Pervasive deficiencies in language, social skills, and imaginary play have also been documented among institutionalized children.[24,26] The contribution of depression to these test results has not been independently assessed.

In institutional settings, numerous factors conspire to delay development (see Chapter 2). The contrast to family life is stark. Young infants are often swaddled or confined to a crib, greatly restricting their physical mobility. Supine sleeping is associated with delayed motor milestones[30]; prolonged restriction in this position likely magnifies these effects. Children are expected to take lengthy naps (Table 13–3). Children without a loving caregiver may be depressed and lack motivation to explore. Social contacts are limited; opportunities for eye contact, touch, and physical closeness are minimal; overtures from the child may not be acknowledged. Monotony and lack of novelty are nearly universal in institutional settings. Toy selection may be limited or inappropriate for the child's age; toys may be kept on display but inaccessible. Children may be limited to a single room, playpen, or area, with rare excursions to other parts of the building or outdoors. Some children have never been off the grounds of the orphanage, and have literally been imprisoned. This monotonous existence and paucity of experience globally impedes development.

Perhaps the most critical environmental factors determining developmental delay are the

> *Goldfarb describes infant life in a family as follows:*
>
> *"The [warm, loving parental] contact is a source of constant stimulation. The child is fondled and handled physically a great deal. He is sung lullabies and talked to. His motor and verbal response receive immediate recognition. He is encouraged to babble, to form sounds and then words, to sit up, to stand up, to walk and climb. He is presented with many multicolored toys. He is carried through a house full of interesting objects, meets children and adults, and is often fascinated by animals about him. He is encouraged to perform various life tasks and to react to problems and frustrations in a way that is pleasing to his parents whom he loves and wants to please."[29]*

quality and quantity of language input received by the children.[31] Children raised in "language-poor" families have reduced vocabulary and syntactic skills and use fewer words and more simplistic speech patterns than children in more "language-enriched" homes.[32] Children's vocabularies increase in relation to the amount of "mother speech" (Table 13–4). Orphanages tend to be exceedingly language-poor environments for young children, with little affect-laden speech or encouragement of verbal production by the child.[31] Orphanage routines do not promote the expression of opinions or preferences by the children, and leave little room for discussion or response to novelty. Indeed, among 3-year-old children residing in Moscow region orphanages, only 14% of children used two-word phrases.[33]

Table 13–3　Schedule for 4- to 7-year-old children in a Romanian orphanage

Time	Activity
7 AM	Waken, wash, dress
7:30–8:30 AM	Breakfast, clean-up
8:30–10 AM	Playroom
10–11:30 AM	Rest, nap
11:30–12:30 PM	Lunch, clean-up
12:30–2 PM	Playroom
2–5 PM	Rest, nap
5–6 PM	Dinner, clean-up
6–7 PM	Playroom
7–8 PM	Bathe, prepare for bed
8 PM	Bedtime, lights out

Note that the same playroom is used throughout the day. Few toys are available, with little or no supervision or organized activities.

Table 13–4　Relation of vocabulary size to maternal talkativeness

Age (months)	*Increase in No. of Vocabulary Words for Children of Most Talkative vs. Least Talkative Mothers*
16	+30
20	+131
26	+290

Source: Data from Huttenlocher.[32]

Malnutrition

Malnutrition or undernutrition also affect development (see Chapter 10). Poor nutrition impairs development by reducing the child's spontaneous physical activity.[34] Among Romanian children residing in institutional care, a strong correlation was found between mental age (but not cognitive potential) and motor age.[24] Motor ability permits the children to experience the environment, poor as it might be, to the fullest. Apathy, depression, and passivity may result from generalized malnutrition or specific micronutrient deficiencies (iron, zinc, iodine) (see Chapter 11), and may diminish the child's ability to interact with the environment.

Medical Conditions

Medical problems are common among children living in institutional care. Recurrent respiratory, gastrointestinal, and skin infections are frequent and may lead to isolation within the orphanage or to a hospital admission. During these times, children are separated from familiar caregivers, peers, and their routine; developmental regression is common. Children may also have unrecognized episodes of otitis media and/or prolonged periods of serous otitis. This functional auditory isolation may severely limit language development; vestibular function may also be impaired. Finally, parasitic infestations (trichuria, geohelminths) may also impair cognitive development,[35,36] even if transient (see Chapter 17). Newly arrived adoptees with concurrent medical conditions are more likely to be developmental delayed.[4,5]

Environmental Enrichment after Developmental Delay

Can developmental delays from environmental deprivation be reduced by improving the child's surroundings? Most studies addressing this question have been conducted in the developing world. Such studies compare the cognitive outcome of malnourished, developmentally delayed children provided with home visitors, maternal educational programs, or similar interventions with that of children who did not receive such assistance. Long-term studies in Jamaica have shown that such stimulation programs globally improve developmental abilities.[34,37–42] Developmental intervention improved IQ scores by about half a standard deviation. Earlier interventions (both dietary and developmental) had more effect than those given later. Nutritional supplementation and educational programs synergistically improve developmental quotients. Sustained effects on IQ, reasoning ability, and vocabulary were found at ages 11 to 12 years, 8 years after the interventions were discontinued.[42] Psychosocial stimulation alone sometimes improved cognitive outcome,[43–45] but other environmental factors, such as the caregiver's verbal IQ, education, and level of stimulation in the home, also contributed to improvement.[46,47]

Several studies have addressed the effects of interventions on developmental outcome of institutionalized children. Among well-nourished, mentally retarded children living in institutional care, participation in an educational program[28] prevented the decline in IQ that nonparticipants experienced. Over 4 years, the enrichment group gained 1.4 IQ points, whereas the deprived group lost 9.65 points. Similarly, young infants in an Iranian orphanage exposed to brief periods of daily stimulation for 6 weeks showed improvement in mental and psychomotor development scores that persisted for 6 months.[48] Overall, the children had less severe decline in development than the control group. In a highly enriched orphanage environment in Iran, developmental abilities of children surpassed "even home-reared American children from predominantly professional families."[49] In the United Kingdom, children in some orphanages had developmental test scores near or above average. These orphanages had small mixed age groups, high staff-to-child ratios, and few household duties for the staff, all factors which increased the frequency of conversation between the adults and the children.[31] Finally, orphans in an enriched program in Eritrea had better cognitive abilities than a group of comparison children.[50]

Adoption is the most dramatic "intervention" for developmental delay due to environmental deprivation. In addition to marked improvement in growth (see Chapter 10), adoption enhances cognition. For example, in one study, all 138 Korean children adopted before age 3 years later achieved above-average IQ scores[51,52] (see Fig. 10–7), and 28 Southeast Asian children adopted in Belgium showed above-average intelligence scores at school age.[10] Studies of Indian children adopted in Sweden and Romanian children adopted in the United Kingdom confirm the links between developmental and growth recovery.[6,15,53] The duration and severity of deprivation are the most significant factors influencing cognitive gains achieved after adoption. Most recovery appears to occur within the first 2 years after placement. Although later-placed children may achieve cognitive scores within the normal range, younger children were more likely to achieve higher scores.[51,15,53] For example, a group of young Romanian children adopted in Canada showed normal or near-normal developmental quotients within 12 months after adoption.[9,13]

Developmental Delay at Arrival

At the time of adoption, many post-institutionalized children display global developmental delays. *Gross motor delays* are the most obvious and may be the most worrisome to parents even though they may be the least serious and shortest lasting. Many children are moderately hypotonic at arrival. Decreased muscle strength is also common. Some have persistent primitive reflexes. Clenched fists and the asymmetric tonic neck reflex often persist past 4 months of age. Absence of the foot placing reflex is common in young infants who rarely have the chance to bounce on someone's lap to practice placing the feet and extending the knees and hips to neutral. Children living in institutional settings are rarely placed prone and therefore lack the opportunity to practice neck and trunk extension[30] or shoulder muscle contraction, resulting in proximal instability. Swaddled infants are unable to practice toes-to-mouth exploration so critical to development of the strength of the abdominal muscles. Children confined to cribs have limited opportunities to practice other mobility skills, such as rolling, creeping, or crawling. Occasionally, children have normal or near-normal gross motor skills. This should not be assumed to be a sign of "intelligence": most children with IQ scores in the range of 55–69 walk on time, and among those with an IQ <55, 40% walk by 15–16 months.[54]

In addition to delays in gross motor skills, *fine motor skills* are also frequently delayed in new arrivals. Lack of experience or practice again contribute to these delays. Toys, if available, may be tied to the crib for visual stimulation but are not available to touch and manipulate. There may be limited toy choices. Older children may not have had the opportunity to play with simple tools, such as crayons or scissors, delaying visual–motor perceptual abilities. Additionally, some children have uncorrected strabismus,[55] making eye–hand coordination difficult.

Although dramatic, delayed motor skills have less prognostic significance than the language and cognitive delays among newly arrived international adoptees. *Language* delays are frequently overlooked or discounted in new arrivals (see Chapter 31). Awareness of the need to learn a new language often overshadows recognition of the nearly universal delay in the child's birth language. In young infants, delays in preverbal skills may not be appreciated, although identification and remediation of this deficiency is exceedingly important. Language ability is often cited as the best predictor of intelligence; the applicability of this to international adoptees is unknown.[54] As with motor delays, environmental deprivation is the most common cause of language deficits among institutionalized children. However, the possibility of hearing im-

> The Jones twins arrived at 4 years of age. Their parents had been told that they spoke "their own language" with each other. Actually, both had severe language impairments with 6-month expressive language skills. The children communicated by grunting and gesturing. Hearing was intact. Cognitive skills were assessed at age 3 years. One year later, expressive language scores were ~12 months, and cognition was 4 years. Childhood apraxia of speech was diagnosed and intensive therapy begun.

pairment as a factor in language delays must never be overlooked: unrecognized or untreated otitis media and serous otitis are frequent among orphanage children. Other possible explanations for language delay include mental retardation, learning disabilities, cerebral palsy, central communication disorders (including autism), mutism, and oral structural or mechanical defects.[54] In general, children with significant language delays in the first 2 years of life rarely develop normal language. A small number of children have developmental language impairment, a focal delay in expressive and/or receptive language in the absence of global cognitive disability, autism, hearing loss, social or emotional problems, or severe environmental deprivation. Some have specific abnormalities on magnetic resonance imaging studies (ventricular enlargement, central volume loss, white-matter abnormalities) suggesting more global neurologic dysfunction.[56]

Problem-solving skills may be difficult to assess shortly after arrival, as children may have no experience or familiarity with the testing materials. Visual interest, curiosity, attention, and exploratory behaviors can be observed, however. Abilities in this area are reliable indicators of nonverbal intelligence; along with language skills these may attest to intellectual strengths. Difficulties in these areas in new arrivals do not necessarily presage later problems.

In contrast to the delays in other domains, *social and self-help skills* are often a particular strength of post-institutionalized children.[24] Children often have been carefully trained in

activities of daily living, and can feed and dress themselves, and wash their hands at surprisingly early ages. Toilet training also is instituted early, although many children regress after adoption. Some children, if given the opportunity, excel in imitation skills. Sharing, taking turns, and cleaning up are also inculcated early. Social skills are highly influenced by environmental exposure. Again, early difficulties do not necessarily predict later problems. Many children are exceptionally engaging and sociable; some are indiscriminately friendly (see Chapter 29). Such adaptive behaviors are reinforced in the orphanage environment.

Attention span is also an important quality to assess in the newly arrived adoptee. Many children in the early days to weeks after adoption display fragmented, distractible, short attention spans. Although this may predict later attentional difficulties, early distractibility is often a reaction to the removal from the monotonous orphanage environment. In the stimulating environment of the adoptive home and the many other environments encountered during normal daily routines, the child may become distractible, inattentive, and overstimulated. This may be commonly observed in a developmental testing situation, where a series of engaging and usually unfamiliar toys is presented within a short time span. With time, regulation of attention span improves. However, hyperactivity, short attention span, and impulsivity may be the first signs of learning disabilities.[54]

Evaluation of Developmental Delay in New Arrivals

Newly arrived internationally adopted children should undergo developmental screening shortly after entry to ascertain their strengths, weaknesses, and need for professional intervention. The assessment must be done at a time most likely to provide an accurate picture (i.e., not the first 48 hours after arrival in the United States!). The child should be comfortable and relaxed, with the preferred caretaker present and assisting. The developmental assessment should be done before painful immunizations, blood tests, or physical examination is attempted.

Most pediatricians are familiar with the Denver Developmental Screening Test. This test has the advantage of familiarity, ease of administration, and reliability but the disadvantage of low specificity and lack of detail. Another manageable option is the Hawaii Early Learning Profile (0–3 years, and 3–6 years, including gross and fine motor, social/emotional, cognition, language, and self-help) (see Appendix 13–1). Developmental screening takes a minimum of 20–30 minutes, more complete testing takes 45–60 minutes; it is therefore useful to schedule specific appointments to accomplish this task. Parent questionnaires may also aid in the identification of children requiring more complete evaluation. Several options are available for different age groups, including the Ages and Stages Questionnaire, the Child Development Inventories, and the Parents' Evaluations of Developmental Status (reviewed in refs. 57 and 58). Asking open-ended questions about development and behavior ("What concerns do you have about the way your child is behaving, learning, developing . . .") is also a validated approach to identifying parental concerns[57,58] but is not as comprehensive as necessary to assess new arrivals. Standardized, multidomain assessments are usually needed to determine eligibility for therapy services. Such evaluations quantify functional age levels and aid parent understanding and perception of the child's abilities, skills, and deficits. Comprehensive developmental testing is available through state early intervention programs (birth to 3 years of age) and local school districts (3–18 years of age) at no cost to families in most locations (they are federally mandated, state funded).

Determination of language competence is a critical part of the developmental assessment on arrival (see Chapter 31). For infants, prespeech utterances may be assessed regardless of the language to which the child was exposed prior to adoption. Older children are best assessed by a

Jason arrived at age 34 months from Russia. His birth mother, said to be schizophrenic, became pregnant while hospitalized in a mental institution. Jason's orphanage had a total of 17 caregivers for 70 children; only 4–5 were on duty at a time. When he arrived, he was covered with (human) bite marks and scratches. He was loud, aggressive, and angry. He weighed 10 kg (weight for age 12 months), was 94 cm tall (height for age 32 months), and had head circumference of 47 cm (average for age 12 months). His developmental skills were assessed at age 17 months for gross and fine motor and cognition. Language was at age 7–10 months, and activities of daily living were at 23 months. His hematocrit was 26%. A positive tuberculin skin test was found, and within several months, a diagnosis of celiac disease was made. With time, his growth and temperament improved dramatically. Development progressed slowly; by age 5 years he could name only five body parts, and erratically identified colors. He had poor articulation. He continued to exhibit the frequent rocking that he displayed on arrival. His behavior stabilized somewhat with clonidine and methylphenidate (Ritalin). He was able to progress in a structured classroom where most of the other children had autism.

bilingual adult shortly after arrival in the United States or, alternatively, by a speech pathologist or educator in the birth country prior to travel. The results of the assessment can then be carefully translated by a competent interpreter. Many children "lose" their birth language quickly, and after immersion in an English-speaking environment, there may be considerable delay before the new language emerges.[59]

Ongoing Developmental Assessment

It is helpful to continue ongoing developmental assessment of the international adoptee during routine follow-up visits. For delayed children, the velocity of developmental progress is more important than scores on standardized developmental tests. Assessment of functional progress may be more useful than reliance on standardized developmental tests (Fig. 13–2).[1] Rather than focusing on specific mile-

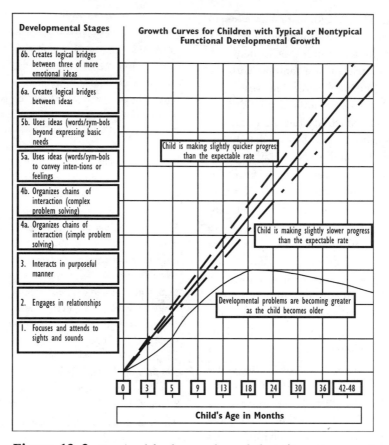

Figure 13–2 *Functional developmental growth chart. (From Greenspan S. Overview and recommendations. In: Greenspan S, Interdisciplinary Council on Developmental and Learning Disorders, eds. Clinical Practice Guidelines. Bethesda, MD: ICDL Press, 2000: 48, with permission.)*

stones, this technique assesses functional development—in other words, the critical building blocks of development, including social interaction, problem solving, and the symbolic and creative use of ideas.[1] Details of this method of developmental assessment are described elsewhere.[1]

Developmental concerns may emerge in some internationally adopted children months or years after arrival in the United States. The pediatrician must guard against some common misconceptions about international adoptees (Table 13–5). Persistent hyperactivity, short attention span, and impulsivity may indicate a learning disability or other problems beyond expected transitional issues. Children deserve a comprehensive evaluation including biomed-

ical assessment, observation of child–caregiver interactions, review of educational program and peer interactions, and assessments of auditory processing, functional language, motor and perceptual motor function, and sensory

Table 13–5 *Misconceptions* about development of internationally adopted children

- Independent ambulation before 18 months = normal intelligence.
- Deaf infants are mute.
- Most mentally retarded infants are dysmorphic.
- Internationally adopted children are language delayed because they need to learn a new language.
- Internationally adopted children will catch-up with time, love, and the care of their parents alone.

processing.[1] Medical evaluation should include neurologic examination (review of serial head circumference measurements, search for dysmorphic features, neurocutaneous examination including Wood's lamp examination), hearing and vision screens, and, for those children with abnormal findings, consideration of more extensive investigation (EEG, metabolic tests [quantitative amino acids and organic acids], urinary uric acid excretion, thyroid studies, and lactate, pyruvate, carnitine, and lead levels). If dysmorphic physical features are found, fragile X testing and high-resolution cytogenetics may be helpful. If a focal lesion is suggested by neurologic examination, cranial magnetic resonance imaging is indicated. Single photon emission computerized tomography (SPECT) or PET scans are presently considered research tools, although they will likely provide useful information in the near future.

In some children, subtle developmental issues become apparent with time. For example, 4-year-old Romanian adoptees demonstrate less interactive role play and imaginary play than adopted British children.[60] Although seemingly minor, this may reflect gaps in understanding the connections between feelings and intentions and actions. In these children, verbal ability also correlated with pretend play skills.

Complex Neurobehavioral Disorders

Some internationally adopted children have complex neurobehavioral disorders. These children usually have global developmental delays, but language and visuomotor perception are most severely affected. Some also have severe attentional, emotional, and behavioral problems, making their management extremely complex (see Chapters 30 and 32). These disorders may be roughly categorized as interactive disorders, regulatory disorders, or disorders of relating and communicating (Table 13–6). Many children have difficulties in more than one area. The category of "disorders of relating and communicating" is the most frustrating for parents, and the most difficult to treat.

Vicky's mom traveled to Romania to collect her. She was dismayed to find her 2-year-old daughter huddled in a corner rocking incessantly and unable to make eye contact. Her growth was at the fifth to tenth percentiles for all parameters. Formal developmental testing on arrival revealed skills in the 6- to 10-month range, except feeding, which was at 4 months. Vicky had frequent self-stimulatory behavior (rocking, head-banging) and often "disappeared into a trance." As she grew older, she became violent and aggressive, was hyperactive, and developed many obsessive behaviors. Multiple medications were prescribed, with varying results as recorded by her mother:

Age (years)	Medication	Result
3.9	Methylphenidate (Ritalin)	Severe agitation
3.9	Clonidine	Extreme emotional lability
3.9	Risperidone (Risperdal)	Helps with mood, anger, aggression
4	Guanfacine (Tenex)	No help with hyperactivity or impulsivity
5.3	Dextroamphetamine (Dexadrine)	Severe agitation, stuttering, poor sleep, upset stomach
5.6	Gabapentin (Neurontin)	Helped with giddiness and rage but was short-lived
5.8	Dextro-/levoamphetamine (Adderall XR)	Helps with hyperactivity and impulsivity
5.10	Paroxetine (Paxil)	Manic/psychotic reaction
5.11	Divalproex (Depakote)	Helps with mania and rage, somewhat sedative

By age 9 years, she had been hospitalized on the children's psychiatry ward twice.

Alice was adopted from China at 7 months of age. Her orphanage had five caregivers for 100 children. Her parents noted that it was extremely quiet and that no toys were evident. After adoption, her parents felt she was very placid. Her growth parameters were all at the fifth percentiles. She was markedly hypotonic on examination. Formal developmental testing disclosed that her skills clustered between age 0 and 2 months. She entered a structured program and received many hours of daily therapy and excellent support from her devoted parents. At 16 months of age, her skills had progressed only to about 6–8 months. By 24 months, she had skills of a 12-month-old. Intensive therapy continued. By 5 years of age, Alice had a 300+ word vocabulary, used two- to four-word sentences with poor syntax and articulation. She had frequent bruxism and was very distractable. She behaved oddly during examination, for example, rubbing the cloth of the doctor's skirt and making no eye contact.

Occasionally, autistic qualities are also present. Of 111 Romanian children adopted in Great Britain, 6% showed autistic-like patterns of behavior (and a further 6% showed isolated autistic features). These children met diagnostic criteria for autism when studied at age 4 years, but 2 years later had showed improvement; in some cases it was remarkable.[61] Apparently, some adoptees with these behavior patterns do surprisingly well after placement within a loving home, intensive interventions, and medications. Precise diagnosis in this population is particularly complicated. For example, hand flapping is a relatively common "orphanage behavior" that persists after adoption. Hand flapping occurs for a variety of reasons.[62] It may be used by a hyperreactive child to gain selective focus and to screen out non-essential parts of the visual environment. In contrast, the hyporeactive child uses the same behavior to increase his or her state of arousal. A third child uses hand flapping to discharge tension. Thus, stereotypy should not be considered diagnostic of autism-spectrum disorders, and even in the same child, the same behavior may have different meanings at different times.[62] The context, frequency, and duration of such behaviors should be considered, as well as their interference with social and environmental interactions.

Multiple complex diagnoses were identified in a study of 30% of Romanian children adopted in Canada. These children had three or more serious problems (IQ <85, atypical insecure attachment pattern to the family, severe behavior problems, or persistent stereotypic behaviors) present more than 3 years after adoption.[14] Recent work by Johnson and col-

Table 13–6 Complex developmental disorders

Type of Disorder	Typical Symptoms	Diagnoses to Consider
Interactive disorders: alterations in the way the child perceives and experiences his or her emotional world	Anxiety, fearful, behavioral controlling, sleeping and eating disorders	Post-traumatic stress disorder, anxiety disorders, mood disorders (including grief, depression), reactive attachment disorder, adjustment disorders
Regulatory disorders: constitutional and maturational deficits	Attentional and behavior problems, irritability, aggression, distractibility, poor frustration tolerance, tantrums, sleeping and eating disorders	Hypersensitive (fearful, cautious, difficult to engage) *or* hyposensitive (withdrawn, self-absorbed, stimulus craving)
Disorders of relating and communicating: impaired social relationships, language, cognition, motor and sensory function	Global disruption in functioning	Multisystem developmental disorder, pervasive developmental delay, neglect, abuse, failure to thrive

Source: Adapted from Greenspan.[1]

Table 13–7 Pre-adoption risk factors for complex developmental delays

Risk Factor	How Determined
Prenatal malnutrition	Head circumference z score <-2 at birth
Prenatal alcohol exposure	Maternal history and/or characteristic facial appearance
Premature birth	Birth weight <2.5 kg
Physically neglected	Weight-for-height z score <-2 or weight and height z scores <-3
Socially neglected	Global developmental delays
Physically abused	History (usually unable to determine)
Prolonged institutionalization	≥ 6 months

Source: Data from Johnson.[63]

leagues determined that the likelihood of complex developmental disorders increases with the number of pre-adoption risk factors identified (Table 13–7).[63] Children with higher numbers of risk factors were more likely to have growth deficits, cognitive delays, and behavior and relationship problems.

Developmental Outcomes of Internationally Adopted Children

Most children rapidly achieve developmental milestones after adoption. Children adopted from difficult circumstances in Romania to the United Kingdom showed remarkable catch-up within 3 years even though more than 50% had developmental quotients <50 when tested on arrival.[15] Similar improvements were found in Romanian children adopted to Canada.[9,13,14] IQs of Southeast Asian children adopted to Belgium surpassed those of locally born children within 4–12 years after adoption.[10] However, long-term cognitive capabilities and academic achievement remain to be explored. The prevalence of learning disabilities, language delays, and associated behavioral problems in this population of children is not yet defined with certainty (see Chapters 31 and 32). As the internationally adopted children who arrived in the United States since the mid- to late 1990s (129,895 children between 1995 and 2002) progress through school, these questions will be answered. For example, a recent survey of parents of 8- to 12-year-old children adopted from Eastern Europe revealed that 61% of children were receiving modified educational programs.[63] All were within one grade level of expected. Thirty-six percent had learning disabilities, and 45% had multiple complex diagnoses, including 38% with attention-deficit hyperactivity disorder, 32% with post-traumatic stress disorder, 19% with depression, 19% with anxiety, 16% with reactive attachment disorder, and 5% with obsessive compulsive disorder. Further investigations delineating the developmental recovery and educational achievements of this group of children are awaited by professionals and by parents.

Key Points for Internationally Adopted Children

- Developmental delay is common in new arrivals.
- Most children display rapid catch-up; motor delays recover quickly.
- Recovery from language delays usually lags behind other areas.
- After initial recovery, many children later have learning disabilities and school-related problems.
- A small group of children have complex neurobehavioral disorders that require intensive management.

FAQs

Q. My 11-month-old patient from Ukraine scores at about 7 months on the Denver. What can I recommend to help her catch-up?

Sally arrived at 15 months. Her growth was at the 10th–25th percentile for all parameters. Her developmental scores ranged from 9 to 11 months, with the lowest scores for expressive language. At follow-up 3 months later, her skills were at 15–16 months of age. By age 2 years, her development was completely age-appropriate.

A. A more complete developmental assessment may be useful to obtain now as a baseline. If you are unable to do this, the local early intervention program ("Birth to Three" program) in your community should be able to perform the assessment. They also offer and supervise ongoing therapy for your patient. Parent education, including recommended therapeutic activities to perform each day with the child, and the expected sequence and rate of progress will also be useful. Frequent follow-up and support by you will also be welcomed by the parents. If a local support group exists for families who have adopted from Ukraine (e.g., FRUA—Families for Russian and Ukrainian Adoption), referral of the parents may also be useful.

Q. Someone told me that for every 3 months in the orphanage, the child loses 1 month developmentally. Is this right?

A. No—a common misconception. This frequent misquote refers to growth. For every 3 months in the orphanage, children lose 1 month of height age.[3,4,7] Development is far too complex to measure in such a simplistic way. Although duration of orphanage confinement clearly contributes to developmental delay, many other factors also influence this.

Q. I think I have one of those "complex developmental delay" kids in my practice. Help!

A. These kids need an enormous amount of help, as do their parents. The first stop should be neurology or developmental pediatrics. Baseline assessment, and "working" diagnoses are needed to direct therapy. MRI and/or PET scans may be needed to identify anatomic abnormalities. Don't forget the hearing screen too. Occupational therapists with sensory processing expertise and other specialized therapists can provide enormous assistance.

Resource

VORT Corporation. Hawaii Early Learning Profile (HELP). Available at: http://www.vort.com/profb3.htm.

Appendix 13–1 Sample items from cognitive section of Hawaii Early Learning Profile for 5- to 6-month-old infants

5 Months	5½ Months	6 Months
Plays with paper	Shows interest in sounds of objects	Plays 2–3 minutes with a single toy
Turns eyes and head to sound of hidden voice	Anticipates visually the trajectory of a slowly moving object	Follows the trajectory of fast-moving object
Reaches for second object purposefully	Works for desired, out of reach object	Retains two of three objects offered
		Slides toy or object on surface
Distinguishes between friendly and angry voices	Responds to facial expressions	Looks for family members or pets when named
Brings feet to mouth		

References

1. Greenspan S. Overview and recommendations. In: Greenspan S et al. (eds.), Interdisciplinary Council on Developmental and Learning Disorders, eds. Clinical Practice Guidelines. Bethesda, MD: ICDLD Press, 2000: 13–55.

2. Jenista JA, Chapman D. Medical problems of foreign-born adopted children. Am J Dis Child 1987; 141:298–302.

3. Johnson DE, Miller LC, Iverson S, et al. The health of children adopted from Romania. JAMA 1992; 268:3446–51.

4. Miller LC, Hendrie NW. Health of children adopted from China. Pediatrics 2000; 105:E76.

5. Miller LC, Kiernan MT, Mathers MI, Klein-Gitelman M. Developmental and nutritional status of internationally adopted children. Arch Pediatr Adolesc Med 1995; 149:40–4.

6. Proos LA, Hofvander Y, Wennqvist K, Tuvemo T. A longitudinal study on anthropometric and clinical de-

velopment of Indian children adopted in Sweden. II. Growth, morbidity and development during two years after arrival in Sweden. Ups J Med Sci 1992; 97:93–106.

7. Albers LH, Johnson DE, Hostetter MK, Iverson S, Miller LC. Health of children adopted from the former Soviet Union and Eastern Europe. Comparison with preadoptive medical records. JAMA 1997; 278:922–4.

8. Smith-Garcia T, Brown JS. The health of children adopted from India. J Community Health 1989; 14:227–41.

9. Benoit TC, Jocelyn LJ, Moddemann DM, Embree JE. Romanian adoption. The Manitoba experience. Arch Pediatr Adolesc Med 1996; 150:1278–82.

10. Wattier P, Frydman M. L'adoption internationale. Enfance 1985; 1:59–76.

11. Nicholson AJ, Francis BM, Mulholland EK, Moulden AL, Oberklaid F. Health screening of international adoptees. Evaluation of a hospital-based clinic. Med J Aust 1992; 156:377–9.

12. Bureau JJ, Maurage C, Bremond M, Despert F, Rolland JC. Children of foreign origin adopted in France. Analysis of 68 cases during 12 years at the University Hospital Center of Tours [in French]. Arch Pediatr 1999; 6:1053–8.

13. Morison SJ, Ames EW, Chisholm K. The development of children adopted from Romanian orphanages. Merrill-Palmer Q 1995; 41:411–30.

14. Ames EW. The Development of Romanian Orphanage Children Adopted to Canada. Burnaby, BC: Human Resources Development Canada, 1997.

15. Rutter M. Developmental catch-up and delay, following adoption after severe global early privation. J Child Psychol Psychiatry 1998; 39:465–76.

16. Greenough WT, Black JE, Wallace CS. Experience and brain development. Child Dev 1987; 58:539–59.

17. Dawson G, Ashman SB, Carver LJ. The role of early experience in shaping behavioral and brain development and its implications for social policy. Dev Psychopathol 2000; 12:695–712.

18. Newport EL. Maturational constraints on language learning. Cog Sci 1990; 14:11–28.

19. Levay S, Weisel TN, Hubel DH. The development of ocular dominancy columns in normal and visually deprived monkeys. J Comp Neurol 1980; 19:11–51.

20. Chugani HT, Behen ME, Muzik O, Juhasz C, Nagy F, Chugani DC. Local brain functional activity following early deprivation: a study of postinstitutionalized Romanian orphans. Neuroimage 2001; 14:1290–301.

21. Colombo M, de la Parra A, Lopez I. Intellectual and physical outcome of children undernourished in early life is influenced by later environmental conditions. Dev Med Child Neurol 1992; 34:611–22.

22. Carlson M, Earls F. Psychological and neuroendocrinological sequelae of early social deprivation in institutionalized children in Romania. Ann N Y Acad Sci 1997; 807:419–28.

23. Castle J, Groothues C, Bredenkamp D, Beckett C, O'Connor T, Rutter M. Effects of qualities of early institutional care on cognitive attainment. E.R.A. Study Team. English and Romanian Adoptees. Am J Orthopsychiatry 1999; 69:424–37.

24. Kaler SR, Freeman BJ. Analysis of environmental deprivation: cognitive and social development in Romanian orphans. J Child Psychol Psychiatry 1994; 35:769–81.

25. Otieno PA, Nduati RW, Musoke RN, Wasunna AO. Growth and development of abandoned babies in institutional care in Nairobi. East Afr Med J 1999; 76:430–5.

26. Tizard B, Joseph A. Cognitive development of young children in residential care: a study of children aged 24 months. J Child Psychol Psychiatry 1970; 11:177–86.

27. Tizard B, Hodges J. The effect of early institutional rearing on the development of eight-year-old children. J Child Psychol Psychiatry 1978; 19:99–118.

28. Vogel W, Kun KJ, Meshorer E. Effects of environmental enrichment and environmental deprivation on cognitive functioning in institutionalized retardates. J Consult Psychol 1967; 31:570–6.

29. Goldfarb W. Effects of psychological deprivation in infancy and subsequent stimulation. Am J Psychiatry 1945; 102:18–33.

30. Davis BE, Moon RY, Sachs HC, Ottolini MC. Effects of sleep position on infant motor development. Pediatrics 1998; 102:1135–40.

31. Tizard B, Cooperman O, Joseph A, Tizard J. Environmental effects on language development: a study of young children in long-stay residential nurseries. Child Dev 1972; 43:337–58.

32. Huttenlocher J. Language input and language growth. Prev Med 1998; 27:195–9.

33. Dubrovina I, et al. Psychological Development of Children in Orphanages (Psichologicheskoe razvitie vospitanikov v detskom dome) [in Russian]. Moscow: Prosveschenie Press, 1991.

34. Meeks Gardner J, Grantham-McGregor SM, Chang SM, Himes JH, Powell CA. Activity and behavioral development in stunted and nonstunted children and response to nutritional supplementation. Child Dev 1995; 66:1785–97.

35. Hutchinson SE, Powell CA, Walker SP, Chang SM, Grantham-McGregor SM. Nutrition, anaemia, geohelminth infection and school achievement in rural Jamaican primary school children. Eur J Clin Nutr 1997; 51:729–35.

36. Callender JE, Walker SP, Grantham-McGregor SM, Cooper ES. Growth and development four years after treatment for the Trichuris dysentery syndrome. Acta Paediatr 1998; 87:1247–9.

37. Grantham-McGregor SM, Powell CA, Walker SP, Himes JH. Nutritional supplementation, psychosocial stimulation, and mental development of stunted children: the Jamaican Study. Lancet 1991; 338:1–5.

38. Grantham-McGregor SM, Walker SP, Chang SM, Powell CA. Effects of early childhood supplementation with and without stimulation on later development in stunted Jamaican children. Am J Clin Nutr 1997; 66:247–53.

39. Gardner JM, Grantham-McGregor SM, Himes J, Chang S. Behaviour and development of stunted and non-stunted Jamaican children. J Child Psychol Psychiatry 1999; 40:819–27.

40. Powell CA, Walker SP, Himes JH, Fletcher PD, Grantham-McGregor SM. Relationships between physical growth, mental development and nutritional supplementation in stunted children: the Jamaican study. Acta Paediatr 1995; 84:22–9.

41. Walker SP, Powell CA, Grantham-McGregor SM, Himes JH, Chang SM. Nutritional supplementation, psychosocial stimulation, and growth of stunted children: the Jamaican study. Am J Clin Nutr 1991; 54:642–8.

42. Walker SP, Grantham-Mcgregor SM, Powell CA, Chang SM. Effects of growth restriction in early childhood on growth, IQ, and cognition at age 11 to 12 years and the benefits of nutritional supplementation and psychosocial stimulation. J Pediatr 2000; 137:36–41.

43. McKay H, Sinisterra L, McKay A, Gomez H, Lloreda P. Improving cognitive ability in chronically deprived children. Science 1978; 200:270–8.

44. Waber DP, Vuori-Christiansen L, Ortiz N, et al. Nutritional supplementation, maternal education, and cognitive development of infants at risk of malnutrition. Am J Clin Nutr 1981; 34:807–13.

45. Grantham-McGregor S, Powell C, Walker S, Chang S, Fletcher P. The long-term follow-up of severely malnourished children who participated in an intervention program. Child Dev 1994; 65:428–39.

46. de Andraca Oyarzun I, Gonzalez Lopez B, Salas Aliaga MI. Characteristics of the family structure of school children with antecedents of severe and early malnutrition which nowadays present different intellectual levels [in Spanish]. Arch Latinoam Nutr 1991; 41:168–81.

47. Ramey CT, Bryant DM, Wasik BH, Sparling JJ, Fendt KH, LaVange LM. Infant Health and Development Program for low birth weight, premature infants: program elements, family participation, and child intelligence. Pediatrics 1992; 89:454–65.

48. Hakimi-Manesh Y, Mojdehi H, Tashakkori A. Effects of environmental enrichment on the mental and psychomotor development of orphanage children. J Child Psychol Psychiatry 1984; 25:643–50.

49. Hunt JM, Mohandessi K, Ghodssi M, Akiyama M. The psychological development of orphanage-reared infants: interventions with outcomes (Tehran). Genet Psychol Monogr 1976; 94:177–226.

50. Wolff PH, Fesseha G. The orphans of Eritrea: a five-year follow-up study. J Child Psychol Psychiatry 1999; 40:1231–7.

51. Lien NM, Meyer KK, Winick M. Early malnutrition and "late" adoption: a study of their effects on the development of Korean orphans adopted into American families. Am J Clin Nutr 1977; 30:1734–9.

52. Winick M, Meyer KK, Harris RC. Malnutrition and environmental enrichment by early adoption. Science 1975; 190:1173–5.

53. O'Connor TG, Rutter M, Beckett C, Keaveney L, Kreppner JM. The effects of global severe privation on cognitive competence: extension and longitudinal follow-up. English and Romanian Adoptees Study Team. Child Dev 2000; 71:376–90.

54. Blasco P. Early developmental indicators of intellectual deficit. Pediatr Rounds 1993; 2:1–3.

55. Ivanov V, Miller LC. Strabismus in institutionalized Russian children. Unpublished. Boston: New England Medical Center, 2004.

56. Trauner D, Wulfeck B, Tallal P, Hesselink J. Neurological and MRI profiles of children with developmental language impairment. Dev Med Child Neurol 2000; 42:470–5.

57. Committee on Children with Disabilities. Developmental surveillance and screening of infants and young children. Pediatrics 2001; 108:192–6.

58. Dworkin PH, Glascoe FP. Early detection of developmental delays: how do you measure up? Contemp Pediatr 1997; 14:158–68.

59. McGuinness T, McGuinness J. Speech and language problems in international adoptees. Am Fam Physician 1999; 60:1322–3.

60. Kreppner JM, O'Connor T, Dunn J, Andersen-Wood L. The pretend and social play of children exposed to severe early deprivation. Br J Dev Psychol 1999; 17:319–32.

61. Rutter M, Andersen-Wood L, Beckett C, et al. Quasi-autistic patterns following severe global privation. J Child Psychol Psychiatry 1999; 40:537–49.

62. Williamson GG, Anzalone ME, Hanft BE. Assessment of sensory processing, praxis, and motor performance. In: Greenspan S, et al. (eds) Interdisciplinary Council on Developmental and Learning Disorders. Clinical Practice Guidelines. ICDLC Press, 2000, 155–175.

63. Johnson D. International adoptee follow-up studies: what have we learned from families and how should this information change adoption practice? presented at Joint Council for International Children's Services, Washington, DC, April 9, 2003.

64. Tirella LG, Miller LC. Educational achievements of 8- to 12-year-old children adopted from Eastern Europe: presented at Joint Council for International Children's Services, Washington, DC, April 10, 2002.

65. Blackman JA, Lindgren SD, Bretthauer J. The validity of continuing developmental follow-up of high-risk infants to age 5 years. Am J Dis Child 1992; 146: 70–5.

V

INFECTIOUS DISEASES

14

TUBERCULOSIS

There is more confusion about tuberculosis (TB) than any other infectious disease of internationally adopted children. Correct application and interpretation of diagnostic criteria for TB have been a source of extensive discussions among practitioners caring for these children. Proper management of potential TB infection among international adoptees is critical: unrecognized TB infection is an enormous risk to public health.[1] A dramatic example of this occurred in 1999 in an outbreak of TB affecting 56 people in a small town in North Dakota.[2] The source was a 9-year-old-boy adopted from the Marshall Islands. His adoptive mother presented with tuberculous hip arthritis, osteomyelitis, obturator myositis, and pelvic abscess 2 years after the adoption. Although tine tests were placed on the boy (and his twin brother) shortly after their arrival in the United States, these had not been read and no further evaluation was performed, even though the patient was 5 cm shorter and 5 kg lighter than his twin. Several other reports document transmission of TB from infants to adults.[3–5]

Because of the complexities and importance of this subject in the management of international adoptees, this section reviews the epidemiology of TB infection, specific aspects of TB in international adoptees, clinical features of disease, and application and interpretation of appropriate diagnostic criteria. The management of children with prior Bacille Camille-Guérin (BCG) vaccination is also discussed, as most American physicians are unfamiliar with this topic.

Epidemiology

Tuberculosis is one of the deadliest diseases in the world.[6] Since antiquity, TB has been associated with crowding, malnutrition, and poverty. Worldwide, about 8 million people develop active TB each year (Figure 14–1).[7] About 3 million die

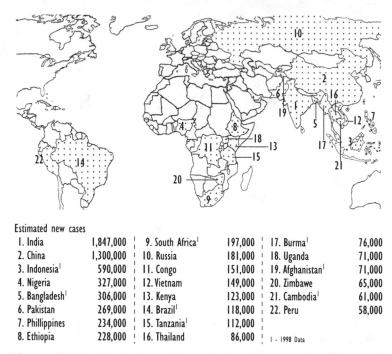

Estimated new cases

1. India	1,847,000	9. South Africa[1]	197,000	17. Burma[1]	76,000
2. China	1,300,000	10. Russia	181,000	18. Uganda	71,000
3. Indonesia[1]	590,000	11. Congo	151,000	19. Afghanistan[1]	71,000
4. Nigeria	327,000	12. Vietnam	149,000	20. Zimbawe	65,000
5. Bangladesh[1]	306,000	13. Kenya	123,000	21. Cambodia[1]	61,000
6. Pakistan	269,000	14. Brazil[1]	118,000	22. Peru	58,000
7. Phillippines	234,000	15. Tanzania[1]	112,000		
8. Ethiopia	228,000	16. Thailand	86,000	1 - 1998 Data	

Figure 14–1 *Distribution of tuberculosis (TB) throughout the world. According to the World Health Organization (WHO), 95% of all TB cases and 99% of all TB deaths are in these 22 countries. Unless noted, data are for 1999. The WHO cautions that the quality of these estimates varies widely. (From Donnelly J. WHO urges $400m for fight against TB. The Boston Globe May 15 2001:A1, A10, with permission.)*

of the disease annually,[6] making it the most frequent infectious cause of death in the world.[8] Nearly 95% of cases occur in the developing world[6]: various sources estimate that between 19% and 43% of the world's population is infected with TB.[6,9] Ninety-five percent of all TB cases and 99% of all TB deaths occur in 22 countries of the world.[10] Many international adoptees arrive in the United States from these countries.

About 15 million people in the United States are infected with TB[6]; nearly half are individuals born outside the United States. In 1999, there were 17,531 new cases of TB reported in the United States: 6% in children under 15 years and 9% in adolescents and young adults 15–24 years of age. Foreign-born children account for ~25% of pediatric cases. Country-specific case rates in foreign-born persons from some common sending countries are shown in Table 14–1.

Table 14–1 Case rate/100,000 by birth country of foreign born in the United States

Birth Country	Rate/1000,000
Vietnam	134.7
Haiti	118.5
Phillipines	95.9
India	75.1
China	62
S. Korea	38.8
Mexico	35.5
Other (186 countries)	18.1

Source: Data from Talbot et al.[7]

Tuberculosis and Internationally Adopted Children

Latent TB infection occurs in ~3% to 19% of internationally adopted children. Most children come from countries with high rates of TB

Table 14–2 Tuberculosis and internationally adopted children

Sending Country (N)	Mean age at arrival (months)	Receiving Country	With tuberculosis[a] (%)
Korea (360)[12]	4	United States	0.5
India (200)[15]	6	United States	2.5
Mostly Korea, Central and South America (293)[13]	14	United States	3 (1.3% with active TB)
Various countries (129)[16]	24	United States	3
China (452)[17]	14.2, 6.5 (2 groups)	United States	3.5
Mostly Korea (101)[14]	6	United States	4
Romania (41)[18]	15.5, 3 (2 groups)	United States	4.8
Mostly Russia (56)[9]	26	United States	5
Mostly Korea and India (100)[20]	33	Australia	9 (3 with active TB)
Mostly Africa and Indian Ocean countries (68)[21]	<12	France	9
Mostly China and Russia (504)[71]	19	United States	19
Refugees from Vietnam, Soviet republics, Africa; *not* adoptees (107)[22]	8 years, 2 months	United States	20

[a]Definitions of infection were not identical in all studies, thus statistics are not strictly comparable.

infection (Table 14–2). Few if any orphanages screen caregivers for TB as a condition for employment, or on an ongoing basis. Furthermore, infants and young children are particularly susceptible to contracting infection. Malnutrition, crowding, and concurrent medical problems further increase the likelihood of infection after exposure in these children. The variable rates among different studies reflect differences in definitions of infection, as well as in the children's countries of origin. For example, Russian origin and orphanage residence correlated highly with TB infection,[11] while infection was infrequent in Korean children who resided in foster care prior to adoption.[12–14]

Clinical Features of Tuberculosis

The course of TB varies enormously after exposure. Malnutrition, young age, close contact with active TB, living or working in congregate settings, residence in a high-prevalence country (China, Southeast Asia, India, Haiti, Domini-

can Republic, Central America, Brazil, Russia and former Soviet Republics, Sub-Saharan Africa), HIV infection, and other medical conditions are all risk factors for development of active disease after exposure.[1] Tuberculosis is highly infectious. It is spread by aerosol generated by coughing, sneezing, spitting, speaking, or singing. Crowded indoor environments with poor ventilation (as found in many orphanages) increase the likelihood of transmission.

Amazingly, about 90% of infected individuals never become ill.[8, 9] Some variation in susceptibility is genetic in origin, although some reflects variation in the virulence of the organism *Mycobacterium tuberculosis*. Host factors, such as age, general health status, nutritional condition, concurrent medical problems, and medications, clearly contribute to disease expression.

Infection results after as few as one to five bacteria are deposited in a terminal alveolus.[9] After phagocytosis, the organism slowly replicates intracellularly over 2–12 weeks to 10^3 or 10^4 organisms. It then travels to regional lymphatics

Table 14–3 Sites of tuberculosis involvement

Lungs
Disseminated or miliary
Lymph nodes (Figure 14-2)
Pleura
Genitourinary tract
Skeleton
Pericardium
Central nervous system (meningitis or tuberculoma)
Abdomen

Jeffrey was adopted from China at age 6 years. He seemed well on arrival, although small (height age was 4 years). At the initial visit, he had knee arthralgias. Knee films were unrevealing, but a chest x-ray showed a large Ghon complex and destructive lesions of the adjacent ribs (Figure 14-3). The TST was 22 mm. Gastric aspirates grew M. tuberculosis. Treatment with isoniazid, rifampin, pyrazinamide, ethambutol, and pyridoxine was given, with resolution of joint symptoms and improvement in growth.

and hilar nodes,[6] and may spread hematogenously to vulnerable areas (Table 14-3).

The clinical course of tuberculosis is designated by stages. After *exposure*, it may take up to 3 months for a positive skin test to develop (see below). During this time, infected individuals cannot be differentiated from noninfected individuals. After the tuberculin skin test (TST) becomes reactive, but before clinical symptoms, children are said to have *latent tuberculosis infection* (LTBI, sometimes called *primary infection*). Risk factors for LTBI in children in New York include foreign birth or travel and contact with an adult with active TB.[23] In some children, LTBI progresses to *active disease*. Young children (<5 years of age) may rapidly develop severe tuberculous meningitis

or disseminated disease.[24] However, most children continue to appear deceptively well. Minimal respiratory symptoms are present; only gradually do persistent fever, poor appetite, weight loss, and reduced activity appear.[25] Air-trapping, hyperinflation, and wheezing may be early signs of pulmonary involvement, often in the absence of fevers.[6] During this time, a chest radiograph may show a Ghon complex, a small parenchymal infiltrate with enlarged hilar lymph nodes. The hilar nodes may be missed if only a posterior–anterior view chest film is done.[26] (A shortage of radiographic supplies often limits film views in adoption sending countries.) Chest films may show areas of atelectasis distal to obstructed segmental bronchi.[24]

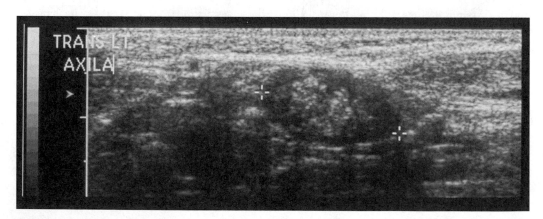

Figure 14–2 *Ultrasound shows enlarged axillary lymph nodes. Culture of excised node was positive for* Mycobacterium tuberculosis. *Ultrasonography shows this to be an ovoid, relatively hypolucent mass with well-defined margins consistent with a lymph node. It measures 1.6 cm in longest diameter and has some irregular areas of echogenicity within. This may represent chronic inflammatory changes or possibly faint calcific deposition. One or two tiny nodes are noted in the surrounding soft tissues.*

During this stage, the x-rays often "look worse than the child." A large pulmonary consolidation in a minimally ill child always suggests TB.[26] Pleural effusions are rare in children under 6 years of age. The combination of fever, cough for more than 2 weeks, and TST ≥ 10 mm is highly predictive of pulmonary TB in some populations.[27]

It may take 12 months or longer after exposure for extrapulmonary involvement of the middle ear/mastoid, joints, bones, skin, or kidneys to become apparent.[28] Skeletal TB occurs in <6% of infected children and does not appear until about 1–3 years after infection. In contrast, miliary disease or tuberculous meningitis may appear within months after infection. Very young children are particularly at risk for miliary tuberculosis, which presents with fever, anorexia, tachypnea, and splenomegaly.[26] Tuberculous meningitis may be difficult to identify in the early stages, which are characterized by low-grade fevers, anorexia, and intermittent vomiting. As the disease progresses, children become irritable and apathetic, then may develop cranial nerve palsies, drowsiness, and seizures. About 40% of

Lisa was adopted from Kazakhstan at 9 months. Her pediatrician was reluctant to place a TST, because the baby had a BCG scar. Lisa showed some catch-up growth and development, but remained somewhat quiet and apathetic. Finally, as part of an evaluation for her incomplete growth recovery, a chest x-ray and TST were done. The x-ray showed enlarged hilar nodes and parenchymal infiltrate, her TST reaction was 19 mm. Her mood improved several weeks after institution of therapy.

children have a negative TST and 25%–50% have normal chest x-rays.[26,29]

Extrapulmonary TB is more common in children than in adults. The most common extrapulmonary form of TB in children is scrofula, or tuberculous cervical adenitis. Children have enlarged, nontender, rubbery cervical and submandibular nodes. These should be completely excised and antimycobacterial therapy given.[26] Nontuberculous mycobacteria cause similar adenopathy, in the absence of a positive TST or in the presence of a TST < 10 mm.[25]

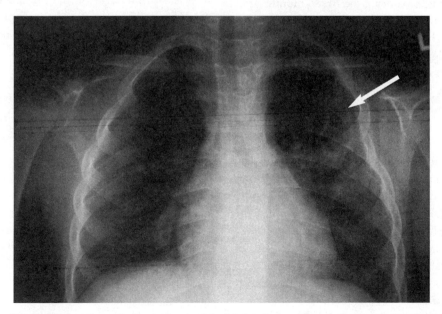

Figure 14–3 *Chest radiograph shows sclerosis of the left fourth posterolateral rib (arrow). Streaky densities are seen within the posterior segment of the left upper lobe in association with prominence of the adjacent left upper hilum. The lungs are markedly hyperinflated. Compression fractures of the T3 through T9 vertebrae were noted on the lateral view. The bones appear osteopenic.*

Tuberculin Skin Test

The TST (sometimes called the PPD, or purified protein derivative test) is the standard method of diagnosing TB infection. It refers to the standard Mantoux skin test in which 5 tuberculin units (TU) in a volume of 0.1 ml are injected intradermally. The reaction (millimeters of induration) is determined 48–72 hours later. Pediatricians who do not regularly care for immigrant children may not be familiar with some of the subtleties of TST use. It takes from 2 to 12 weeks after exposure for the test to become positive.[30] The interpretation of the TST is not straightforward: different criteria are applied depending on risk factors identified in the individual patient. These risk factors are intended to identify individuals at risk for active disease (Table 14–4). Although the TST may someday be replaced by molecular biological techniques[32] or T-lymphocyte release of γ-interferon in response to PPD,[33] it presently remains the standard for TB diagnosis.

Tuberculin skin test results are categorized on the basis of dimensions of induration (<5 mm, ≥5–9 mm, ≥10–14 mm, or ≥15 mm) at 48–72 hours (Table 14–5). The appropriate category used for interpretation should be determined prior to application of the TST. These

---

Dima arrived at age 2 years from Russia, along with his unrelated sister Katya. He was small (height, weight, and head circumference were below the fifth percentile). An initial TST was 12 mm, and 9 months of INH was prescribed. Unfortunately, no increase in dose was given, although he gained more than 7 kg. Near the end of his (inadequate) treatment, large axillary nodes were detected. His chest x-ray remained negative. A lymph node biopsy showed caseating granulomas, consistent with TB. Possibly because of the concurrent INH treatment, cultures were negative. Therapy with isoniazid, pyrazinamide, and rifampin was given.

Why do some children progress from LTBI to active disease? The risk factors for progression of disease are incompletely understood. Children, especially those less than 2 years of age, are at high risk to acquire TB and to develop progressive disease (with the potential for disseminated TB).[6,30] Forty percent of infants with untreated TB infection develop clinical disease within 1 to 2 years.[24] The risk of progression is highest during the first 6 months after infection and remains high for at least 2 years (although it can be many years).[28] In a survey of immigrants to Australia, the highest rate of progression occurred among those with a strongly positive TST on arrival, regardless of BCG vaccination status.[31]

Concurrent HIV infection or other immunodeficiency, various medical conditions, malnutrition, pulmonary fibrotic lesions on chest x-ray, and recent TST conversion all increase the risk of disease progression.[6,28,30] Overall, individuals with LTBI have a lifetime risk of 5%–10% of developing TB, but if they are immunocompromised this increases to 5%–10% *per year*.[1] Virtually all children with LTBI should be treated to prevent future disease.[24] Prophylactic treatment with isoniazid is 98%–100% protective against the development of tuberculous disease for at least 20 years[28] in the absence of new exposures.

Table 14–4 Risk factors for tuberculosis in international adoptees

Risk Factors for Infection
Born in country with high prevalence
Poor access to health care
Live or spend time in institution
Close contact with persons with infectious TB

Risk Factors for Developing Active Disease
    if Infected
Children <4 years of age
HIV infected
Recent skin test conversion
Concurrent medical conditions (including malnutrition)

Source: Adapted from Diagnostic Standards and Classification of Tuberculosis in Adults and Children.[6]

Table 14–5 Interpretation of the tuberculin skin test

≥5 mm induration is considered a positive TST result if child
  is HIV positive
  has recent contact with active tuberculosis (cannot rule out)[a]
  has an abnormal chest x-ray
  is immunosuppressed
  is at high risk of developing active TB (see Table 14–4)
≥10 mm induration is considered a positive TST result if child
  is born or whose parents were born in high prevalence countries[a]
  is resident of institution (orphanage)[a]
  is exposed to high-risk adults (resident or employee of jail, nursing home, etc., illicit drug user)[a]
  is <4 years of age[a]
  has certain medical conditions (Hodgkin disease, lymphoma, diabetes, malnutrition[a])
  from high-prevalence regions of the world[a]
>15 mm induration is considered a positive TST result if child
  is 4 years of age or older without any risk factors

[a]Particularly relevant to international adoptees. Source: Adapted from American Academy of Pediatrics.[28]

categories apply *regardless* of prior BCG vaccination.[6,28] A TST <5 mm is considered negative.

Administration of the Tuberculin Skin Test

There are many pitfalls in the administration of the TST. The PPD should be drawn up as needed, not transferred from container to container, and should be given as soon as possible after the syringe is filled. The reagent should be stored refrigerated (not frozen) and kept mostly in the dark.[6] If the first test is given improperly (not intradermal), it should be repeated a few centimeters away immediately. After injection, the reaction usually starts to emerge at 5–6 hours and then peaks at 48–72 hours. Occasionally, it may not peak until after 72 hours[6,24]: this should not alter interpretation of the result. A positive reaction may persist as long as 1 week.[30] The optimal method to read the skin test results is shown in Figure 14–4.[26] The dimension of the maximal diameter of induration should be recorded in millimeters (not as "positive" or "negative"). Parents should not be relied upon to read TST results correctly.[34,35]

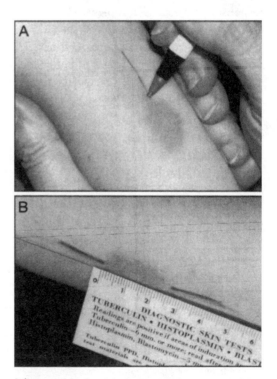

Figure 14–4 *A. Drawing the initial line in a ballpoint pen reading of a tuberculin skin test. B. Reading the skin test results in millimeters with the ballpoint pen method. (Reproduced with permission from Pediatrics in Review, Vol. 18, pp. 50–58, Figure 3A, 3B, Copyright 1997.)*

The TST can be placed concurrently with live-virus vaccines (measles, mumps, rubella, oral polio, varicella, yellow fever),[6] but should be deferred for 4–6 weeks *after* live virus administration, as a false negative may result.[6,28] In addition, false negative results occur because of concurrent viral or bacterial infection, serious diseases, malnutrition, young age, or immunosuppression.[28,26] Between 5% and 10% of children with culture-positive disease have persistently negative skin tests[26,28]; this can be as high as 25% in the initial phases of infection.[6] Thus a negative skin test should never rule out TB if other findings support the diagnosis.

The "two-step" method of TST identifies infected individuals who have lost the ability to respond to the TST (and consequently have a false negative result). An initial test "primes" the appropriate delayed-type hypersensitivity responses to a second test placed 2–3 weeks later. A reactive response on the second test suggests long-standing infection. This method probably has little utility in young children, but serves as a reminder that repeat testing may be useful when clinical suspicion suggests infection. Repeated TST application cannot induce induration in an uninfected, unvaccinated person.[9]

False positive reactions occur with cross-reactions to nontuberculous mycobacterial infections or following vaccination with BCG (see below). Reaction to the TST after BCG vaccination rarely exceeds 5 mm by age 3 to 5 years,

and usually has disappeared altogether by 6 months of age in children receiving BCG at birth.[36,37] Reactions to nontuberculous mycobacterial infections rarely exceed 10 mm.[26] Prior BCG vaccination should not be considered when evaluating results of TST (see below).

Interpretation of TST results in internationally adopted children is difficult, as details of their medical histories are usually incomplete (Table 14–6). These children must first be recognized as a high-risk group. Most experts concur that detection of all TB infections in high-risk groups is more important than concern about treating some false positive reactors.[1] For example, only 5% of children in the general U.S. population with a ≥5–9 mm TST are infected with TB. However, children with the same size reaction who have had contact with an adult with contagious TB have a 50% chance of having TB infection.[28] The likelihood that a positive skin test represents a true infection is influenced by the prevalence of infection with *M. tuberculosis* in the population.[6] Thus, conservative management of internationally adopted children is warranted.

Bacille Calmette-Guérin Vaccine

Bacille Calmette-Guérin vaccine is used in more than 100 countries of the world. Since 1921, more than 3 billion doses have been given, although the efficacy of the vaccine has not been firmly es-

---

Table 14–6 Difficulties in TB management in internationally adopted children

Difficulty	Treatment
Lack of information about possible exposure to active TB	Conduct careful evaluation and follow-up in children with any TST reaction or any suggestive symptoms.
Possibility of recent exposure just before adoption	Repeat TST 3–6 months after arrival.
Uncertain date and number of BCG vaccinations	Examine for BCG scars; if fresh, defer TST. Otherwise, do not consider BCG in interpretation of TST results.
Inability to identify source case; may therefore be unable to establish drug susceptibilities. Possible multiple-drug–resistant TB	Make a vigorous attempt to isolate organism from children with active infection.

tablished.[6] Studies show efficacy ranging from "detrimental" to as much as "80% benefit" in vaccine recipients.[38,39] Several recent meta-analyses of BCG efficacy clearly showed that it reduces the risk of some forms of TB by ~50%,[26,39,40] possibly by reducing bacillemia after infection.[41] Specific benefits to vaccinees include reduction of disseminated TB (78%), meningitis (64%), and death from TB (71%). Some of the variability has to do with the strain used for vaccination, genetic variability of the vaccinees, and the nature of endemic mycobacteria in different parts of the world.[6] Curiously, BCG-induced tuberculin reactivity does not correlate with protection against tuberculosis.[6,30,42]

Vaccination with BCG, usually given on the left deltoid, causes a small superficial ulcer in most recipients which heals within several months (Fig. 14–5). However, 25%–50% of vaccinees fail to develop a scar.[42] Occasionally, the vaccine causes a suppurative adenitis (4%), abscess (Fig. 14–6), or, very rarely, osteomyelitis.[43] Skin lesions and lymphadenitis usually do not require treatment, as most spontaneously resolve. Occasionally, a course of INH and Rifampin is recommended for prolonged or painful adenitis. Disseminated BCG infection is a rare complication.[44] More problematic is the TST reactivity that results from vaccination in some recipients, which may interfere with diagnosis of TB infection. Because of this, some countries with low prevalence of TB prefer not to use the vaccine, thus preserving the ability to screen the population for TB infection without this confounding factor.

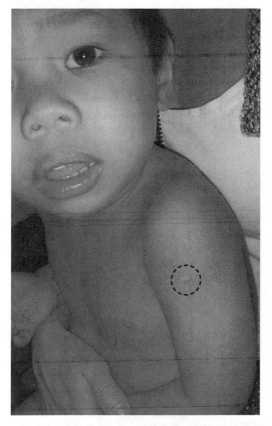

Figure 14–5 *Typical, well-healed BCG scar. (With permission.)*

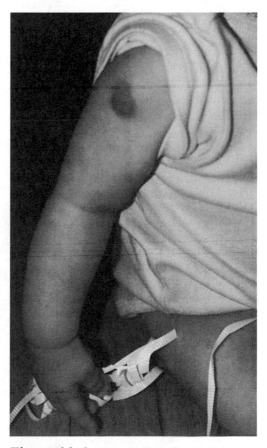

Figure 14–6 *BCG sites may become deeply indurated. This usually resolves spontaneously, although secondary infection may occur.*

Joseph was adopted from Colombia at age 5. When he moved to a new town at age 6, his pediatrician noted that no TST had been done on arrival. Joseph's TST was indurated 18 mm; his chest x-ray was normal. His pediatrician investigated the entire family and found that Joseph's adoptive grandfather, age 72, also had a positive TST (24 mm) and an abnormal chest x-ray with extensive calcifications. Since his grandfather lived in the home, it seemed likely that he had infected Joseph, rather than the other way around. Both were treated with good results.

Many physicians have the mistaken notion that BCG-vaccinated individuals will always test positive when TST is performed. Others mistakenly believe that TST is dangerous in BCG-vaccinated individuals. Although some individuals become TST reactive after BCG vaccination, this is far from a universal response. The TST reaction size after BCG is usually <10 mm and usually wanes over time (although it can be "boosted" by serial testing).[6,30,42] Fewer than 50% of infants given BCG shortly after birth have a reactive TST at 6–12 months of age; reactivity usually has disappeared altogether by 6 months of age in children receiving BCG at birth.[36] Virtually all vaccinated infants have nonreactive skin tests by 5 years of age.[24,42,45] Individuals vaccinated later in childhood may maintain skin test reactivity longer.[24] The size of skin test reaction after BCG varies with strain and dose of vaccine, route of administration, age of patient, nutritional status of the recipient, number of years since vaccination, and frequency of skin testing.[24] Tuberculin skin test reactions >15–20 mm are unlikely to be attributable to BCG. In general, a positive TST is more likely due to BCG if the individual has multiple BCG scars[46,47] (Figure 14–7) or a recent (<12 weeks) BCG. From 10% to 25% of BCG-vaccinated individuals have a positive TST if retested within 1 to 4 weeks after an initial negative test.[42,47] However, such studies have all been performed in adults; results in infants and children may differ.

In contrast, a positive TST is more likely due to TB infection if the individual has had known contact with a contagious adult,[48] has emigrated from a country with a high prevalence of TB, or has not had a BCG vaccine for some time[28]—the usual circumstances for international adoptees. As there is *no* reliable method of distinguishing tuberculin reactions caused by vaccination with BCG from those

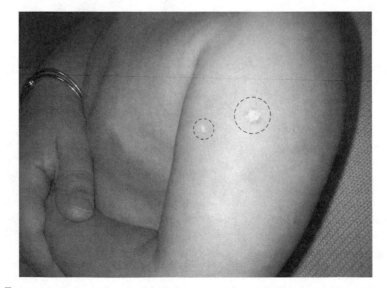

Figure 14–7 *Some children receive multiple BCG vaccinations. A positive TST is more likely in recipients of multiple BCG vaccinations. (With permission.)*

caused by infection, prior vaccination should *not* influence the interpretation of the reaction or the decision of whether or not to treat.[6,24,30] It is hoped that new diagnostic tests for TB will allow identification of active infection.

Other Diagnostic Tests

Children with a positive TST should undergo careful clinical evaluation for signs of pulmonary and extrapulmonary TB infection.[24] A posterior–anterior and lateral chest radiograph should be obtained. Usually these films are normal. Most children with TB are infected with few organisms and seldom cough or produce sputum. If pulmonary TB is suspected, three early-morning gastric aspirates should be obtained, although the likelihood of positive results ranges from <10% to 40% of children with radiographic evidence of significant pulmonary disease.[6,24] Detailed guidelines for obtaining clinical samples are described in the Diagnostic Standards and Classification of Tuberculosis in Adults and Children.[6] After collection, molecular amplification techniques are sometimes used to hasten mycobacterial identification and drug sensitivity patterns.[32] Genotyping of *M. tuberculosis* isolates may prove useful in the future management of clinical disease.[49]

Treatment

Children with LTBI should be treated with isoniazid (INH) for 9 months (see Multidrug-resistant Tuberculosis, below). This reduces the risk of clinical disease by 90% during the first year after treatment; the protective effect can last at least 30 years.[24,25] Most experts agree that routine monitoring of liver function tests is not necessary for otherwise healthy children.[24–26] Exceptions include children with chronic medical problems (diabetes, uremia, seizures, hepatic disease) and those taking other potentially hepatotoxic medications. Elevation of transaminases occurs in fewer than 2% of children taking

INH and clinical hepatitis occurs in <1%.[24] However, children should be seen, evaluated clinically, and compliance reviewed every 4–6 weeks, and families should be instructed to discontinue the INH if the child develops vomiting, abdominal pain, or jaundice.[24] Parents must be informed of the importance of treatment compliance and the dangers of missed doses.

Although INH is available as a syrup, crushed pills are usually a better choice if accurate dosing can be achieved. Some children experience bloating, diarrhea, and flatulence while taking the syrup because of the sorbitol it contains; this problem is usually temporary as the intestine "accommodates" to the osmotic load. The syrup bottle must be shaken vigorously to resuspend the medication prior to each use. Supplemental pyridoxine is generally not necessary unless the child has other medical problems or significant malnutrition. It is sensible to prescribe a standard multivitamin preparation. The dose of INH must be increased commensurate with the child's growth.

Children with active TB should be managed by a pediatric infectious disease specialist. Multiple medications are required; general guidelines for treatment are reviewed in refs. 6, 24, 28, 50, and 51. A diagram of treatment decisions is shown in Figure 14–8.

Multidrug-Resistant Tuberculosis

About 9% of *M. tuberculosis* isolates in the United States are resistant to INH.[24] In some countries, however, as many as 50% are resistant to one or more drugs.[52] Multidrug-resistant TB "hot-spots" have been identified in Estonia, Latvia, the Oblasts of Ivanovo and Tomsk in Russia, and the provinces of Henan and Zhejiang in China.[53] In Texas, isolates from foreign-born patients were more likely to be resistant to at least one drug (15.4% vs. 8.4%) and to be multidrug resistant (2.4% vs. 0.7%) than isolates from U.S.–born patients. Identification of drug-resistant organisms in children usually de-

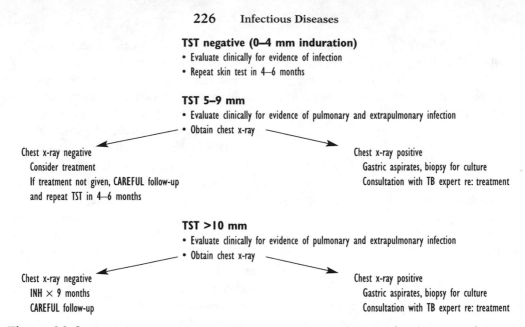

TST negative (0–4 mm induration)
- Evaluate clinically for evidence of infection
- Repeat skin test in 4–6 months

TST 5–9 mm
- Evaluate clinically for evidence of pulmonary and extrapulmonary infection
- Obtain chest x-ray

Chest x-ray negative
Consider treatment
If treatment not given, CAREFUL follow-up
and repeat TST in 4–6 months

Chest x-ray positive
Gastric aspirates, biopsy for culture
Consultation with TB expert re: treatment

TST >10 mm
- Evaluate clinically for evidence of pulmonary and extrapulmonary infection
- Obtain chest x-ray

Chest x-ray negative
INH × 9 months
CAREFUL follow-up

Chest x-ray positive
Gastric aspirates, biopsy for culture
Consultation with TB expert re: treatment

Figure 14–8 *Treatment decisions in assessing internationally adopted children for tuberculosis infection.*

pends on identification of the adult source case[54,55]: for internationally adopted children this is an impossibility. Therefore, every effort must be made to isolate and culture the organism in an internationally adopted child with active TB. A recent decision-analysis model suggests that rifampin plus pyrazinamide is the preferred treatment for treating latent TB infection in adult immigrants from Vietnam, Haiti, and the Phillipines, while INH alone is preferred for immigrants from most other regions.[56] The applicability of this analysis to children is uncertain.

Key Points for Internationally Adopted Children

- Tuberculosis exposure is common in children residing in orphanages throughout the world.
- Between 0.5% and 19% of internationally adopted children have LTBI.
- Many children are vaccinated with BCG; this is *not* a contraindication to TST.
- Because of the unknown possible exposure, internationally adopted children must be con-

sidered a high-risk group when the TST is interpreted.
- Identification and treatment of infected children is important for public and personal health.

FAQs

Q. What is the best way to be sure my newly arrived patient doesn't have tuberculosis infection?

A. TST at entry and then again at 4–6 months later. Although comprehensive data have not yet been published to document the utility of follow-up tuberculosis skin testing, many international adoption medicine specialists have identified children with positive skin tests at follow-up.

Q. Should I obtain a gastric aspirate if my patient's TST is positive? She has a negative chest x-ray and no respiratory symptoms.

A. No, if you've searched carefully for signs of clinical TB, this child would be classified as LTBI. Nine months of treatment with INH are recommended.

Q. My patient finished his 9 months of INH treatment. Should he have further TSTs? What if they are required for school or camp? Is any special follow-up necessary?

A. Additional TSTs are not necessary. Possible signs of TB activation should be sought at regular annual physicals. Parents should be encouraged to retain documents describing the child's treatment; these often need to be submitted to camps and schools.

Q. Is "directly observed therapy" necessary for INH treatment in an extremely compliant family?

A. No—as long as you have carefully explained the importance of treatment for LTBI and the need to restart if doses are missed. An office visit every 6 weeks or so during treatment may be advisable to answer questions. Check for any untoward effects of therapy, and encourage ongoing compliance.

Q. Because of the chance of drug-resistant TB, is it appropriate for children with LTBI to receive INH alone?

A. Children with LTBI should be treated with INH alone. This recommendation may change as more is learned about global patterns of multidrug-resistant TB.

Resources

Division of Tuberculosis Elimination, National Center for HIV, STD and TB prevention. Core Curriculum on Tuberculosis. Available at: http://www.cdc.gov/nchstp/tb/pubs/corecurr.

Phone advice from TB experts for physicians with questions about TB (funded in part by the CDC): 415-502-4700 or 800-4TB-DOCS.

National Jewish Center for Immunology and Respiratory Medicine Tel: 800-423-8891, ext. 1279 for clinical consultation, ext. 1427 for pharmacology.

Local public health departments and tuberculosis control programs.

References

1. Medical Advisory Committee for the Elimination of Tuberculosis. Latent Tuberculosis Infection: A Guide for Massachusetts Providers. Boston: Massachusetts Department of Health, 2000.

2. Curtis A, Ridzon R, Vogel R, et al. Extensive transmission of *Mycobacterium tuberculosis* from a child. N Engl J Med 1999; 341:1491–5.

3. Cantwell MF, Shehab ZM, Costello AM, et al. Brief report: congenital tuberculosis. N Engl J Med 1994; 330:1051–4.

4. Lee LH, LeVea CM, Graman PS. Congenital tuberculosis in a neonatal intensive care unit: case report, epidemiological investigation, and management of exposures. Clin Infect Dis 1998; 27:474–7.

5. Rabalais G, Adams G, Stover B. PPD skin test conversion in health-care workers after exposure to *Mycobacterium tuberculosis* infection in infants. Lancet 1991; 338:826.

6. Diagnostic Standards and Classification of Tuberculosis in Adults and Children. [This official statement of the American Thoracic Society and the Centers for Disease Control and Prevention was adopted by the ATS Board of Directors, July 1999. This statement was endorsed by the Council of the Infectious Disease Society of America, September 1999.] Am J Respir Crit Care Med 2000; 161:1376–95.

7. Talbot EA, Moore M, McCray E, Binkin NJ. Tuberculosis among foreign-born persons in the United States, 1993–1998. JAMA 2000; 284:2894–900.

8. Bloom BR, Small PM. The evolving relationship between humans and *Mycobacterium tuberculosis*. N Engl J Med 1998; 338:677–8.

9. Small PM, Fujiwara PI. Management of tuberculosis in the United States. N Engl J Med 2001; 345:189–200.

10. Donnelly J. WHO urges $400m for fight against TB. The Boston Globe May 15, 2001:A1, A10.

11. Saiman L, Aronson J, Zhou J, et al. Prevalence of infectious diseases among internationally adopted children. Pediatrics 2001; 108:608–12.

12. Lange WR, Warnock-Eckhart E. Selected infectious disease risks in international adoptees. Pediatr Infect Dis J 1987; 6:447–50.

13. Hostetter MK, Iverson S, Thomas W, McKenzie D, Dole K, Johnson DE. Medical evaluation of internationally adopted children. N Engl J Med 1991; 325:479–85.

14. Jenista JA, Chapman D. Medical problems of foreign-born adopted children. Am J Dis Child 1987; 141:298–302.

15. Smith-Garcia T, Brown JS. The health of children adopted from India. J Community Health 1989; 14:227–41.

16. Miller LC, Kiernan MT, Mathers MI, Klein-Gitelman M. Developmental and nutritional status of internationally adopted children. Arch Pediatr Adolesc Med 1995; 149:40–4.

17. Miller LC, Hendrie NW. Health of children adopted from China. Pediatrics 2000; 105:E76.

18. Johnson DE, Miller LC, Iverson S, et al. The health of children adopted from Romania. JAMA 1992; 268: 3446–51.

19. Albers LH, Johnson DE, Hostetter MK, Iverson S, Miller LC. Health of children adopted from the former Soviet Union and Eastern Europe. Comparison with preadoptive medical records. JAMA 1997; 278:922–4.

20. Nicholson AJ, Francis BM, Mulholland EK, Moulden AL, Oberklaid F. Health screening of international adoptees. Evaluation of a hospital based clinic [see comments]. Med J Aust 1992; 156:377–9.

21. Bureau JJ, Maurage C, Bremond M, Despert F, Rolland JC. Children of foreign origin adopted in France. Analysis of 68 cases during 12 years at the University Hospital Center of Tours [in French]. Arch Pediatr 1999; 6:1053–8.

22. Meropol SB. Health status of pediatric refugees in Buffalo, N.Y. Arch Pediatr Adolesc Med 1995; 149:887–92.

23. Saiman L, San Gabriel P, Schulte J, Vargas MP, Kenyon T, Onorato IM. Risk factors for latent tuberculosis infection among children in New York City. Pediatrics 2001; 107:999–1003.

24. Starke JR, Correa AG. Management of mycobacterial infection and disease in children. Pediatr Infect Dis J 1995; 14:455–69; quiz 469–70.

25. de La Rosa JM, Escobedo M. Tuberculosis and other infectious diseases in the adolescent immigrant. Adolesc Med 2000; 11:453–66.

26. Abernathy RS. Tuberculosis: an update. Pediatr Rev 1997; 18:50–8.

27. Salazar GE, Schmitz TL, Cama R, et al. Pulmonary tuberculosis in children in a developing country. Pediatrics 2001; 108:448–53.

28. American Academy of Pediatrics. Tuberculosis. In: Pickering L, ed. 2003 Red Book: Report of the Committee on Infectious Diseases. Elk Grove Village, IL: American Academy of Pediatics, 2003:642–60.

29. Yaramis A, Gurkan F, Elevli M, et al. Central nervous system tuberculosis in children: a review of 214 cases. Pediatrics 1998; 102:e49.

30. Targeted tuberculin testing and treatment of latent tuberculosis infection. Am J Respir Crit Care Med 2000; 161:S221–47.

31. Marks GB, Bai J, Simpson SE, Sullivan EA, Stewart GJ. Incidence of tuberculosis among a cohort of tuberculin-positive refugees in Australia: reappraising the estimates of risk. Am J Respir Crit Care Med 2000; 162:1851–4.

32. Smith KC, Starke JR, Eisenach K, Ong LT, Denby M. Detection of *Mycobacterium tuberculosis* in clinical specimens from children using a polymerase chain reaction. Pediatrics 1996; 97:155–60.

33. Jasmer RM, Nahid P, Hopewell PC. Latent tuberculosis infection. N Engl J Med 2002; 347:1860–6.

34. Halsey NA. for the Committee on Infectious Diseases. American Academy of Pediatrics. Update on tuberculosis skin testing of children. Pediatrics 1996; 97:282–4.

35. Froelich H, Ackerson LM, Morozumi PA. Targeted testing of children for tuberculosis: validation of a risk assessment questionnaire. Pediatrics 2001; 107:e54.

36. Lifschitz M. The value of the tuberculin skin test as a screening test for tuberculosis among BCG-vaccinated children. Pediatrics 1965; 36:624–7.

37. Nemir RL, Teichner A. Management of tuberculin reactors in children and adolescents previously vaccinated with BCG. Pediatr Infect Dis J 1983; 2:446–51.

38. Brewer TF. Preventing tuberculosis with bacillus Calmette-Guérin vaccine: a meta-analysis of the literature. Clin Infect Dis 2000; 31 (Suppl 3):S64–7.

39. Colditz GA, Brewer TF, Berkey CS, et al. Efficacy of BCG vaccine in the prevention of tuberculosis. JAMA 1994; 271:698–702.

40. Colditz GA, Berkey CS, Mosteller F, et al. The efficacy of Bacillus Calmette-Guérin vaccination of newborns and infants in the prevention of tuberculosis: meta-analyses of the published literature. Pediatrics 1995; 96:29–35.

41. Wittes RC. Bacille Calmette-Guérin vaccine. Clin Infect Dis 2000; 31(Suppl 3):S115–31.

42. Menzies D. What does tuberculin reactivity after bacille Calmette-Guérin vaccination tell us? Clin Infect Dis 2000; 31 (Suppl 3):S71–4.

43. Bannon MJ. BCG and tuberculosis. Arch Dis Child 1999; 80:80–3.

44. Casanova JL, Blanche S, Emile JF, et al. Idiopathic disseminated bacillus Calmette-Guérin infection: a French national retrospective study. Pediatrics 1996; 98:774–8.

45. Zhang LX, Tu DH, He GX, et al. Risk of tuberculosis infection and tuberculous meningitis after discontinuation of Bacillus Calmette-Guérin in Beijing. Am J Respir Crit Care Med 2000; 162:1314–7.

46. Ildirim I, Hacimustafaoglu M, Ediz B. Correlation of tuberculin induration with the number of Bacillus Calmette-Guérin vaccines. Pediatr Infect Dis J 1995; 14: 1060–3.

47. Sepulveda RL, Ferrer X, Latrach C, Sorenson RU. The influence of Calmette-Guérin Bacillus immunization on the booster effect of tuberculin testing in healthy young adults. Am Rev Respir Dis 1990; 142:24–8.

48. Lienhardt C, Sillah J, Fielding K, et al. Risk factors in tuberculosis infection in children in contact with infectious tuberculosis cases in The Gambia, West Africa. Pediatrics 2003; 111:e608–14.

49. Barnes PF, Cave MD. Molecular epidemiology of tuberculosis. N Engl J Med 2003; 349:1149–56.

50. Treatment of childhood tuberculosis: Consensus Statement of IAP Working Group. Indian Academy of Pediatrics. Indian Pediatr 1997; 34:1093–6.

51. Starke JR. Tuberculosis in children. Prim Care 1996; 23:861–81.

52. Sahly HM, Adams GJ, Soini H, Teeter L, Musser JM. Epidemiologic differences between United States- and foreign-born tuberculosis patients in Houston, Texas. J Infect Dis 2001; 183:461–8.

53. Espinal MA. The global situation of MDR-TB. Tuberculosis (Edinb) 2003; 83:44–51.

54. Schaaf HS, Gie RP, Kennedy M, Beyers N, Hesseling PB, Donald PR. Evaluation of young children in contact with adult multidrug-resistant pulmonary tuberculosis: a 30-month follow-up. Pediatrics 2002; 109: 765–71.

55. Schaaf HS, Gie RP, Beyers N, Sirgel FA, de Klerk PJ, Donald PR. Primary drug-resistant tuberculosis in children. Int J Tuberc Lung Dis 2000; 4:1149–55.

56. Khan K, Muennig P, Behta M, Zivin JG. Global drug-resistance patterns and the management of latent tuberculosis infection in immigrants to the United States. N Engl J Med 2002; 347:1850–9.

15

HEPATITIS B

Hepatitis B virus (HBV) is the most common serious infection in internationally adopted children. Nearly all children are tested in their birth countries for HBV; very few children who test positive are offered for international adoption. Exceptions include a single infected member of a sibling group. Despite negative HBV test results from the birth country in virtually all children placed for international adoption, about 5%–7% of new arrivals are infected. This discrepancy is due to tests done in the birth country being inaccurate or infection occurring after testing was completed. Infection with HBV represents risks to the infected child, the child's family, and the community. Physicians caring for internationally adopted children should recognize the risk factors for HBV infection, appropriate diagnostic tests, their timing and interpretation, clinical features of HBV infection, need for vaccination to prevent HBV, and the basic principles of management of the HBV carrier. This chapter reviews these features of HBV infection.

Epidemiology

Hepatitis B virus is one of the most common chronic viral infections in the world, affecting about 300 million people worldwide.[1] Most internationally adopted children come from areas of high or moderate prevalence; thus it is not surprising that some have HBV infection. The prevalence of chronic HBV infection (Fig. 15–1) is high (>8%) in all socioeconomic groups in Africa, Southeast Asia (including China, Korea, Indonesia, and the Philippines), the several countries of the Middle East, South and Western Pacific Islands, interior Amazon Basin, and certain parts of the Caribbean (Haiti and the Dominican Republic). Nearly 75% of infected people reside in Asia. Prevalence of HBV is moderate (2%–7%) in South Central and Southwest Asia, Israel, Japan, Eastern and

Hepatitis B, 2002

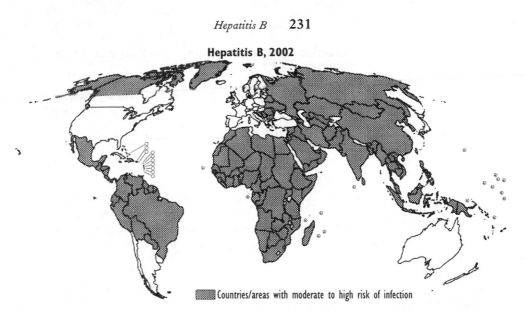

Countries/areas with moderate to high risk of infection

Figure 15–1 *Distribution of hepatitis B throughout the world. Shaded ares indicate countries with moderate to high risk of infection. (From the World Health Organization, 2002, with permission.)*

Southern Europe and Russia, and most of Central and South America. In comparison, in Northern and Western Europe, North America, Australia, and New Zealand, chronic HBV infection prevalence is low (<2%) in the general population.

Hepatitis B Virus and Internationally Adopted Children

The prevalence of HBV infection among internationally adopted children is about 5%–7%, with several notable exceptions (Table 15–1). However, many more children show evidence of exposure to HBV. Most of the surveys (listed chronologically) cited in Table 15–1 were compiled before the widespread use of HBV vaccine, thus the presence of hepatitis B surface antibody (HbsAb) represents natural immunity. Dramatically higher prevalences of HBV infection were reported in several studies that evaluated children adopted in the late 1970s–1980s. At that time, Romanian orphanages had an extraordinarily high prevalence of HBV infection, some as high as 85%.[2] The reasons for the higher prevalence of HBV reported in

the other three studies listed[3–5] is not fully understood.

Timing and accuracy of HBV tests in birth countries are questionable. Results may be obtained months or even years prior to adoption. Perhaps the needle used to obtain the blood for testing may itself transmit HBV. For these reasons, testing in birth countries is of limited value.

Although most internationally adopted children infected with HBV are asymptomatic carriers, some have more active disease. Some investigators suggest that multiple exposures to HBV or concomitant malnutrition augment the disease expression.[24]

Clinical Spectrum

The clinical manifestations of HBV infection vary widely, from asymptomatic carriage to fatal fulminant hepatitis (about 1% of infections).[25–27] The incubation period ranges from 60 to 180 days after infection. Most patients have nonspecific constitutional symptoms and remain anicteric. Some patients have prominent extrahepatic manifestations including fever, arthropathy, and rash. Young children most commonly

Table 15–1 Hepatitis B virus infection among internationally adopted children

Country of Origin, Year, (N)	sAg+ (%)	sAb+[a] (%)	Comments
Vietnam, 1976 (33)[5]	27	30	HBV serology tested as part of an investigation of hepatitis A outbreak among adoptive families
Korea and India, 1978 (400)[6]	5	—	Adopted in Sweden
Korea, 1985 (140)[7]	4.3	—	Ages from 6 months to 16 years; all were also eAg+
Various countries, 75% Korea, 1987 (128)[8]	6	22	—
Korea, 1987 (360)[9]	2.8	—	Mean age was 5 months
Korea, 1988 (884)[10]	4.5	—	Tested 1–2 weeks prior to adoptive placement. Follow-up tests in U.S. confirmed results for most children (3 additional found sAg+, 2 sAg+ in Korea were negative in U.S.)
Korea 85% and India 15%, 1988 (511)[11]	7	—	75% of sAg+ children were also eAg+
India, 1989 (200)[12]	6	—	25 had received blood transfusions
Various countries, 50% Korea, 1989 (52)[3]	19	—	—
Korea, 1990 (2300)[13]	3.3	—	—
Romania, 1991 (169)[14]	35	53	Children in orphanages or in hospitals in remote region of Romania
Romania, 1991 (11)[15]	27	18	—
Phillipines, 1991 (218)[16]	5	—	20% had core Ab (some maternal Ab). Compared with 360 Korean adoptees, of whom 2.8% were sAg+
Various countries, Korea 41%, Central and South America 31%, 1991 (293)[17]	5	—	Risk associated with Asian origin, transfusion in birth country (15 times the risk), date of entry into study (earlier more likely to be infected)
Romania, 1992 (65)[18]	20	53	Infection correlated with older age and longer time in orphanage
Various countries, Korea 36% India 21%, 1992 (100)[19]	2	—	Adopted in Australia —
Romania, 1996 (22)[20]	27	—	—
Russia, 1997 (56)[21]	2	14	—
Various countries (Africa, Indian Ocean, Southeast Asia), 1999 (68)[4]	16	—	Adopted in France
China, 2000 (452)[22]	6	22	—
Various countries, 48% China, 2001[23]	2.8	35	19% of all children in study had received ≥1 HBV vaccine

Ab, antibody; sAb, surface antibody; sAg, surface antigen.

[a]Suggestive of prior infection rather than vaccination for most cases.

are asymptomatic carriers. The risk of chronic carriage relates to the age at the time of infection. Chronic hepatitis develops in ~90% of infants infected perinatally, 20%–30% of children infected between ages 1 and 5 years, and only 2%–10% of older children and adults. Although most chronically infected children are asymptomatic, some have chronic active hepatitis. About 20%–25% of chronically infected individuals develop cirrhosis or hepatocellular carcinoma, usually after the third or fourth decade of life, although these complications may occur earlier, even during childhood. Hepatitis B virus has various subtypes and genotypes. According to some investigators, specific viral subtypes may determine clinical manifestations. For example, Giannotti-

Crosti skin papules are most common with HBV subtype ayw. Subtypes show variable geographic distribution.[28] Genotypes may also influence clinical course: HBV-infected Taiwanese patients most often had severe disease if infected with genotype C, although hepatocellular carcinoma occurred most commonly with genotype B.[29] Replication and incorporation of HBV into the genome of infected hepatocytes are most active during the first few years after infection.

Diagnosis of Hepatitis B Virus

The diagnosis of HBV infection depends upon the demonstration of HBV surface antigen (HBsAg) in the circulation. The serologic tests used to evaluate HBV and their interpretation are shown in Table 15–2. Many commercial laboratories offer an "HBV panel," usually consisting of tests for sAg and immunoglobulin M (IgM) core antibody (Ab), designed to identify recent infection. This is inadequate to assess internationally adopted children, in whom screening should include HBsAg, HBsAb, HB core Ab, and hepatic transaminases.

A *carrier* is an individual in whom HBsAg is found at two intervals separated by at least 6 months. Surface antigen usually appears in the serum several weeks after exposure (range, 7 days to 4 months) and about 1 month before clinical evidence of infection (Fig. 15–2).[25]

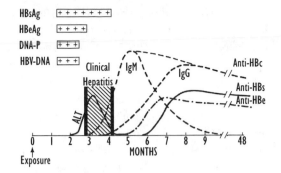

Figure 15–2 *Sequence of events in acute hepatitis B virus infection. Clinically evident hepatitis is preceded by hepatitis B surface antigen (HBsAg) serum positivity. Anti-HBc seroconversion occurs during the clinical phase of illness, whereas anti-HBs usually appears 1–3 months after recovery. Anti-HBc circulates as IgM during the first 6–12 months after appearance. DNA polymerase (DNA-P) and HBeAg disappear as anti-HBC appears. (Reprinted from* Textbook of Pediatric Infectious Diseases, *Vol. 1, Feigin RD, Cherry JD, et al. p 619, Copyright 1998, with permission from Elsevier.)*

Appearance of HBV DNA and HBV antigen (HbeAg) follow shortly thereafter. Transaminases increase about 1–4 weeks after appearance of surface antigen, and peak with the development of clinical hepatitis. The HBV core Ab appears during the phase of clinical hepatitis; IgM core Ab persists for 4 to 6 months and is followed by IgG core Ab. IgM core Ab alone may be present in infected children during the

Table 15–2 Diagnostic tests for hepatitis B virus infection

Test	Usage
HB surface antigen (HBsAg)	Detects infection (may be transiently present after vaccine administration)
HB surface antibody (HBsAb)	Present after immunization or natural infection; indicates immunity to HBV
HB core antibody (HB core Ab)	Present during acute, resolved, or chronic infection; *not* found after vaccination
HBV IgM antibody to core antigen (HB IgM core Ab)	Acute or recent HBV infection (may be found in the absence of HBsAg during seronegative window after infection)
HB e antibody (HBeAb)	Marker for lower risk of infectivity
HB e antigen (HBeAg)	Marker for increased risk of infectivity, hepatocellular necrosis, and inflammation
HB viral DNA	Quantification of circulating levels of HBV DNA by PCR technique

Neither eAb nor core Ab indicate immunity to HBV.

Source: Modified from American Academy of Pediatrics.[26]

"seronegative window period" when HBsAg levels fall below the detection limit of most commercial assays.[30] HBV DNA and eAg disappear from the circulation during recovery. HBsAb usually appears 1–3 months after disappearance of HBsAg. In patients who become carriers, surface antigenemia persists and IgG HB core Ab is found, often in high titer, but anti-HBs does not develop. Interpretation of some common patterns of HBV test results are shown in Table 15–3.

Of these patterns, isolated core Ab most commonly causes confusion. Except in infants in whom antibody may represent maternal antibody, core Ab alone may indicate that sAb has waned or, alternately, that sAg is below the detection limit of conventional assays. Polymerase chain reaction (PCR) techniques to amplify circulating HBV DNA can identify the latter group. Some investigators recommend administration of a "booster" dose of HBV vaccine to identify the former group: immune individuals should have an anamnestic response.

Development of eAb, although a favorable prognostic sign, does not confer immunity. Children with eAb who lack sAb likely have active viral infection, although this may be limited to the liver or other intracellular compartments. These individuals must still be considered infectious; PCR may demonstrate circulating HBV in low levels. They should be monitored prospectively for the development of sAb.

Internationally adopted children should be tested for HBV infection upon arrival to the United States (HBsAg, HBsAb, HB core Ab, liver function tests). Because of the potential for exposure just prior to travel and the long incubation of HBV, children should also be tested again 6 months after arrival in the United States.

Hepatitis B Virus Variants

Rarely, patients may be infected with HBV variants that are not detected by standard assays for surface antigen. These variants have been reported from Europe and Asia and likely are underrecognized. Most commonly, "surface antigen negative HBV" is due to infection with virus that has undergone mutations in the major hydrophilic loop of surface antigen (amino

Table 15–3 Interpretation of hepatitis B virus test results

Surface Antigen	Core Antibody	Surface Antibody	Interpretation and Recommendations
−	−	−	Not infected, or very early infection with no markers yet present. Repeat testing in 6 months if patient is newly arrived child.
−	−	+	Immune (either via natural infection or vaccine) or maternal antibody. If infant is <8–10 months, retest serially to verify absence of infection and determine need for vaccine.
−	+	+	Immune after natural infection, or maternal antibody, or combination. If infant is <8–10 months, retest serially to verify absence of infection and determine need for vaccine.
−	+	−	Recovering from acute HBV infection *or* distantly immune with nondetectable levels of HbsAb *or* false positive core Ab *or* nondetectable levels of HBsAg (actually a carrier). Retest in 1–2 months.
+	−	−	Infected, without demonstrable antibody response. Check liver function tests, eAg, eAb, viral DNA, and follow closely. May be seen transiently after vaccination.
+	+	−	Early infection, may be carrier. Check liver function tests, eAg, eAb, viral DNA, and follow closely.
+	+/−	+	Lab error *or* early response to chronic HBV infection *or* infection with 2 strains of HBV: one elicited anti-HBS response, and second strain is antibody-resistant and caused a chronic infection.

Source: Modified from American Academy of Pediatrics.[26]

acids 98–156). This site is the main target for antibodies used in diagnostic tests. Individuals infected with these variants may have core Ab in the circulation as the only obvious marker of disease, although at least 10%–40% are viremic as demonstrated by PCR. Other reasons for "surface antigen negative HBV" include early infection, co-infection with hepatitis C (which down-regulates HBV replication and protein synthesis), or the presence of circulating immune complexes that interfere with immunoassays.

Variants of eAg expression also occur, most commonly because of mutations of the precore region of the HBV genome. These mutations decrease eAg expression and may cause more serious disease.[31,32]

Transmission of Hepatitis B Virus

The main routes of transmission of HBV are vertical (perinatal) transmission, blood, and sexual contact. Vertical transmission occurs when the mother develops acute HBV infection during the third trimester, or if she is a chronic carrier.[27] Some birth mothers acquire HBV as a consequence of their injection drug use. Transmission risk to the infant is increased if the mother is eAg positive. Transplacental infection is unusual; most vertical transmission occurs at the time of delivery via exposure to blood and cervical or vaginal secretions. Surface antigen usually cannot be detected in infected newborns until several weeks of age: peak antigenemia after neonatal infection occurs around 3 months of age, but may not appear until 6 months or later. Although HBsAg may be found in breast milk, several studies show no difference in risk of transmission between breast and bottle-fed infants born to HBsAg-positive mothers.[26]

Among adoptees, vertical transmission accounts only for a portion of all infected children. Risk of HBV in internationally adopted children relates to prevalence in the birth country as well as exposures prior to adoption. Transmission of

Vicki was adopted from Russia. She arrived in the United States in September, and shortly afterwards had negative test results for HB sAg and sAb. When seen in follow-up for developmental delays in March, a second blood sample showed the presence of HBsAg. Further evaluation confirmed HBV (e Ag positive, hepatitis viral DNA >30,000 pg/ml). No history of exposure was elicited during her time in the United States, but on further questioning her mother remembered that the orphanage doctors gave Vicki a special vitamin shot prior to her travel to the United States. "I didn't even notice if they used a sterile needle," said her mom, "My mind was on so many other things." Vicki probably got infected just as she was leaving Russia, and was in the seronegative window period when her first blood tests were done.

HBV is common during institutional life. Exposure to reused, improperly sterilized needles or other medical equipment is frequent in some settings. Parenteral injections are common, sometimes because of lack of palatable oral medications formulated for children. Transfusion of (inadequately screened) blood or blood products is frequent in some countries and may not be recorded in the child's medical record. Blood products may be given to ill neonates, infants or children in lieu of other types of volume expanders or medications that would be used in the United States for similar conditions.

Because HBV survives in the environment for at least 1 week,[9] indirect inoculation via environmental contamination may also occur. Hepatitis B virus is not readily transmitted by oral exposure to saliva. However, percutaneous or permucosal contact with saliva (via a bite or open skin lesion, for example) may transmit HBV. It may be transmitted within the orphanage or household via shared toothbrushes, nail-clippers, razors, or hair-clippers contaminated with blood from an infected individual. Transmission may also occur through open skin lesions (such as impetigo or excoriated scabies) either directly or via shared washcloths, towels, or clothing. Percutaneous or permucosal transmission is more likely in a heavily contaminated environment.

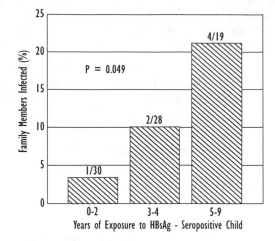

Margie was adopted from Kazahkstan at 22 months of age. On arrival in the United States, she was found to have HBV infection with transaminases in the range of 300–400. Review of her complete medical file from Kazakhstan revealed that Margie had been given 287 parenteral injections prior to adoption: antibiotics, vitamins, vaccines, and various other compounds. Most of the injections were series of vitamin treatments for "perinatal encephalopathy" and consisted of repeated series of 40 injections of vitamin B_1, B_6, B_{12}, and "aloe." This series had been repeated four times in the first 19 months of life.

Figure 15–3 *Risk of infection with hepatitis B for family members of infected Asian adoptees. Percent of family members infected relates to duration of exposure to an HbsAg-seropositive child. (Friede A, Harris JR, Kobayashi JM, Shaw FE Jr, Shoemaker-Nawas PC, Kane MA. Transmission of hepatitis B virus from adopted Asian children to their American families. 1988; 78:26–9. ©1988, American Public Health Association.)*

Among children living in residential care in South Africa, about 80% became infected with HBV by age 5 years.[33]

Hepatitis B Virus and Adoptive Families

Although the main routes of HBV transmission are via blood or sexual contact, transmission via ordinary household contact may occur after inapparent permucosal or percutaneous exposures. Several surveys carried out before the availability of HBV vaccine clearly demonstrate the risk of transmission within the family. For example, among the families of 40 adopted Vietnamese children, 6% of adults and 23% of American-born siblings had HBsAb.[5] One mother developed clinical hepatitis. Among 309 families of 511 Korean or Indian children, 9% of relatives exposed to a seropositive child had evidence of present or past HBV infection.[11] The relative risk for HBV among family members was 5.3, and the risk increased with years of exposure to the seropositive child (Fig. 15–3). In a third study, 64% of parents exposed to seropositive children developed acute HBV, and another 27% had serological evidence of exposure.[34] Similar results have been reported among adoptive families in Sweden. In one study, 61% of family members had evidence of exposure from their adopted Korean, Indian, or Thai children, including 19% with clin-

ical HBV or surface antigen.[6] In another survey, 36 seropositive adopted children transmitted HBV to 54 family members.[35] The risk of transmission was greatest during the first year after adoption (67% of cases).

Natural History of Hepatitis B Virus Infection

Longitudinal studies of untreated HBV acquired in childhood indicate that some individuals achieve remission. These children lose circulating eAg and develop eAb; markers of HBV replication disappear and liver disease remits. Seroconversion rates range from 4% to 10% per year, and 33%–80% over longer periods of follow-up.[36–46] However, reactivation may occur in as many as 35% of cases, particularly within the first few years after development of eAb. Reactivation may be associated with exacerbation of liver disease. Ethnic background of the host or specific infecting HBV genotype influences the likelihood of clearance.[29] Some patients in whom eAg disappears remain at risk for hepatocellular carcinoma; continued monitoring is essential even among those with normal transaminases.

About 5%–6% of carriers eventually lose HBsAg as well. Viral DNA may not be completely eradicated, however. PCR techniques may demonstrate HBV viral DNA in peripheral blood mononuclear cells and serum of some sAg-negative patients, even in the presence of sAb. About 30% of Chinese patients and 50% of Japanese patients with serological markers of past HBV infection have detectable serum viral DNA.[47] Thus clearance of sAg followed by emergence of antibodies does not necessarily indicate termination of viremia. Some of these individuals may develop hepatocellular carcinoma or cirrhosis even after seroconversion.[48]

The incidence of hepatocellular carcinoma has been greatly reduced by implementation of universal vaccination in some countries. Taiwan introduced universal vaccination in 1984 and reduced the HBV carrier rate from 10% to <1%.[49] Since virtually all children with hepatocellular carcinoma have HBsAg, this likely will result in reductions in future cases of hepatocellular carcinoma.

Prevention of Hepatitis B Virus Infection

Universal vaccination of newborns has greatly reduced the incidence of HBV in many countries. However, in some countries that send children to the United States for adoption, these programs are neither well established nor correctly implemented. Vaccine may be improperly manufactured or stored, administered incorrectly (via subcutaneous instead of intramuscular injection, gluteal instead of deltoid, for example), or given too late after birth to be effective in preventing vertical transmission. Furthermore, infants may not receive second and third doses of vaccine, especially if they are transferred to several institutions prior to admission to the orphanage. Financial constraints are a large bar-

Greg was adopted from Russia at 32 months of age. Although his family had been advised to receive the HBV vaccine series prior to the adoption, they were dissuaded by physicians at a travel clinic they consulted. Greg turned out to be an active, rambunctious toddler. After he'd been home for about 7 months, his live-in, 76-year-old grandmother developed severe HBV with serum bilirubin rising to 29 mg/dl. She recovered after months of illness. Although no definite exposure could be identified by the family, presumably his grandmother had inapparent blood contact with Greg, perhaps after a scrape or cut.

rier to availability of HBV vaccine, as its cost rivals that of the six other recommended infant vaccines combined. Prospective adoptive parents and adoption agencies may be misinformed that vaccination prevents disease even if the series is incomplete or was administered several months after birth.[30]

In general, vaccination has been extremely effective in reducing the incidence of transmission of HBV within ordinary household contact. The vaccine is among the safest vaccines licensed in the United States. Protective titers (>10 mIU/ml) develop after three vaccines in 90%–95% of teens and adults and in >98% of infants.[50] However, some individuals do not respond to the conventional series of three vaccines given at 0, 1, and 6 months with measurable titers of sAb. Smoking, obesity, and age >40 years may reduce immune responses. Specific genetic and ethnic factors may also contribute to the limited responses, which seem to be specific for HBsAg. Individuals with the HLA haplotype B8-SC01-DR3 appear to have a specific defect in response to HBV vaccine,[51] as do some aboriginal residents of China.[52] Family contacts of children positive for HBsAg should have titers checked 1 to 6 months after completion of their third dose of vaccine to determine immune status. From 15% to 25% of nonresponders gain immunity after one additional dose, and 30% to 50% respond after three additional doses. Thus nonresponders should receive an additional one to three vaccine doses and then be reevaluated for sAb.

There have been rare reports of "escape mutants" of HBV for which vaccine and HBIg are not protective. Possession of certain single amino acid substitutions may confer this trait.[53]

Transient Positivity after Vaccination

Vaccination itself may cause transient antigenemia.[54,55] Positive tests for HBsAg have been found in patients immunized with Engerix B® or Gen Hevac B® vaccine for as long as 21 days after vaccination. This is an important consideration in adoptees whose recent vaccine history may not be known when testing occurs shortly after adoption.

Management of Hepatitis B Virus

Once the diagnosis of HBV infection is established, hepatic transaminases, bilirubin, and alkaline phosphatase are measured to assess the degree of liver inflammation. Additional useful tests include IgM and total core antibody, e antigen and e antibody, and quantitative viral DNA and α-fetoprotein levels. Screening for hepatitis A, hepatitis C, and HIV should also be done. If available, screening for hepatitis D (delta virus) may provide additional useful information, especially in children from Mediterranean countries, Romania, South America, Africa, and the Middle East.[30] A liver ultrasound should also be obtained.

In newly diagnosed children, biochemical reevaluation should be repeated on several occasions within 2–10 weeks to monitor for signs of progression. If transaminases remain normal, monitoring intervals can gradually be lengthened. At a minimum, assessments should be completed annually and include measurement of transaminases, bilirubin, alkaline phosphatase, HBV sAg, sAb, eAg, eAb, core Ab, α-fetoprotein, as well as liver ultrasound. Hepatitis A vaccine should be administered to nonimmune individuals. Counseling about vaccination recommendations for household contacts, transmission risks, and household precautions should be offered. Adequate HBsAb titers should be verified among regular household contacts.

Children with elevated transaminases should be referred for biopsy, treatment, and specialized follow-up.

Treatment

Antiviral treatment of HBV is evolving rapidly. Ongoing clinical trials are posted by the National Institutes of Health.[56] For most drug trials, remission has been defined as absent HB viral DNA and loss of eAg.[57,58] Responses occasionally occur months after treatment. Some patients also eventually lose sAg as well. Interferon-α (IFN-α) has been widely used but is reserved for patients with persistent elevation of transaminases and chronic hepatitis on biopsy. Treatment is generally three times a week via subcutaneous administration. About 25%–40% of adult patients gain remission after 4–6 months of treatment with IFN-α.[59] Meta-analysis of six randomized clinical trials of IFN-α involving 240 children showed clearance of HBV DNA in 35% of treated patients.[60] Transaminases returned to normal in 39% of children, and eAg cleared in 23%. Improvement persisted after completion of therapy in many children: 29% continued with nondetectable HBV DNA. Prolonged therapy (>6 months) was associated with a better response, as were patients with high alanine aminotransferase (ALT) at entry.[61] The best responders are those with high ALT, low HBV DNA levels, and active inflammation, necrosis, and fibrosis on liver biopsy, with no other underlying diseases.[39]

Patients with normal levels of ALT usually have immune tolerance to the virus (and usually have been infected via vertical transmission), and generally don't respond to IFN-α. Likewise, patients without eAg may be infected by variant strains that don't respond to IFN-α.

Many patients have further elevation of transaminases during treatment. Children usually tolerate IFN-α well, although side effects include initial reactions that can be severe, as well as long-term reactions (fatigue, myalgias, headaches, irritability, anorexia, depression, hair loss).[57] Neutropenia and thrombocytopenia occur occasionally but are dose related. About 2% of adults have severe reactions: bacterial infection, autoimmune disease, severe depression, seizure, acute cardiac or renal failure, and pneumonitis.

An alternate drug is lamivudine, a nucleoside analogue which interferes with DNA polymerase involved in viral replication.[62] Early data on lamivudine suggest that this may also be effective and well tolerated.[63] However, it does not prevent the incorporation of HBV genome into hepatocyte DNA, and thus does not prevent the long-term risks of hepatocellular carcinoma. The new nucleotide analogue, adefovir dipivoxil, has recently been shown to improve liver histology, reduce circulating HBV DNA levels, and normalize ALT levels in significantly more adult patients than among those receiving placebos.[64–66] Combination therapies will likely offer benefits over single agents. Other drugs under investigation include non-nucleoside antivirals (these block protein synthesis involved in viral replication) and non-interferon immune enhancers (which promote T-cell activation).

Key Points for Internationally Adopted Children

- About 5% of internationally adopted children are infected with HBV.
- Virtually all HBV-infected international adoptees had negative tests for this virus in their birth countries.
- Test results in birth countries are no guarantee that children are HBV negative.

- Most infected children are asymptomatic, chronic carriers of HBV.
- Recommended tests on arrival include HBsAg, HBsAb, HB core Ab, and ALT/AST; these should be repeated 6 or more months after entry to the United States.
- Some infected children develop active hepatitis and benefit from treatment.
- Household members should receive HBV vaccine prior to arrival of the child.

FAQs

Q. My newly adopted patient had a negative test for HBsAg in Russia just 1 month ago! Do I really need to test her again?

A. She must not only be tested now, but again in 6 months. The many reasons include the following facts: *(1)* not all lab tests are reliable in countries from which children are adopted, *(2)* she may have gotten infected after the test was done (it's very common for children to receive parenteral exposures in most countries, or she could even have gotten infected by the needle used to draw the blood for her hepatitis test), *(3)* she could have been in the "seronegative window period" when the test was originally done. Surface antigen may not appear for several months after infection.

Q. My 2-year-old patient's HBsAb came back positive. Does he need further HBV vaccinations?

A. If your lab gives a quantitative result that suggests the child is immune, no further vaccines are necessary. Immunity usually correlates with a titer of $\geq$ 10 mIU/ml.

Q. My patient is HBsAg positive. Which family members should receive the HBV vaccine? What about day care?

A. Anyone in regular household contact should receive the vaccine. This could include relatives, close friends, and babysitters. The safety and efficacy of the HBV vaccines make pre-exposure prophylaxis very important. The *Red Book*[26] states that HBV-infected children may not be restricted from day care. Exceptions include children with open skin lesions or behavioral problems (biting). Hepatitis B virus status is private information. Licensed child care facilities should practice universal precautions. However, parents may want to review their personal situation with you to discuss this further.

Q. Some prospective adoptive parents just consulted me. They are traveling to get their child in about 4 weeks! I know they need the HBV vaccine, but isn't it too late to give it?

A. The vaccine may be given on an accelerated schedule. About 30% of healthy adults will develop antibody after a single dose, and 75%–80% after a second dose given 1 month later. In cases when an accelerated schedule is used, a fourth dose is usually suggested (0, 1, 2, and 6 months). Family members should at least receive the first two doses of vaccine before travel, and blood precautions should be reviewed.

Q. Must I wait out the incubation period to vaccinate my new patient from Guatemala with HBV vaccine? I'd like her to be protected quickly, but wonder if the vaccine would be harmful if she turns out to be a carrier.

A. It's okay to begin the vaccine series. Vaccination of carriers is not harmful; in fact it was tested as a means of boosting their immune systems in hopes of aiding clearance of the virus. Go ahead and vaccinate, but remember you must retest her for sAg ~6 months after her arrival in the United States.

Q. My 3-year-old Romanian patient is HBsAg positive. His parents and siblings all received three doses of the HBV vaccine. They all have titers of HBsAb reported as "immune" except for his dad (age 33) and 6-year-old sister. What now?

A. The dad and sister should be screened for HBsAg. If negative for HBsAg and HBsAb are <10 mIU/ml, they should each receive an additional one to three vaccines and be reassessed. Meanwhile, blood precautions must be followed (cleaning blood spills with dilute bleach solution [1/2 cup per gallon of water], HBIg prophylaxis for blood exposures).

Q. I have a family who adopted 14-month-old Chinese twins, then found out that both babies are HBsAg positive. The parents both are immune to HBV, but should they receive a booster shot sometime?

A. At present, booster doses are not recommended, as immune memory persists for more than 10 years. However, this should be reviewed periodically, and in high-risk situations a booster could be considered.

Q. How long do passively transferred antibodies persist? My 6-month-old Chinese patient has HB core Ab, and I have a 10-month-old Kazakh patient with HBsAb. What now?

A. Passively transferred IgG antibodies in general have a half life of 20–30 days and reach their lowest levels about 4 months of age. However, the level of antibody in the mother's circulation and other factors affect the concentration in the infant's blood. Both patients should be followed at intervals to determine their status of antibodies as well as sAg.

Q. From a practical point of view, what should I do about the possibility of HBV variants? My 4-year-old patient from India has had core Ab since she was adopted at age 1 year. She's never developed sAb. What should I do?

A. Start by testing for HBV DNA by PCR. This will amplify low levels of antigen that may be present. Also, it's important to check for eAg and eAb, as well as transaminases. It's likely she's either immune after natural infection but has low levels of sAb (sometimes a dose of vaccine can identify these patients), or is a carrier with low levels of circulating antigen, or infected with an escape mutant.

Resources

Immunization Action Coalition. Available at: http://www.immunize.org/.

National Center for Infectious Diseases. Viral Hepatitis B. Available at: http://www.cdc.gov/ncidod/diseases/hepatitis/b.

Hepatitis B Foundation. Available at: http://www.hepb.org/.

National Digestive Diseases Information Clearinghouse. What I need to know about hepatitis B. Available at: http://www.niddk.nih.gov/health/digest/pubs/hep/hepb/hepb.htm.

HepNet: The Hepatitis Information Network. Hepatitis B. Available at: http://www.hepnet.com/hepb.html.

References

1. National Center for Infectious Diseases. Traveler's Health. Hepatitis, viral, type B. Available at: cdc.gov/travel/diseases/hbv.htm.

2. Haukenes G, Brinchmann-Hansen K, Macovei O. Prevalence of hepatitis B and C and HIV antibodies in children in a Romanian orphanage. APMIS 1992; 100:757–61.

3. Hostetter MK, Iverson S, Dole K, Johnson D. Unsuspected infectious diseases and other medical diagnoses in the evaluation of internationally adopted children. Pediatrics 1989; 83:559–64.

4. Bureau JJ, Maurage C, Bremond M, Despert F, Rolland JC. Children of foreign origin adopted in France. Analysis of 68 cases during 12 years at the University Hospital Center of Tours [in French]. Arch Pediatr 1999; 6:1053–8.

5. Vernon TM, Wright RA, Kohler PF, Merrill DA. Hepatitis A and B in the family unit. Nonparenteral transmission by asymptomatic children. JAMA 1976; 235:2829–31.

6. Nordenfelt E, Dahlquist E. HBsAg positive adopted children as a cause of intrafamilial spread of hepatitis B. Scand J Infect Dis 1978; 10:161–3.

7. Greenblatt M, Khoo EC. Incidence of hepatitis B carriers among adopted Korean children [letter]. N Engl J Med 1985; 312:1639.

8. Jenista JA, Chapman D. Medical problems of foreign-born adopted children. Am J Dis Child 1987; 141: 298–302.

9. Lange WR, Warnock-Eckhart E. Selected infectious disease risks in international adoptees. Pediatr Infect Dis J 1987; 6:447–50.

10. Murray DL, Lynch M, Doughty A, Cho BK. Results of screening adopted Korean children for HBsAg [letter]. Am J Public Health 1988; 78:855–6.

11. Friede A, Harris JR, Kobayashi JM, Shaw FE Jr, Shoemaker-Nawas PC, Kane MA. Transmission of hepatitis B virus from adopted Asian children to their American families. Am J Public Health 1988; 78:26–9.

12. Smith-Garcia T, Brown JS. The health of children adopted from India. J Community Health 1989; 14: 227–41.

13. Murray DL. International adoptees and hepatitis B virus infection. Am J Dis Child 1990; 144:523–4.

14. Rudin C, Berger R, Tobler R, Nars P, Just M, Pavic N. HIV-1, hepatitis (A, B, and C), and measles in Romanian children. Lancet 1990; 336:1592–3.

15. Kurtz J. HIV infection and hepatitis B in adopted Romanian children. BMJ 1991; 302:1399.

16. Ascher DP, Montez M. Infectious disease risks among Filipino adoptees. J Trop Pediatr 1991; 37:318–9.

17. Hostetter MK, Iverson S, Thomas W, McKenzie D, Dole K, Johnson DE. Medical evaluation of internationally adopted children. N Engl J Med 1991; 325:479–85.

18. Johnson DE, Miller LC, Iverson S, et al. The health of children adopted from Romania. JAMA 1992; 268:3446–51.

19. Nicholson AJ, Francis BM, Mulholland EK, Moulden AL, Oberklaid F. Health screening of international adoptees. Evaluation of a hospital-based clinic. Med J Aust 1992; 156:377–9.

20. Benoit TC, Jocelyn LJ, Moddemann DM, Embree JE. Romanian adoption. The Manitoba experience. Arch Pediatr Adolesc Med 1996; 150:1278–82.

21. Albers LH, Johnson DE, Hostetter MK, Iverson S, Miller LC. Health of children adopted from the former Soviet Union and Eastern Europe. Comparison with preadoptive medical records. JAMA 1997; 278:922–4.

22. Miller LC, Hendrie NW. Health of children adopted from China. Pediatrics 2000; 105:E76.

23. Saiman L, Aronson J, Zhou J, et al. Prevalence of infectious diseases among internationally adopted children. Pediatrics 2001; 108:608–12.

24. Zwiener RJ, Fielman BA, Squires RH Jr. Chronic hepatitis B in adopted Romanian children. J Pediatr 1992; 121:572–4.

25. Broderick A, Jonas MM. Hepatitis B and D viruses. In: Feigin RD, Cherry JD, Demmler GJ, Kaplan SL (eds). Textbook of Pediatric Infectious Diseases. Philadelphia: Saunders, 2004: vol. 2: 1863–83.

26. American Academy of Pediatrics. Committee on Infectious Diseases. Hepatitis B. In: Pickering LK, ed. 2003 Red Book: Report of the Committee on Infectious Diseases. Elk Grove Village, IL: The American Academy of Pediatrics, 2003: 318–36.

27. Sanchez PJ, Siegel JD. Hepatitis viruses. In: McMillan JA, DeAngelis CD, Feigen RD, Warshaw B. (eds.) Oski's Pediatrics: principles and practice. Philadelphia: Lippincott-Williams & Wilkins, 1999: 447–50.

28. Snitbhan R, Scott RM, Bancroft WH, Top FH Jr, Chiewsilp D. Subtypes of hepatitis B surface antigen in Southeast Asia. J Infect Dis 1975; 131:708–11.

29. Kao J, Chen P, Lai M, Chen D. Hepatitis B genotypes correlate with clinical outcomes in patients with chronic hepatitis B. Gastroenterology 2000; 118:554–9.

30. Hostetter MK. Infectious diseases in internationally adopted children: findings in children from China, Russia, and Eastern Europe. Adv Pediatr Infect Dis 1999; 14:147–61.

31. Sato S, Suzuki K, Akahane Y, et al. Hepatitis B virus strains with mutations in the core promoter in patients with fulminant hepatitis. Ann Intern Med 1995; 122:241–8.

32. Hawkins AE, Gilson RJ, Beath SV, et al. Novel application of a point mutation assay: evidence for transmission of hepatitis B viruses with precore mutations and their detection in infants with fulminant hepatitis B. J Med Virol 1994; 44:13–21.

33. Solarsh GC, McKerrow N, Mlisana KP, Loening WE, Gouws E. Hepatitis B infection in black children from residential care facilities in KwaZulu-Natal. Implications for adoption and foster care. S Afr Med J 1996; 86:345–9.

34. Sokal EM, Van Collie O, Buts JP. Horizontal trans-

mission of hepatitis B from children to adoptive parents [letter]. Arch Dis Child 1995; 72:191.

35. Christenson B. Epidemiological aspects of the transmission of hepatitis B by HBsAg-positive adopted children. Scand J Infect Dis 1986; 18:105–9.

36. Bortolotti F, Cadrobbi P, Crivellaro C, et al. Long-term outcome of chronic type B hepatitis in patients who acquire hepatitis B virus infection in childhood. Gastroenterology 1990; 99:805–10.

37. Fujisawa T, Komatsu H, Inui A, et al. Long-term outcome of chronic hepatitis B in adolescents or young adults in follow-up from childhood. J Pediatr Gastroenterol Nutr 2000; 30:201–6.

38. Di Marco V, Lo Iacono O, Camma C, et al. The long-term course of chronic hepatitis B. Hepatology 1999; 30:257–64.

39. Bortolotti F, Jara P, Barbera C, et al. Long-term effect of alpha interferon in children with chronic hepatitis B. Gut 2000; 46:715–8.

40. Chang MH. Natural history of hepatitis B virus infection in children. J Gastroenterol Hepatol 2000; 15 Suppl:E16–9.

41. Bortolotti F, Jara P, Crivellaro C, et al. Outcome of chronic hepatitis B in Caucasian children during a 20-year observation period. J Hepatol 1998; 29:184–90.

42. Lok AS, Lai CL. A longitudinal follow-up of asymptomatic hepatitis B surface antigen–positive Chinese children. Hepatology 1988; 8:1130–3.

43. Chang MH, Chen DS, Hsu HC, Hsu HY, Lee CY. Maternal transmission of hepatitis B virus in childhood hepatocellular carcinoma. Cancer 1989; 64:2377–80.

44. Hsu HC, Wu MZ, Chang MH, Su IJ, Chen DS. Childhood hepatocellular carcinoma develops exclusively in hepatitis B surface antigen carriers in three decades in Taiwan. Report of 51 cases strongly associated with rapid development of liver cirrhosis. J Hepatol 1987; 5:260–7.

45. Moyes CD, Milne A, Waldon J. Liver function of hepatitis B carriers in childhood. Pediatr Infect Dis J 1993; 12:120–5.

46. Chan CY, Lee SD, Yu MI, Wang YJ, Tsai YT, Lo KJ. Long-term follow-up of hepatitis B virus carrier infants. J Med Virol 1994; 44:336–9.

47. Kato J, Hasegawa K, Torii N, Yamauchi K, Hayashi N. A molecular analysis of viral persistence in surface antigen-negative chronic hepatitis B. Hepatology 1996; 23:389–95.

48. Adachi H, Kaneko S, Matsushita E, Inagaki Y, Unoura M, Kobayashi K. Clearance of HBsAg in seven patients with chronic hepatitis B. Hepatology 1992; 16:1334–7.

49. Chang MH, Chen CJ, Lai MS, et al. Universal hepatitis B vaccination in Taiwan and the incidence of hepatocellular carcinoma in children. Taiwan Childhood Hepatoma Study Group. N Engl J Med 1997; 336: 1855–9.

50. Lemon SM, Thomas DL. Vaccines to prevent viral hepatitis. N Engl J Med 1997; 336:196–204.

51. Alper CA, Kruskall MS, Marcus-Bagley D, et al. Genetic prediction of nonresponse to hepatitis B vaccine. N Engl J Med 1989; 321:708–12.

52. Hsu LC, Lin SR, Hsu HM, et al. Ethnic differences in immune responses to hepatitis B vaccine. Am J Epidemiol 1996; 143:718–24.

53. Okamoto H, Yano K, Nozaki Y, et al. Mutations within the S gene of hepatitis B virus transmitted from mothers to babies immunized with hepatitis B immune globulin and vaccine. Pediatr Res 1992; 32:264–8.

54. Koksal N, Altinkaya N, Perk Y. Transient hepatitis B surface antigenemia after neonatal hepatitis B immunization. Acta Paediatr 1996; 85:1501–2.

55. Lunn ER, Hoggarth BJ, Cook WJ. Prolonged hepatitis B surface antigenemia after vaccination. Pediatrics 2000; 105:E81.

56. ClinicalTrials.gov.http://www.clinicaltrials.gov/ct/search?term=hepatitistb.

57. Hoofnagle JH, di Bisceglie AM. The treatment of chronic viral hepatitis. N Engl J Med 1997; 336:347–56.

58. Omata M. Treatment of chronic hepatitis B infection. N Engl J Med 1998; 339:114–5.

59. Niederau C, Heintges T, Lange S, et al. Long-term follow-up of HBeAg-positive patients treated with interferon alfa for chronic hepatitis B. N Engl J Med 1996; 334:1422–7.

60. Torre D, Tambini R. Interferon-alpha therapy for chronic hepatitis B in children: a meta-analysis. Clin Infect Dis 1996; 23:131–7.

61. Ozen H, Kocak N, Yuce A, Gurakan F. Retreatment with higher dose interferon alpha in children with chronic hepatitis B infection. Pediatr Infect Dis J 1999; 18:694–7.

62. Lai CL, Chien RN, Leung NW, et al. A one-year trial of lamivudine for chronic hepatitis B. Asia Hepatitis Lamivudine Study Group. N Engl J Med 1998; 339:61–8.

63. Dienstag JL, Schiff ER, Wright TL, et al. Lamivudine as initial treatment for chronic hepatitis B in the United States. N Engl J Med 1999; 341:1256–63.

64. Mailliard ME, Gollan JL. Suppressing hepatitis B without resistance—so far, so good. N Engl J Med 2003; 348:848–50.

65. Marcellin P, Chang TT, Lim SG, et al. Adefovir dipivoxil for the treatment of hepatitis B e antigen–positive chronic hepatitis B. N Engl J Med 2003; 348:808–16.

66. Hadziyannis SJ, Tassopoulos NC, Heathcote EJ, et al. Adefovir dipivoxil for the treatment of hepatitis B e antigen–negative chronic hepatitis B. N Engl J Med 2003; 348:800–7.

16

HEPATITIS C

Hepatitis C virus (HCV) is an endemic viral infection throughout the world: approximately 3% (170 million) of the world's population is infected.[1] Although HCV is uncommon among international adoptees,[2] it is important to identify infected children for proper monitoring and in some cases, treatment. Evidence of HCV exposure or infection is found on ~5%–10% of pre-adoption medical referrals from Russia and Eastern Europe. Such records do not reliably identify infected children. Differentiation of maternal antibody from infection is usually not possible on the basis of information provided in pre-adoptive medical records. Thus, advising prospective parents is difficult. This section reviews the epidemiology, clinical features, diagnostic tests, and current treatments of HCV, as they relate to the internationally adopted child.

Epidemiology

The prevalence of HCV varies in different geographic regions (Fig. 16–1). In Eastern Europe, the Middle East, and Asia, prevalence is about 1%–5%. In western Europe, North America, and most of Central America, the prevalence is considerably less, about 0.2%–0.5%. Table 16–1 shows some selected prevalence studies in regions from Russia and China. These two sending countries accounted for nearly half of all international adoptions to the United States in 2002. Differences in the populations studied and methodologies account for the variability in prevalence.

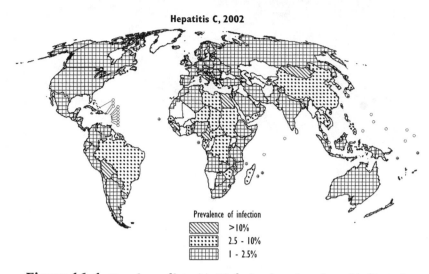

Hepatitis C, 2002

Prevalence of infection
>10%
2.5 - 10%
1 - 2.5%

Figure 16–1 *Prevalence of hepatitis C infection throughout the world. (From the World Health Organization, 2002, with permission.)*

Table 16–1 Prevalence of hepatitis C virus in various populations

Site	No. and Description of Subjects	Subjects with HCV infection (%)
Russia		
Siberia[3]	348 from general population	1.4
Daghestan (Russia)[4]	10,682 volunteer blood donors	0.9
	267 paid blood donors	7.5
	97 "high-risk" patients	50–80
	87 with chronic liver disease	40–50
Russia[5]	4216 from general population	
	Central Euro-Russian	0.7
	Mongolian	10.7
Russia[6]	2217 from general population	
	Central Asian Republics	3–5
	Moscow region	1.3
China		
Nanjing (southern China)[7]	998 individuals	
	600 from general population	0.5 (all <12 years old with prior transfusion)
	398 with liver disease	5
Lanzhou (western China)[8]	Volunteer blood donors	2.5
	Paid blood donors	35
Wuhan (east-central China)[9]	637 children, including	
	65 post-transfusion	30.8
	103 healthy children in day care	2.9
	50 with "infantile hepatitis"	6
China[10]	100 women	3
Shenyang China[11]	3902 from general population	0.4–1.7
Shaanxi China[12]	150 women	3
China[13]	494 women	2.4

Table 16–2 Prevalence of hepatitis C virus antibodies or infection in internationally adopted children

Reference	n/N	%	Sending Country
16	0/6	0	Not specified
17	1/452	0.2	China
18	4/496	0.8	16 countries
19	2/129	1.5	22 countries
2	2/89	2.2	20 countries
Miller, unpublished	17/670	2.5	Russia, Ukraine, China, Vietnam, Guatemala, Kazakhstan

Studies are not directly comparable as different definitions of HCV infection were used.

Hepatitis C Virus and International Adoptees

Hepatitis C virus screening of newly arrived internationally adopted children has not been routinely recommended in standard references,[14–15] even though some of these children are infected with HCV (Table 16–2). Many clinics specializing in evaluation of international adopted children screen all new arrivals, as risk factors are rarely disclosed in available medical history.

International adoptees may acquire HCV from various sources. Some birth mothers are infected via injection drug use or other routes and may transmit the infection vertically. Thus HCV antibody may be a proxy marker for prenatal drug exposure. International adoptees may also be exposed to HCV-contaminated needles, blood products, or medical equipment in hospitals or orphanages. Acquisition from infected peers or via sexual abuse is also possible, but these are less likely sources of infection.

Transmission of Hepatitis C Virus

Hepatitis C virus is transmitted vertically or parenterally[20] (Table 16–3). About 5% of infants born to HCV-infected mothers become infected. The risk increases to 10%–11% if the mother has HCV RNA in the serum at the time

In pre-adoptive counseling, Ms. G., a single mother, emphatically insisted that she could not handle a child with special medical needs. Michael's medical referral was carefully scrutinized to identify any hint of problems. Sure enough, when he arrived at age 9 months from Romania, his initial evaluation revealed antibody to hepatitis C and moderate to severe sensorineural hearing loss. An engaging and delightful baby, Michael charmed everyone, especially his mom. By age 18 months, his antibody had disappeared (presumably maternal antibody) and he was speaking age-appropriately, thanks to his hearing aids.

of delivery;[21] risk relates to HCV titer[22,23] and genotype.[24] Unlike hepatitis B, prophylactic measures to reduce perinatal transmission are not available. The rate of perinatal transmission is considerably enhanced in mothers concurrently infected with HIV, even without transmission of HIV. It is not certain if transmission is more likely to occur in utero[24] or at delivery.[21] Breast feeding does not appear to be a major route of transmission.

Parenteral exposures (blood products or contaminated needles) of HCV are the most common route of infection.[25] HCV is 10-fold less likely to be transmitted after accidental needle-stick than hepatitis B.[1] Sexual transmission between monogamous spouses is relatively uncommon. Compared to HBV, HCV transmission within normal household contact is un-

Table 16–3 Risk factors for hepatitis C virus infection in children

Exposure to blood products
Exposure to contaminated medical supplies/equipment
Maternal HCV infection
High-risk behaviors (injection drug use, body piercing or tattooing)

Source: Data from Jonas.[21]

usual, but may occur via inapparent blood exposures (such as shared toothbrushes, razors, etc.). About 4% (range, 0% to 11%) of household contacts of HCV-infected individuals become infected.[15,25–27]

Hepatitis C Virus Genotypes

Six distinct HCV genotypes have been characterized. Genotypes 1 and 2 are broadly distributed, with types 1a and 1b being most common in the United States and western Europe, followed by genotypes 2 and 3. Genotype 4 is common in Egypt and Africa, 5 is common in South Africa, and 6 is found in Southeast Asia.[1,28] (Others describe somewhat different distributions of genotypes: 1a, North and South America, Europe, and Asia; 1b, Asia; 3b, Japan, Nepal, Thailand, Bangladesh, and Indonesia; 4, Africa; 5, Southern Africa; 6, Hong Kong, and Vietnam.[25]) Genotype determines some aspects of clinical expression of disease response to therapy. Hepatitis C genotype 1, especially 1b, is most likely to be associated with progression to advanced liver disease and to be refractory to therapy.[28,29] Genotype also influences vertical transmission: genotypes 1b and 3a were more readily transmitted in one Italian study.[24] Immunity is also genotype-specific; infection with more than one genotype is therefore possible.

Clinical Features

Hepatitis C in children is usually asymptomatic. After exposure, the incubation period is usually 6–7 weeks, with a range from 2 weeks to 6 months. Some children have abdominal pain, anorexia, and mild flu-like symptoms. Jaundice occurs only in 4%–25% of children; few have elevated transaminases.[20,25] Fulminant hepatitis is rare.[25]

The progression of liver disease after infection is highly variable.[1] About one-third of infected persons have no progression for 30 years or more. Serious liver disease develops in one-third of persons 20 years or less after infection. Most individuals infected as adults (~80%) become HCV carriers. Most (60%–70%) later develop chronic hepatitis. From 10% to 20% develop cirrhosis over several decades, but <3% die from the consequences of long-term infection. Once cirrhosis develops, hepatocellular carcinoma develops at a rate of 1%–4% per year.[1] After 20 years, hepatocellular carcinoma will develop in 1.9%–6.7% of patients with chronic HCV infection.[30] The incidence of hepatocellular carcinoma is highest among Asians, Hispanics, Native Americans, and Pacific Islanders.[30]

The long-term outcome of infected children is less well defined; young age at infection may be somewhat protective.[29] Hepatitis C may be milder after vertical than horizontal transmission. Some children develop only a transient viremia after vertical transmission, without development of liver disease.[21] Occasionally, elevated aminoalanine transferase (ALT) levels in infected children return to normal. However, liver biopsies usually reveal chronic hepatitis. Thus vertical transmission of HCV, although frequently associated with biochemical evidence of hepatic injury early in life, appears to cause only mild liver disease in the first one to two decades of life.[21,22,28]

Similarly, the outcome of HCV infection acquired via exposure to blood products may be better in children than adults.[23,28,29] Some children spontaneously clear the infection. Of 458 children who received blood transfusions during cardiac surgery before implementation of blood-donor screening,[31] 14.6% had antibodies to HCV, but only 55% of these had detectable circulating HCV RNA. All but one of the antibody-positive children had normal transaminase levels.

Other factors also influence the course of disease. Particular viral genotypes (see above) or co-infection with HBV or HIV increase the morbidity of HCV infection. Some patients with HCV have "occult" HBV infections (surface antigen–negative HBV). Of 200 patients with HCV-related chronic liver disease, 33% had detectable HBV genomes in the serum or liver, despite the absence of circulating hepatitis B surface antigen (HBsAg).[32] Infection with HCV thus may alter the gene expression of HBsAg or promote production of an antigenically modified sAg protein not readily detectable by usual assays. Co-infection with both viruses accelerates the evolution to cirrhosis, reduces the response to interferon, and may favor neoplastic transformation.

Diagnosis of Hepatitis C Virus

Diagnostic testing for HCV has many pitfalls. The antibody tests currently licensed to diagnose infection do not distinguish between current and resolved infection.[25,28] Current screening assays, (enzyme immunoassays, or ELISAs), measure antibody to one or more antigens (c100–3 and c33c) in nonstructural regions (NS3 and NS4) and the core region (c22–3) of the HCV genome. These assays detect antibody in 90%–95% of patients with infection within about 5–6 weeks after infection and remain positive for many years. About 5%–10% of infected individuals are not identified by these assays, although some seroconvert after a long interval.[33] False negatives may occur early in the course of disease. False positive results from these ELISAs may be considerable, and should be confirmed by recombinant immunoblot assays, which have better sensitivity and specificity. No antibody test distinguishes between acute, chronic, or resolved infection, or between maternally transmitted antibody and infection-induced antibody. Maternal antibody may persist as long as 12–15 months.[2,34,35] Infants co-infected with HIV may not seroconvert until 26 months or later.[36]

Molecular diagnostic techniques such as polymerase chain reaction (PCR) enhancement of HCV RNA or branched-chain DNA assays are now available in many laboratories. Qualitative HCV RNA assays are useful to confirm infection in patients with HCV antibodies or to identify early infection before the appearance of antibodies. Quantitative tests are most useful to monitor response to treatment. They are not as sensitive as qualitative tests; negative results cannot be used as assurance that no virus is present. PCR tests are costly and not well standardized. False negative and false positive rates may be unacceptably high. In one study of 86 American laboratories, only 16% correctly determined the results of all samples submitted as part of a quality control investigation.[25] Results of HCV PCR tests performed in birth countries of internationally adopted children should therefore be interpreted with extreme caution.

Normal ALT levels and undetectable HCV RNA usually indicate resolution of infection in patients with positive antibody assay results; however, chronic persistent subclinical hepatitis cannot be definitively excluded.[37] Long-term follow-up using multiple primers in PCR assays may be necessary to identify fluctuations in viremia and HCV variants.[37]

Because of these difficulties, a single negative or positive RNA result should not be considered diagnostic. Serial samples should be assayed in antibody-positive individuals. Persons with antibodies or HCV RNA in blood are considered infectious until proven otherwise. Children with elevated ALT levels and equivocal testing results should be referred to a pediatric gastroenterologist for further evaluation. Assays for specific HCV genotype should be limited to patients requiring antiviral treatment. Liver ultrasound and biopsy can provide helpful additional information and help assess the need for treatment.

Nadia, age 4 years, arrived from Russia. Hepatitis C antibody was found, and further investigation revealed high levels of circulating HCV RNA. A liver biopsy showed mild fibrosis and activity. She remained asymptomatic. Therapy will be considered in the future when more effective modalities (pegylated interferon and ribivarin) are available for children.

- Many more children have maternally transmitted antibodies to HCV.
- Because of the prolonged incubation period and lack of symptoms of HCV, children should be tested at entry and again 6 or more months later.
- Compared to HBV, HCV presents a lower risk of transmission to adoptive family members.

Treatment of Hepatitis C Virus

Treatment of HCV infection is rapidly evolving. Currently, therapy with pegylated interferon alone or in combination with ribavirin is recommended for treatment of HCV-infected adults. The combination results in a sustained response in about 40% of treated individuals. A lower response rate is seen among patients infected with genotype 1, the most common form in the United States.[28] Responses seem to be better among those with shorter duration of disease (possibly reflecting a lower viral load) and younger age at treatment. In 33%–56% of children treated with interferon alone, sustained virologic response occurred, although the number of children studied and reported is small.[21,38] No reports of combination therapy in children have yet been published. Dose, duration, drug formulation, and schedules of treatment are likely to be refined over the coming years. Current protocols are available at the National Institutes of Health (NIH) Web site.[39,40]

Infected individuals should be immunized against hepatitis A and hepatitis B to prevent further injury to the liver.

Key Points for Internationally Adopted Children

- A small proportion of internationally adopted children are infected with HCV.

Resources

Hepatitis C: What Clinicians and Other Health Professionals Need To Know. Available at: http://www.cdc.gov/ncidod/diseases/hepatitis/c_training/edu/default.htm.

National Center for Infectious Diseases. Viral Hepatitis. Available at: http://www.cdc.gov/ncidod/diseases/hepatitis/index.htm.

HepNet: The Hepatitis Information Network. National Institutes of Health Consensus Conference. Available at: http://www.hepnet.com/nih/contents.html.

FAQs

Q. Prospective parents just consulted me about a 9-month-old baby in Russia whose birth mother has hepatitis C. What do I advise?

A. This is difficult, and comes up fairly often. It is first important to recognize that the accuracy of the information about the birth mother may be questionable. If she is truly infected, the source of her hepatitis C is rarely known with certainty. She may have become infected from injection drug use (most likely), exposure to contaminated medical supplies, or an infected sexual partner (less likely), etc. It's important to think of these sources that may indicate co-infection with other agents and other prenatal exposures. Only about 5% of infants born to mothers with hepatitis C are themselves infected, or about 10% if the mother is HIV infected. As with the birth mother's test results, any diagnostic testing on the child may or may not be correct. Occasionally, such children undergo testing at specialized diagnostic centers, as arranged by the adoption agencies. These private laboratories have a variety of tests available—usually the anti-HCV Ab result is reported, although occasionally HCV-RNA PCR results are provided. This is somewhat reassuring; however, it should be recognized that these are technically difficult tests and have poor interlaboratory agreement. Thus, although this situation seems alarming, it is not drastically different from most of the other referrals from this region in terms of actual risk. Just because HCV isn't mentioned in the pre-adoptive medical record certainly does not guarantee that the birth mother is not infected. Indeed, in our International Adoption Clinic, few children with HCV infection were identified as such on their pre-adoptive records.

Q. My 4-year-old patient from Kazakhstan has a positive antibody screen for hepatitis C. What next?

A. This should be investigated further with a more sophisticated test (recombinant immunoblot assay) [RIBA] and qualitative HCV RNA PCR assays. Liver function tests should be checked, as well as serology for hepatitis B and hepatitis A. Negative and positive results should be repeated on several occasions to confirm. Meanwhile, the child should be immunized for hepatitis B and hepatitis A to prevent further assaults on the liver. The utility of further testing, such as liver ultrasound and measurement of α-fetoprotein, has not been established. In the presence of normal liver function tests, a period of "watchful waiting" is usually in order. However, as treatments for hepatitis C improve, it is possible that earlier intervention may result in a better outcome, and normal liver function tests do not always exclude active inflammation that may require treatment. Consultation with a pediatric gastroenterologist experienced in the management of liver disease will clarify parameters for monitoring and treatment.

Q. From a practical point of view, how much should I worry about "missing" hepatitis C because of difficulties with test reliability, timing, etc.? The child arrived in the United States from Vietnam 3 months ago.

A. Screening for anti-HCV at arrival and 6 months after arrival is recommended for all children. Screening with liver function tests (ALT) at

these times may indicate the need for closer follow-up and more detailed testing.

References

1. Lauer GM, Walker BD. Hepatitis C virus infection. N Engl J Med 2001; 345:41–52.

2. Johansson PJ, Lofgren B, Nordenfelt E. Low frequency of hepatitis C antibodies among children from foreign countries adopted in Swedish families. Scand J Infect Dis 1990; 22:619–20.

3. Ohba K, Mizokami M, Kato T, et al. Seroprevalence of hepatitis B virus, hepatitis C virus and GB virus-C infections in Siberia. Epidemiol Infect 1999; 122:139–43.

4. Abdourakhmanov DT, Hasaev AS, Castro FJ, Guardia J. Epidemiological and clinical aspects of hepatitis C virus infection in the Russian Republic of Daghestan. Eur J Epidemiol 1998; 14:549–53.

5. Lvov DK, Samokhvalov EI, Tsuda F, et al. Prevalence of hepatitis C virus and distribution of its genotypes in Northern Eurasia. Arch Virol 1996; 141:1613–22.

6. Iashina TL, Favorov MO, Shakhgil'dian IV, et al. The spread of hepatitis C markers among the population of regions of Russia and Central Asia [in Russian]. Zh Mikrobiol Epidemiol Immunobiol 1993:46–9.

7. Suzuki K, Mizokami M, Cao K, et al. Prevalence of hepatitis C virus infection in Nanjing, southern China. Eur J Epidemiol 1997; 13:511–5.

8. Wu RR, Mizokami M, Lau JY, et al. Seroprevalence of hepatitis C virus infection and its genotype in Lanzhou, western China. J Med Virol 1995; 45:174–8.

9. Fang F, Dong YS, Zhang M. Hepatitis C virus infection in different groups of children in Wuhan area. J Tongji Med Univ 1993; 13:239–43.

10. Zhang ZW, Shimbo S, Qu JB, et al. Hepatitis B and C virus infection among adult women in Jilin Province, China: an urban–rural comparison in prevalence of infection markers. Southeast Asian J Trop Med Public Health 2000; 31:530–6.

11. Huang F, Dong Y, Wang Z. Study on HCV infection and the distribution of HCV genotypes in different populations in Shenyang area [in Chinese]. Zhonghua Liu Xing Bing Xue Za Zhi 1998; 19:134–7.

12. Shimbo S, Zhang ZW, Gao WP, et al. Prevalence of hepatitis B and C infection markers among adult women in urban and rural areas in Shaanxi Province, China. Southeast Asian J Trop Med Public Health 1998; 29:263–8.

13. Qu JB, Zhang ZW, Shimbo S, et al. Urban–rural comparison of HBV and HCV infection prevalence in eastern China. Biomed Environ Sci 2000; 13:243–53.

14. American Academy of Pediatrics. Medical evaluation of internationally adopted children for infectious diseases. In: Pickering LK, ed. 2003 Red Book: Report of the Committee on Infectious Diseases. Elk Grove Village, IL: American Academy of Pediatrics, 2003: 173–4.

15. American Academy of Pediatrics Committee on Infectious Diseases. Hepatitis C virus infection. Pediatrics 1998; 101:481–5.

16. Choulot JJ, Mechain S, Saint Martin J, Doireau V, Mensire A. Adoption and chronic hepatitis B carrier state [in French]. Arch Pediatr 1998; 5:869–72.

17. Miller LC, Hendrie NW. Health of children adopted from China. Pediatrics 2000; 105:E76.

18. Saiman L, Aronson J, Zhou J, et al. Prevalence of infectious diseases among internationally adopted children. Pediatrics 2001; 108:608–12.

19. Miller LC, Kiernan MT, Mathers MI, Klein-Gitelman M. Developmental and nutritional status of internationally adopted children. Arch Pediatr Adolesc Med 1995; 149:40–4.

20. American Academy of Pediatrics. Hepatitis C. In: Pickering LK, ed. 2003 Red Book: Report of the Committee on Infectious Diseases. Elk Grove Village, IL: American Academy of Pediatrics, 2003: 336–40.

21. Jonas MM. Treatment of chronic hepatitis C in pediatric patients. Clin Liver Dis 1999; 3:855–67.

22. Bortolotti F, Resti M, Giacchino R, et al. Hepatitis C virus infection and related liver disease in children of mothers with antibodies to the virus. J Pediatr 1997; 130:990–3.

23. Hoshiyama A, Kimura A, Fukisawa T, Kage M, Kato H. Clinical and histologic feature of chronic hepatitis C infection after blood transfusion in Japanese children. Pediatrics 2000; 105:62–65.

24. Zein NN. Vertical transmission of hepatitis C: to screen or not to screen. J Pediatr 1997; 130:859–61.

25. Mayer AN, Jonas MM. Hepatitis C virus. In: Feigin RD, Cherry JD, Demmler GJ, Kaplan SL. eds. Textbook of Pediatric Infectious Diseases, Vol. 2. Philadelphia: W.B. Saunders Company, 2004: 2237–51.

26. Camerero C, Martos I, Delgado R, et al. Horizontal transmission of hepatitis C virus in households of infected children. J Pediatr 1994; 123:98–99.

27. Vegnente A, Iorio R, Saviano A, et al. Lack of intrafamilial transmission of hepatitis C virus in family members of children with chronic hepatitis C infection. Pediatr Infect Dis J 1994; 13:886–9.

28. Aach RD, Yomtovian RA, Hack M. Neonatal and pediatric post-transfusion hepatitis C: a look back and a look forward. Pediatrics 2000; 105:836–42.

29. Jonas MM. Hepatitis C infection in children. N Engl J Med 1999; 341:912–3.

30. El-Serag HB, Mason AC. Rising incidence of hepatocellular carcinoma in the United States. N Engl J Med 1999; 340:745–50.

31. Vogt M, Lang T, Dlindler C. Prevalence and clinical outcome of hepatitis C infection in children who underwent cardiac surgery before the implementation of blood-donor screening. N Engl J Med 1999; 341:866–70.

32. Cacciola I, Pollicino T, Squadrito G, Cerenzia G, Orlando ME, Raimondo G. Occult hepatitis B virus infection in patients with chronic hepatitis C liver disease. N Engl J Med 1999; 341:22–6.

33. Maggiore G, Caprai S, Cerino A, Silini E, Mondelli MU. Antibody-negative chronic hepatitis C virus infection in immunocompetent children. J Pediatr 1998; 132: 1048–50.

34. Dunn DT, Gibb DM, Healy M, et al. Timing and interpretation of tests for diagnosing perinatally acquired hepatitis C virus infection. Pediatr Infect Dis J 2001; 20:715–6.

35. Hostetter MK. Infectious diseases in internationally adopted children: findings in children from China, Russia, and Eastern Europe. Adv Pediatr Infect Dis 1999; 14:147–61.

36. Granovsky MO, Minkoff HL, Tess BH, et al. Hepatitis C virus infection in the mothers and infants cohort study. Pediatrics 1998; 102:355–9.

37. Matsuoka S, Tatara K, Hayabuchi Y, Taguchi Y, et al. Serologic, virologic, and histologic characteristics of chronic hepatitis C virus disease in children infected by transfusion. Pediatrics 1994; 94:919–22.

38. Fujisawa T, Inui A, Ohkawa T, Komatsu H, Miyakawa Y, Onoue M. Response to interferon therapy in children with chronic hepatitis C. J Pediatr 1995; 127:660–2.

39. Abstracts from NIH Consensus Development Conference on Management of Hepatitis C, Bethesday, MD, March 24–26, 1997. Available at: http://www.hepnet.com/nih/contents.html.

40. ClinicalTrials.gov available at http://www.clinicaltrials.gov/ct/search?term=hepatitis+c.

17

INTESTINAL PARASITES AND OTHER ENTERIC INFECTIONS

Intestinal parasites are found in ~25% of internationally adopted children after arrival in the United States (Table 17–1). Parasites are spread by poor hygiene in crowded environments, conditions common in many orphanages. Infection with *Giardia lamblia* is most frequent (especially in children from Eastern Europe),[1] but other parasites are often found. The incidence of parasite infection and likelihood of multiple parasites increases with the duration of institutionalization[2] (Fig. 17–1).

Intestinal parasite infections are ubiquitous throughout the world. The distribution varies depending on climate, topography, and other factors (Table 17–2). Although parasites may cause anemia, diarrhea, poor growth, and other clinical problems, most infected children in the developing world are not treated, because the rate of reinfection is so high. In some populations of children, parasite infection is universal.[14] Infection with multiple parasites is common (Fig. 17–2). Parasitized children are usually smaller and more likely to be anemic than their noninfected peers. Children with recurrent childhood diarrhea due to parasites had reduced overall fitness and impaired cognitive function in one study;[15] eradication of

Table 17–1 Prevalence of intestinal parasites among international adoptees

Country (N)	%
Korea (360)[3]	0
Korea 41%, other 59% (293)[4]	14
Various countries (129)[5]	21
Korea 36%, India 21%, other 43% (100)[6]	23
Romania (22)[7]	23
China 48%, Russia 31%, other 21% (504)[1]	23[a]
Asia or Latin America (128)[8]	29
Romania (65)[2]	33
Various countries (68)[9]	38
India (114)[10]	44[a]
Russia, Eastern Europe (56)[11]	51[a]
Korea 50%, other 50% (52)[12]	6
China (452)[13]	9

[a]Includes bacterial pathogens.

251

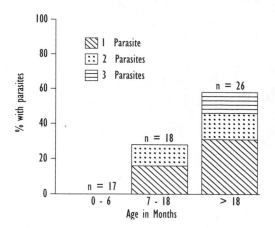

Figure 17–1 *Age-related incidence of infection with single or multiple parasites in Romanian adoptees (n = 61). Age is a proxy marker for duration of institutionalization. (From Johnson DE, Miller LC, Iverson S, et al. The health of children adopted from Romania. JAMA 1992; 268:3446–51, Copyright © 1992, American Medical Association. All rights reserved.)*

parasites is sometimes accompanied by improved neuropsychiatric function.[16–18]

This section reviews the clinical manifestations and recommendations for diagnosis and treatment of some of the common intestinal parasites isolated from international adoptees. Additional details are readily available elsewhere.[34,35]

Diagnosis of Intestinal Parasites

All newly arrived internationally adopted children should be screened for intestinal parasites by microscopic examination of stool samples. Three samples collected 2–3 days apart are recommended to increase detection rate.[36] These should be collected in a polyvinyl alcohol kit (or examined fresh) and submitted to an experienced parasitology laboratory. First morning stool samples that have been in the diaper for several hours are not optimal for examination. Supplemental assay of fecal *Giardia* antigen by immunoassay should be performed if available. Children with persistent signs or symptoms should be evaluated more thoroughly if initial stool screening does not yield a satisfactory ex-

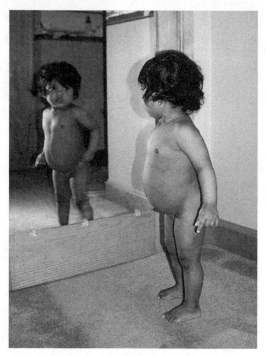

Figure 17–2 *This 21-month-old adopted from India had multiple parasites on arrival to the United States (With permission.)*

planation; screening for *Cryptosporidium parvum* antigen may be helpful in some children.[34] Late presentation of intestinal parasites sometimes occurs, even among children adequately screened at arrival. Parasites may not be identified during initial stool screening because of laboratory errors, improper sample collection or handling, low parasite load, intermittent shedding, interfering substances (such as concurrent antibiotics), or other factors. Thus the possibility of parasitic infection should be considered months or even years after arrival in symptomatic children. Eosinophilia is *not* a reliable marker of intestinal parasitic infection; only some parasites induce eosinophilia (most notably hookworm, *Strongyloides*, and *Toxocara*).

Household spread may create a reservoir of infection that is difficult to eradicate. If this is suspected, concurrent screening of all household members (and treatment of infected individuals) is necessary.

Table 17-2 Prevalence of parasitic infections among children worldwide[a]

Country, N	Overall (%)	Ascaris (%)	Trichuris (%)	Hookworms (%)	Dientamoeba (%)	Giardia (%)	Strongyloides (%)	Enterobius (%)	Ent. coli (%)
Argentina, 139 orphanage children[19]	—	13	—	—	—	23	—	43	45
Bolivia, 558 school children[14]	99	—	—	—	—	—	—	—	—
Brazil, 360 school children[20]	42	29	16	1.7	—	—	13	—	—
Brazil, 300 nursery school children[21]	88	15	0.7	6	—	78	—	4	—
Brazil, 520 rural children[22]	—	41	40	—	—	44	—	—	16
Calgary Canada, 1532 hospital in- and out-patients[23]	7	—	—	—	23	31	—	2	—
Ecuador, school children[24]	—	33	6.5	24	—	—	—	—	—
Egypt, 1844 school children[25]	—	—	—	—	—	25	—	—	—
Indonesia, 348 school children[26]	44	44	76	9	—	—	—	3	—
Kenya, 460 preschool children[27]	20	15	28	—	—	—	—	—	—
Laos, 669 villagers[28]	82	31	24	29	—	—	10	3.4	—
Malaysia, 291 school children[29]	70	63	39	13	—	—	—	—	—
Nepal, 300 school children[30]	44	—	3	13	—	14	—	—	21
United States, 104 pediatric clinic patients[31]	40	—	—	—	21	17	—	—	—
United States, 107 refugee children[32]	22	8	2	5	2	3	—	—	—
Thailand, 169 villagers[33]	46–72	—	—	—	—	—	—	—	—

[a]Studies varied in aims and techniques.

Nicholas was adopted from the Phillipines at 15 months of age. Although he had no gastrointestinal symptoms or eosinophilia, he had three stool samples tested for parasites. All were negative. When the family changed pediatricians, the new doctor requested three more samples, which were also negative. Nicholas grew well, had no gastrointestinal symptoms, and thrived in every way. Two years later, he coughed up a 10-inch Ascarid worm (at the Thanksgiving dinner table, of course!).

Clinical Signs of Parasitic Infection

Various clinical symptoms suggest parasitic infection. Gastrointestinal symptoms, such as diarrhea, bloating, vomiting, or malabsorption, may indicate parasite infection, but these may also reflect enteric bacterial infection, intro- duction of new foods into the diet, lactose intolerance (see Chapter 28), food allergies, or other problems. Parasites may cause prominent extraintestinal symptoms such as irritability and behavior changes, pulmonary symptoms, or eosinophilia. Particular clinical symptoms suggest specific parasites (Table 17–3).

Intestinal Parasites: What to Do

Some authors suggest empiric broad-spectrum antiparasite treatment (albendazole) for newly arrived immigrants[41] as an effective method to decrease morbidity. This approach has not yet been studied in children, and albendazole is still considered an investigational drug in young children. Furthermore, albendazole is ineffective against many common parasites (including *Giardia, Entamoeba histolytica, Dientamoeba fragilis, Schistosomia*).

Parasites commonly identified in newly arrived international adoptees include *Giardia*

Table 17–3 Clinical symptoms suggestive of specific parasite infections

Symptoms	Possible Parasite(s)
Diarrhea most common, also behavioral changes, growth arrest, chronic abdominal pain, fecal incontinence	*Giardia*
Large-volume, thick, formless, and odiferous stools, flatulence	*Giardia*[31]
Diarrhea, abdominal pain (often severe), blood and mucus	*Ent. histolytica*
Right upper-quadrant abdominal pain, high fever, abdominal distention, irritability, tachypnea	*Ent. histolytica* liver abscess
Leukocytosis and elevated alkaline phosphatase with normal transaminases	*Ent. histolytica* liver abscess[37]
Diarrhea and anal pruritis	*Dientamoeba* and *Ent. vermicularis*[38]
Acute watery diarrhea	*Dientamoeba fragilis*
Chronic recurrent abdominal pain	*Dientamoeba fragilis*[31]
Intestinal obstruction	*Entamoeba* or *Ascaris*
Pneumonia and eosinophilia	*Ascaris*, hookworms, *Strongyloides, Toxocara*
Hepatic abscess	*Entamoeba* or *Ascaris*
Biliary obstruction	*Ascaris*
Radiographic findings or clinical symptoms resembling inflammatory bowel disease (without elevated ESR)	*Strongyloides*[39] or *Trichuris*
Isolated eosinophilia	*Strongyloides, Filaria, hookworms, Schistosomia, Toxocara*
Protein-losing enteropathy	*Strongyloides*
Mucoid diarrhea, vague abdominal pain, distention, voluminous stools	*Strongyloides*
Bloody diarrhea	Parasite ± *Shigella*[40]

lamblia, Entamoeba histolytica, Dientamoeba fragilis, and the nematodes (*Ascaris lumbricoides, Trichuris trichiura,* hookworms, pinworms, and *Strongyloides*). Diagnosis and management of each are discussed below.

In some children, less familiar parasites are identified. Many of these are non-pathogens and do not require specific treatment (Table 17–4). However, their presence should alert the physician to the possibility that other pathogenic parasites are present.

Giardia lamblia

Giardia lamblia is the most commonly isolated intestinal parasite from international adoptees. *Giardia* is readily spread by fecal–oral contact, person-to-person contact, communal toys, or bathwater in heavily contaminated environments. Children in schools or institutions frequently share *Giardia* (Table 17–5). *Giardia* cysts remain viable for 3 months in a moist environment and are resistant to chlorination. Infants

Table 17–4 Less familiar parasites

Parasite	Need to Treat?
Blastocystis hominis	No, unless symptomatic and no other cause is determined (metronidazole)
Entamoeba coli (may be mistaken for *Ent. histolytica* and vice versa)	No, unless symptomatic and no other cause is determined (diloxanide furoate or metronidazole)
Entamoeba hartmanii, polecki, dispar	No
Hymenolepsis nana (dwarf tapeworm)	Yes, praziquantal 25 mg/kg × 1 (investigational)
Cryptosporidium	No, unless immunocompromised
Microsporidia	No, unless immunocompromised
Cyclospora	Usually self-limited, but could try trimethopirm-sulfamethoxzole if persistent and symptomatic
Isospora	No, unless immunocompromised
Iodamoeba butschlii	No
Endolimax nana	No

Table 17–5 Prevalence of *Giardia* infections in children

Country, Setting	Frequency of Giardia infection (%)	Comments
Malaysia, school children[49]	1–11	—
Australia, school children[50]	2.6	—
India, children with diarrhea for >2 weeks[51]	15	—
Sweden, refugees[52]	17	—
Italy, mentally retarded in institution[53]	17	—
International adoptees from Eastern Europe (Russia, Moldova, Romania, Bulgaria, Hungary)[1]	28	Children with *Giardia* were older than those without (22 months vs. 15.5 months, $p < 0.001$)
Honduras, barrio-dwelling infants[54]	36	Accounted for 29% of diarrheal episodes, but 47% of children had multiple parasites (as many as 10!)
Egypt, school children[55]	62	Also infected with *Ascaris* (20%) and *Ent. histolytica* (19%). Infected children more likely to be underweight.
Romania, institutionalized children[56]	72	Associated with HIV infection
Argentina, orphans and homeless children[19]	84	Many with multiple parasites

Anita was adopted from Honduras. Height and weight were both below the third percentile. She had somewhat poor appetite but no diarrhea. Her first stool sample showed Giardia. After this was treated with furazolidone, a repeat sample was examined. This showed Trichuris trichuria and Ascaris lumbricoides. After repeated sampling, four more parasites were identified (Hymenolepsis nana, Strongyloides stercoralis, Necator americanus, and Blastocystis hominis)—a total of seven parasites. After several months, all were eradicated and her growth velocity accelerated greatly.

may become infected with *Giardia* as early as 3 months of age; 86% of infants have diarrhea with their first infection.[42] Infection with *H. pylori*, common among international adoptees,[43] may increase susceptibility to *Giardia*.[44–46]

Although diarrhea is the most common sign of *Giardia* infection, many children have nonspecific symptoms such as anorexia, irritability, and flatulence.[31] Other children have behavioral changes, chronic abdominal pain, anemia, or fecal incontinence. Reduced weight gain is common among infected infants, especially during prolonged infections and periods of diarrhea.[47,48] Infected individuals usually pass copious amounts of formless, odiferous stools. Eosinophilia is rare, as in other parasitic infections limited to the intestinal tract. Many children with *Giardia* infection are asymptomatic. Giardiasis should be considered in any internationally adopted child with 7 or more days of unexplained diarrhea, even after long residence in the United States.

Diagnosis. Examination of three stool samples identifies *Giardia* in >90% of those infected.[57] Immunoassay to detect cyst and trophozoite antigens (*Giardia* antigen test) shed in the feces supplements microscopic examination; sensitivities are equal to or superior to microscopic examination.[58,59]

Occasionally, *Giardia* cannot be isolated despite high clinical suspicion. In some cases,

empiric treatment may be warranted. Endoscopy with sampling of duodenal contents and small bowel biopsy is sometimes necessary to verify the diagnosis.

Treatment. Metronidazole (15 mg/kg divided tid for 5–7 days) or furazolidone (6 mg/kg divided qid for 10 days; currently unavailable) are recommended for treatment of *Giardia* in children. In spite of its widespread and accepted use for the treatment of *Giardia*, metronidazole has not been approved by the U.S. Food and Drug Administration (FDA) for this indication.[57] Metronidazole must be compounded into a palatable solution; it is not commercially available as a liquid in the United States and is extremely bitter. It should not be given with ethanol-containing medications or digoxin. At a dose range of 15–22.5 mg/kg per day $\times$ 5–10 days, median efficacy is about 94%.[57] Some infectious-disease experts suggest doses as high as 35–50 mg/kg per day. Furazolidone is a palatable substitute, but must be given with caution in children with G6PD deficiency and is not recommended for children <1 month of age. Median efficacy is about 92% when given at 8 mg/kg per day for 7–10 days.[57] (It is also effective against *Klebsiella* spp., *Clostridium* spp., *Escherichia coli*, *Campylobacter* spp., and *Staphylococcus aureus*.) Availability of this drug, however, has recently been problematic. Tinidazole, also not FDA approved for this indication, is another possible choice, and is given as a single dose (50 mg/kg).[35,60] Quinacrine, while effective in eradicating *Giardia*, is poorly tolerated, especially in children. Nitazoxanide (Alinia™) was recently approved for treatment of *Giardia* in children; recommended doses are 100 mg bid, ages 2–3 years, and 200 mg bid, ages 4–11 years for 3 days. This agent likely has broad antiparasitic effects that have not yet been fully studied.[61]

Although some experts[34] suggest that asymptomatic individuals do not require treatment, it seems prudent to treat international adoptees. Most of these children have growth delays, possibly due to *Giardia* infection. Infected children may serve as vectors for household or day care spread. Some have multiple parasites, which may not become evident until the *Giardia* is eradicated.

Giardia is difficult to eradicate in some children. Management options for these children are listed in Table 17–6. Careful history and repeat stool analysis are necessary to differentiate between drug resistance, reinfection, and post-*Giardia* lactose intolerance.[57] The latter responds to a lactose-free diet within several weeks.

Further detailed recommendations for management of *Giardiasis* are readily available.[62]

Entamoeba histolytica

Entamoeba histolytica is found occasionally among internationally adopted children; it may cause significant morbidity if not recognized. This parasite is common in Africa, South and Central America, and Asia: about 500 million people worldwide are colonized with *Ent. histolytica* (or the similar-appearing but nonpathogenic *Ent. dispar*).[63] Most individuals become infected by about age 3 years. Only about 1% of people with *Ent. histolytica* develop clinical symptoms, although most have failure to thrive (75%) and anemia (94%).[64] *Ent. histolytica* causes painful, bloody, mucoid diarrhea and ulcerations of the intestinal mucosa, which may perforate. Some patients develop pseudomembranous colitis or fulminant necrotizing colitis, stricture, or ob-

struction. In fulminant disease, the parasite disseminates to the liver, usually causing a single abscess in the right lobe. Susceptibility to liver abscess appears to be linked to the presence of the genetic marker HLA-DR3.[65] Although liver abscesses are more common in adults, they may occur in children as young as 3 weeks of age.[64] Most patients do not have diarrhea or dysentery before presentation with liver abscess.[37] From the liver, *Ent. histolytica* may travel to the lungs, heart, brain, spleen, larynx, aorta, and stomach.

Ent. histolytica is difficult to identify in stool samples, as cysts are shed only intermittently. Water and urine destroy the trophozoites, and concurrent antibiotic therapy often renders the cysts nonidentifiable. Examination of stool samples collected in polyvinyl alcohol kits is most likely to reveal *Ent. histolytica*. Antigen detection assays will likely become available to improve diagnostic yield.[66]

Iodoquinol 30–40 mg/kg per day divided tid for 20 days (maximum 1950 mg/day) is recommended for treatment. Paromomycin may also be used for asymptomatic infection (25–35 mg/kg per day divided tid for 7 days) and may be preferred.[67] Other alternatives are available through the Centers for Disease Control and Prevention (CDC) Drug Service (tel: 404-639-3670). Extraintestinal amebiasis should be managed by an infectious diseases expert. Usually, combination therapy with metronidazole and an intraluminal agent such as iodoquinol is recommended.

Table 17–6 Management of recurrent or persistent *Giardia*

- Switch from metronidazole to furazolidone or vice versa.
- Treat with metronidazole or furazolidone at higher dose (see text).
- Treat with metronidazole for 10–14 days.
- Treat with nitazoxanide or tinidazole.
- Test all family members and household contacts, treat all those infected concurrently.
- Review hygiene precautions.
- Consider alternative drugs (e.g., albendazole + metronidazole. See Gardner and Hill[57] for details).
- Test for other pathogens or other diagnoses (e.g., lactose intolerance).
- Consider concurrent immunodeficiency (hypogammaglobulinemia, HIV infection).

Dientamoeba fragilis

D. fragilis is also occasionally identified in stool samples from international adoptees (2.2% of 455 children in a recent study[1]). *D. fragilis*, an intestinal flagellate protozoan (like *G. lamblia*), infects mucosal crypts from the cecum to the rectum. The route of transmission is unknown; however, because patients are frequently coinfected with *E. vermicularis*, some investigators have speculated that *D. fragilis* may be transmitted in the eggs of the pinworm.[38,68]

Symptoms are present in 15%–85% of infected individuals. Acute, watery diarrhea,[68,69] abdominal pain, anal pruritis,[38] irritability, weight loss, fatigue, flatulence, and anorexia[70] are most common. Some patients report alternating diarrhea and constipation. Stools are "mushy," with foul odor, and bloody or mucoid. Crampy or colicky abdominal pain with tenderness in the lower quadrants may be found. Eosinophilia occurs in 30%–60% of children with *D. fragilis*.[68–70] Nearly all infected individuals can be identified if three stool specimens collected in polyvinyl alcohol are submitted. Samples should be collected on alternate days, as *D. fragilis* is excreted in a cyclical pattern.[38] Antibiotics interfere with the identification of *D. fragilis* for several weeks after completion of treatment.

Treatment is recommended with iodoquinol (30–40 mg/kg per day, divided tid for 20 days, maximum 2 grams/day). Alternative therapy with paromomycin,[35] metronidazole,[70] tetracycline or doxycycline (for older children), or erythromycin[68,69] is sometimes recommended.

Nematodes

Nematodes, including *Ascaris lumbricoides*, *Trichuris*, *Enterobius*, hookworms, and *Strongyloides stercoralis*, are acquired by egg ingestion or penetration of the skin by larval forms in the soil. The organisms are resistant to chemical disinfectants and remain viable in soil for several months. After skin penetration, hookworms and *Strongyloides* travel via lymphatics to the liver, right heart, and lungs. Worldwide, nematode infections, especially hookworms, significantly impair growth and neurocognitive development. In some studies, intellectual function improved after eradication.[16,18,71–73] In other studies, slight or no improvement was found.[74–76] Limited exposure to the outdoors reduces the likelihood of nematode infection in children residing in orphanages. However, some children are exposed and infected. Although infrequently found in international adoptees, these parasites must be properly identified and treated.

Ascaris lumbricoides

Ascaris infections afflict more than 1 billion people in the world. Infections are extremely common in China, Africa, and Central and South America: more than 7% of slum children in India are infected.[77] Infection may offer some as yet ill-defined protection from cerebral malaria.[78] The organism is resistant to disinfectants, freezing, and sewage treatment (Fig. 17–3). Clinical symptoms include constitutional symptoms, malabsorption, intestinal obstruction, and poor growth.[79] The malabsorption results from ascaris-secreted peptides which that block pancreatic digestive enzymes. Treatment with albendazole 400 mg once (investigational for this indication) or mebendazole 100 mg bid for 3 days or 500 mg once[35] is recommended.

Trichuris trichiura

Trichuris infects an estimated 800 million people globally. The organisms embed in colonic mucosa. Most infected individuals are asymptomatic; some develop anemia, bloody mucoid diarrhea, tenesmus, rectal prolapse, and failure to thrive. Intestinal symptoms can be acute or more chronic. Treatment with mebendazole 100 mg bid for 3 days or 500 mg once[35] or albendazole 400 mg once (investigational for this indication) is recommended.

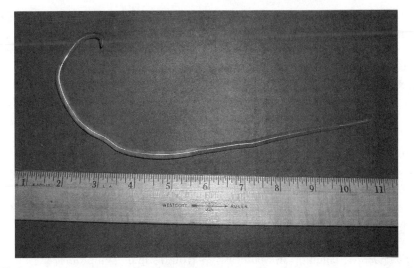

Figure 17–3 *Ascarid worm. (Courtesy of David Hamer, M.D.)*

Hookworms

Hookworms cause a great deal of misery throughout the world. Hookworms are responsible for ~1 million liters of blood loss each day, resulting in widespread iron deficiency anemia. Furthermore, hookworm-induced protein-losing enteropathy contributes directly to malnutrition. In India, China, the Mediterranean region, and South America, *Ancylostoma duodenale* is the common hookworm; in the Western Hemisphere, Southeast Asia, and the Pacific, *Necator americanus* is more common. Mixed infections can occur. Infections occur more commonly in agricultural regions.

Signs of hookworm infection include pruritis of the soles (often minor), followed by abdominal pain, diarrhea, nausea, and anorexia. These symptoms usually resolve, but children may nonetheless experience delays in physical and intellectual growth. Some delays are irreversible. Indonesian children infected with hookworm had lower scores on cognitive and memory tests (fluency, digit span, number choice, picture search, and mazes) independent of hemoglobin level.[80] Curiously, hookworm infection prevalence, incidence, and intensity were reduced in BCG-vaccinated children in Brazil compared to those without this vaccine.[81]

Diagnosis is difficult as the organism undergoes periods of developmental arrest when no eggs appear in the feces. Albendazole (400 mg once, investigational for this indication) or mebendazole 100 mg bid for 3 days or 500 mg once[35] is effective against *N. americanus*; mebendazole is preferred for *A. duodenale*.

Enterobius vermicularis

Pinworms *(Ent. vermicularis)* are common among institutionalized children and also in children post-adoption. In a recent study, 29% of children in a Thai orphanage were infected.[82] The possible relationship to *D. fragilis* is described above. Pinworms should be considered in children with nocturnal anal pruritis, vulvitis, perianal granuloma,[83] and possibly urinary tract infections.[84] Isolated pinworm infections are associated with lower serum copper, zinc, and magnesium levels,[85] and with reduced IQ among Egyptian school children (possibly due to lower socioeconomic status?).[86] Eosinophilia does not occur. Reinfection via self-inoculation can occur. Treatment with mebendazole (100 mg once, repeat in 2 weeks) or pyrantel pamoate (11 mg/kg once, not to exceed 1 gram) is recommended. All household members should be treated; some experts recommend retreatment after 2–3 weeks.

Strongyloides

Strongyloides stercoralis is the most virulent helminth infection. Thankfully, it is less common than *Ascaris* or hookworms. Unlike other helminths, *Strongyloides* has the capacity to replicate in humans.[87] This can result in hyperinfection, especially if the individual is immunosuppressed. *Strongyloides*, common in Southeast Asia and the Caribbean, occurs worldwide.

Clinically, patients have watery, mucoid diarrhea, which is often severe. Diarrhea may alternate with constipation. Protein-losing enteropathy can result in growth stunting and failure to thrive. Recurrent abdominal pain and anorexia may occur, along with pneumonitis, urticaria, depression,[88] and eosinophilia.

Diagnosis of *Strongyloides* is difficult; the organism is tricky to isolate and identify. Efforts should be made, however, to exclude the possibility of *Strongyloides* infection in patients from endemic areas who must be treated with corticosteroids or immunosuppressive agents. Specific techniques (serology, examination of duodenal fluid, Baermann's fecal extraction, or Haradi-Mori stool culture method) may be required for diagnosis.[89] Serology should be obtained in children with unexplained eosinophilia. Treatment of choice is ivermectin (200 μg/kg per day for 1–2 days).[35,87]

Enteric Bacterial Infections

Bacterial enteric infections also cause gastrointestinal symptoms in internationally adopted children. Diarrheogenic *E. coli, Salmonella, Shigella*, and *Campylobacter* infections occur in orphanages, sometimes in epidemic form.[90–95] These pathogens are sometimes identified in stool cultures from symptomatic new arrivals (see also Chapter 20). The prevalence of infection with these pathogens in these children is not well known, as screening is not routinely performed (Table 17–7). Stools should be cultured for bacterial pathogens if children have gastrointestinal symptoms (diarrhea, abdominal pain, flatulence). Antimicro-

Table 17–7 Prevalence of enteric bacterial pathogens in newly arrived internationally adopted children

Country of origin (N)	Adoptees with Enteric Bacterial Pathogens (%)	Description (N)
China (86)[13]	8	2 *Salmonella*
		2 *Campylobacter*
		2 both
		1 *Clostridium difficile*
Various countries (504)[1]	Number screened not indicated	5 *Campylobacter*
		3 *Shigella*
		2 *Salmonella*
Various countries (293)[4]	Number screened not indicated	4 *Salmonella*
		3 *Campylobacter*
Various countries (100)[6]	7	5 *Salmonella*
		2 *Campylobacter*
India (121)[96]	61	4 *Shigella*
		61 *Salmonella*
India (114) (in Sweden)[10]	16	18 *Salmonella*
	1.8	2 *Shigella*

bial treatment for acute bacterial enteritis caused by diarrhea-associated *Salmonella* or *Campylobacter* is usually reserved for young infants, malnourished children, or those with serious underlying conditions. In most others, these are self-limiting conditions, although they can be readily spread within the household. Children infected with non-typhoidal *Salmonella* sometimes become asymptomatic carriers for several months after the infection and may transmit it to others during this time. Children infected with *Shigella* or diarrheogenic *E. coli* should be treated with antibiotics; treatment of *E. coli* 0157:H7 is controversial.[34] *Shigella* usually responds to ampicillin, cefixime, or ceftriaxone. Drug sensitivity testing is needed to select the most appropriate drug for diarrheogenic *E. coli*. Infection with *Helicobacter pylori* is discussed in Chapter 20.

Key Points for Internationally Adopted Children

- Intestinal parasites are common in newly arrived international adoptees.
- *Giardia* is most frequently identified and may be transmitted within the household if not treated.
- Multiple parasites are commonly found.
- Stool examinations for ova and parasites miss infections in some children.
- Repeat testing in children after treatment or in those with suggestive symptoms is helpful.

References

1. Saiman L, Aronson J, Zhou J, et al. Prevalence of infectious diseases among internationally adopted children. Pediatrics 2001; 108:608–12.

2. Johnson DE, Miller LC, Iverson S, et al. The health of children adopted from Romania. JAMA 1992; 268: 3446–51.

3. Lange WR, Warnock-Eckhart E. Selected infectious disease risks in international adoptees. Pediatr Infect Dis J 1987; 6:447–50.

4. Hostetter MK, Iverson S, Thomas W, McKenzie D, Dole K, Johnson DE. Medical evaluation of internationally adopted children. N Engl J Med 1991; 325:479–85.

5. Miller LC, Kiernan MT, Mathers MI, Klein-Gitelman M. Developmental and nutritional status of internationally adopted children. Arch Pediatr Adolesc Med 1995; 149:40–4.

6. Nicholson AJ, Francis BM, Mulholland EK, Moulden AL, Oberklaid F. Health screening of international adoptees. Evaluation of a hospital based clinic. Med J Aust 1992; 156:377–9.

7. Benoit TC, Jocelyn LJ, Moddemann DM, Embree JE. Romanian adoption. The Manitoba experience. Arch Pediatr Adolesc Med 1996; 150:1278–82.

8. Jenista JA, Chapman D. Medical problems of foreign-born adopted children. Am J Dis Child 1987; 141:298–302.

9. Bureau JJ, Maurage C, Bremond M, Despert F, Rolland JC. Children of foreign origin adopted in France. Analysis of 68 cases during 12 years at the University Hospital Center of Tours [in French]. Arch Pediatr 1999; 6:1053–8.

10. Proos LA, Hofvander Y, Wennqvist K, Tuvemo T. A longitudinal study on anthropometric and clinical development of Indian children adopted in Sweden. Ups J Med Sci 1992; 97:93–106.

11. Albers LH, Johnson DE, Hostetter MK, Iverson S, Miller LC. Health of children adopted from the former Soviet Union and Eastern Europe. Comparison with preadoptive medical records. JAMA 1997; 278: 922–4.

12. Hostetter MK, Iverson S, Dole K, Johnson D. Unsuspected infectious diseases and other medical diagnoses in the evaluation of internationally adopted children. Pediatrics 1989; 83:559–64.

13. Miller LC, Hendrie NW. Health of children adopted from China. Pediatrics 2000; 105:E76.

14. Esteban JG, Flores A, Aguirre C, Strauss W, Angles R, Mas-Coma S. Presence of very high prevalence and intensity of infection with *Fasciola hepatica* among Aymara children from the Northern Bolivian Altiplano. Acta Trop 1997; 66:1–14.

15. Guerrant DI, Moore SR, Lima AA, Patrick PD, Schorling JB, Guerrant RL. Association of early childhood diarrhea and cryptosporidiosis with impaired physical fitness and cognitive function four–seven years later in a poor urban community in northeast Brazil. Am J Trop Med Hyg 1999; 61:707–13.

16. Boivin MJ, Giordani B. Improvements in cognitive performance for schoolchildren in Zaire, Africa, following an iron supplement and treatment for intestinal parasites. J Pediatr Psychol 1993; 18:249–64.

17. Nokes C, McGarvey ST, Shiue L, et al. Evidence for an improvement in cognitive function following treat-

ment of *Schistosoma japonicum* infection in Chinese primary schoolchildren. Am J Trop Med Hyg 1999; 60:556–65.

18. Nokes C, Grantham-McGregor SM, Sawyer AW, Cooper ES, Bundy DA. Parasitic helminth infection and cognitive function in school children. Proc R Soc Lond B Biol Sci 1992; 247:77–81.

19. Guignard S, Arienti H, Freyre L, Lujan H, Rubinstein H. Prevalence of enteroparasites in a residence for children in the Cordoba Province, Argentina. Eur J Epidemiol 2000; 16:287–93.

20. Tsuyuoka R, Bailey JW, Nery Guimaraes AM, Gurgel RQ, Cuevas LE. Anemia and intestinal parasitic infections in primary school students in Aracaju, Sergipe, Brazil. Cad Saude Publica 1999; 15:413–21.

21. Machado ER, Costa-Cruz JM. *Strongyloides stercoralis* and other enteroparasites in children at Uberlandia city, state of Minas Gerais, Brazil. Mem Inst Oswaldo Cruz 1998; 93:161–4.

22. Saldiva SR, Silveira AS, Philippi ST, et al. *Ascaris–Trichuris* association and malnutrition in Brazilian children. Paediatr Perinat Epidemiol 1999; 13:89–98.

23. Kabani A, Cadrain G, Trevenen C, Jadavji T, Church DL. Practice guidelines for ordering stool ova and parasite testing in a pediatric population. The Alberta Children's Hospital. Am J Clin Pathol 1995; 104:272–8.

24. San Sebastian M, Santi S. Control of intestinal helminths in schoolchildren in Low-Napo, Ecuador: impact of a two-year chemotherapy program. Rev Soc Bras Med Trop 2000; 33:69–73.

25. Curtale F, Nabil M, el Wakeel A, Shamy MY. Anaemia and intestinal parasitic infections among school-age children in Behera Governorate, Egypt. Behera Survey Team. J Trop Pediatr 1998; 44:323–8.

26. Pegelow K, Gross R, Pietrzik K, Lukito W, Richards AL, Fryauff DJ. Parasitological and nutritional situation of school children in the Sukaraja district, West Java, Indonesia. Southeast Asian J Trop Med Public Health 1997; 28:173–90.

27. Brooker S, Peshu N, Warn PA, et al. The epidemiology of hookworm infection and its contribution to anaemia among pre-school children on the Kenyan coast. Trans R Soc Trop Med Hyg 1999; 93:240–6.

28. Vannachone B, Kobayashi J, Nambanya S, Manivong K, Inthakone S, Sato Y. An epidemiological survey on intestinal parasite infection in Khammouane Province, Lao PDR, with special reference to *Strongyloides* infection. Southeast Asian J Trop Med Public Health 1998; 29:717–22.

29. Zulkifli A, Anuar AK, Atiya AS, Yano A. The prevalence of malnutrition and geohelminth infections among primary schoolchildren in rural Kelantan. Southeast Asian J Trop Med Public Health 2000; 31:339–45.

30. Yong TS, Sim S, Lee J, Ohrr H, Kim MH, Kim H. A small-scale survey on the status of intestinal parasite infections in rural villages in Nepal. Korean J Parasitol 2000; 38:275–7.

31. Spencer MJ, Millet VE, Garcia LS, Rhee L, Masterson L. Parasitic infections in a pediatric population. Pediatr Infect Dis 1983; 2:110–3.

32. Meropol SB. Health status of pediatric refugees in Buffalo, NY. Arch Pediatr Adolesc Med 1995; 149:887–92.

33. Triteeraprapab S, Nuchprayoon I. Eosinophilia, anemia and parasitism in a rural region of northwest Thailand. Southeast Asian J Trop Med Public Health 1998; 29:584–90.

34. American Academy of Pediatrics. Drugs for parasitic infections. In: Pickering LK, ed. 2003 Red Book: Report of the Committee on Infectious Diseases. Elk Grove Village, IL: American Academy of Pediatrics, 2003: 744–70.

35. Drugs for parasitic infections. Med Lett 2002; April:1–12.

36. Staat MA. Infectious disease issues in internationally adopted children. Pediatr Infect Dis J 2002; 21:257–8.

37. Shamsuzzama SM, Haque R, Hasin SK, Petri WA, Hashiguchi Y. Socioeconomic status, clinical features, laboratory and parasitological findings of hepatic amebiasis patients—a hospital-based prospective study in Bangladesh. Southeast Asian J Trop Med Public Health 2000; 31:399–404.

38. Yang J, Scholten T. *Dientamoeba fragilis*: a review with notes on its epidemiology, pathogenicity, mode of transmission, and diagnosis. Am J Trop Med Hyg 1977; 26:16–22.

39. Dallemand S, Waxman M, Farman J. Radiological manifestations of *Strongyloides stercoralis*. Gastrointest Radiol 1983; 8:45–51.

40. Townes JM, Quick R, Gonzales OY, et al. Etiology of bloody diarrhea in Bolivian children: implications for empiric therapy. Bolivian Dysentery Study Group. J Infect Dis 1997; 175:1527–30.

41. Muennig P, Pallin D, Sell RL, Chan MS. The cost-effectiveness of strategies for the treatment of intestinal parasites in immigrants. N Engl J Med 1999; 340:773–9.

42. Islam A, Stoll BJ, Ljungstrom I, Biswas J, Nazrul H, Huldt G. *Giardia lamblia* infections in a cohort of Bangladeshi mothers and infants followed for one year. J Pediatr 1983; 103:996–1000.

43. Miller LC, Kelly N, Tannamaat M, Grand RJ. Serologic prevalence of *H. pylori* infection in internationally adopted children. *Helicobacter* 2003; 8:173–8.

44. Oberhuber G, Kastner N, Stolte M. Giardiasis: a histologic analysis of 567 cases. Scand J Gastroenterol 1997; 32:48–51.

45. Sanad MM, Darwish RA, Nasr ME, el-Gammal NE, Emara MW. *Giardia lamblia* and chronic gastritis. J Egypt Soc Parasitol 1996; 26:481–95.

46. Doglioni C, De Boni M, Cielo R, et al. Gastric giardiasis. J Clin Pathol 1992; 45:964–7.

47. Lunn PG, Erinoso HO, Northrop-Clewes CA, Boyce SA. *Giardia intestinalis* is unlikely to be a major cause of the poor growth of rural Gambian infants. J Nutr 1999; 129:872–7.

48. Farthing MJ, Mata L, Urrutia JJ, Kronmal RA. Natural history of *Giardia* infection of infants and children in rural Guatemala and its impact on physical growth. Am J Clin Nutr 1986; 43:395–405.

49. Shekhar KC, Prathapa S, Gurpreet K. Prevalence of giardiasis among Malaysian primary school children. Med J Malaysia 1996; 51:475–9.

50. Hellard ME, Sinclair MI, Hogg GG, Fairley CK. Prevalence of enteric pathogens among community-based asymptomatic individuals. J Gastroenterol Hepatol 2000; 15:290–3.

51. Rastogi A, Malhotra V, Uppal B, Aggarwal V, Kalra KK, Mittal SK. Aetiology of chronic diarrhoea in tropical children. Trop Gastroenterol 1999; 20:45–9.

52. Benzeguir AK, Capraru T, Aust-Kettis A, Bjorkman A. High frequency of gastrointestinal parasites in refugees and asylum seekers upon arrival in Sweden. Scand J Infect Dis 1999; 31:79–82.

53. Gatti S, Lopes R, Cevini C, et al. Intestinal parasitic infections in an institution for the mentally retarded. Ann Trop Med Parasitol 2000; 94:453–60.

54. Kaminsky RG. Parasitism and diarrhoea in children from two rural communities and marginal barrio in Honduras. Trans R Soc Trop Med Hyg 1991; 85:70–3.

55. Shubair ME, Yassin MM, al-Hindi AI, al-Wahaidi AA, Jadallah SY, Abu Shaaban Na-D. Intestinal parasites in relation to haemoglobin level and nutritional status of school children in Gaza. J Egypt Soc Parasitol 2000; 30:365–75.

56. Brannan DK, Greenfield RA, Owen WL, Welch DF, Kuhls TL. Protozoal colonization of the intestinal tract in institutionalized Romanian children. Clin Infect Dis 1996; 22:456–61.

57. Gardner TB, Hill DR. Treatment of giardiasis. Clin Microbiol Rev 2001; 14:114–28. Available at: http://cmr.asm.org/cgi/reprint/14/1/114.pdf.

58. Maraha B, Buiting AG. Evaluation of four enzyme immunoassays for the detection of *Giardia lamblia* antigen in stool specimens. Eur J Clin Microbiol Infect Dis 2000; 19:485–7.

59. Goldin AJ, Apt W, Aguilera X, Zulantay I, Warhurst DC, Miles MA. Efficient diagnosis of giardiasis among nursery and primary school children in Santiago, Chile by capture ELISA for the detection of fecal *Giardia* antigens. Am J Trop Med Hyg 1990; 42:538–45.

60. Pengsaa K, Limkittikul K, Pojjaroen-anant C, et al. Single-dose therapy for giardiasis in school-age children. Southeast Asian J Trop Med Public Health 2002; 33:711–7.

61. Juan JO, Lopez Chegne N, Gargala G, Favennec L. Comparative clinical studies of nitazoxanide, albendazole and praziquantel in the treatment of ascariasis, trichuriasis and hymenolepiasis in children from Peru. Trans R Soc Trop Med Hyg 2002; 96:193–6.

62. Centers for Disease Control and Prevention. Parasites and Health. Giardiasis. Available at: http://www.dpd.cdc.gov/dpdx/HTML/Giardiasis.htm

63. Haque R, Huston CD, Hughes M, Houpt E, Petri WA. Amebiasis. N Engl J Med 2003; 348:1565–73.

64. Moazam F, Nazir Z. Amebic liver abscess: spare the knife but save the child. J Pediatr Surg 1998; 33:119–22.

65. Arellano J, Perez-Rodriguez M, Lopez-Osuna M, et al. Increased frequency of HLA-DR3 and comploltype SCO1 in Mexican mestizo children with amoebic abscess of the liver. Parasite Immunol 1996; 18:491–8.

66. Haque R, Faruque AS, Hahn P, Lyerly DM, Petri WA. *Entamoeba histolytica* and *Entamoeba dispar* infection in children in Bangladesh. J Infect Dis 1997; 175:734–6.

67. Blessman J, Tannich E. Treatment of asymptomatic intestinal *Entamoeba histolytica* infection [letter]. N Engl J Med 2002; 347:1384.

68. Preiss U, Ockert G, Bromme S, Otto A. *Dientamoeba fragilis* infection, a cause of gastrointestinal symptoms in childhood. Klin Padiatr 1990; 202:120–3.

69. Spencer MJ, Garcia LS, Chapin MR. *Dientamoeba fragilis*. An intestinal pathogen in children? Am J Dis Child 1979; 133:390–3.

70. Cuffari C, Oligny L, Seidman EG. *Dientamoeba fragilis* masquerading as allergic colitis. J Pediatr Gastroenterol Nutr 1998; 26:16–20.

71. Kvalsvig JD, Cooppan RM, Connolly KJ. The effects of parasite infections on cognitive processes in children. Ann Trop Med Parasitol 1991; 85:551–68.

72. Boivin MJ, Giordani B, Ndanga K, et al. Effects of treatment for intestinal parasites and malaria on the cognitive abilities of schoolchildren in Zaire, Africa. Health Psychol 1993; 12:220–6.

73. Levav M, Mirsky AF, Schantz PM, Castro S, Cruz ME. Parasitic infection in malnourished school children: effects on behaviour and EEG. Parasitology 1995; 110:103–11.

74. Callender JE, Walker SP, Grantham-McGregor SM, Cooper ES. Growth and development four years after treatment for the *Trichuris* dysentery syndrome. Acta Paediatr 1998; 87:1247–9.

75. Simeon DT, Grantham-McGregor SM, Wong MS. *Trichuris trichiura* infection and cognition in children: results of a randomized clinical trial. Parasitology 1995; 110:457–64.

76. Gardner JM, Grantham-McGregor S, Baddeley A.

Trichuris trichiura infection and cognitive function in Jamaican school children. Ann Trop Med Parasitol 1996; 90:55–63.

77. Paul I, Gnanamani G. Quantitative assessment of *Ascaris lumbricoides* infection in school children from a slum in Visakhapatnam, south India. Southeast Asian J Trop Med Public Health 1999; 30:572–5.

78. Nacher M, Gay F, Singhasivanon P, et al. *Ascaris lumbricoides* infection is associated with protection from cerebral malaria. Parasite Immunol 2000; 22:107–13.

79. Watkins WE, Pollitt E. Effect of removing *Ascaris* on the growth of Guatemalan schoolchildren. Pediatrics 1996; 97:871–6.

80. Sakti H, Nokes C, Hertanto WS, et al. Evidence for an association between hookworm infection and cognitive function in Indonesian school children. Trop Med Int Health 1999; 4:322–34.

81. Barreto ML, Rodrigues LC, Silva RC, et al. Lower hookworm incidence, prevalence, and intensity of infection in children with a Bacillus Calmette-Guerin vaccination scar. J Infect Dis 2000; 182:1800–3.

82. Sirivichayakul C, Pojjaroen-anant C, Wisetsing P, Lalitphiphat A, Chanthavanich P, Kabkaew K. Prevalence of enterobiasis and its incidence after blanket chemotherapy in a male orphanage. Southeast Asian J Trop Med Public Health 2000; 31:144–6.

83. Avolio L, Avoltini V, Ceffa F, Bragheri R. Perianal granuloma caused by *Enterobius vermicularis*: report of a new observation and review of the literature. J Pediatr 1998; 132:1055–6.

84. Ok UZ, Ertan P, Limoncu E, Ece A, Ozbakkaloglu B. Relationship between pinworm and urinary tract infections in young girls. APMIS 1999; 107:474–6.

85. Koltas IS, Ozcan K, Tamer L, Aksungur P. Serum copper, zinc and magnesium levels in children with enterobiosis. J Trace Elem Med Biol 1997; 11:49–52.

86. Bahader SM, Ali GS, Shaalan AH, Khalil HM, Khalil NM. Effects of *Enterobius vermicularis* infection on intelligence quotient (I.Q) and anthropometric measurements of Egyptian rural children. J Egypt Soc Parasitol 1995; 25:183–94.

87. Liu LX, Weller PF. Strongyloidiasis and other intestinal nematode infections. Infect Dis Clin North Am 1993; 7:655–82.

88. Haggerty JJ, Sandler R. Strongyloidiasis presenting as depression: a case report. J Clin Psychiatry 1982; 43:340–1.

89. Burke JA. Strongyloidiasis in childhood. Am J Dis Child 1978; 132:1130–6.

90. Ringertz S, Rockhill RC, Ringertz O, Sutomo A. *Campylobacter* fetus subsp. *jejuni* as a cause of gastroenteritis in Jakarta, Indonesia. J Clin Microbiol 1980; 12:538–40.

91. Reiff A, Jacobs E, Kist M. Seroepidemiological study of the immune response to *Campylobacter pylori* in potential risk groups. Eur J Clin Microbiol Infect Dis 1989; 8:592–6.

92. Taylor DN, Blaser MJ, Echeverria P, Pitarangsi C, Bodhidatta L, Wang WL. Erythromycin-resistant *Campylobacter* infections in Thailand. Antimicrob Agents Chemother 1987; 31:438–42.

93. *Shigella dysenteriae* type 1—Guatemala, 1991. MMWR Morb Mortal Wkly Rep 1991; 40:421, 427–8.

94. Yamada S, Ohta K, Obata H, Matsushita S, Hirata I, Kudoh Y. On the outbreak of shigellosis in Tokyo, 1992 [in Japanese]. Kansenshogaku Zasshi 1993; 67:1183–9.

95. Fagarasan S, Borza T, Ionescu M, Sasca IC, Radulescu A, Bocsan I. Plasmid profile analysis and restriction enzyme analysis in characterizing *Shigella flexneri* isolates from an outbreak. Roum Arch Microbiol Immunol 1996; 55:305–12.

96. Smith-Garcia T, Brown JS. The health of children adopted from India. J Community Health 1989; 14:227–41.

18

HUMAN IMMUNODEFICIENCY VIRUS

Human immunodeficiency virus infection (HIV) is now endemic in many countries of the world. One of the principal concerns of parents adopting internationally is that their child will have unrecognized HIV infection. Physicians counseling prospective adoptive parents may also wonder how to assess the risks of HIV infection in an individual child. Such concerns are valid. Medical information about a prospective child rarely contains detailed information about the birth mother's HIV status or associated risk factors. Although most children are tested for HIV antibodies on one or more occasions in the birth country, test results may not be reliable. The timing of tests for HIV infection in relation to possible exposures and adoptive placement is also problematic: a negative test result does not prevent subsequent exposure. Furthermore, HIV infection may not be recognized clinically prior to adoption as the child's physicians may lack training, experience, or access to suitable diagnostic tests. Moreover, some characteristics of HIV infection overlap with the effects of institutionalization, making differentiation of these conditions difficult. Finally, the prevalence of HIV infection in many of the sending countries is increasing rapidly, statistically increasing the risk of infection.

In this section, the epidemiology of HIV infection among internationally adopted children in the United States and in some of the frequent sending countries is reviewed. This chapter also addresses risk factors for the child, diagnostic pitfalls in the pre-adoptive medical referral, overlapping clinical signs of HIV infection and institutionalization, and management at arrival to the United States. Detailed discussions of the virology, transmission, clinical course, and treatment of HIV are found in standard textbooks.[1-3]

HIV and Internationally Adopted Children

Despite widespread concern about HIV infection in international adoptees, the actual risk is low. Among published surveys of infectious disease risks among various populations of internationally adopted children, no child with HIV infection was identified (Table 18–1). A recent unpublished multicenter survey of 7299 children adopted since the early 1990s and evaluated in 17 international adoption clinics throughout the United States revealed that only 12 children (0.16%) were infected with HIV (Table 18–2).[4] The actual proportion of HIV-infected children is likely somewhat less; the survey included only some of the internationally adopted children entering the United States during that time and may have been biased toward those with more medical problems who underwent evaluation in specialized clinics. Although the prevalence of HIV among international adoptees is low, this will undoubtably increase in the future as HIV epidemics expand.

HIV and Immigration

HIV testing is not required for medical clearance of children less than 15 years of age to enter the United States. Testing may be requested, however, at the discretion of the overseas examining physician (see Chapter 9). The physician is mandated to request this testing if "there is reason to suspect infection."[12]

Epidemiology of HIV Infection in Sending Countries

Global patterns of HIV infection have changed greatly since the first reports of acquired immunodeficiency syndrome (AIDS) 20 years ago.[13] Spread via heterosexual contact and shared needles and syringes by injection drug users now account for most new cases worldwide. Updated statistics and country-by-country trends can be found at the UNAIDS Web site[13] (see Chapter 3 for adult prevalence rates for sending countries). Country-wide statistics may be misleading; for example, Myanmar re-

Table 18–1 HIV among internationally adopted children

Receiving Country	N	+HIV ELISA	Sending Country
United States[5]	504	2 Ab positive, both PCR negative	48% from China, 31% from Russia
United States[6]	64 (293 total, initially only high risk tested; later all tested)	1 Ab positive, PCR negative	Child with positive HIV Ab from Colombia; most children were from Korea and Central and South America
United States[7]	60	0	Romania
Australia[8]	100	0	36% from Korea, 21% from India
France[9]	68	0	48.5% from Africa or Indian Ocean countries
United States[10]	56	0	Former Soviet Union and Eastern Europe
United States[11]	237	0	China
United States[4]	7299	59 Ab positive. 12 infected. (10 had negative tests in birth countries; 2 were known to be HIV positive)	Various (see Table 18–2)

Ab, antibody; ELISA, enzyme-linked immunoadsorbent assay; PCR, polymerase chain reaction.

Table 18–2 Countries of origin for 59 HIV-seropositive internationally adopted children and infection status

Country of Origin	ELISA Positive	Infected
Cambodia	20	4
China	9	0
Russia	9	1
India	6	0
Romania	4	4
Vietnam	3	2
Thailand	3	0
Guatemala	1	0
Panama	1	1
Ethiopia	1	0
Ukraine	1	0
South Korea	1	0

Source: Data from Aronson.[4]

ports a national prevalence rate of 2% but among injection drug users and sex workers the rates are 60% and 40%, respectively. It is difficult to extrapolate such data to birth mothers of children later placed for international adoption, as the social characteristics of these women have not been comprehensively surveyed. These mothers may be more likely to be injection drug users (or sexual partners of such individuals), commercial sex workers, and/or co-infected with other sexually transmitted diseases (enhancing HIV transmission) than are pregnant women in the general population. Thus the risk of vertical transmission to children later placed in international adoptions is greater than that indicated by prevalence rates in the general population of the country.

Eastern Europe and Central Asia

Eastern Europe and Central Asia are experiencing the fastest-growing HIV epidemic in the world.[14,15] There was a fivefold increase between 1995 and 1997,[16] and about 250,000 new infections in 2000. The number of new diagnoses doubled annually between 1998 and 2001. In Russia, 523 new infections were reported in 1991 and over 129,000 in 2001 (Fig. 18–1). About 700,000 individuals are currently infected with HIV; about half of reported cases occur among injection drug users. Overall adult prevalence is 0.9%; among high-risk populations prevalence is 15.3%.[17] Prevalence rates vary by region; in Murmansk region the rate is 51/100,000, whereas in St. Petersburg the rate is 241/100,000.[15]

Rapid spread of infection has also occurred in Belarus, Kazakhstan, Moldova, and Ukraine.[18] In Ukraine, the adult HIV prevalence rate is 1% (highest in region), and the number of reported cases skyrocketed from <50 per year before 1994 to 12,000 in 1996.[19,20]

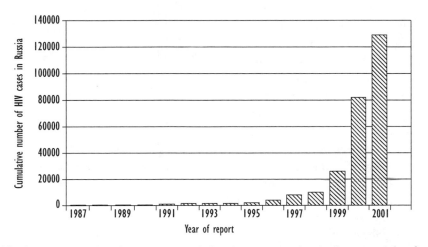

Figure 18–1 *Annual number of HIV cases reported in the Russian Federation 1987–2001 (as of June 2001). (Reprinted with permission from UNAIDS.)*

The contributing factors to this epidemic include the increasing rate of injection drug users (about 1% of the population) and widespread needle sharing. An explosive increase in syphilis infections (from 4.2 per 100,000 in 1987 to an estimated 157 per 100,000 in 2000) has also fueled the rapid increase in HIV infection.[13]

Romania

Romania has the highest number of pediatric HIV cases in Europe:[17,21,22] 9022 cases since 1985 (compared to 2014 adults). In 1989, large numbers of HIV-infected children were discovered, mostly residing in institutions. The medical practice of administering "micro-transfusions" of unscreened blood as treatment for anemia or malnutrition was the source for most of these infections.[21] Seventy-seven percent of cases were found in 5 of Romania's 41 districts[22]; 94% of infections occurred in children <13 years of age. There are currently ~7000 infected individuals; 5000 of them are children. The prevalence rate among adults is at least 0.2%, mostly commercial sex workers and injection drug users.[17]

China

About ~600,000 Chinese have HIV infection, including 4800 children. Reported infections increased 67% in the first 6 months of 2001 compared with the previous year.[23] Drug users account for 60%–70% of reported infections;[23] between 50% and 70% of these individuals are infected. Coincident with the rise in injection drug use, the number of patients with sexually transmitted diseases rose almost 30%. Infection among sex workers varies greatly, from 0.1% to 5% in some areas to as high as 10.7% in other regions (notably Guangxi).

Serious epidemics in Henan Province in central China have recently emerged. In this region, tens of thousands (or more) rural villagers became infected after selling blood to collection centers that did not follow sterile techniques.[24]

Vietnam

By 1999, a cumulative total of 17,046 cases of HIV infection were reported in Vietnam, with a cumulative incidence rate of 22.5 per 100,000.[25] Injection drug users account for nearly 90% of the total. HIV prevalence among commercial sex workers ranges from 0% to 13.2%.

India

HIV infection varies greatly among different regions of India. Overall, prevalence is estimated at 2% of pregnant women but >10% among women with other sexually transmitted diseases.

Guatemala

The prevalence of HIV infection in Guatemala is estimated at 1.38%—among the highest rate in Central America.[26] About 73,000 persons were infected as of 1999, the highest total for the region. Pregnant women with HIV infection may receive free antiretroviral therapy through the public health system.

Other Latin America and Caribbean Countries

The Caribbean region has the second highest prevalence rate of HIV infection in the world, second only to Sub-Saharan Africa. In Haiti, the prevalence rate exceeds 4%. In Brazil, an estimated 600,000 individuals are infected, but prevention efforts among injection drug users appear to be decreasing the rate of infection.

Risk Factors for HIV Infection in the Internationally Adopted Child

In the United States, "infants who have been abandoned, are in the custody of the state, or have positive toxicology screens should be considered high risk for exposure to HIV."[2] Similarly, abandoned children from other countries are at increased risk for HIV exposure compared with other children. The internationally adopted child may become infected via various routes (Table 18–3). As with hepatitis B and hepatitis C, HIV is transmitted vertically or horizontally. Vertical transmission is the most common route of infection for children worldwide, and is enhanced if the birth mother is co-infected with syphilis or other sexually transmitted diseases. A high viral load in the birth mother increases the likelihood of transmission of HIV. Transmission is also increased in the presence of chorioamnionitis, maternal illicit drug use, or smoking during pregnancy.[1] Exposure to cervical secretions (prolonged rupture of membranes) and vaginal delivery increase risk of transmission to the newborn. Such obstetric details are usually missing from referral packets. Lack of prenatal care, unfortunately common among international adoptees, precludes administration of antiretroviral therapy prior to delivery, if such treatment is available.

Other potential sources of infection are listed in Table 18–3. Some abandoned infants are nursed by other lactating mothers in the maternity hospital. Although breast milk and breast feeding are desirable, it is doubtful that these "wet nurses" are screened for HIV infection. Use of banked milk from unscreened women is another potential source of exposure. Abandoned infants, born without prenatal care, are more likely to become ill than infants who remain with their mothers. Neonatal illness increases the chances of exposure to needles, syringes, medical equipment, and blood products. In some countries, transfusions of whole blood, blood components, or other blood products are administered to infants and children with anemia or malnutrition. This practice, common in Romania in the 1980s, was responsible for the enormous epidemic of HIV among institutionalized children in that country. Finally, internationally adopted children may be victims of sexual abuse, either prior to institutionalization or within the institution by staff or older children.

Diagnosis of HIV Infection

Pre-Adoption

Information about the HIV status of relinquishing birth mothers is rarely available for children placed for international adoption. An occasional exception is Guatemala, where the birth mother's laboratory test results for HIV (as well as hepatitis B and syphilis) are sometimes included in the referred child's medical dossier. Other than this, specific laboratory test results on the birth mother are generally unavailable.

Most internationally adopted children are screened for the presence of antibodies to HIV on one or more occasion prior to adoption. Most commonly, an enzyme-linked immunoadsorbent assay (ELISA) is performed. More sophisticated virologic tests (HIV culture, p 24 antigen, DNA or RNA polymerase chain reaction [PCR]) are seldom available, although in some countries (Cambodia, Vietnam, Guatemala) these tests may be performed in children whose antibody screening is positive. The accuracy and timing of any of these tests may be questionable. The accuracy of results from laboratories with inadequate quality control practices and supervision may be poor. More complicated tests, such as PCR, may be prone to inaccurate results (both false positive and false negative results). Timing is also a potential source of confusion. HIV virologic tests done in the first 7 days of life may be negative in as many as 20%–60% of

Table 18–3 Potential routes of transmission of HIV infection in internationally adopted children

- Vertical transmission
- Breast milk from infected mother (or from milk bank or "wet nurse")
- Needles, syringes, medical equipment
- Transfusion of blood or blood products
- Blood exposure within the institution
- Sexual abuse by HIV-positive individual

The Smiths felt they could handle any issue in their child-to-be except HIV infection. Once they identified their child in Russia, they arranged with their adoption agency to have a local contact hire a special physician to visit the orphanage and draw a blood sample from the child for HIV testing. They then arranged for the sample to be shipped to a lab in Chicago to be tested for HIV by culture, DNA PCR, RNA PCR, and ELISA. All results were negative. Upon their arrival in Russia to finalize the adoption, they were concerned to learn when they arrived that he had been hospitalized for a serious diarrheal infection. When they arrived at the hospital to meet their child, they found him receiving a blood transfusion.

vertically infected infants.[1] In adequate laboratories, tests become progressively more accurate by about 3–6 months of age. Problems with timing of laboratory tests in children exposed via other routes are discussed below.

Only some children born to infected mothers are themselves infected. Thus, children with positive ELISAs due to maternal antibody must be differentiated from those with actual infection. The proportion of infected infants born to HIV-infected mothers varies among different studies,[1] from as high as 48% in India and 42.8% in Africa to about 14%–33% in the United States. Maternal antibody IgG is usually undetectable by about 10–13 months of age but occasionally may remain as long as 18 months.[1] For children <18 months of age, diagnosis of HIV infection requires specific virological confirmation (HIV culture, HIV PCR [DNA PCR preferred to RNA PCR] or p24 antigen). Such tests are sometimes available in birth countries in specialized labs; the accuracy may vary greatly. In addition, some methods (PCR and culture) may show false negative results in early blood specimens from some infected infants, due to infection late in gestation or low viral load. By 3–6 months of age, HIV culture or PCR tests have >90% sensitivity in detecting vertically acquired infection in infants. Additional tests may be helpful to confirm the diagnosis.

In older children (>18 months of age), ELISA testing and a confirmatory Western blot are adequate to confirm a diagnosis of HIV. However, because of the risk of horizontally acquired infection, it must be recognized that a negative test does not exclude disease with certainty. Children may be incubating the infection when the test is performed or may be infected after the test is completed. Exposure to contaminated medical supplies or equipment, blood products, or sexual abuse may infect children waiting for adoptive placement. An exposure may occur literally hours or minutes prior to the placement of the child with adoptive parents. Thus it must be recognized that HIV testing—even sophisticated virologic assays—may have been done prior to infection or during a seronegative window. Even the most sensitive and specific fourth-generation assays (which detect both HIV antibody and antigen) have seronegative windows after exposure, emphasizing that repeated tests over time are necessary to identify infection.[27,28]

Role of Specialized Laboratories

Because of concern about accuracy of laboratory test results in some countries, some adoption agencies and facilitators have identified specialized laboratories to test prospective adoptees for HIV (and other infections). These laboratories are usually private facilities where testing is done on a fee-for-service basis. Examples include the Pasteur Institutes in Vietnam and Cambodia, Euromed Clinic in St. Petersburg, Russia, and the American Medical Centers in Russia and other Eastern European countries. These laboratories offer several advantages, including likely sterile technique used to obtain sample and availability of more sophisticated tests (i.e., virologic assays such as PCR for HIV infection). Quality control even in these laboratories is not guaranteed, however. It must be remembered that negative test results often occur shortly after infection and furthermore, that a negative test does not preclude later infection.

Post-Adoption

No data yet indicate that some infected children are missed if screened only at arrival. This is theoretically possible. As a practical approach, it is recommended that children be tested at arrival to the United States and again 6 months later to ensure that the incubation period for HIV infection has (likely) elapsed.[29] (Rarely, seroconversion is very delayed after infection; intervals of >30 months have been reported in adults.[30])

Shared Clinical Manifestations of HIV Infection and Institutionalization

Clinical signs of HIV infection may mimic common findings among institutionalized children (Table 18–4). Failure to thrive, developmental delay, and recurrent infections occur in both conditions. In the absence of reliable laboratory data and reports of physical findings, it is difficult to differentiate complications related to HIV infection from those due to institutionalization. Growth delay and failure to thrive are prominent features of HIV infection in children and may predate other symptoms of infection. Wasting, defined as *(1)* persistent weight loss >10% of baseline *or (2)* downward crossing of at least 2 percentile lines on weight-for-age chart in child ≥1 year *or (3)* less than the fifth percentile on weight-for-height chart on two consecutive measurements, plus chronic diarrhea or fevers, is an AIDS-defining condition.[1] These criteria are also fulfilled by many children with institutional failure-to-thrive. Malabsorption, micronutrient deficiencies, and diarrhea also frequently occur in both groups of children.

Developmental delay may also result from HIV infection or from institutionalization. Progressive HIV encephalopathy may not be difficult to differentiate from orphanage-acquired developmental delays, but lack of precise information and sequential evaluations may confuse this assessment during pre-adoptive evaluations. HIV-encephalopathy, defined as *(1)* failure to attain developmental milestones (or loss of them) or loss of intellectual ability, *(2)* impaired brain growth or acquired microcephaly, or *(3)* acquired symmetric motor deficit (paresis, pathologic reflexes, ataxia, gait disturbance), is also an AIDs-defining condition. In particular, many institutionalized children have acquired microcephaly (see Chapter 12). Other conditions often seen in institutionalized or post-institutionalized children, expressive language delays and attention-deficit disorder, also occur with HIV infection.[1]

Finally, opportunistic infections are AIDS-defining conditions but are not specific for this disease. Immune dysfunction associated with malnutrition may also increase the risk of opportunistic infections (Table 18–4).

Other manifestations of HIV infection, such as lymphoproliferative lung disorders, malignancy, cardiac or renal dysfunction, and bone marrow suppression (see Chapter 22 for exception), are more specific for this condition and less likely to occur in the uninfected institutionalized child.

HIV-2

Most diagnostic ELISA tests in the United States currently recognize antibodies to HIV-1 and HIV-2; however, this may not be true of tests used in sending countries. HIV-2 is most prevalent in West Africa (Guinea-Bissau, Burkina Faso, Gambia, Cape Verde, Senegal, Ivory Coast) and southern Africa (Angola, Mozambique),[1] countries which seldom send children to the United States. Some children arrive in the United States each year from Ethiopia, South Africa, and Sierra Leone. Furthermore, HIV-2 has been identified in North America, South America, Europe, India, and Korea,[62] usually among immigrants from West Africa or their sexual partners. Vertical transmission is less common than with HIV-1.

Table 18–4 Shared manifestations: HIV infection and institutionalization

Central Nervous System

Attention-deficit disorder[31]

Developmental delay

Acquired microcephaly

Encephalopathy, as defined by one or more of the following for at least 2 months:

   Loss of or failure to attain developmental milestones or loss of intellectual ability

   Impaired brain growth or acquired microcephaly

   Acquired symmetric motor deficit (paresis, pathologic reflexes, ataxia, gait disturbance)

Gastrointestinal Complications

Wasting or failure to thrive

   Persistent weight loss <10% of baseline *or*

   Downward crossing of at least 2 percentile lines on weight-for-age chart in child ≥1 year *or*

   Less than the fifth percentile on weight-for-height chart on two consecutive measurements plus chronic diarrhea or fevers

Opportunistic Infections (may occur secondary to malnutrition)

Pneumocystis carinii (jiroveci) pneumonia[32–46] (see Chapter 22)

Mycobacterium avium-intracellulare[47]

Disseminated cytomegalovirus infection[41,45]

Chronic candidiasis[37,48,49]

Severe bacterial infections (bacteremia, pneumonia, osteomyelitis, meningitis, sinusitis)[43,45,48,50–53]

Tuberculosis[43,52,54–58]

Chronic herpes simplex[43,58–61]

Other findings[1]

Recurrent respiratory infections

Chronic otitis media

Intestinal parasites (*B. hominis*)

Enteric pathogens (*Salmonella, Shigella, Campylobacter, Cryptosporidia, Isospora, Microsporidia*)

Delayed dental development

Dental caries

Anemia (iron and vitamin B_{12} deficiencies)

Skin conditions

   Molluscum contagiosum

   Seborrheic dermatitis

   Norwegian scabies

   Atopic dermatitis

   Eczema

Key Points for Internationally Adopted Children

- HIV infection is rare among international adoptees.
- The prevalence of infection is expected to increase.
- Children have many risk factors for HIV infection.
- It may be difficult to identify HIV infection in an institutionalized child; institutionalization may cause problems similar to those seen in HIV infection.
- Children should be tested at arrival and ≥6 months later; young infants should have specialized testing for HIV infection.

FAQs

Q. A 4-year-old from Thailand just came to my office with her new adoptive parents. She has no vaccine records whatsoever. She's a smart kid and her parents are anxious to enroll her in a part-time preschool. She needs vaccines before she can enter preschool. Do I need to wait to vaccinate her until her HIV status is completely "cleared" in 6 months?

A. Don't hesitate to vaccinate her. Vaccines are recommended for children with actual or suspected infection. Feel free to administer IPV, DTaP, MMR, HBV, Hib, pneumococcal conjugate vaccine, and influenza (i.e., all but OPV) vaccines as per *Red Book* recommendations. Varicella vaccine should be withheld until results of initial HIV testing are available. As usual, it's best to spread this over a reasonable time frame, and not start immediately at the child's first visit with you. Meanwhile, it is important to test for HIV antibodies at entry and again 6 months later.

Q. I saw a 9-month-old from Cambodia who has a positive ELISA for HIV. We are waiting for the results of the more specific virologic tests. What about his vaccination schedule?

A. This boy can get DTaP, IPV, HIB, hepatitis B, pneumococcal, and influenza vaccines. Varicella and MMR are suggested at 12 months unless he is severely immunocompromised (check CD4 count). If he truly is infected, he may have a poor immunologic response to these vaccines. You should consult an expert in pediatric HIV to guide your management.

Q. With the epidemics of HIV in some of the sending countries, why are so few internationally adopted children infected?

A. Although the numbers are presently small, it is likely that there will be a significant increase in the next decade. Meanwhile, it is likely that many infected children do not survive long enough to be placed for international adoption. Survival is quite limited in untreated children who become symptomatic during the first year of life. Furthermore, local physicians undoubtably identify many infected children and withdraw them from consideration. Although laboratory test accuracy in individual cases may be questionable, in general, these tests identify most infected children, thereby precluding their consideration as possible adoptees. Finally, even if HIV infection is not specifically diagnosed, related problems may supervene and prevent adoption.

Q. I have a 14-month-old in my practice with tuberculosis, failure to thrive, and developmental delay. She also has almost constant oral thrush. I did an ELISA for HIV shortly after she arrived from China, at age 11 months, and it was negative. Should I do some other more sophisticated tests for HIV too? Or just wait and repeat the ELISA in a few more months?

A. That's a lot going on for one baby. However, if HIV is responsible for all these difficulties, the antibody screen should be positive already. It's important to repeat it as scheduled, just to be sure there isn't another problem to add to the list.

Useful Web Sites

U.S. Department of Health and Human Services. AIDS info. Available at: http://www.aidsinfo.nih.gov.

National Center of HIV, STD, and TB Prevention. Divisions of HIV/AIDS Prevention. Available at: http://www.cdc.gov/hiv.

UNAIDS. The Joint United Nations Program on HIV/AIDS. Up-to-date statistics by country; difficulties in data collection; overall epidemiological situation. Available at: http://www.unaids.

References

1. Hanson IC, Shearer WT. AIDS and other acquired immunodeficiency diseases. In: Feigin RD, Cherry JD, eds. Textbook of Pediatric Infectious Diseases. Philadelphia: W.B. Saunders, 1998: 954–79.

2. Working Group on Antiretroviral Therapy. Antiretroviral therapy and medical management of pediatric HIV infection. Pediatr 1998; 102 (Suppl):1005–1085.

3. American Academy of Pediatrics. Human immunodeficiency virus infection. In: Pickering L, ed. 2000 Red Book: Report of the Committee on Infectious Diseases. Elk Grove Village, IL: American Academy of Pediatrics, 2000: 360–82.

4. Aronson J. HIV in Internationally Adopted Children. Washington, DC: Joint Council for International Children's Services, 2002.

5. Saiman L, Aronson J, Zhou J, et al. Prevalence of infectious diseases among internationally adopted children. Pediatrics 2001; 108:608–12.

6. Hostetter MK, Iverson S, Thomas W, McKenzie D, Dole K, Johnson DE. Medical evaluation of internationally adopted children. N Engl J Med 1991; 325:479–85.

7. Johnson DE, Miller LC, Iverson S, et al. The health of children adopted from Romania. JAMA 1992; 268: 3446–51.

8. Nicholson AJ, Francis BM, Mulholland EK, Moulden AL, Oberklaid F. Health screening of international adoptees. Evaluation of a hospital based clinic. Med J Aust 1992; 156:377–9.

9. Bureau JJ, Maurage C, Bremond M, Despert F, Rolland JC. Children of foreign origin adopted in France. Analysis of 68 cases during 12 years at the University Hospital Center of Tours [in French]. Arch Pediatr 1999; 6: 1053–8.

10. Albers LH, Johnson DE, Hostetter MK, Iverson S, Miller LC. Health of children adopted from the former Soviet Union and Eastern Europe. Comparison with preadoptive medical records. JAMA 1997; 278:922–4.

11. Miller LC, Hendrie NW. Health of children adopted from China. Pediatrics 2000; 105:E76.

12. U.S. Citizenship and Immigration Services. Frequently asked questions for Form 1-693. Available at: http://uscis.gov.

13. The Joint United Nations Program on AIDS. Epidemiology. Available at: http://www.unaids.org/EN/resources/epidemiology.asp.

14. Stephenson J. HIV/AIDS surging in Eastern Europe. JAMA 2000; 284:3113–4.

15. Stephenson J. Researchers wrestle with spread and control of emerging infections. JAMA 2002; 287:2061–3.

16. Dehne KL, Khodakevich L, Hamers FF, Schwartlander B. The HIV/AIDS epidemic in Eastern Europe: recent patterns and trends and their implications for policy-making. AIDS 1999; 13:741–9.

17. U.S. Agency for International Development. HIV/AIDS in Russia. Available at: http://www.usaid.gov/our_work/global_health/aids/countries/eande/russiabrief.pdf.

18. Rhodes T, Ball A, Stimson GV, et al. HIV infection associated with drug injecting in the newly independent states, Eastern Europe: the social and economic context of epidemics. Addiction 1999; 94:1323–36.

19. Hamers FF. HIV infection in Ukraine (1987–96). Rev Epidemiol Sante Publique 2000; 48:1S3–15.

20. The Joint United Nations Program on AIDS. World AIDS Day 2003. Available at: http://www.unaids.org/en/events/world+aids+day+2003.asp.

21. Kozinetz C, Matusa R, Cazazu A. The changing epidemic of pediatric HIV infection in Romania. Ann Epidemiol 2000; 10:474–475.

22. Kozinetz CA, Matusa R, Cazacu A. The burden of pediatric HIV/AIDS in Constanta, Romania: a cross-sectional study. BMC Infect Dis 2001; 1:7.

23. Zhang Kl KL, Ma SJ. Epidemiology of HIV in China. BMJ 2002; 324:803–4.

24. Gill B, Chang J, Palmer S. China's HIV crisis. Foreign Affairs 2002; 81: Mar/Apr 96–103.

25. Quan VM, Chung A, Long HT, Dondero TJ. HIV in Vietnam: the evolving epidemic and the prevention response, 1996 through 1999. J Acquir Immune Defic Syndr 2000; 25:360–9.

26. Wheeler DA, Arathoon EG, Pitts M, et al. Availability of HIV care in Central America. JAMA 2001; 286:853–60.

27. Meier T, Knoll E, Henkes M, Enders G, Braun R. Evidence for a diagnostic window in fourth generation assays for HIV. J Clin Virol 2001; 23:113–6.

28. Weber B, Fall EH, Berger A, Doerr HW. Reduction of diagnostic window by new fourth-generation human immunodeficiency virus screening assays. J Clin Microbiol 1998; 36:2235–9.

29. Horsburgh CRJ, Ou CY, Jason J, et al. Duration of human immunodeficiency virus infection before detection of antibody. Lancet 1989; 2:637–40.

30. Imagawa DT, Lee MH, Wolinsky SM, et al. Human immunodeficiency virus type 1 infection in homosexual men who remain seronegative for prolonged periods. N Engl J Med 1989; 320:1458–62.

31. Cesena M, Lee DO, Cebollero AM, Steingard R. Case study: behavioral symptoms of pediatric HIV-1 encephalopathy successfully treated with clonidine. J Am Acad Child Adolesc Psychiatry 1995; 34:302–6.

32. Nordin J, Myers MG. *Pneumocystis carinii* in a Vietnamese foundling. Am J Dis Child 1975; 129:1361.

33. Redman JC. *Pneumocystis carinii* pneumonia in an adopted Vietnamese infant. A case of fulminant disease with recovery. JAMA 1974; 230:1561–3.

34. Dutz W, Jennings-Khodadad E, Post C, Kohout E, Nazarian I, Esmaili H. Marasmus and *Pneumocystis carinii* pneumonia in institutionalised infants. Observations during an endemic. Z Kinderheilkd 1974; 117:241–58.

35. Dutz W, Post C, Vessal K, Kohout E. Endemic infantile *Pneumocystis carinii* infection: the Shiraz study. Natl Cancer Inst Monogr 1976; 43:31–40.

36. Gleason WA, Roodman ST. Reversible T cell depression in malnourished infants with *Pneumocystis pneumonia*. J Pediatr 1977; 90:1032–3.

37. Goldbach PD, Mohsenifar Z, Medici MA, Lee S, Smith S. *Pneumocystis carinii* pneumonia in an apparently nonimmunocompromised patient. South Med J 1982; 75:1256–8.

38. Gretillat F, Mselati JC, Lavaud J, et al. Congenital syphilis, malnutrition and *Pneumocystis carinii* pneumonia [in French]. Arch Fr Pediatr 1979; 36:813–7.

39. Hodson EM, Springthorpe BJ. Medical problems in refugee children evacuated from South Vietnam. Med J Aust 1976; 2:747–9.

40. Hughes WT, Price RA, Sisko F, et al. Protein-calorie malnutrition. A host determinant for *Pneumocystis carinii* infection. Am J Dis Child 1974; 128:44–52.

41. Leung TF, Ng PC, Fok TF, et al. *Pneumocystis carinii* pneumonia in an immunocompetent infant with congenital cytomegalovirus infection. Infection 2000; 28:184–6.

42. Paes RA, Chieffi PP, D'Andretta Neto C, Nascimento Mde F. *Pneumocystis carinii* interstitial pneumonia in malnourished children. Report of 4 cases [in Portuguese]. Rev Inst Med Trop Sao Paulo 1982; 24:188–92.

43. Purtilo DT, Connor DH. Fatal infections in protein-calorie malnourished children with thymolymphatic atrophy. Arch Dis Child 1975; 50:149–52.

44. Russian DA, Levine SJ. *Pneumocystis carinii* pneumonia in patients without HIV infection. Am J Med Sci 2001; 321:56–65.

45. Tomashefski JF Jr, Butler T, Islam M. Histopathology and etiology of childhood pneumonia: an autopsy study of 93 patients in Bangladesh. Pathology 1989; 21:71–8.

46. Wang NS, Huang SN, Thurlbeck WM. Combined *Pneumocystis carinii* and cytomegalovirus infection. Arch Pathol 1970; 90:529–35.

47. Cathebras PJ, Bouchou K, Rousset H. Pulmonary *Mycobacterium avium* intracellulare with transient CD4+ T-lymphocytopenia without HIV infection. Eur J Med 1993; 2:509–10.

48. Klingspor L, Stitzing G, Johansen K, Murtaza A, Holmberg K. Infantile diarrhoea and malnutrition associated with *Candida* in a developing community. Mycoses 1993; 36:19–24.

49. Matee MI, Simon E, Christensen MF, et al. Association between carriage of oral yeasts and malnutrition among Tanzanian infants aged 6–24 months. Oral Dis 1995; 1:37–42.

50. Berman S. Epidemiology of acute respiratory infections in children of developing countries. Rev Infect Dis 1991; 13:S454–62.

51. Johnson AW, Osinusi K, Aderele WI, Adeyemi-Doro FA. Bacterial aetiology of acute lower respiratory infections in pre-school Nigerian children and comparative predictive features of bacteraemic and non-bacteraemic illnesses. J Trop Pediatr 1993; 39:97–106.

52. Melaku A, Lulseged S. Chronic suppurative otitis media in a children's hospital in Addis Ababa, Ethiopia. Ethiop Med J 1999; 37:237–46.

53. Tupasi TE, Lucero MG, Magdangal DM, et al. Etiology of acute lower respiratory tract infection in children from Alabang, Metro Manila. Rev Infect Dis 1990; 12:S929–39.

54. Adegbola RA, Falade AG, Sam BE, et al. The etiology of pneumonia in malnourished and well-nourished Gambian children. Pediatr Infect Dis J 1994; 13:975–82.

55. Caksen H, Arslan S, Oner AF, Kuru M, Karakok M, Odabas D. Multiple metastatic tuberculous abscesses in a severely malnourished infant. Pediatr Dermatol 2002; 19:90–1.

56. Ibadin MO, Oviawe O. Trend in childhood tuberculosis in Benin City, Nigeria. Ann Trop Paediatr 2001; 21:141–5.

57. Karyadi E, Schultink W, Nelwan RH, et al. Poor micronutrient status of active pulmonary tuberculosis patients in Indonesia. J Nutr 2000; 130:2953–8.

58. Orren A, Kipps A, Moodie JW, Beatty DW, Dowdle EB, McIntyre JP. Increased susceptibility to herpes simplex virus infections in children with acute measles. Infect Immun 1981; 31:1–6.

59. Brooks SE, Taylor E, Golden MH, Golden BE. Electron microscopy of herpes simplex hepatitis with hepatocyte pulmonary embolization in kwashiorkor. Arch Pathol Lab Med 1991; 115:1247–9.

60. Templeton AC. Generalized herpes simplex in malnourished children. J Clin Pathol 1970; 23:24–30.

61. Tinaztepe K, Saatci U, Tinaztepe B, Ogus H. Fatal disseminated herpes simplex virus infection in malnourished infants. Turk J Pediatr 1971; 13:40–8.

62. Kim S, Kim E, Park K, et al. Introduction of human immunodeficiency virus 2 infection into South Korea. Acta Virol 2000; 44:15–22.

19

SYPHILIS

Syphilis is seldom diagnosed in newly arrived international adoptees (Table 19–1). Most infected children are asymptomatic and are identified by routine screening. Many additional children have been diagnosed and treated in their birth countries prior to adoption, most of them from Russia and countries of the former Soviet Union. Although an infrequent problem, unrecognized syphilis has severe consequences. This section reviews the epidemiology of syphilis in sending countries, specific concerns for international adoptees, diagnosis and clinical features of congenital syphilis presenting after the newborn period, and current recommendations for treatment and follow-up. Management of acquired syphilis has been recently reviewed elsewhere.[1–6]

Epidemiology

Worldwide, each year approximately 900,000 pregnancies occur among women infected with syphilis; 40% of these infants die. Congenital syphilis contributes to 29% of perinatal and infant deaths and 26% of stillbirths.[16] Although syphilis cases declined in many countries in the 1960–1970s, this disease has been epidemic in

Table 19–1 Prevalence of syphilis in internationally adopted children

Country of Origin	Number Positive/ Total Number	%
Russia[7]	0/56	0
Various countries, 79% Russia or China[8]	0/478	0
China[9]	1/335	0.30
Various[10]	1/293	0.34
Korea[11]	2/360	0.6
Various countries[12]	1/100	1
Various countries[13]	2/129	1.5
Romania[14]	1/59	1.7
Various countries[15]	4/68	5.8

the former Soviet Union (Table 19–2), China and the United States in the last 10–12 years.

The republics of the former Soviet Union report enormous increases in cases of syphilis[17] (Fig. 19–1). In 1990 in Russia there were 7931 cases registered; in 1996, there were 387,704 cases. Overall, the case rate for syphilis is about 277/100,000 inhabitants. These numbers represent a 15-fold increase among adults and 20-fold among children.[18] In the Novosibirsk region of Russia, rates increased rapidly from 15/100,000

in 1993 to 311/100,000 in 1997.[19] Case rates were as high as 1500/100,000 in the Tuva region in 1998, with congenital syphilis found in 41.8/10,000 newborns.[20] Rates recently increased as much as 175-fold in Kazakhstan.[20]

Although syphilis screening is provided free of charge in prenatal clinics in most countries of the former Soviet Union, young teenage, homeless, or marginalized mothers often avoid prenatal care.[20] Other reasons cited for these alarming increases include scarcity of condoms, lack of knowledge, use of outdated treatment techniques,[21] proliferation of poor-quality private-sector treatment centers for sexually transmitted diseases, and other sociocultural changes.[17]

China also reports increases in rates of syphilis: as much as 25-fold between 1989 and 1998 (0.17/100,000 to 4.31/100,000).[22] More international travel, increased migration of people from rural to urban areas, and rapid changes in sexual beliefs and practices have led to greater transmission of syphilis and other sexually transmitted diseases in China.[22] World Health Organization sentinel sites document increases in prevalence of syphilis from 1.4/100,000 to 31.1/100,000, and in cases of congenital syphilis from 2 to 73 between 1993 and 1998.[23]

Globally, about 12 million new cases of syphilis occur annually (Table 19–3). The

Table 19–2 Congenital syphilis cases in Eastern Europe (1998)

Country	Cases (n)
Armenia	12
Azerbaijan	11
Belarus	23
Georgia	20
Kazakhstan	294
Kyrgyzstan	67
Latvia	16
Moldova	4
Russian Federation	840
Tajikistan	4
Turkmenistan	5
Ukraine	79
Uzbekistan	3

Source: Data from Riedner et al.[20]

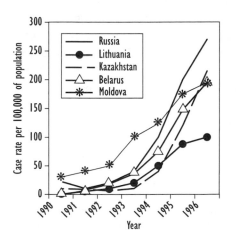

Figure 19–1 *Syphilis prevalence rates in Baltic countries, 1990–96. Data from World Health Organization.*[25]

Table 19–3 Global distribution of new syphilis cases (1999)

Region	Estimated No. of New Cases
Sub-Saharan Africa	4 million
South and Southeast Asia	4 million
Latin America and Caribbean	3 million
North Africa and Middle East	370,000
Eastern Asia and Pacific region	240,000
Western Europe	140,000
Eastern Europe and Central Asia	100,000
North America	100,000
Total	~12 million

Source: Data from World Health Organization.[25]

World Health Organization, United States Agency for International Development, and the Pan-American Health Organization, working in Africa and Central and South America, have targeted maternal and congenital syphilis for improved clinical management.

In the United States, mothers of syphilitic infants are more likely to be of lower socioeconomic status, use cocaine, and have fewer prenatal visits[4,24] than mothers of healthy infants. Similar information about mothers of syphilitic infants in adoption-sending countries is not available, but may be comparable.

Syphilis and Internationally Adopted Children

Evaluation of syphilis status of prospective adoptees prior to placement is confounded by several factors. Not all countries routinely screen birth mothers and/or newborns for syphilis. Even if syphilis screening is routinely offered as a part of prenatal care, few birth mothers of international adoptees receive such care. Medical records of international adoptees contain little or no information about maternal status. Even if a history of maternal syphilis is indicated, specific information about the adequacy and timing of treatment is usually unavailable. Children born at home (rather than a hospital) may never be tested for syphilis. Incorrectly timed or single determinations of syphilis exposure (in infant or mother) may not detect maternal infection occurring late in pregnancy.[26,27] Prozone effects (antibody excess prevents formation of antigen–antibody complexes necessary for the test) may occasionally cause false negative results. Moreover, negative test results do not preclude later exposure (via sexual abuse). Finally, the accuracy of the laboratory test results in the birth country may be questionable. Thus, it is essential to test all new arrivals for serologic evidence of syphilis infection.

Additional concerns regarding children with congenital syphilis include the risks of co-infection with HIV, hepatitis B, and/or hepatitis C. Syphilis greatly enhances HIV transmission.[16,28] The risk of exposure to possibly contaminated needles (HIV, hepatitis B, hepatitis C) during treatment for congenital syphilis has not been fully assessed.

Russia and the Former Soviet Union

Syphilis screening protocols are generally well established in the countries of the former Soviet Union. Certain occupational groups are screened annually, including food workers, nursery, obstetric, and pediatric staff, and school and hotel workers.[17] Newborns are routinely tested regardless of maternal history with the "RW" (occasionally listed as "WR" in preadoptive records), or Wasserman, test (a nontreponemal test, see below). Some Russian terminology related to congenital syphilis is described in Chapter 4. Some indication of exposure to syphilis is found on ~15% of medical records of international adoptees from the former Soviet Union. In some cases, the birth mother had adequately treated syphilis years before the conception of this child; in other cases, the newborn has obvious signs of congenital syphilis. Generally, newborns with any indication of possible syphilis exposure are treated with antibiotics under the direction of a "dermato-venereologist." Although details of the type, route, dose, and duration of treatment are rarely provided, serologic and clinical evaluations of these children after arrival in the United States suggest that most have been adequately treated. Because of the social stigma associated with syphilis, local adopting families often decline adoption of these children.

China

For many years, no pre-adoptive information about syphilis testing was available for children from China. Recently, results of syphilis screening have been included on many pre-adoptive medical reports. These tests are listed as

"TRUST" or RPR. Prenatal and maternal histories are unavailable for Chinese adoptees. If children with congenital syphilis are identified and treated prior to adoption, this information is not habitually included with medical referrals.

Guatemala

Medical referrals of infants from Guatemala often include results of maternal laboratory tests for syphilis (and for HIV and hepatitis B), as well as those of the child. Documentation of treatment is usually available for infected children. Results of standard laboratory tests (RPR) are usually provided for older children.

Korea

Syphilis screening results are usually included in pre-adoptive medical records from Korea. Occasionally, medical records indicate a diagnosis of congenital syphilis; details of evaluation and treatment are also recorded.[11]

Other Countries

Information about syphilis from other countries is sporadic. Even if screening protocols for congenital syphilis are well established, children placed for international adoption may have missed testing, have unavailable or unreliable results, or have been infected after testing (through sexual abuse).

Clinical Features of Congenital Syphilis

Syphilis is readily transmitted from an infected mother to her unborn child. Recently infected mothers (primary or secondary syphilis) have 70%–100% likelihood of transmitting the disease to the fetus.[28] Infants are usually infected transplacentally; this can occur at any stage of pregnancy and during any stage of maternal syphilis.[29] The fetus is infected hematogenously, resulting in widespread involvement. Less commonly, the infant becomes infected at the time of delivery via contact with an active syphilitic lesion.[4,28]

Judith was adopted from Romania. Her parents had to make two trips to complete the adoption. At age 2 months, she seemed perfectly healthy. When they returned 1 month later, she had an odd rash on her trunk, palms, and soles. A Romanian pediatrician told her parents that Judith had syphilis. Lab work proved this was correct, and appropriate therapy was begun immediately.

Only about one-third to one-half of infected infants are symptomatic at birth;[16,28] the remainder are asymptomatic and may not come to medical attention for months or years unless serology is tested. Early and late congenital syphilis have variable manifestations (Tables 19–4 and 19–5). Clinical findings of late congenital syphilis result from further hematogenous spread of the organism[28] and occur in about 40% of untreated infants. Failure to thrive, persistent fevers, hepatitis/hepatomegaly, aseptic meningitis, and nonspecific skin rashes all may appear after the newborn period.[4,26] Laboratory clues to diagnosis include elevated alkaline phosphatase (out of proportion to aminotransferases) and monocytosis.[26]

In general, adequate therapy in the neonatal period prevents complications of late congenital syphilis.[28] However, incomplete treatment may delay disease expression. Early treatment does not completely protect against the development of Hutchinson teeth,[33] keratitis, or saber shins.[4,6,30] Multiple courses of treatment may be needed to treat children co-infected with HIV.

Diagnosis

The diagnosis of congenital syphilis is usually based on results of the mother's serologic tests.[28] Ideally, the mother is tested several times during pregnancy and also at delivery.

Table 19–4 Early congenital syphilis: first 2 years of life[a]

Area Affected	Symptoms
General	Low birth weight, lymphadenopathy
Mucocutaneous	Maculopapular or vesiculobullous rash including palms and soles, followed by desquamation, fissures around the oral, nasal, and anal mucous membranes[4,29]
Gastrointestinal	Hepatomegaly with or without splenomegaly, abnormal liver function tests (may have isolated elevation in alkaline phosphatase[26] hyperbilirubinemia, pancreatitis
Respiratory	Rhinitis, coryza, "snuffles" (profuse nasal drainage lasting longer than a cold, can be bloody and can contain live spirochetes), abnormal chest x-ray: "pneumonia alba"
Hematologic	Coombs-negative hemolytic anemia, thrombocytopenia, leukocytosis or leukopenia, monocytosis
Renal	Nephrotic syndrome
Bone	Osteochondritis, periostitis (abnormal x-rays in 90% of symptomatic and 20% of asymptomatic infants) (Fig. 19–2)
Neurologic	Abnormal cerebrospinal fluid in 80%, cranial nerve palsies, hydrocephalus, cerebral infarction, seizure disorders, mental retardation

[a]Usual presentation is within 15 weeks of birth.

Source: Data from refs. 3, 4, 26, 28.

Table 19–5 Late congenital syphilis: after 2 years of age

Area Affected	Symptoms
Ocular	Interstitial keratitis (usually appears close to puberty, ground-glass appearance in the cornea with vascularization of the sclera, can cause blindness)
Neurologic	Paresis, eighth-nerve deafness (~8–10 years of age), developmental delays, hydrocephalus
Dental	Hutchinson's teeth (notched central incisors, seen in deciduous and permanent teeth), mulberry molars (abnormal development of cusps of first molars), or Moon's molars (small, domed first molars) (Fig. 19–3); perioral fissures, tongue lesions[31]
Musculoskeletal	Painless knee arthritis (Clutton's joints) and saber shins. Rarely, unilateral and asymmetrical,[32] sternoclavicular thickening, flaring scapulae
Bone	Saddle nose, frontal bossing, short maxilla, perforation of the hard palate, protruding mandible

Source: Data from refs. 28–30.

She *and* her infant may be seronegative early after infection. Results of syphilis testing of birth mothers of international adoptees are seldom available, except for some infants from Guatemala. Diagnosis thus rests on the results of the child's tests.

Screening tests for syphilis, or nontreponemal antigen tests, detect antibody to the cell membrane glycolipid cardiolipin. Examples include the Venereal Disease Research Laboratory (VDRL) microscopic slide test or rapid plasma reagin (RPR). Titers of these tests are useful to follow response to treatment. Positive screening tests must be confirmed with treponemal tests such as fluorescent treponemal antibody absorption (FTA-ABS) and microag-glutination–*T. pallidum* (MHA-TP). These tests usually remain reactive for life[28]; antibody titers do not correlate with disease activity.[29] Although non-treponemal tests rarely give false negative results, it is worthwhile to consider testing all new arrivals with a treponemal test as well (usually MHA-TP).[34,35] False positives occasionally occur.

Neither nontreponemal nor treponemal tests distinguish maternal IgG from antibody produced by the fetus in response to infection.[28] Comparison of mother's and infant's titers to differentiate maternal antibody from passive transfer is not possible for international adoptees. Newer diagnostic tests may allow discrimination of maternal antibody from active infection.[28]

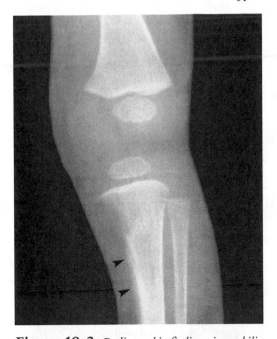

Figure 19–2 *Radiographic findings in syphilis. Typical features include thickened cortex over the metaphysis, symmetrical lateral metaphyseal defects of the proximal tibia (Windberger's sign), and subperiosteal cortical thickening.*

Neurosyphilis is difficult to diagnose.[36] The combination of physical examination, conventional laboratory tests, radiographic studies, and IgM immunoblotting and PCR testing (if available) of serum and cerebrospinal fluid (CSF) best identifies infants with neurosyphilis.[37] Treatment

Erin, a Chinese 15-month-old, had a positive VDRL, 1:16, on her first blood test after arrival. Her FTA-ABS and MHA-TP tests were negative. She was clinically well. Over 3 months, her titer decreased to nondetectable, suggesting that this was maternal antibody.

regimens for newborns are thus designed to eradicate neurosyphilis, as ascertainment of infection remains difficult. Lumbar puncture should be performed in any child with positive treponemal antibody tests.

Darkfield microscopic examination of nasal discharge or exudate from skin lesions may reveal *T. pallidum* organisms.[29]

Management

New arrivals should all undergo serologic testing for syphilis with a nontreponemal antigen test. Children whose test results are negative need no further evaluation. Those with a history of treated congenital syphilis should have careful clinical examination and follow-up RPR testing at 1, 2, 3 or 4, 6, and 12 months of age. Ophthalmologic and audiologic evaluations should be obtained. Nontreponemal antibody

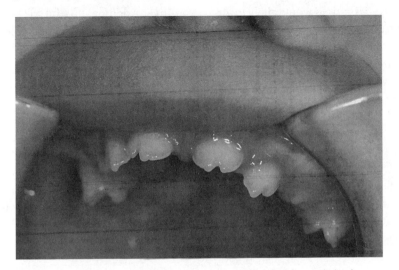

Figure 19–3 *Dental anomalies in a child with congenital syphilis. (With permission.)*

titers should be nonreactive by 6 months of age if the infant was adequately treated or was not infected and initially seropositive due to maternal antibody.[3,28] If sexual abuse is suspected, testing should be repeated 1 or more months after arrival in the United States to identify children infected just prior to departure. Children adopted at <3 months of age should be screened at the time of adoption, and then again at 10–12 weeks of age.[27,28]

Children with positive nontreponemal screening tests should have confirmatory treponemal antigen tests performed. If positive, more complete evaluation should be undertaken, including CSF analysis (cells, protein, VDRL), long-bone films, CBC with platelet count, liver function tests, ophthalmologic exam, auditory brain stem evoked responses, and chest radiograph. Sufficient serum should be collected prior to treatment so that serial titers can be determined in the same assay.

The Centers for Disease Control and Prevention (CDC)[36] define high-risk children as those whose mother's syphilis was *(1)* untreated or inadequately treated during pregnancy; *(2)* treated with non-penicillin regimen; *(3)* treated, but antibody titers did not decrease after therapy as expected; *(4)* treated less than 1 month prior to delivery; *(5)* treated, but details are undocumented; or *(6)* was not adequately serologically followed after treatment to judge response. These definitions would apply to virtually all internationally adopted children with a maternal history of syphilis. Furthermore, a history of maternal syphilis may be unknown. Thus, syphilis must be carefully considered in all international adoptees.

Treatment

Treatment of children with congenital syphilis varies greatly throughout the world. Parenteral antibiotic treatment is usually limited to intramuscular injections; maintenance of long-term intravenous access in infants is uncommon in some settings.

Details of treatment protocols for congenital syphilis are available in standard pediatric references. The *Red Book*[3] recommends that children older than 4 weeks of age with possible congenital syphilis (or who have neurologic involvement) should be treated with aqueous crystalline penicillin, 200,000 to 300,000 U/kg per day intravenously (administered every 6 hours) for 10 days. This regimen also should be used to treat children older than 1 year of age who have late and previously untreated congenital syphilis. Some experts also suggest giving such patients benzathine penicillin G, 50 000 U/kg intramuscularly in three weekly doses following the 10-day course of intravenous aqueous penicillin.[3] If the patient has minimal clinical manifestations of disease, normal CSF examination, and negative CSF VDRL, three weekly doses of benzathine penicillin G, 50,000 U/kg intramuscularly, may suffice.

After treatment, children should be followed up at 1, 2, 3, 6, and 12 months with careful physical examination and repeat serology.[3,28] Children should have a fourfold decrease in VDRL by 3 months and an eightfold decrease (or nonreactive) by 6 months.[28] Follow-up CSF assay should be done at 6 months of age, and retreatment should be considered if the VDRL is positive. Additional useful follow-up includes annual hearing and ophthalmologic evaluations, and screening for neurologic, dental, and developmental disorders.

Key Points for Internationally Adopted Children

- Undiagnosed syphilis is uncommon in international adoptees but critically important to recognize.
- All new arrivals should be tested for syphilis.

- Some children arrive with previously treated congenital syphilis; these children deserve close attention and follow-up.
- Some children with congenital syphilis present with late complications, even if adequately treated. Dental anomalies are most common, but ocular or auditory complications may occur.

FAQs

Q. *Valerie was adopted from Russia. She was born at home, and apparently didn't have any medical assessment until she was 5 months old and entered institutional care. At that time, she was diagnosed with syphilis. It looks like she probably got reasonable treatment, according to her records from Russia—28 days of penicillin injections, although there is no information about the dose. What are her risks of long-term complications? Her prospective parents are especially worried about the late development of deafness or eye problems.*

A. Interstitial keratitis and dental abnormalities may rarely occur even after adequate treatment in infancy. She should have annual ophthalmologic, hearing, and neurologic examinations along with general follow-up.

Q. *Even worse, Roberto just arrived at 15 months of age from El Salvador and has strongly positive VDRL and FTA-ABS results. I presume he's had untreated congenital syphilis all this time. What about risks of future complications for him?*

A. This is a higher-risk situation, as his disease was untreated for so long. He should have a complete assessment to determine the extent of disease (see above) and treatment should be started immediately.

Q. *Is there such a thing as maternal antibodies for syphilis that don't mean infection in the child?*

A. Yes. Both nontreponemal (RPR and VDRL) and treponemal tests (FTA-ABS and MHA-TP) detect both IgM and IgG class of antibodies. Thus, these cannot distinguish between passively transferred maternal IgG antibody and polyclonal IgG and IgM antibodies produced in response to active infection. Without access to the mother's

serum for comparison, it is prudent to assume that these antibodies represent infection. Infants with positive results should be fully evaluated and treated. An exception would be a clinically well infant with extremely low titers. This child may be closely monitored with serial blood tests. If titers disappear, it may be presumed that this represented maternal antibody.

Q. *The VDRL I ordered on my new patient from Lithuania came back positive. The sample was automatically forwarded to the State Board of Health and a MHA-TP test was done on it. That test was negative. What does it all mean, and what do I do now?*

A. This most likely is a false positive test, which may be due to autoimmune disease, tuberculosis, infectious mononucleosis, endocarditis, or recent febrile illness. A follow-up of both tests in a few weeks should be done, and other diagnoses considered in the interim.

Q. *Harry was treated in El Salvador for congenital syphilis. I don't have the details of his treatment. His VDRL and FTA-ABS IgG are positive here in the United States. Does he need a lumbar puncture?*

A. Yes. He should also have roentgenograms of his long bones and auditory and visual testing. If any evidence of syphilis is found or test results are equivocal, aggressive antibiotic treatment should be given.

Q. *I've been taking care of Janine for 3 years, since she arrived from Bulgaria. She's now 9 years old, and I've become convinced from what her mother reports and what Janine says that she had been sexually abused in Bulgaria. Luckily, I had done a VDRL when she was first adopted, which was negative, and a follow-up one last week was also negative. Her case makes me wonder if all kids should have a follow-up VDRL sometime after adoption, and not just the initial test that is usually recommended. What if a child was sexually abused—and exposed to syphilis — just prior to the adoption? Testing within a few days or weeks might not identify a recent exposure. Should follow-up tests be routinely done for syphilis like we do for HIV, hepatitis B, and hepatitis C?*

A. This is worth considering, but at present no standard recommendations for follow-up testing of syphilis serology have been established. Initial and follow-up testing should certainly be obtained in situations where sexual abuse is suspected or proven.

Useful Web Sites

National Center for HIV, STD and TB Prevention, Division of Sexually Transmitted Diseases. Some facts about syphilis. Available at: http://www.cdc.gov/nchstp/dstd/Fact_Sheets/syphilis_Facts.htm.

National Institute of Allergy and Infectious Diseases. Syphilis. Available at: http://www.niaid.nih.gov/factsheets/stdsyph.htm.

References

1. Glaser JH. Centers for Disease Control and Prevention guidelines for congenital syphilis. J Pediatr 1996; 129:488–90.

2. Hollier LM, Cox SM. Syphilis. Semin Perinatol 1998; 22:323–31.

3. American Academy of Pediatrics. Syphilis. In: Pickering L, ed. 2003 Red Book: Report of the Committee on Infectious Diseases. Elk Grove Village, IL: American Academy of Pediatrics, 2003: 595–607.

4. Starling SP. Syphilis in infants and young children. Pediatr Ann 1994; 23:334–40.

5. Sung L, MacDonald NE. Syphilis: a pediatric perspective. Pediatr Rev 1998; 19:17–22.

6. Gutman LT. Syphilis. In: Feigin RD, Cherry JD, eds. Textbook of Pediatric Infectious Diseases. Philadelphia: W.B. Saunders, 1998: 1543–56.

7. Albers LH, Johnson DE, Hostetter MK, Iverson S, Miller LC. Health of children adopted from the former Soviet Union and Eastern Europe. Comparison with preadoptive medical records. JAMA 1997; 278:922–4.

8. Saiman L, Aronson J, Zhou J, et al. Prevalence of infectious diseases among internationally adopted children. Pediatrics 2001; 108:608–12.

9. Miller LC, Hendrie NW. Health of children adopted from China. Pediatrics 2000; 105:E76.

10. Hostetter MK, Iverson S, Thomas W, McKenzie D, Dole K, Johnson DE. Medical evaluation of internationally adopted children. N Engl J Med 1991; 325:479–85.

11. Lange WR, Warnock-Eckhart E. Selected infectious disease risks in international adoptees. Pediatr Infect Dis J 1987; 6:447–50.

12. Nicholson AJ, Francis BM, Mulholland EK, Moulden AL, Oberklaid F. Health screening of interna-tional adoptees. Evaluation of a hospital based clinic. Med J Aust 1992; 156:377–9.

13. Miller LC, Kiernan MT, Mathers MI, Klein-Gitelman M. Developmental and nutritional status of internationally adopted children. Arch Pediatr Adolesc Med 1995; 149:40–4.

14. Johnson DE, Miller LC, Iverson S, et al. The health of children adopted from Romania. JAMA 1992; 268:3446–51.

15. Bureau JJ, Maurage C, Bremond M, Despert F, Rolland JC. Children of foreign origin adopted in France. Analysis of 68 cases during 12 years at the University Hospital Center of Tours [in French]. Arch Pediatr 1999; 6:1053–8.

16. Finelli L, Berman SM, Koumans EH, Levine WC. Congenital syphilis. Bull World Health Organ 1998; 76 Suppl 2:126–8.

17. Tichonova L, Borisenko K, Ward H, Meheus A, Gromyko A, Renton A. Epidemics of syphilis in the Russian Federation: trends, origins, and priorities for control. Lancet 1997; 350:210–3.

18. Ingram M. Syphilis soars in Russia. BMJ 1995; 311:78.

19. Lycova SG, Khryanin AA. Trends in the incidence of syphilis and gonorrhoea in Novosibirsk region, western Siberia. Sex Transm Infect 1999; 75:448–9.

20. Riedner G, Dehne KL, Gromyko A. Recent declines in reported syphilis rates in Eastern Europe and central Asia: are the epidemics over? Sex Transm Infect 2000; 76:363–5.

21. Waugh MA. Epidemics of syphilis in the Russian Federation. Lancet 1997; 350:595.

22. Chen XS, Gong XD, Liang GJ, Zhang GC. Epidemiologic trends of sexually transmitted diseases in China. Sex Transm Dis 2000; 27:138–42.

23. World Health Organization. Status and Trends of STI, HIV/AIDS in Western Pacific 1999. China. Available at: http://www.wpro.who.int/Technical/unit/STD/pdf/sti-part2_04_china.pdf.

24. Sison CG, Ostrea EMJ, Reyes MP, Salari V. The resurgence of congenital syphilis: a cocaine-related problem. J Pediatr 1997; 130:289–92.

25. World Health Organization. Estimated new cases of syphilis among adults. 1999. Available at: http://www.who.int/docstore/hiv/GRSTI/pdf/figure09.pdf.

26. Dorfman DH, Glaser JH. Congenital syphilis presenting in infants after the newborn period. N Engl J Med 1990; 323:1299–302.

27. Jonna S, Collins M, Abedin M, Young M, Milteer R, Beeram M. Postneonatal screening for congenital syphilis. J Fam Pract 1995; 41:286–8.

28. Stoll BJ. Congenital syphilis: evaluation and management of neonates born to mothers with reactive sero-

logic tests for syphilis. Pediatr Infect Dis J 1994; 13:845–52; quiz 853.

29. Ikeda MK, Jenson HB. Evaluation and treatment of congenital syphilis. J Pediatr 1990; 117:843–52.

30. Azimi PH. Interstitial keratitis in a five-year-old. Pediatr Infect Dis J 1999; 18:299, 311.

31. Ulmer A, Fierlbeck G. Oral manifestations of secondary syphilis. N Engl J Med 2002; 347:1677.

32. Gadea A, Figueredo M, Bowen JR. Persistent bony lesions in congenital syphilis. A report of three cases. Int Orthop 1993; 17:43–7.

33. Christian CW, Lavelle J, Bell LM. Preschoolers with syphilis. Pediatrics 1999; 103:E4.

34. Birnbaum NR, Goldschmidt RH, Buffett WO. Resolving the common clinical dilemmas of syphilis. Am Fam Physician 1999; 59:2233–40, 2245–6.

35. Muic V, Ljubicic M, Vodopija I. Bayes' theorem–based assessment of VDRL syphilis screening miss rates. Sex Transm Dis 1999; 26:12–6.

36. Beeram MR, Chopde N, Dawood Y, Siriboe S, Abedin M. Lumbar puncture in the evaluation of possible asymptomatic congenital syphilis in neonates. J Pediatr 1996; 128:125–9.

37. Michelow IC, Wendel GDJ, Norgard MV, et al. Central nervous system infection in congenital syphilis. N Engl J Med 2002; 346:1792–8.

20

HELICOBACTER PYLORI

Helicobacter pylori (HP) infection is perhaps the most common infection of humankind.[1–3] At least 1 billion people are infected;[4] most acquire the infection in infancy or early childhood.[5] Infection with HP may contribute to the poor growth of institutionalized children[6,7] and to the failure to thrive of some international adoptees after arrival to the United States. In a recent serosurvey, 31% of 226 children from 18 countries had antibodies to HP.[7] Antibodies were common among children who had previously resided in an orphanage (vs. foster care) (Fig. 20–1), were older at adoption (43.4 months ± 4.3 vs. 17.2 months ± 1.8, p <0.0001), and were co-infected with intestinal parasites (44% vs. 19%, p = 0.002). International adoptees are at high risk for acquisition of HP infection in early life and thus also for the long-term problems associated with infection.

This chapter reviews the epidemiology, gastrointestinal manifestations, effects on growth, anemia, diagnostic tests, and treatment of HP infection for internationally adopted children.

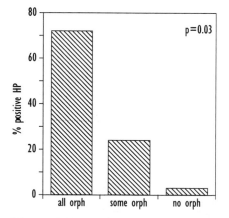

Figure 20–1 *Seroprevalence of* H. pylori *(HP) infection relates to residence prior to adoption in orphanage (orph), foster care (no orph), or mixed. (Reprinted with permission from Blackwell Publishing, Ltd. Miller LC, Kelly N, Tannemaat M, Grand R. Serologic prevalence of antibodies to* Helicobacter pylori *in internationally adopted children.* Helicobacter *2003; 8(3): 173.)*

Epidemiology

The incidence of HP infection varies enormously throughout the world (Fig. 20–2).[4] The infection clusters within families with young children, especially those residing in crowded conditions.[4] Infection is more common among poor children and in developing countries.[5] The highest prevalence of infection occurs among residents of institutions, submarine crews, crowded households, and orphanages.[6] Young children with faltering growth in developing countries also have very high prevalence of infection.[8] Most children in high-risk groups become infected by the first or second year of life.[6,9] The route of transmission is unknown but is suspected to be fecal–oral or oral–oral.[4] Breast milk IgA antibodies protect infants from infection.[1,10]

Gastrointestinal Manifestations of Helicobacter pylori Infection

Infected individuals have lifelong chronic gastritis; spontaneous resolution of infection is infrequent. Some individuals are asymptomatic for

Elizabeth, an 8-year-old developmentally delayed and non-verbal child adopted from Romania at age 4, had progressive and severe behavior problems. As she became more violent and aggressive, her mother became convinced that her daughter was in pain. Serologic tests for H. pylori *were negative, but eventually endoscopy was done and revealed "the worst case of* H. pylori *I've ever seen," according to the gastroenterologist. Treatment corresponded with marked improvement in Elizabeth's behavior. Cultures of the* H. pylori *organism revealed multiple drug resistance.*

decades,[4] however, morbidity increases with duration of infection.[10] Symptoms suggesting HP infection include epigastric pain, nocturnal abdominal pain, hematemesis, recurrent vomiting, and protein-losing enteropathy.[4,11] Most infected children have no obvious symptoms, although chronic gastritis is found pathologically. Some children have duodenal ulcer disease. Eradication of infection promotes healing of chronic gastritis and duodenal ulcers.[5] It is unknown whether infants and young children have transient infections.[9,12]

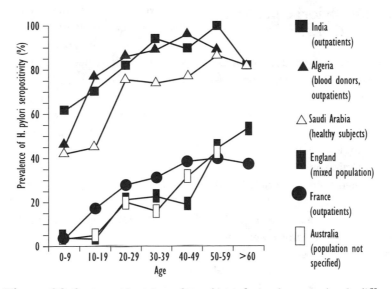

Figure 20–2 *Seroepidemiology of* H. pylori *infection demonstrating the difference in disease prevalence between developing and developed countries. (Reprinted from Textbook of Pediatric Infectious Diseases, Vol. 2, Feigin RD, Cherry JD, p 1490. Copyright 1998, with permission from Elsevier.)*

Kenny arrived at 18 months of age from Russia. He was healthy, though small. A handsome and engaging boy who seemed well adjusted and happy, he awoke frequently at night with loud crying. His parents suspected night terrors and tried a behavioral approach. Little improvement occurred. A sleep expert suggested more stringent responses by the parents, which they attempted to no avail. Discouraged and worried, they tried to think of other reasons for Kenny's wakening. As Kenny developed more language, he was able to tell them, "My tummy hurts." Further investigation led to identification of moderately severe gastritis and HP infection. Shortly after treatment, Kenny began to sleep through the night without disturbance.

A small subset of untreated patients develop gastric cancers (adenocarcinoma or lymphoma).[2,4,13] Individuals infected with *cagA*-producing strains are the most susceptible.[14] The International Agency for Research on Cancer designates HP as a "group 1 human carcinogen."[14] Gastic cancer is a leading cause of death in the developing world, where early childhood infection with HP is the rule.[10,13,14]

Helicobacter pylori *Infection and Growth*

Infection with HP may cause dyspepsia, decreased energy intake, malnutrition, chronic gastritis, and cytokine release (possibly IL-8[15]). These factors, alone or in combination, may adversely affect growth.

Intriguing studies from the developing world link HP infection and malnutrition. In the Gambia, elevated titers of anti-HP antibodies were strongly associated with malnutrition in children less than 30 months of age. Children with marasmus and diarrhea were more likely to be infected than those with marasmus alone. Children in Korea or West Africa with persistent diarrhea and malnutrition had more than twice the prevalence of HP infection than that of healthy controls.[1,11,16] Similarly, HP infection was more common in malnourished

children in Colombia and Peru.[17,18] However, no relation was found between either brief or persistent diarrhea and HP infection among infants in Peru.[19]

Infection with HP may cause gastric achlorhydria,[16] which can predispose to enteric infections. Loss of the gastric acid barrier at critical times allows passage of enteric pathogens to the small intestine, resulting in persistent diarrhea, malnutrition, and failure to thrive (see Chapters 17 and 10). *Helicobacter pylori* infection, depressed urine acid output, malnutrition, and growth failure were strongly associated in Gambian infants.[8] Infection with HP was also associated with reduced gastric acid secretion for at least 3 months after infection. Infants with HP infection had poor growth compared with uninfected children: the authors suggest that HP may open the door to other infections that more directly impact growth.

Among privileged children in the Western world, HP infection is associated with growth delay in older children,[10,15,20,21] although this is not supported in all studies.[22] Serosurveys in Guatemala and Bangladesh detected no relation of HP infection to height,[23,24] possibly because many other factors contributed to short stature. Lengthy follow-up may be needed to identify the effects of HP infection on linear growth.[15] In a serologic survey of elderly people, the highest infection rate was found in men who had failed to thrive at 1 year of age. The authors speculate that HP may directly cause growth failure in infancy, or that smaller infants are more susceptible to infection.[10]

Helicobacter pylori *Infection and Iron Deficiency Anemia*

Helicobacter pylori infection is also associated with iron deficiency anemia (see Chapter 11), probably a consequence of gastric achlorhydria, which reduces iron absorption. Refractory iron deficiency anemia improves after treatment of HP infection. In Korean preadolescents, those with iron deficiency anemia had twice as many HP infections as those who were non-anemic; height was reduced in children who had both anemia and HP infection.[11]

Diagnosis of Helicobacter pylori Infection

Definitive diagnosis of HP infection is difficult without endoscopy, especially in young children who are not able to cooperate with [13]-C-urea breath testing. Serology, although readily available, is not the preferred method to diagnose infection, especially in children.[5] IgG antibody does not appear for more than 9 months after infection in infants.[9] Infected children may not achieve maximal antibodies to HP until age 7 or 8 years.[5] Young children have low titers after infection. Furthermore, their antibodies may recognize different immunodominant proteins than those produced by adults, affecting the sensitivity of screening tests.[2] Antibodies do not eliminate the infection and remain positive for a variable period of time after infection.[4] In most patients, antibody titers decrease over 6–12 months but remain detectable.[25] Spontaneous clearance of infection may occur even in children with persistent antibody.[26] Thus, the sensitivity and specificity of antibody testing are suboptimal in children. In a comparison of seven diagnostic methods in 53 children with abdominal pain,[26] 27 children were identified with HP infection by means of gold-standard methods (either culture, or two of three tests positive: histology, biopsy urease test, or [13]-C-urea breath test). The accuracy of the other tests evaluated were stool antigen test, 96%; biopsy urease test, 96%; histology, 98%; polymerase chain reaction, 94%; culture, 98%; urea breath test, 100%; and serology, 85%. Others confirm that the [13]-C-urea breath test is both sensitive and specific in children over 6 years.[5] In another report, stool antigen tests had 100% sensitivity, 70% specificity, 54% positive predictive value, and 100% negative predictive value; application of the test to samples obtained from children must still be refined before widespread clinical use.[27] Therefore, noninvasive diagnosis in young children remains problematic.

Who Should Be Tested?

Some investigators suggest that testing be done only among those in whom the symptoms are severe enough to justify the risks of therapy.[5] Decision analysis in adult populations suggests the most efficient, cost-effective strategy is to check serology in dyspeptic patients under age 45 and treat accordingly.[28] The conclusion of the European Consensus Conference on HP in 1998 was that screening should not be performed routinely in children with gastrointestinal symptoms (including abdominal pain) but only if symptoms suggested peptic ulcer or esophagitis.[5] However, these recommendations were based on clinical experience with European children from low-risk environments. Internationally adopted children come from high-risk environments. A high index of suspicion should be maintained in this group of children. The diagnosis of HP infection should be vigorously pursued if symptoms warrant. When noninvasive testing methods improve (e.g., stool antigen tests or PCR), screening all newly arrived international adoptees will be worth consideration.

Treatment of Helicobacter pylori

About 90% of HP infections are cured when medications are used properly.[2] General recommendations for treatment are two antibacterial agents (e.g., amoxicillin and clarithromycin) and a proton-pump inhibitor (omeprazole) for 14 days.[29–35] Unfortunately, drug resistance is becoming more frequent and may be more common in organisms acquired in the developing world.[36] There are marked geographic differences in the frequency of resistant organisms.[37–40] Management of drug-resistant HP usually requires consultation with infectious disease and gastroenterology specialists.

Key Points for Internationally Adopted Children

- International adoptees are at high risk for HP infection.
- *H. pylori* infection may contribute to the poor growth of international adoptees prior to arrival in the United States.
- Infection with HP should be considered in internationally adopted children with epigastric pain, nocturnal abdominal pain, hematemesis, recurrent vomiting, protein-losing enteropathy, poor growth, other intestinal infections, or resistant iron deficiency anemia.
- Infection with HP is associated with increased long-term risk of gastric cancer.

FAQs

Q. Which children should be evaluated for HP infection?

A. Besides those children with obvious symptoms suggesting HP infection, children with poor growth, multiple intestinal infections (bacterial and/or parasitic), and resistant iron deficiency anemia would be good candidates for screening.

Q. What screening tests are appropriate?

A. Serology plus one or more additional methods should be used. Stool antigen tests are becoming more available and more reliable. If children are old enough, the ^{13}-C-urea breath test is another excellent noninvasive method to identify infections. If necessary, children should undergo endoscopy to confirm the diagnosis.

Q. What should be done with children whose test results are positive for HP?

A. Infected children should be treated. In some cases (for example, a symptomatic child with positive serology), "empiric" treatment with triple therapy may be offered, although definitive diagnosis is preferable. Close follow-up is necessary, with further investigations if symptoms do not resolve. Serology is unlikely to correlate with disease activity or cure; other follow-up tests are more useful, especially if symptoms continue.

References

1. Weaver LT. Royal Society of Tropical Medicine and Hygiene Meeting at Manson House, London, 16 February 1995. Aspects of *Helicobacter pylori* infection in the developing and developed world. *Helicobacter pylori* infection, nutrition and growth of West African infants. Trans R Soc Trop Med Hyg 1995; 89:347–50.

2. Czinn S. Serodiagnosis of *Helicobacter pylori* in pediatric patients. Pediatr Gastroenterol Nutr 1999; 28:132–4.

3. Suerbaum S, Michetti P. *Helicobacter pylori* infection. N Engl J Med 2002; 347:1175–86.

4. Gilger M. *Helicobacter pylori*. In: Feigin RD, Cherry JD, eds. Textbook of Pediatric Infectious Disease. Philadelphia: W.B. Saunders Company, 1998: 1488–93.

5. Drumm B, Koletzko S, Oderda G. *Helicobacter pylori* infection in children: a consensus statement. European Paediatric Task Force on *Helicobacter pylori*. J Pediatr Gastroenterol Nutr 2000; 30:207–13.

6. Lewindon PJ, Lau D, Chan A, Tse P, Sullivan PB. *Helicobacter pylori* in an institution for disabled children in Hong Kong. Dev Med Child Neurol 1997; 39:682–5.

7. Miller LC, Kelly N, Tannemaat M, Grand RJ. Serologic prevalence of antibodies to *Helicobacter pylori* in internationally adopted children. *Helicobacter* 2003; 8:173–8.

8. Dale A, Thomas JE, Darboe MK, Coward WA, Harding M, Weaver LT. *Helicobacter pylori* infection, gastric acid secretion, and infant growth. J Pediatr Gastroenterol Nutr 1998; 26:393–7.

9. Rothenbacher D, Inceoglu J, Bode G, Brenner H. Acquisition of *Helicobacter pylori* infection in a high-risk population occurs within the first 2 years of life. J Pediatr 2000; 136:744–8.

10. Fall CH, Goggin PM, Hawtin P, Fine D, Duggleby S. Growth in infancy, infant feeding, childhood living conditions, and *Helicobacter pylori* infection at age 70. Arch Dis Child 1997; 77:310–4.

11. Choe YH, Kim SK, Hong YC. *Helicobacter pylori* infection with iron deficiency anaemia and subnormal growth at puberty. Arch Dis Child 2000; 82:136–40.

12. Gold BD, Goodman K. *Helicobacter pylori* infection in children: to test or not to test . . . what is the evidence? [editorial; comment]. J Pediatr 2000; 136:714–6.

13. Wong BCY, Ching CK, Lam SK. *Helicobacter pylori* infection and gastric cancer. Hong Kong Med J 1999; 5:175–9.

14. Parsonnet J. *Helicobacter pylori* in the stomach—a paradox unmasked. N Engl J Med 1996; 335:278–280.

15. Perri F, Pastore M, Leandro G, et al. *Helicobacter pylori* infection and growth delay in older children. Arch Dis Child 1997; 77:46–49.

16. Sullivan PB, Thomas JE, Wight DG, et al. *Helicobacter pylori* in Gambian children with chronic diarrhoea and malnutrition. Arch Dis Child 1990; 65:189–91.

17. Goodman KJ, Correa P, Tengana Aux HJ, DeLany JP, Collazos T. Nutritional factors and *Helicobacter pylori* infection in Colombian children. J Pediatr Gastroenterol Nutr 1997; 25:507–15.

18. Klein PD, Graham DY, Gaillour A, Opekun AR, Smith EO. Water source as risk factor for *Helicobacter pylori* infection in Peruvian children. Gastrointestinal Physiology Working Group. Lancet 1991; 337:1503–6.

19. Castro-Rodriguez JA, Leon-Barua R, Penny M. *Helicobacter pylori* is not a determinant factor of persistent diarrhoea or malnutrition in Peruvian children. Trans R Soc Trop Med Hyg 1999; 93:537–9.

20. Patel P, Mendall MA, Khulusi S, Northfield TC, Strachan DP. *Helicobacter pylori* infection in childhood: risk factors and effect on growth. BMJ 1994; 309:1119–23.

21. Raymond J, Bergeret M, Benhamou PH, Mensah K, Dupont C. A 2-year study of *Helicobacter pylori* in children. J Clin Microbiol 1994; 32:461–3.

22. Oderda G, Palli D, Saieva C, Choiorboli E, Bona G. Short stature and *Helicobacter pylori* infection in Italian children: prospective multicentre hospital-based case–control study. BMJ 1998; 317:514–5.

23. Clemens J, Albert MJ, Rao M, et al. Sociodemographic, hygienic and nutritional correlates of *Helicobacter pylori* infection of young Bangladeshi children. Pediatr Infecti Dis J 1996; 15:1113–8.

24. Quinonez JM, Chew F, Torres O, Begue RE. Nutritional status of *Helicobacter pylori*–infected children in Guatemala as compared with uninfected peers. A J Trop Med Hyg 1999; 61:395–8.

25. Walsh J, Peterman W. The treatment of *Helicobacter pylori* infection in the management of peptic ulcer disease. N Engl J Med 1995; 333:984–91.

26. Ni YH, Lin JT, Huang SF, Yang JC, Chang MH. Accurate diagnosis of *Helicobacter pylori* infection by stool antigen test and 6 other currently available tests in children. J Pediatr 2000; 136:823–7.

27. Roggero P, Bonfiglio A, Luzzani S, et al. *Helicobacter pylori* stool antigen test: a method to confirm eradication in children. J Pediatr 2002; 140:775–7.

28. Friedman L. *Helicobacter pylori* and nonulcer dyspepsia. N Engl J Med 1998; 339:1928–30.

29. Teo EK, Fock KM, Ng TM, Khor CJ, Tan AL. Metronidazole-resistant *Helicobacter pylori* in an urban Asian population. J Gastroenterol Hepatol 2000; 15:494–7.

30. Rowland M, Imrie C, Bourke B, Drumm B. How should *Helicobacter pylori*–infected children be managed? Gut 1999; 45:136–9.

31. Covacci A, Telford JL, Del Giudice G, Parsonnet J, Rappuoli R. *Helicobacter pylori* virulence and genetic geography. Science 1999; 284:1328–33.

32. Robinson DM, Abdel-Rahman SM, Nahata MC. Guidelines for the treatment of *Helicobacter pylori* in the pediatric population. Ann Pharmacother 1997; 31:1247–9.

33. Sherman PM, Hunt RH. Why guidelines are required for the treatment of *Helicobacter pylori* infection in children. Clin Invest Med 1996; 19:362–7.

34. Malaty HM. *Helicobacter pylori* infection and eradication in paediatric patients. Paediatr Drugs 2000; 2:357–65.

35. Oderda G, Rapa A, Bona G. A systematic review of *Helicobacter pylori* eradication treatment schedules in children. Aliment Pharmacol Ther 2000; 14:59–66.

36. Houben MH, Van Der Beek D, Hensen EF, Craen AJ, Rauws EA, Tytgat GN. A systematic review of *Helicobacter pylori* eradication therapy—the impact of antimicrobial resistance on eradication rates. Aliment Pharmacol Ther 1999; 13:1047–55.

37. Banatvala N, Davies GR, Abdi Y, et al. High prevalence of *Helicobacter pylori* metronidazole resistance in migrants to east London: relation with previous nitroimidazole exposure and gastroduodenal disease. Gut 1994; 35:1562–6.

38. Gupta VK, Dhar A, Srinivasan S, Rattan A, Sharma MP. Eradication of *H. pylori* in a developing country: comparison of lansoprazole versus omeprazole with norfloxacin, in a dual-therapy study. Am J Gastroenterol 1997; 92:1140–2.

39. Ahuja V, Dhar A, Bal C, Sharma MP. Lansoprazole and secnidazole with clarithromycin, amoxycillin or pefloxacin in the eradication of *Helicobacter pylori* in a developing country. Aliment Pharmacol Ther 1998; 12:551–5.

40. Vasquez A, Valdez Y, Gilman RH, et al. Metronidazole and clarithromycin resistance in *Helicobacter pylori* determined by measuring MICs of antimicrobial agents in color indicator egg yolk agar in a miniwell format. The Gastrointestinal Physiology Working Group of Universidad Peruana Cayetano Heredia and the Johns Hopkins University. J Clin Microbiol 1996; 34:1232–4.

21

IMMUNIZATIONS AND VACCINE-PREVENTABLE DISEASES

On February 14, 2001, a group of Chinese girls returned to the United States with their new adoptive parents. One of the children, a 10-month-old girl, was ill upon arrival at the airport in Houston, Texas. She went directly to the Emergency Room at Texas Children's Hospital, where she was found to have fever, cough, coryza, Koplik spots, and rash. Measles was suspected and later confirmed. Public health investigation revealed measles infections in 14 other Chinese adoptees in nine states, from the same travel group.[1] One secondary case of measles also occurred. The outbreak was traced to a ceremony held at the Guangzhou Consulate General Office, where 54 adopting families met to receive their travel visas. Other exposures included Consulate staff (including one pregnant Chinese woman), hotel personnel, and flight attendants and passengers on numerous flights. A similar outbreak occurred in April 2004.[1a]

These outbreaks illustrate several points. First, vaccine-preventable diseases can and do occur among internationally adopted children. Indeed, in the first publication describing the comprehensive health problems of internationally adopted children, 4/128 children developed vaccine-preventable diseases within 30 days of arrival (2 with varicella, and 1 each with mumps and rubeola).[2] Second, these vaccine-preventable diseases can quickly spread to susceptible contacts. Most important, although the vaccine status of these children was not known, it has become apparent that immunization records of internationally adopted children may not denote immunity to vaccine-preventable diseases.

One of the first tasks of the physician caring for newly arrived international adoptees is to review vaccination records. Interpreting these records and formulating a plan for vaccine administration has been problematic. This area remains a topic of active research, and new findings and recommendations are likely to emerge over the next several years. This section reviews the adequacy of immunity to vaccine-preventable diseases, the interpretation of the vaccine record, and current recommendations for management of immunizations in internationally adopted children (see Chapter 9 and refs. 3–8 for recommendations of vaccines for adult and child international travelers).

Adequacy of Immunity: Is There a Problem?

Hostetter and Johnson[9] first emphasized the possible problems in vaccine-induced immunity among internationally adopted children. They state that their interest was piqued when they noted that some records indicated that vaccines had been administered prior to the child's birth date! On further scrutiny, other obvious flaws became apparent in vaccine records of some children adopted internationally. For example, "too perfect" dates of vaccine administration (Fig. 21–1), incorrect intervals of administration, and incorrect number of doses are common (Table 21–1). Although some investigators suggest that records in the "same handwriting/same ink color" should be considered fraudulent, this can occur when records are recopied in preparation for adoption.

Table 21–1 Immunization record from Russian orphanage showing excessive administration of polio vaccine in 32-month-old child (date, dose, lot number)

Poliomyelitis
December 22, 2000—2 drops 6012
February 25, 2001—2 drops 6017
March 25, 2001—2 drops 6735
April 24, 2001—2 drops 6738
August 15, 2001—2 drops 7112
December 19, 2001–2 drops 7118
June 12, 2002—2 drops 7129
October 5, 2002—2 drops 7139
June 28, 2003—2 drops 7228

Investigations of the immune status of international adoptees upon arrival to the United States have yielded somewhat different results. Hostetter and Johnson tested the immune status of 26 children adopted from China, Russia, and other Eastern European countries.[9] All children had received at least three diphtheria–tetanus–pertussis (DTP) vaccines. Titers of antibody to diptheria and tetanus were then determined. Adequacy of immunity was linked to the locale where the children had received their vaccines: only 12% of children vaccinated in orphanages had protective titers, compared

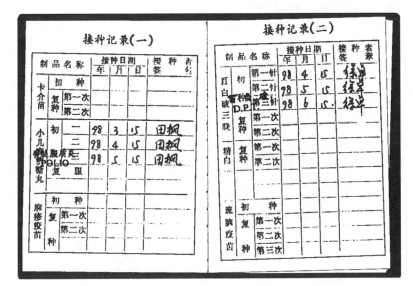

Figure 21–1 *Immunization record from China showing "too perfect" dates of vaccine administration.*

with 78% of those vaccinated in the community. Overall, only 35% of children with written records of age-appropriate immunizations had protective titers. When this study was extended to a larger group of children ($n = 55$), similar results were found.

Several follow-up studies have been reported. Some internationally adopted children with written documentation of three to six polio vaccines had inadequate titers of neutralizing antibodies to one or more serotypes of polio.[10, 11] Incomplete immunity to a broad panel of antigens was found in 70 international adoptees from 13 countries (43% from Russia or China) who had received ≥3 DTP or polio vaccines, or vaccination against measles, mumps, and rubella in their birth countries[11] (Table 21–2). No relation was found between immune status, the age of the child, the location of vaccine administration (orphanage vs. community), nutritional status, or associated medical problems.

A further study assessed the immune status of 51 children from 11 countries (Russia 39%, China 20%, Romania 10%, Korea 8%, Vietnam 6%, India 6%).[12] Strikingly better immune responses were detected. Of children who had received ≥2 DTP injections, 100% had protective titers against diphtheria toxin and 82% had protective titers against tetanus (most of the remainder had indeterminate immunity). Similarly, 67% of children who had received ≥2 hepatitis B virus (HBV) vaccines had hepatitis B surface antibody (HbsAb).

In the Netherlands, 133 internationally adopted children with ≥3 DPT and polio vaccinations recorded were tested for protective antibodies.[13] Only about three-fifths of the Chinese children were fully protected against tetanus and diphtheria; this is considerably lower than the children adopted from other countries (Table 21–3). Protection against polio was also lower in the Chinese children (71%–94% were immune for the different serotypes of polio vs. 82%–100% of children adopted from other countries and 96%–100% of British control children).[13]

Possible explanations for the variable results among these reports include differences in patient populations, methods and timing of ascertaining immunity, and inclusion criteria. Although exact results differ, it is clear that some internationally adopted children may have in-

Table 21–2 Immunity in internationally adopted children after vaccination in birth countries

Status	Percent with Immunity							
	Tetanus	Diphtheria	Polio-1	Polio-2	Polio-3	Measles	Mumps	Rubella
Immune	61	88	58	65	62	90	66	79
Borderline	35	9	0	0	0	0	14	4
Not immune	3	3	42	35	38	10	19	16

Source: Data from Miller et al.[11] Numbers are rounded.

Table 21–3 Immunity of children from China or other countries adopted in the Netherlands, compared with Dutch-born children

	Tetanus				Diphtheria			
	China	Other	Dutch[a]	Dutch[b]	China	Other	Dutch[a]	Dutch[b]
Immune	58	94	95	100	61	71	64	100
Borderline	29	6	5	0	23	26	31	0
Not immune	13	0	0	0	15	3	5	0

Numbers are rounded. [a]Tested 6 months after dose 3. [b]Tested 1 month after dose 4.

Source: Reprinted with permission from Elsevier.[13]

adequate immunity despite recorded vaccines. This may reflect falsification of written certificates, blunting of the immune response due to prolonged institutionalization, or decreased potency of vaccine lots used in orphanages.[9] Malnutrition may diminish immune responses to vaccines, although this is not confirmed in all studies.[14–19] Stress also reduces humoral immune responses after immunization.[20, 21] Improper vaccine storage and handling may be even more common in orphanages than in private practices in the United States,[22] where a recent survey detected storage problems in 44% of practices surveyed.

Interpretation of the Vaccine Record

Correct interpretation of the child's vaccine record is necessary to plan sensible management of vaccinations. An accurate translation is essential (Table 21–4). Many physicians rely on the vaccine record prepared as part of the child's medical visa evaluation. This form (Supplemental Form to OF-157, Visa Applicant's Documentation of Immunization, to be completed by panel physician only) was developed to fulfill the requirements of the U.S. Immigration and Nationality Act of 1996. This act mandates that applicants for permanent U.S. residency submit documentation that they have received all vaccines required by the Advisory Committee on Immunization Practices (ACIP). A waiver to this requirement was instituted in 1997 to exempt internationally adopted children <10 years of age, if new parents agree to ensure that the child receives needed vaccinations within 30 days of entry into the United States. This waiver spares children the burden of receiving multiple vaccinations just prior to travel to the United States. Although this form

Table 21–4 Vaccine terminology in Russian, Chinese, Romanian, and Spanish

Language	Diphtheria, Pertussis, Tetanus	Polio	Measles, Mumps, Rubella	Hepatitis B	Other
Russian	Дифтерия Коклюш Столбняк ,АКДС	Полиомиелит	Корь Эпидемический паротит Краснуха	Гепатит Б	Ветряная оспа = Varicella
Chinese	白喉 百日咳 破傷風	小兒麻痹	麻疹 腮腺炎 德國麻疹	乙型肝炎	日本乙型腦炎 "Encephalitis" or "cerebrospinal meningitis" usually refers to Japanese encephalitis but occasionally refers to meningococcal vaccine
Romanian	Tetracoq	AP (although occasionally this refers to antiparotitis)	AR (anti-rubeola)	AH	
Spanish	Difteria Tos ferina Tetanós	Polio	Sarampión Parótidas Rubeóla	Hepatitis B	"Meningitis" usually indicates *H. influenzae B* (HIB)

is widely used, its accuracy may be questionable. On this (and other forms), monovalent measles vaccine (commonly administered in many countries) may be recorded incorrectly in the space for MMR (measles, mumps, rubella), which is seldom administered in adoption sending countries.

A recent large study assessed the acceptability and completeness of overseas immunization records of internationally adopted children.[23] The criteria for a valid record included documentation of the type of vaccine and date of administration. Acceptability of overseas immunizations under the U.S. schedule required that the age of administration and intervals of administration meet the recommendations of the ACIP.[24] Of 504 children, only 178 had preadoption immunization records. Eleven of these were considered invalid. Children born in China were twice as likely to lack a valid immunization record. Only 9% of children with valid overseas immunization records were considered completely up to date according to the U.S. schedule; not surprising, as most countries use World Health Organization schedules which recommend fewer vaccines. More than two-thirds of the children were up to date for at least one vaccine series. Thus, deficiencies in the vaccine records of international adoptees are common by U.S. standards.

Management of Immunizations in the Internationally Adopted Child

As demonstrated by the studies cited above, a valid immunization record does not guarantee that a child has adequate immunity to vaccine-preventable diseases. The 2003 *Red Book* states the following:

Immunization records for certain children, especially for those from an orphanage, may not accurately reflect protection because of inaccuracies, lack of vaccine potency, or other problems, such as recording MMR but giving a product that did not contain one of the components (e.g., rubella).

Therefore, it may be reasonable to ascertain antibody titers for these children . . . if any question exists about whether immunizations were administered or were immunogenic, the best course is to repeat the injection of the immunizations in question.[8] The ACIP formulated a more detailed statement with essentially the same conclusions.[24] These recommendations are summarized in Table 21–5.

The potential for overadministering DTaP vaccine is the most significant risk if vaccinations are given without prior assessment of immunity. The fourth and fifth DTaP doses may be associated with localized arm swelling (which can be severe but resolves completely without sequelae).[25] Otherwise, ACIP recommendations indicate that vaccination (if, in fact, it is revaccination) is unlikely to cause complications.

At present, these ACIP recommendations are applicable to *all* internationally adopted children (and also to most immigrant children, except those from industrialized countries). However, the present recommendations are not based on large-scale peer-reviewed research. Published reports to date have not addressed the immune status of internationally adopted children from regions other than Russia, China, and Eastern Europe. Many practitioners believe that vaccines administered in South Korea, India, and Central and South America are more reliable.[26] No data yet address this important query. Based on the quality of medical care offered to Korean children awaiting adoption and Guatemalan children in foster care, it seems reasonable to assume that vaccines are properly administered. Thus valid immunization records (see above) can probably be accepted. Likely other exceptions will be identified.

There are several pitfalls with the use and interpretation of titers to verify immunity (Table 21–6). Most important, the correct test must be ordered. Neutralizing antibodies determine immunity to polio. Such antibodies persist lifelong and correlate with immunity; complement-fixing antibodies (often the "default test" in laboratories when further specifications are not provided) are elevated only briefly after exposure. Hemagglutination assays underestimate

Table 21–5 Approaches to evaluation of immunizations of internationally adopted children

Disease(s)	*Recommended Approach*	*Alternative Approach*
Measles, mumps, rubella	(Re)vaccinate with MMR	Conduct serologic testing for IgG antibodies to measles, mumps, rubella (as indicated in vaccine record)

Comments: If record indicates receipt of monovalent measles or measles-rubella vaccine at age ≥1 year, and child has protective antibody against measles and rubella, give a single dose of MMR as age-appropriate to ensure protection against mumps (and rubella if measles vaccine alone had been used). If record indicates receipt of MMR at age ≥12 months, and child has protective concentration of antibody to measles, no additional vaccination is needed unless required for school entry.

HIB	Age-appropriate vaccination	—
Hepatitis B	Serologic testing	

Comments: If records indicate receipt of ≥3 doses of vaccine, child may be protected. Additional doses are not needed if ≥1 doses were administered at age ≥6 months. Children who received their last hepatitis B vaccine dose at age ≤6 months should receive an additional dose at age ≥6 months. Those who have received ≤3 doses should complete the series at the recommended intervals and ages.

Poliovirus	(Re)vaccinate with IPV	Serologic testing for neutralizing antibodies

Comments: Because the booster response after a single dose of IPV is excellent among children who previously received OPV, a single dose of IPV can be administered initially with serologic testing performed 1 month later.

DTaP	(Re)vaccinate with DTaP, with serologic testing for specific IgG antibody to tetanus and diptheria toxins in the event of a severe local reaction	If records indicate receipt of ≥3 doses, conduct serologic testing for IgG antibody to diphtheria and tetanus toxins before administering additional doses, or administer a single booster dose of DTaP, followed by serologic testing after 1 month for specific IgG antibody to diphtheria and tetanus toxins with revaccination as appropriate.

Comments: One can revaccinate with DTaP vaccine without regard to recorded doses; however, there may be increased rates of local adverse reactions after the fourth and fifth doses of DTP or DTaP. If a severe local reaction occurs, serologic testing for specific IgG antibody to tetanus and diphtheria toxins can be measured before administering additional doses. Protective concentration indicates that further doses are unnecessary and subsequent vaccination should occur as age-appropriate. No established serologic correlates exist for protection against pertussis.

If record indicates receipt of ≥3 doses of DTP or DTaP, serologic testing for specific IgG antibody to both diphtheria and tetanus toxin before additional doses is reasonable. If a protective concentration is present, recorded doses can be considered valid, and the vaccination series should be completed as age-appropriate. Indeterminate antibody concentration might indicate immunologic memory but antibody waning; serology can be repeated after a booster dose if the vaccination provider wishes to avoid revaccination with a complete series.

Alternately, if records indicate receipt of ≥3 doses, a single booster dose can be administered, followed by serologic testing after 1 month for specific IgG antibody to both diphtheria and tetanus toxins. If a protective concentration is obtained, the recorded doses can be considered valid and the vaccination series completed as age-appropriate. Children with indeterminate concentration after a booster dose should be revaccinated with a complete series.

Varicella	Age-appropriate vaccination if child lacks medical history of varicella	Serologic testing for child >15 months (history of varicella often not provided)
Pneumococcal vaccines	Age-appropriate vaccination	—

DTaP, diphtheria–tetanus–acellular pertussis; DTP, diphtheria–tetanus–pertussis; HIB, *Haemophilus influenzae* type B; IPV, inactivated poliomyelitis vaccine; MMR, measles, mumps, rubella; OPV, oral polio vaccine.

Source: Adapted from American Academy of Pediatrics[8] and Atkinson et al.,[24] reprinted with permission.

Table 21–6 Difficulties with use of titers to verify immunity

Cost
Volume of blood required
Ordering the right test
Appropriate time to test related to prior vaccination
Confounding maternal antibodies
Lack of quantitative information

protective antibody against diptheria toxin.[24] The interval from most recent vaccination to assessment of antibody titers must also be considered; results may be artifactually high if tested too soon after immunization[26] and may wane if tested late.[13] Recommendations for the proper time to test range from 6 weeks to 6 months post-vaccination. Quantitative antibody titers are more useful than reports of positive or negative to assure long-lasting immunity. In infants, the presence of maternal antibodies should not be misinterpreted to represent immunity. The cost of checking titers is considerable, but this must be weighed against the cost of the vaccinations and associated expenses. Given these concerns, some practitioners recommend revaccination of all children. However, a more individualized approach, taking into account the child's age, country of origin, and validity of vaccination record, is probably more sensible.

Late Complications of Vaccine-Preventable Diseases

For pediatricians trained in the last 20 years, late complications of vaccine-preventable diseases are seldom encountered and may be difficult to recognize. Unfortunately, international adoptees who had natural disease in their birth countries prior to adoption may develop these complications. For example, in 2000, a 13-year-old Thai boy adopted at age 4 years died of subacute sclerosing panencephalitis (SSPE).[27] Investigation determined that he had likely acquired wild-type measles in Thailand prior to adoption, then developed this devastating complication after a prolonged latent period. The authors of this report speculate that "further cases of SSPE are likely to occur among internationally adopted children," as the risk of this complication of measles is 100–200 times higher in nonimmunized children.

Key Points for Internationally Adopted Children

- Some internationally adopted children are unprotected from vaccine-preventable diseases.
- Vaccine records from birth countries may be unreliable.
- Revaccination or measurement of antibody titers to administered antigens is recommended to ensure adequate immunity to vaccine-preventable diseases.

FAQs

Q. I've had trouble getting insurance companies to cover the cost of the vaccine titers. It's expensive! What should I do?

A. This has been a big problem in many places. If possible, it's best to try to discuss this with the insurance company in advance. The cost of administering vaccines is usually substantially less than the titers, therefore many third-party payors balk at coverage. Explaining the special situation of the child sometimes helps. Parents may also be willing to assume the cost of this testing when the alternative of multiple shots and doctor visits is outlined.

Q. It makes sense to me to restart the vaccines of a 10-month-old from China with a questionable record. But, it seems excessive to redo all the vaccines or even to check the titers of a 5-year-old from Guatemala with a very valid-appearing vaccine record. Do I really have to do one or the other?

A. Unfortunately, the detailed investigations needed to answer this question have not yet been completed. Vaccines administered in a community clinic may be more valid than those given in an orphanage. However, it's best to be conservative rather than risk susceptibility to a vaccine-preventable disease.

Resources

Association of Regional and University Pathologists (Salt Lake City), 800-242-2787. Antibody titers to verify immunity. http://www.aruplab.com for details of available tests.

References

1. Gomez M. Measles without borders. Texas Department of Health. Available at: http://www.tdh.state.tx.us/immunize/uparch/sp01meas.htm.

1a. Measles among adoptees from China. Available at: http://www.cdc.gov/mmwr/preview.

2. Jenista JA, Chapman D. Medical problems of foreign-born adopted children. Am J Dis Child 1987; 141: 298–302.

3. Hostetter MK. Epidemiology of travel-related morbidity and mortality in children. Pediatr Rev 1999; 20: 228–33.

4. Cappello M. Immunizations for children traveling abroad. Pediatr Infect Dis J 1998; 17:157–8.

5. World Health Organization. International travel and health. Available at: http://www.who.int/ith.

6. U.S. Department of State. The Bureau of Consular Affairs. Travel Health information. Available at: http://www.travel.state.gov.

7. National Center for Infectious Disease. Travelers' Health. Available at: http://www.cdc.gov/travel.

8. American Academy of Pediatrics. Immunization in special clinical circumstances. International travel. In: Pickering LK, ed. Red Book: 2003 Report of the Committee on Infectious Diseases. Elk Grove Village, IL: American Academy of Pediatrics, 2003: 938.

9. Hostetter MK, Johnson DJ. Immunization status of adoptees from China, Russia, and Eastern Europe [abstract]. Pediatr Res 1998; 43:147A.

10. Miller LC. Internationally adopted children—immunization status [letter]. Pediatrics 1999; 103:1078.

11. Miller LC, Comfort K, Kelly N. Immunization status of internationally adopted children. Pediatrics 2001; 108:1050–1.

12. Staat MA, Daniels D. Immunization verification in internationally adopted children [abstract]. Pediatr Res 2001; 49:468A.

13. Schulpen TW, van Seventer AH, Rumke HC, van Loon AM. Immunisation status of children adopted from China. Lancet 2001; 358:2131–2.

14. el-Gamal Y, Aly RH, Hossny E, Afify E, el-Taliawy D. Response of Egyptian infants with protein calorie malnutrition to hepatitis B vaccination. J Trop Pediatr 1996; 42:144–5.

15. Bahl R, Bhandari N, Kant S, Molbak K, Ostergaard E, Bhan MK. Effect of vitamin A administered at Expanded Program on Immunization contacts on antibody response to oral polio vaccine. Eur J Clin Nutr 2002; 56:321–5.

16. Chandra RK. Reduced secretory antibody response to live attenuated measles and poliovirus vaccines in malnourished children. BMJ 1975; 2:583–5.

17. McMurray DN, Loomis SA, Casazza LJ, Rey H. Influence of moderate malnutrition on morbidity and antibody response following vaccination with live, attenuated measles virus vaccine. Bull Pan Am Health Organ 1979; 13:52–7.

18. McMurray DN, Loomis SA, Casazza LJ, Rey H, Miranda R. Development of impaired cell-mediated immunity in mild and moderate malnutrition. Am J Clin Nutr 1981; 34:68–77.

19. Greenwood BM, Bradley-Moore AM, Bradley AK, Kirkwood BR, Gilles HM. The immune response to vaccination in undernourished and well-nourished Nigerian children. Ann Trop Med Parasitol 1986; 80:537–44.

20. Cohen S, Miller GE, Rabin BS. Psychological stress and antibody response to immunization: a critical review of the human literature. Psychosom Med 2001; 63:7–18.

21. Snyder BK, Roghmann KJ, Sigal LH. Effect of stress and other biophysical factors on primary antibody response. J Adoles Health Care 1990; 11:472–9.

22. Bell KN, Hogue CJR, Manning C, Kendal AP. Risk factors for improper vaccine storage and handling in private provider offices. Pediatrics 2001; 107:e100.

23. Schulte J, Maloney S, Aronson J, Gabriel PS, Zhou J, Saiman L. Evaluating acceptability and completeness of overseas immunization records of internationally adopted children. Pediatrics 2002; 109:e22.

24. Atkinson WL, Pickering LK, Schwartz B, Weniger BG, Iskander JK, Watson JC. General Recommendations on Immunization: Recommendations of the Advisory Committee on Immunization Practices (ACIP) and the American Academy of Family Physicians (AAFP). MMWR Recomm Rep. 2002; 51:1–35.

25. Advisory Committee on Immunization Practices. Use of diptheria toxoid-tetanus toxoid-acellular pertussis vaccine as a five-dose series. Available at: http://www.cdc.gov/mmwr/preview/mmwrhtml/rr4913a1.htm.

26. Hostetter MK. Infectious diseases in internationally adopted children: the past five years. Pediatr Infect Dis J 1998; 17:517–8.

27. Bonthius DJ, Stanek N, Grose C. Subacute sclerosing panencephalitis, a measles complication, in an internationally adopted child. Emerging Infect Dis 2000; 6:377–81.

22

UNUSUAL AND OTHER
INFECTIOUS DISEASES

Some practitioners caring for international adoptees expect to encounter frequent exotic infectious diseases among their patients, but such conditions are uncommon. Intestinal parasites, latent tuberculosis, and hepatitis B occur routinely in internationally adopted children (see Chapters 14, 15, and 17). Otherwise, serious "exotic" infections seldom occur. However, persistent fever, splenomegaly, respiratory tract infection, anemia, or eosinophilia in new arrivals should prompt further evaluation based on diseases likely to occur in the country of origin.[1] Occasionally, vaccine-preventable diseases (measles, pertussis) appear in new arrivals[2,3] (see Chapter 21). These can be challenging diagnoses for American pediatricians, most of whom have never seen a case.

Scabies and cytomegalovirus (CMV) infection are infections of more general concern. These infections are relatively common in international adoptees; they are important because they may spread to other family members. Pediculosis also occurs occasionally[4,5]; management is generally straightforward.[1] This section reviews scabies, CMV, and the few rarities reported in international adoptees. An update on the recent emergence of severe acute respiratory syndrome (SARS) is also provided.

Scabies

Scabies is a common infection in orphanages. About 10% of newly arrived international adoptees have scabies. Scabies is spread by skin-to-skin transmission, but in heavily contaminated environments it may be transmitted by fomites.[6–8] Scabies sometimes occurs in epidemic form in institutions; risk factors include residents' ages, size of the institution, and the caregiver/resident ratio.[9] Clinical signs lag several weeks behind initial infestation. Thus scabies may not appear until the newly adopted child has been home for some time. Scabies should be strongly suspected in *any* new arrival with a pruritic rash, especially if itching is worse at night. Some children are irritable and feed poorly (Table 22–1). Typical dermal mite burrows are difficult to identify in young children because of excoriation, crusting, or eczematization.[8] In some young children, vesicles, nodules, or pustules are the predominant lesions (Fig. 22–1). Occasionally, post-scabetic nodules (skin folds, diaper area) persist after infection is eradicated. Infantile acropustulosis sometimes appears after scabies. Diagnosis of scabies by skin scraping is sometimes difficult (Table 22–2); empiric treatment of suspicious rashes is sometimes confirmatory.[10]

Crusted (Norwegian) scabies presents as crusted scaling plaques, either generalized or localized to the hands and feet. This condition occurs in heavily infested individuals with concurrent immunodeficiency or malnutrition. Treatment of primary scabies with topical corticosteroids may induce crusted scabies.[11] Some authors suggest treatment of

Table 22–1 Clinical distribution of scabies lesions in children <3 years

Palms
Soles
Scalp
Face
Posterior auricular
Generalized

Source: Data from Peterson and Eichenfield.[8]

Table 22–2 Differential diagnosis of scabies[6–8,10]

Atopic dermatitis
Dishidrotic eczema
Acropustulosis of infancy
Impetigo (but may be secondary to scabies)
Seborrheic dermatitis
Contact dermatitis
Papular urticaria
Recurrent pyoderma
Lichen planus
Syphilis
Human immunodeficiency virus–related dermatosis
Drug reaction
Other insect bites
Rarities (e.g., histiocytosis X)

Source: Data from refs. 6, 8, and 10.

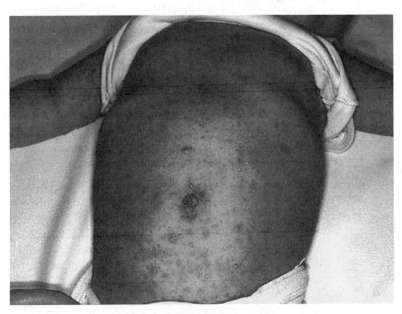

Figure 22–1 *Scabies. (Courtesy of the New Zealand Dermatological Society.)*

these individuals with a single dose of oral ivermetin (which also eradicates nematodes such as stronglyoides).

The treatment of choice for infants and young children is 5% permethrin lotion (Elimite).[6–8,10] This is approved for use in patients as young as 2 months of age. Principles of treatment are listed in Table 22–3; treatment failure usually results from lack of adherence to recommendations. Families must be educated that pruritis may persist for several weeks after treatment.

Cytomegalovirus Infection

Children residing in orphanages, like others in group care settings,[12–14] frequently become infected with CMV (Table 22–4). In a survey of 293 internationally adopted children,[15] 45% had

Table 22–3 Treatment of scabies in young children

Treat all family members and contacts simultaneously.

For infants and toddlers, apply lotion from head to toe, including soles and web spaces. For older children and adults, apply from the neck down. Include under trimmed nails.

Remove lotion by bathing after 8–14 hours.

Launder all intimate clothing and bedding in hot water. Alternatives include dry cleaning or storage for 1 week.

Source: Data from Peterson and Eichenfield.[8]

Table 22–4 Cytomegalovirus in internationally adopted children (positive urine cultures)

Country of Origin	Positive urine culture for CMV (%)
Haiti	81
India	77
Phillipines	75
Central and South America	46
Korea	29
Total	45 (111/247)

Source: Data from Hostetter et al.[15]

positive urine cultures for CMV. Three of the children with positive urine cultures had presumptive evidence of congenital CMV, including one child with deafness, intracranial calcifications, and seizures, and two children had previous perinatal hepatitis. The need to identify children with CMV infection and the management of those with positive results have been controversial.[16–18] Although the proportion of internationally adopted children with CMV is high, it is comparable to North American children of similar ages who attend group day care.[12–14] Differentiation of asymptomatic carriage from occult congenital CMV is difficult in the international adoptee, in whom accurate perinatal information is usually lacking.

Cytomegalovirus conveys several risks to children and their families. Children with congenital CMV may develop later intellectual deficits and hearing impairment. Children with CMV may also transmit the virsus to their adoptive mothers. About 50% of North American women in middle and upper income groups are not immune; thus exposure to a CMV-excreting child might result in primary infection in the adoptive mother.[15] If CMV is acquired during pregnancy, the mother may transmit the virus to her fetus with dire consequences. Some investigators have suggested that CMV immune status be determined in adoptive mothers so that counseling may be provided to those who are not CMV immune if their adopted children are CMV carriers.[16,17] Alternatively, counseling may be provided to all adoptive mothers.[16,17] Others have objected that screening of select groups of children is unlikely to diminish the risks of congenital CMV.[18] At present, specific testing of adoptees is not recommended;[1] however counseling of adoptive mothers and/or determination of CMV immunity should be considered.[12]

Unusual Infections

Some internationally adopted children arrive from countries with many endemic tropical diseases. Practitioners should be aware of unusual symptoms or signs and remain aware of the country of origin of the child. The longer the interval from arrival to presentation, the less likely the symptoms are to be attributable to infections acquired in the birth country.[1] Although largely directed toward Westerners who travel abroad, several Web sites may assist in identification of unusual symptoms in newly arrived children[19–21] (the World Health Organization's "International Travel and Health" or the CDC's "Yellow Book"). The *Red Book*[1] is also a useful resource. The Centers for Disease Control and Prevention also offers telephone advice at 877-FYI-TRIP (toll-free). A few unusual infections that have been identified in internationally adopted or immigrant children are listed in Table 22–5.

Beatrice was 6 months old when adopted from Vietnam. She seemed healthy but a bit lethargic when her mom traveled with her back to the United States. The new family stopped to visit relatives in California for a few days before returning to the East Coast. She began to cough and became more irritable. By the time the plane landed in Boston, Beatrice was in severe respiratory distress. The family went directly to the emergency room. Beatrice was admitted to the intensive care unit and intubated. Pneumocystis carinii pneumonia was diagnosed. Her CD4 count was so low that HIV infection was assumed to be present. However, all tests for HIV were negative. A comprehensive search for other causes of pediatric immunodeficiency was made, but no specific diagnosis could be found. She remained critically ill and immunosuppressed; a bone marrow transplant was planned. The day before the scheduled transplant, a CBC showed a rising CD4 count. Within a few days, all counts and all tests of immune function were normal. Ten weeks after admission, she was discharged. One year later, she is healthy and thriving.

Severe Acute Respiratory Syndrome

Severe acute respiratory syndrome (SARS), an atypical pneumonia characterized by high rate of transmission to health care workers, began in Guangdong Province, China, in November 2002. The disease quickly spread to Hong Kong, Singapore, Taiwan, and Canada, and global travel was devastated (Table 22–6). As the epidemic progressed, many parents adopting from China became anxious about travel to Asia to receive their children. By spring 2003, Chinese authorities adjusted the regulations for adoptive parents, reducing the amount of in-country travel necessary. Increasingly strict health advisories limiting travel were posted by the Centers for Disease Control and Prevention and the World Health Organization. Initially, adopting parents were exempted from these regulations, as their travel was considered essential. However, on May 15, 2003, the Chinese government temporarily closed international adoption in an effort to contain the ongoing epidemic of SARS.

In the initial stages of the epidemic, children (and especially infants) appeared to be relatively unaffected by SARS.[29] Nonetheless, several children adopted from China were hospitalized in the United States with presumed SARS. All children recovered and in several, other causes of their respiratory symptoms were determined (respiratory syncytial virus, RSV). Nonetheless, new developments in this outbreak should be monitored,[20,30] by clinicians caring for children adopted from affected areas.

Key Points for Internationally Adopted Children

- The prevalence of latent tuberculosis infection, intestinal parasites, and hepatitis B far exceeds that of exotic infectious diseases.
- Persistent or unusual symptoms (fever, splenomegaly, anemia, rash, eosinophilia) should prompt appropriate investigations.
- Scabies and lice are common and sometimes difficult to eradicate.

Table 22–5 Unusual infectious diseases in internationally adopted or immigrant children

	Endemic Regions	Clinical Signs	Diagnosis	Comments
Tungiasis (cutaneous infestation caused by gravid sand flea)[22]	Central and South America, Sub-Saharan Africa, India, Pakistan	Localized skin lesions, secondary cellulitis, autoamputation, gas gangrene	Histology	—
Neurocysticercosis (brain infection with Taenia solium)[23,a]	Latin America, Asia, Africa	Seizures	Characteristics CT findings: ring-enhancing lesion surrounded by edema; serology	May have long incubation after infection (7 years)
Pneumocystis carinii pneumonia[24–27]	Asia (especially Vietnam?)	Progressive interstitial pneumonia with normal auscultation	Histology, serology	7 cases found among Vietnamese children transported to U.S. during "Operation Babylift" (1975); other cases found subsequently
Malaria[28]	Central and South America, Africa, Indian subcontinent, Southeast Asia, Middle East, Oceania	Episodic fevers, flu-like illness, shaking chills, headache, myalgias, fatigue, nausea, vomiting, diarrhea. Hemolytic anemia, jaundice. Plasmodium falciparum may cause kidney failure, seizures, mental confusion, coma, death	Peripheral blood smear	2/200 children adopted from India diagnosed after arrival
Leprosy[28]	Indian subcontinent, Western Pacific (Marshall Islands)	Range in severity: Mild cases may have one or more hypopigmented skin macules. More severe cases have symmetric skin lesions, nodules, plaques, thickened dermis, and involvement of nasal mucosa resulting in nasal congestion and epistaxis. Skin lesions have loss of sensation.	Skin smears	—

[a]Children were not international adoptees but immigrants or exposed to travelers.

Table 22–6 Cumulative number of reported probable cases of severe acute respiratory syndrome (SARS) in common sending countries, Asian transit countries, United States, and Canada

Country	Cumulative number of cases (total)[a]	Number of deaths[a]
Canada	251	43
China	5327	349
Colombia	1	0
Hong Kong	1755	299
India	3	0
Mongolia	9	0
Philippines	14	2
Republic of Korea	3	0
Romania	1	0
Russia	1	0
Singapore	238	33
Taiwan	346	37
Thailand	9	2
United States	29	0
Vietnam	63	5
Total	8098	774

Data for November 1, 2002 to July 31, 2003.

[a]Includes countries not shown.

Source: Data from the World Health Organization.[30]

References

1. American Academy of Pediatrics. Medical evaluation of internationally adopted children. In: Pickering L, ed. Red Book: 2003 Report of the Committee on Infectious Diseases. Elk Grove Village, IL: American Academy of Pediatrics, 2003: 173–80.

2. Johns L, Rowe-West B, MacCormack J, et al. Pertussis in an infant adopted from Russia. MMWR Morbid Mortal Wkly Rep 2002; 51:394–5.

3. Reynolds A, Gong T, Li H, et al. Measles outbreak among internationally adopted children arriving in the United States. MMWR Morbid Mortal Wkly Rep 2001; 51: 1115–6.

4. Morsy TA, el-Ela RG, Morsy AT, Nassar MM, Khalaf SA. Two contagious ectoparasites in orphanage children in Nasr City, Cairo. J Egypt Soc Parasitol 2000; 30:727–34.

5. Ozturkcan S, Ozcelik S, Saygi G, Ozcelik S. Spread of scabies and pediculus humanus among the children at Sivas orphanage. Indian Pediatr 1994; 31:210–3.

6. Angel TA, Nigro J, Levy ML. Infestations in the pediatric patient. Pediatr Clin North Am 2000; 47:921–35.

7. Chosidow O. Scabies and pediculosis. Lancet 2000; 355:819–26.

8. Peterson CM, Eichenfield LF. Scabies. Pediatr Ann 1996; 25:97–100.

9. Holness DL, DeKoven JG, Nethercott JR. Scabies in chronic health care institutions. Arch Dermatol 1992; 128:1257–60.

10. Potts J. Eradication of ectoparasites in children. Postgrad Med 2001; 110:57–64.

11. Marliere V, Roul S, Labreze C, Taieb A. Crusted (Norwegian) scabies induced by use of topical corticosteroids and treated successfully with ivermectin. J Pediatr 1999; 135:122–4.

12. Balc JF, Zimmerman B, Dawson JD, Souza IE, Petheram SJ, Murph JR. Cytomegalovirus transmission in child care homes. Arch Pediatr Adol Med 1999; 153:75–9.

13. Pass RF, Hutto SC, Reynolds DW, Polhill RB. Increased frequency of cytomegalovirus infection in children in group day care. Pediatrics 1984; 74:121–6.

14. Pass RF, Hutto SC, Ricks R, Cloud GA. Increased rate of cytomegalovirus infection among parents of children attending day-care centers. N Engl J Med 1986; 314:1414–8.

15. Hostetter MK, Iverson S, Thomas W, McKenzie D, Dole K, Johnson DE. Medical evaluation of internationally adopted children. N Engl J Med 1991; 325:479–85.

16. Hostetter M, Johnson DE. International adoption. An introduction for physicians. Am J Dis Child 1989; 143:325–32.

17. Hostetter MK. Internationally adopted children and cytomegalovirus. Pediatrics 1989; 84:937–8.

18. Barton LL, Friedman AD. Internationally adopted children and cytomegalovirus. Pediatrics 1989; 84:937.

19. The Yellow Book. Health information for international travel, 2003–04. Available at: http://www.cdc.gov/travel/yb/.

20. National Center for Infections Diseases. Travelers' Health. Available at: http://www.cdc.gov/travel/.

21. World Health Organization. International Travel and Health. Available at: http://www.who.int/ith/.

22. Fein H, Naseem S, Witte DP, Garcia VF, Lucky A, Staat MA. Tungiasis in North America: a report of 2 cases in internationally adopted children. J Pediatr 2001; 139: 744–6.

23. Stamos JK, Rowley AH, Hahn YS, Chadwick EG, Schantz PM, Wilson M. Neurocysticercosis: report of unusual pediatric cases. Pediatrics 1996; 98:974–7.

24. Giebink GS, Sholler L, Keenan TP, Franciosis RA, Quie PG. *Pneumocystis carinii* pneumonia in two Vietnamese refugee infants. Pediatrics 1976; 58:115–8.

25. Gleason WA, Roden VJ, DeCastro F. Pneumocystis pneumonia in Vietnamese infants. J Pediatr 1975; 87:1001–2.

26. Nordin J, Myers MG. *Pneumocystis carinii* in a Vietnamese foundling. Am J Dis Child 1975; 129:1361.

27. Redman JC. *Pneumocystis carinii* pneumonia in an adopted Vietnamese infant. A case of fulminant disease with recovery. JAMA 1974; 230:1561–3.

28. Smith-Garcia T, Brown JS. The health of children adopted from India. J Community Health 1989; 14:227–41.

29. Hon KLE, Leung CW, Cheng WTF, et al. Clinical presentations and outcome of severe acute respiratory syndrome in children. Lancet 2003; 361: 1701–3.s

30. World Health Organization. Cumulative number of reported probable cases of SARS. Available at: http://www.who.int/csr/sars/country/table2003_09_23/en/.

VI

OTHER MEDICAL CONDITIONS

23

INHERITED DISORDERS OF ERYTHROCYTES

nemia is the most common noninfectious medical condition in newly arrived international adoptees (Table 23–1). Most cases are due to iron deficiency (see Chapter 11); however, a number of inherited erythrocyte disorders also occur among internationally adopted children. Thalassemias, hemoglobinopathies, and glucose-6-phosphate dehydrogenase (G6PD) deficiency are relatively common disorders in the countries of origin of many international adoptees. Thalassemias and hemoglobinopathies are disorders of hemoglobin synthesis; G6PD deficiency is an enzymatic defect of erythrocytes.

About 3%–35% of newly arrived children have anemia detected in their initial complete blood counts. Usually this is a hypochromic, microcytic anemia. Once iron deficiency is excluded, other causes of the anemia should be considered. Thalassemia and other hemoglobinopathies are strongly suspected if the mean cell volume/red blood cell count (MCV/RBC) index is <12 (the Mentzer Index). Many states include hemoglobin electrophoresis in newborn screen panels. This is an efficient way to identify children with hemoglobin variants and may be obtained on older children by special arrangement with State Screening Laboratories.

This section will review the epidemiology and fundamental clinical and pathologic features of the more common forms of thalassemia, hemoglobinopathy, and G6PD deficiency, all of which occur frequently among international adoptees.

Thalassemias

The thalassemias are a hereditary group of hypochromic anemias, resulting from defective synthesis of the α- or β-globin chains of hemoglobin. Adult hemoglobin, hemoglobin A, is composed of two α and two β globins ($\alpha^2\beta^2$). In α-thalassemias, there is decreased or absent α-globin chain synthesis; in β-thalassemia, there is decreased or absent β-globin chain synthesis.

309

Table 23–1 Prevalence of anemia among newly arrived international adoptees

Adoptees with Anemia (%)	Sending Country (N)	Comments
3.4	Various, mostly Korea and Colombia (128)[1]	—
3.8	Mostly Korea (52)[2]	—
8.8	Various countries (68)[3]	—
12	Mostly Korea and India (99)[4]	—
18.5	India (200)[5]	—
31	Various countries (129)[6]	—
35	China (152)[7]	10/192 had thalassemia trait
N = 17 of those >6 months old (No. or % not specified)	Various countries, mostly Korea (293) (but only results of those >6 months old given)[8]	1 with G6PD deficiency

Definitions of anemia are not strictly comparable among studies.

Epidemiology

Like the sickle cell gene, thalassemia genes are found in areas where *P. falciparum* malaria is common. The α-thalassemia trait, perhaps the most common single gene disorder in the world, may protect from severe forms of malaria as well as other infections.[9] The α-thalassemias are widespread. The single α-globin gene deletion (–α/αα) is prevalent across tropical Africa, the Mediterranean region, the Middle East, India, Southeast Asia, and southern China. The αα-thalassemia trait (—/αα) is more common in Southeast Asia, including southern China, and more rarely in the Mediterranean region. Hemoglobin H disease, in which three of the four α-globin genes are deleted (—/–α) or mutated, is highly prevalent in southern China and Southeast Asia.[10] The β-thalassemias are common around the Mediterranean Sea (Greece and Italy), Arabian Peninsula, Turkey, Iran, Africa, Indian subcontinent, and Southeast Asia, including southern China, Malay Peninsula, and Indonesia.[11] (Fig. 23–1). There are probably fewer than 1000 children in the United States with homozygous β-thalassemia.

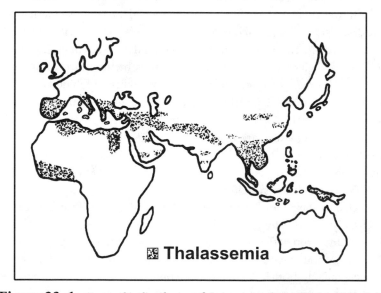

Figure 23–1 *Geographic distribution of thalassemia. (From Nathan DG, Oski FA, eds. Hematology of Infancy and Childhood, Vol. 1. Philadelphia: W.B. Saunders, 1993:784, with permission from Elsevier.)[13]*

Table 23–2 Homozygous β-thalassemia in the United States (major and intermediate)

Ethnicity	% (rounded)
Italian	44
Greek	18
Indian/Pakistani	11
Middle East	9
Chinese	8
African American	4
Southeast Asian	4
Other	2

Source: Data adapted from Pearson et al.[12]

Most are of Greek or Italian ancestry (Table 23–2).

Clinical Features

The severity of disease reflects the degree of impairment of α- or β-globin synthesis. Heterozygotes for α- or β-thalassemia may be hematologically normal silent carriers or have mild microcytic hypochromic anemia. Hemolysis and ineffective erythropoiesis occur in homozygotes. β-Thalassemia tends to be more severe, as each chromosome contains only one β-globin gene; in contrast, there are two copies of the α-globin gene. Thalassemia intermedia is applied to patients with β-thalassemia whose disease falls between severe transfusion-dependent thalassemia major and asymptomic thalassemia trait. Over 150 different mutations may cause β-thalassemia.

Thalassemia becomes clinically apparent as fetal hemoglobin wanes, usually within the first year of life. Rarely, children present as late as 3–5 years of age if compensatory production of fetal hemoglobin (Hb F) is prolonged. A comparison of some common hematologic parameters in α- and β-thalassemia and iron deficiency anemia is shown in Table 23–3.

Diagnosis

Thalassemia should be considered when microcytosis and hypochromia are present. A trial of iron therapy is often helpful in distinguishing iron deficiency anemia from thalassemia. Because both conditions may coincide, it is important to treat underlying iron deficiency rather than assuming that microcytosis is due to thalassemia alone (see Chapter 11). Transferrin saturation or ferritin should be measured to verify or exclude the diagnosis of iron deficiency anemia. Determination of iron status is critical; iron deficiency artificially lowers Hb A2 levels and can thus alter interpretation of test results. After iron repletion, hemoglobin electrophoresis should be performed. Elevated levels of Hb A2 (>3.5%) establish the diagnosis of heterozygous β-thalassemia; markedly elevated levels of fetal hemoglobin (Hb F) are found in homozygotes. In patients with microcytosis, hypochromia, and erythrocytosis who have normal Hb A2 and Hb F, but no iron deficiency, α-thalassemia is most likely. Rarely, α- and β-thalassemia coexist. In transfusion de-

Table 23–3 Comparison of α- and β-thalassemias and iron deficiency: typical findings

	α-thalassemia	β-thalassemia	Iron Deficiency
Hemoglobin (gm %)	12.6	11.3	10.2
RBC count ($\times 10^6$/μl)	5.6	4.7	4.6
MCV (fl)	65	60	67
MCH (pg)	23	20	21
RDW	Increased	Increased	Increased
Hemoglobin A2 (2–3.5%)	Normal or decreased	5%	Normal or decreased
Hemoglobin F (<1%)	<1%	2%	<1%

MCH, mean cell hemoglobin; MCV, mean cell volume; RCB, red blood cell count; RDW, red blood cell distribution width.

Source: Modified from McDonagh et al.[13]

pendent children, iron chelation treatment can prevent long-term organ system damage from iron overload.

The Web site http://www.thalassemia.com, published by the Division of Hematology-Oncology of Oakland Children's Hospital, is an excellent resource for additional information about thalassemia.

Hemoglobinopathies

Epidemiology

The hemoglobinopathies are qualitative disorders of hemoglobin production. The geographic distributions and clinical features of some of the more common hemoglobinopathies (trait or disease) are shown in Table 23–4. A letter designation is given for each chain of hemoglobin (e.g., HB SS is a homozygote for HB S, HB AS is a heterozygote). As with thalassemia, heterozygotes for some of the hemoglobinopathies are resistant to more severe forms of malaria. The widespread geographic distribution of hemoglobin S, associated with sickle cell trait and disease, is usually surprising to American pediatricians.

The compound heterozygous condition, hemoglobin E/β-thalassemia, is now recognized with increasing frequency among Asian immigrants.[14] Clinically, this condition ranges from mild, asymptomatic anemia to severe, life-threatening disease. If concurrent iron deficiency is present, it may be difficult to distinguish between homozygous hemoglobin E and heterozygous hemoglobin E/β thalassemia without family studies.

Table 23–4 Selected hemoglobinopathies[11-13]

Abnormal Hemoglobin	Geographic Distribution	Hemoglobin Profile	Clinical Manifestations
Hemoglobin S	Equatorial Africa, Caribbean, Panama, Guyana, Brazil, Italy, Greece, Middle East, India	SS	Severe hemolytic anemia; vaso-occlusive, sequestration, and aplastic crises; susceptibility to infections
		AS	Rare symptoms under extreme conditions (unpressurized aircraft, high-altitude strenuous exercise, etc.); some inability to concentrate urine
Hemoglobin C	West Africa	CC	Moderate hemolytic anemia, splenomegaly, target cells and spherocytes
		AC	Target cells
Hemoglobin SC	Africa	SC	Target cells, moderate anemia, splenomegaly, occasional vaso-occlusive crises, aseptic necrosis of femoral head, retinal damage. Some susceptibility to pneumococcus or *H. influenzae*
Hemoglobin D	NW India	DD	Mild hemolytic anemia, splenomegaly
		AD	Rare symptoms; usually none
Hemoglobin E	Southeast Asia, especially Thailand (>50% in some regions), Laos (lowlands), Cambodia	EE	Mild to moderate hemolytic anemia, prominent target cells, microcytosis, splenomegaly
		AE	Target cells

Clinical Features

Hemoglobinopathy should be suspected in children with anemia, hemolysis, and splenomegaly. Fever or certain drug exposures may exacerbate hemolysis. Red blood cells are hypochromic, often with basophilic stippling. Heinz bodies may sometimes be found.

Diagnosis

Hemoglobin electrophoresis identifies most hemoglobin variants. As fetal hemoglobin disappears, these disorders become easier to define.

Glucose 6-Phosphate Dehydrogenase Deficiency

Glucose 6-phosphate dehydrogenase deficiency results in acute hemolysis after infection or certain drug exposures. There are more than 10 variants of the enzyme; those which result in hemolysis are found among individuals with African, Mediterranean, or Asian backgrounds (Fig. 23–2). Like the hemoglobinopathies and thalassemias, the "malaria resistance hypothesis" has been invoked to explain the persistence of the G6PD deficiency genetic variants. The G6PD gene is located on the X chromosome. Males are either normal or affected hemizygotes; females may be normal or deficient homozygotes, or heterozygotes. The heterozygote has two populations of red blood cells: normal and deficient in G6PD. Most female heterozygotes are asymptomatic. Those who happen to have a high proportion of deficient cells resemble the male hemizygotes.

Some patients have mild anemia, due to shortened erythrocyte survival. Most have no problems unless subjected to environmental stress. Bacterial or viral infections, drugs (including the *Giardia* treatment furazolidone), certain foods, or metabolic acidosis can induce

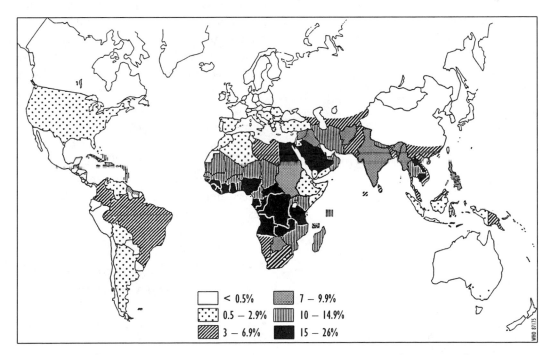

Figure 23–2 *Geographic distribution of G6PD deficiency, % of population affected. (From Nathan DG, Oski FA, eds. Hematology of Infancy and Childhood, Vol. 1. Philadelphia: W.B. Saunders, 1993:689, with permission from Elsevier.)*

hemolysis in susceptible individuals (Table 23–5). Thus, G6PD deficiency must be excluded before certain drugs are given.

Table 23–5 Drugs and foods inducing hemolysis in G6PD-deficient individuals[a]

Antimalarials
Primaquine
Pamaquine
Dapsone
Chloroquine

Sulfonamides
Sulfamethoxazole (Gantanol)
Sulfafurazole (Gantrisin)[*]
Sulfanilamide
Sulfapyridine
Co-trimoxazole (Septrin)
Bactrim

Analgesics
Acetanilid
Acetylsalicyclic acid (aspirin); moderate doses may be used
Acetophenetidin (phenacetin)

Antiparasitic agents
Furazolidone (Furoxone)

Foods
Fava beans
Red wine[b]
All legumes[b]
Blueberries[b]
Soy products[b]
Tonic water[b]
Camphor[b]

Miscellaneous
Nitrofurantoin
Chloramphenicol
Vitamin K (water-soluble form)
Methylene blue
Nalidixic acid
Doxorubicin
Naphthalene (moth balls)
Pyridium

[a]This is a partial list of such foods and drugs. Complete lists of foods and drugs to be avoided can be found at the Web site http://rialto.com/g6pd/ or http://www.favism.org/favism/english/index.mv?pgid=avoid.
[b]Reported by some individuals.

Rare Hematologic Disorders

Thousands of rare hematologic disorders have been described. Two in particular that may be encountered in international adoptees are described below.

Southeast Asian Ovalocytosis

Like most of the other conditions discussed in this section, this red cell membrane disorder is also prominent in malarial regions. It is frequently recognized in Malaysia, Melanesia, and the Philippines. Southeast Asian ovalocytosis is inherited in an autosomal dominant pattern. The presence of prominent ovalocytes on peripheral smear raises the possibility of this diagnosis.

Chuvash Polycythemia

A number of internationally adopted children from the Chuvash area of Russia have been placed in the United States. An autosomal recessive polycythemia is common in this region,[15] located on the west bank of Volga River in central European Russia. About 70% of residents are of Chuvash ethnicity. About 22% of affected patients are diagnosed before age 10 years. Patients have markedly elevated hemoglobin levels (22.6 + 1.4 grams/dl), but normal leukocytes and platelets. The disorder has a mortality rate greater than 10% over 10 years of observation; survival beyond age 40 years appears to be uncommon.

Key Points for Internationally Adopted Children

- Anemia is common in newly arrived international adoptees
- Iron deficiency is a common cause of anemia (see Chapter 11) but inherited erythrocyte disorders may coexist.

- Iron repletion is necessary prior to diagnostic evaluation.
- Children with hypochromic, microcytic anemia, and MCV/RBC index <12 should be further evaluated (hemoglobin electrophoresis after iron repletion).
- Because of the young age of many children at the time of adoption (and the presence of fetal hemoglobin), it may be difficult to identify specific hemoglobin disorders.

FAQs

Q. Should I screen all internationally adopted children for these hemoglobin rarities?

A. A complete blood count at arrival is all that is needed to start; a fingerstick hematocrit is not adequate. The red blood cell indices should be scrutinized carefully and further work-up planned depending on the findings. G6PD screens should be done before administration of drugs that might trigger hemolysis, or may be included as part of initial screening tests obtained in newly arrived children. Most state screening programs for newborns include a hemoglobin electrophoresis: for 4 drops of blood a lot of information is obtained. Annual CBCs until age 2 or 3 are useful in children who arrive as young infants, especially those from Asia.

Q. My 10-month-old patient from China has the following lab results: Hgb 9.7, Hct 30%, MCV 58, RDW 19, RBC 5.77. Now what?

A. With this initial information, it is impossible to differentiate between iron deficiency, thalassemia, or hemoglobinopathy (or a combination). The Mentzer Index (MCV/RBC) = 10.05 is suggestive of thalassemia. Treat with iron supplements for at least 2 months. (Orange juice aids iron absorption.) Then, repeat the lab work and obtain a hemoglobin electrophoresis. It is also useful to obtain iron levels, TIBC, and ferritin and to review the blood smear. Remember that most international adoptees are undergoing many biochemical and metabolic changes within the first months after arrival, and this may indicate recovering iron deficiency rather than any hemoglobinopathy.

Q. My patient's blood work showed Hgb 10.4, Hct 33%, MCV 57, iron 54 (normal 50–150), transferrin 290 (normal 200–400), and TIBC 348 (240–480). Hemoglobin electrophoresis showed Hgb H "positive", Hgb A2 2.5% (normal 1.5–3.5), and Hgb F 4.2% (NI 0.4–2.0). She's an 8-month-old from China. What now?

A. These results suggest that the baby has α-thalassemia trait. She does not need iron supplementation. The tests should be repeated in 6 months to reassess the Hgb F level—presently it is probably normal for age.

Q. This 12-month-old from Lebanon has Hgb 10.1, Hct 32%, MCV 64, and RDW 34. The smear shows microcytosis, anisocytosis, and some ovalocytes, target cells, and bizarre red cell forms. Examination by the pathologist showed a "bimodal" population of erythrocytes. A hemoglobin electrophoresis showed normal Hgb A2 but Hgb F was slightly elevated. What does this mean?

A. This is most suggestive of iron deficiency anemia that is responding to therapy. There may be an associated hemoglobinopathy; the electrophoresis should be repeated in 6 months. She should be treated with iron meanwhile.

References

1. Jenista JA, Chapman D. Medical problems of foreign-born adopted children. Am J Dis Child 1987; 141: 298–302.

2. Hostetter MK, Iverson S, Dole K, Johnson DE. Unsuspected infectious diseases and other medical diagnoses in the evaluation of internationally adopted children. Pediatrics 1989; 83:559–64.

3. Bureau JJ, Maurage C, Bremond M, Despert F, Rolland JC. Children of foreign origin adopted in France. Analysis of 68 cases during 12 years at the University Hospital Center of Tours [in French]. Arch Pediatr 1999; 6: 1053–8.

4. Nicholson AJ, Francis BM, Mulholland EK, Moulden AL, Oberklaid F. Health screening of international adoptees. Evaluation of a hospital based clinic [see comments]. Med J Aust 1992; 156:377–9.

5. Smith-Garcia T, Brown JS. The health of children adopted from India. J Community Health 1989; 14: 227–41.

6. Miller LC, Kiernan MT, Mathers MI, Klein-Gitelman M. Developmental and nutritional status of interna-

tionally adopted children. Arch Pediatr Adolesc Med 1995; 149:40–4.

7. Miller LC, Hendrie NW. Health of children adopted from China. Pediatrics 2000; 105:E76.

8. Hostetter MK, Iverson S, Thomas W, McKenzie D, Dole K, Johnson DE. Medical evaluation of internationally adopted children. N Engl J Med 1991; 325:479–85.

9. Allen SJ, O'Donnell A, Alexander ND, et al. $\alpha+$-Thalassemia protects children against disease caused by other infections as well as malaria. Proc Natl Acad Sci USA 1997; 94:14736–41.

10. Chen FE, Ooi C, Ha SY, et al. Genetic and clinical features of hemoglobin H disease in Chinese patients. N Engl J Med 2000; 343:544–50.

11. Olivieri NF. The beta-thalassemias. N Engl J Med 1999; 341:99–109.

12. Pearson HA, Cohen AR, Giardina PJ, Kazazian HH. The changing profile of homozygous beta-thalassemia. Pediatrics 1996; 97:352–6.

13. McDonagh KT, Nienhuis AW. The thalassemias. In: Nathan DG, Oski FA, eds. Hematology of Infancy and Childhood, Vol. 1. Philadelphia: W.B. Saunders, 1993: 783–879.

14. Krishnamurti L, Chui DHK, Dallaire M, LeRoy B, Waye JS, Perentesis JP. Coinheritance of alpha-thalassemia-1 and hemoglobin E/beta-thalassemia. J Pediatr 1998; 132:863–5.

15. Sergeyeva A, Gordeuk VR, Tokarev YN, Sokol L, Prchal JF, Prchal JT. Congenital polycythemia in Chuvashia. Blood 1997; 89:2148–54.

24

LEAD AND OTHER ENVIRONMENTAL TOXINS

Pediatricians throughout the world recognize the impact of environmental exposures on the health and well-being of children.[1] Doctors working in orphanages are no different, and frequently cite "poor ecology" or "bad air and water" as primary problems of the children in their care.

Adoptive parents often are dismayed to discover that their child-to-be resides in a heavily polluted, industrialized city. Prior to travel, some families research their child's birth city or region and discover proximity to nuclear power stations, mining pits (e.g., nickel, copper, coal), or other potential sources of environmental toxins. They wonder if there will be any long-term effects on the child from possible exposures. For example, the potential risks to children adopted from the areas surrounding Chernobyl, the site of the 1986 nuclear power disaster, remain a frequent concern nearly 20 years later.

Exposures to environmental toxins are not unique to institutionalized children. However, such exposures may act synergistically with other adverse environmental factors to increase the likelihood of problems. Concurrent iron or zinc deficiency, malnutrition, and lack of developmental stimulation—all problems that may occur in the orphanage setting—make children more vulnerable to neurotoxicants. For example, negative effects on cognitive and motor abilities were found among Dutch children prenatally exposed to PCB and dioxin only if parental and home characteristics were suboptimal.[2] Similarly, the effects of lead exposure on fine motor and visual motor function were ameliorated to some extent by a favorable home environment.[3] This suggests that children reared in institutions may be more vulnerable to the detrimental effects of toxins than children in a protective family environment.

Isolating the effects of specific environmental exposures is virtually impossible. Children may be exposed through air, water, food, or dust. In the United States, about 80,000 chemicals are presently in commercial use.[4] The numbers in other countries vary widely. Little is known about the developmental toxicology of these chemicals alone or in combination. Genetic vulnerability, timing and magnitude of dose, and other biological factors undoubtably influence the effects in individuals. Children have special vulnerability to these substances, compared with adults.[5] Asthma, cancer, compromised immune function, endocrine disruption (see Chapter 27), and developmental disorders have all been linked to toxic environmental exposures.[5,6]

The risks of lead and other environmental exposures for internationally adopted children are reviewed in this chapter, with a focus on developmental and behavioral disorders. (For more in-depth reviews of developmental neurotoxicology, see refs. 4–7.)

Developmental Neurotoxicants

Developmental neurotoxicants are chemical substances found in the environment that adversely affect neurobehavioral function in the child. Their presence may be suspected in children with various neurodevelopmental problems; proof of causality is difficult. Developmental problems are common among the general population of children in the United States: ~17% of children under age 18 suffer from one or more learning, developmental, or behavioral disabilities.[4] Attention-deficit disorder affects 3%–6% of all school children, although the prevalence may be considerably higher.[4] Learning disabilities affect approximately 5%–10% of school children, and autism affects about 0.2% of children (double the number 10 years ago).[4] The incidence of these disorders has been increasing; some investigators speculate that this reflects increasing exposure to developmental neurotoxicants. These neurobehavioral diagnoses are even more common among internationally adopted chil-

dren. In a survey of 81 children ages 8–12 years of age adopted from Eastern Europe, 52% had language disorders, 38% had attention-deficit disorder, 36% had learning disabilities, and 32% had sensory processing dysfunction.[8] In most cases, the causes of these problems are unknown. Although genetic susceptibility contributes to the development of these problems, certain environmental exposures may increase expression of these disorders.

Most children likely experience multiple exposures to environmental toxins throughout development, beginning in fetal life. Known developmental neurotoxicants such as lead, mercury, cadmium, manganese, nicotine, pesticides, dioxin and PCBs, and solvents (including ethanol, see Chapter 5) are common throughout the world.[4] Some of the effects on children of exposure to these substances are listed in (Table 24–1).

Subclinical exposures, although minor for the individual, may have profound implications for the population.[5] For example, a five-point drop in IQ may not have a discernable effect on an individual, but a five-point drop in population mean IQ reduces the number of gifted children by 50% and increases the number of children with borderline IQ by 50%.[4,5]

In the next section, specific information about lead exposure in China and other countries will be reviewed and other country-specific risks discussed.

Lead

Very few "country-specific" risks for health problems occur among internationally adopted children. Rather, most children share the risks conferred by the institutional environments from which they were adopted—environments that are strikingly similar from country to country. An exception to this generalization is the increased risk of lead exposure among children from China (Table 24–2). Although some chil-

Table 24–1 Neurodevelopmental effects of some environmental toxins

Toxin	Effects
Lead	Attention deficits, increased impulsiveness, reduced school performance, aggression, delinquent behavior
Mercury	Mental retardation, gait and visual disturbances
	Language, attention and memory impairments after small prenatal exposures (such as resulting from regular maternal fish consumption)
Manganese	Hyperactivity
	Learning disabilities
Nicotine	Prenatal: IQ deficits (see Chapter 7), learning disorders, attention deficits
	Postnatal (i.e., passive smoke): impaired speech, language skills, intelligence
Dioxins and PCBs	Learning disabilities
	IQ deficits, hyperactivity, attention deficits
Pesticides	Impaired stamina, coordination, memory, representational drawing abilities
	Hyperactivity (seen in animals after one small dose on a single critical day of development)
Solvents	Structural birth defects, hyperactivity, attention deficits, reduced IQ, learning and memory deficiencies
	Alcohol—one drink a day during pregnancy may cause impulsive behavior, deficits in memory, IQ, school performance, and social adaptability in the child (see Chapter 5)

Source: Adapted from Schettler et al.,[4] reprinted with permission.

Table 24–2 Elevated blood lead levels in internationally adopted children

Country (N)	Adoptees with Elevated Blood Lead Level (%)
China (883)	1–13
Cambodia (71)	7
Other Asia (47)	2
Russia (557)	1–5
Other Eastern Europe (107)	3–7
Central and South America (95)	1

Source: Adapted from Aronson et al.[9]

dren from other countries have elevated blood lead levels,[9] the prevalence of lead toxicity among children adopted from China is notable. Elevated lead levels were found in 14% of 492 children adopted from China.[10] Some regions of Russia have excessive lead exposure as well. In a survey of Krasnouralsk, Volgograd, and Eka-terinburg, 23% of kindergarteners had elevated blood lead levels.[11]

Lead poisoning occurs globally. In one survey, 11% of refugee children (not adoptees) from Asia, Africa, and the Near East had lead poisoning.[12] Refugee children from some countries and regions were more likely to have elevated lead levels, specifically Vietnam (27%), Africa (27%), and the Near East (25%). A refugee child from Sudan was the first child to die from lead poisoning in the United States in 10 years; her lead level was 392 μg/dl 5 weeks after arrival in the United States.[12] Lead exposure for refugee children and adoptees may come from leaded gasoline, industrial emissions, traditional medicines, or foods contaminated through ceramic bowls, lead pots, or cooking utensils. Children with poor dietary intake of iron and calcium may have increased absorption of lead.[6,13,14]

The adverse effects of lead exposure on cognitive function is well established.[15–22] Even "low levels" (<10 μg/dl) of lead reduce intellectual function.[23–25] Multiple other adverse effects also occur, even at relatively low levels.[26] Some of these effects are listed in Table 24–3. Many of these effects are long-lasting and persist despite treatment. Indeed, cranial magnetic resonance spectroscopy demonstrates altered metabolism in frontal gray matter in lead-exposed individuals even several years after

Table 24–3 Effects of lead exposure on young children

Effects on Growth

Inverse correlations with stature and head circumference (even at low levels)[30]

Prenatal exposure associated with low birth weight, early postnatal exposure decreases early weight gain[31]

Prenatal exposure associated with lower birth weight and infant body mass index[32]

Decreased height, delayed puberty in girls (3 μg/dl)[33]

Effects on Behavior

Increased somatic complaints, delinquency, aggression, anxious/depressed behavior, social problems, attention problems, internalizing and externalizing behaviors (reported by parents, teachers, and children) in 12-year-olds with elevated lead burden[34]

Increased externalizing behavior scores in boys and internalizing behavior scores in girls[35]

More fear, withdrawal, and disinterest behaviors in young preschoolers with levels 10–25 μg/dl[36]

Dose–response between hair lead levels (even at low levels) and negative teacher ratings for behavior and attention[37]

Adjudicated delinquency associated with elevated bone lead levels[38]

Effects on Attention

Slower reaction time, less flexibility in changing focus of attention[39]

Less ability to "focus-execute" and shift attention[40]

Effects on School Performance

Decreased language processing performance[41]

Impaired psychometric intelligence, language function, attention, classroom behavior (levels as low as 15 μg/dl)[42]

More school dropouts, reading disability, lower vocabulary and grammatical reasoning scores, poorer eye–hand coordination, longer reaction times in young adults with history of elevated dentin lead levels at ages 6–7 years[43]

Significantly lower IQ scores, impaired auditory and language processing, increased reaction times, increased classroom behavior problems[18]

Decreased IQ, impaired attention, and impaired speech performance[44]

Intellectual and academic performance deficits at age 57 months and 10 years[16,45]

Decreased scores for arithmetic, reading, nonverbal reasoning, and short-term memory (even at levels <5 μg/dl)[25]

Decreased fine motor and visual motor function[3,6]

Decreased performance on neuropsychological tests (even at levels <5 μg/dl)[46]

Decreased language processing abilities associated with elevated bone lead levels[41]

Hearing impairment[6]

---

exposure.[27] Improvement in lead level does not invariably restore IQ.[28]

As in studies of prenatal exposure to drugs, alcohol, and tobacco (see Chapters 5–7), additional environmental confounders may contribute to the adverse outcomes of lead-exposed children. Such children are often born after poor or no prenatal care and are raised in families with lower income, education, and more crowded conditions.[29] Co-exposure to other neurotoxicants may also occur. Nutritional factors also contribute to lead absorption. Fat, vitamin C, calcium, iron, and zinc status all influence lead bioavailability.[30] Similarly, children residing in orphanage care may be more vulnerable to the effects of lead because of concurrent dietary deficiencies and suboptimal environment (Fig. 24–1).

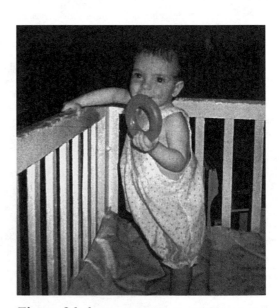

Figure 24–1 *Notice chew marks and chipped paint on railing of playpen. (With permission.)*

Chernobyl and the Risks of Radiation Exposure

On April 26, 1986, the nuclear reactors in Chernobyl, Ukraine caught fire, and radioactive fission products were released into the atmosphere for 7 days, until the smoke and fire were finally contained (Fig. 24–2). The radioactive plume was detected in Ukraine, Belarus, Russia, Scandinavia, the Netherlands, Belgium, and Great Britain. Later the plume shifted to central Europe, the northern Mediterranean, and the Balkans. The isotopes iodine-131, tellurium-iodine-132, cesium-137, and cesium-134 were deposited throughout these areas. Although this accident occurred nearly 20 years ago, the consequences are still emerging among children throughout Belarus, Ukraine, and parts of the Russian Federation.[47–51] Children in other parts of Europe, as far away as the north of England, also have been affected.[48,52]

The most dramatic effect of the Chernobyl disaster on child health has been a dramatic increase in the number of cases of papillary thyroid cancer. This cancer is typically more aggressive at presentation than other forms of thyroid cancer, and is frequently associated with thyroid autoimmunity and activation of the *RET* proto-oncogene.[53] Among exposed children without thyroid cancer, there appears to be an increase in benign thyroid nodules, hypothyroidism, autoimmune thyroiditis, and increase in circulating thyroid antibodies. Exposed children who migrated to Israel have increased circulating "clastogenic" factors (chromosome-damaging substances); their Israeli-born siblings do not.[54]

Nutritional deficiencies may exacerbate the health risks of exposure.[55] In utero exposure is linked to mental retardation and behavioral and emotional deviations.[6] Little information is available to assess the risks to children born after the disaster. Some of the children placed for international adoption from these regions likely were born to parents who were themselves irradiated as children. An increase in the incidence of hematopoietic malignancies has been found in children born after the accident to irradiated parents.[56] The full sequelae and long-term health risks of this "second genera-

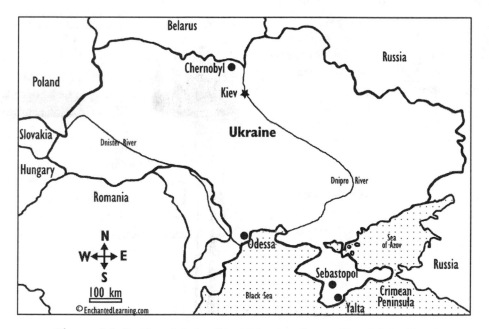

Figure 24–2   *Chernobyl, site of the 1986 nuclear disaster. (Copyright Enchanted Learning.com. Used by permission.)*

Table 24-4 Environmental threats in Asian countries

Region	Toxic Agents	Effects
Bangladesh (extreme), Cambodia, China, India, Nepal, Phillipines, and Vietnam	Groundwater widely contaminated with arsenic[a]	Hyperkeratosis, skin and other cancers
Phillipines	Mercury, cadmium, lead contamination, of fish	Neurotoxins
Cambodia (and others)	DDT, PCBs, dioxins, furans	Neurotoxins
Vietnam	Agent Orange	Birth defects, cancers, adverse reproductive outcomes
India, Thailand, China	Groundwater fluoride contamination, airborne fluoride from burning fluoride-laden coal	Dental (discolored, blackened, mottled teeth) and skeletal fluorosis (spine, bone, joint deformities)

[a]Also in Argentina, Chile, Mexico, Canada, and the United States.

Source: Adapted from UNEP, UNICEF, WHO[6] and Carpenter et al.[59]

tion" of Chernobyl victims are not completely known at present. Children at highest risk include (*1*) those exposed in utero, (*2*) those living in radioactivity contaminated territories, (*3*) those evacuated from resettlement zones, (*4*) those influenced by radioactive iodine emitted by the accident, and (*5*) those born to liquidators of the accident.[57] Few international adoptees fall into these categories.

Although the risks are not well-defined, children adopted from this region deserve regular scrutiny for thyroid problems and hematopoietic problems.

Other Ecological Disasters and Child Health

Sadly, many parts of the world are troubled by ecological disasters. Another notable site for international adoption is the Aral Sea region in Kazakhstan. Child health in this area has been compromised by the excessive environmental pollution with organochlorines resulting in birth defects, growth delays, and psychoneurological retardation.[58] An extremely high prevalence of hypercalciuria (due to renal tubular damage or to excessive intake of calcium and

sodium) has also been reported.[59] Notable problems in other Asian sending countries for international adoption are listed in Table 24-4).

Key Points for Internationally Adopted Children

- Developmental neurotoxicants are widespread throughout the world.
- Internationally adopted children may encounter these prenatally and/or postnatally.
- Other adverse environmental factors likely potentiate the harmful effects of neurotoxicants.
- Developmental neurotoxicants contribute to behavioral and cognitive problems.
- Children from the Chernobyl region should be monitored for thyroid and hematopoietic problems at annual physical examinations, supplemented by laboratory testing if indicated.

Resources

Alliance to End Childhood Lead Poisoning. Available at: www.globalleadnet.org.

Children in the New Millennium: Environmental Impact on Health. New York: United Nations, 2002. Available at: www.unep.org, www.unicef.org, and www.who.int.

References

1. Shea KM. Global environmental change and children's health: understanding the challenges and finding solutions. J Pediatr 2003; 143:149–54.

2. Vreugdenhil HJ, Lanting CI, Mulder PG, Boersma ER, Weisglas-Kuperus N. Effects of prenatal PCB and dioxin background exposure on cognitive and motor abilities in Dutch children at school age. J Pediatr 2002; 140:48–56.

3. Wasserman GA, Musabegovic A, Liu X, Kline J, Factor-Litvak P, Graziano JH. Lead exposure and motor functioning in 4(1/2)-year-old children: the Yugoslavia prospective study. J Pediatr 2000; 137:555–61.

4. Schettler T, Stein J, Reich F, Valenti M. In Harm's Way: Toxic Threats to Child Development. Boston: Greater Boston Physicians for Social Responsibility, 2000. Available at: http://psr.igc.org/ihw-project.htm

5. Landrigan P, Garg A. Chronic effects of toxic environmental exposures on children's health. J Toxicol 2002; 40:449–57.

6. UNEP, UNICEF, WHO. Children in the New Millennium; Environmental Impact on Health. New York: United Nations, 2002.

7. McCally M, Hu H, Chivian E. Critical condition: Human Health and the Environment—A Report by Physicians for Social Responsibility. Boston: MIT Press, 1993.

8. Tirella LG, Miller LC. Educational Outcomes in Post-Institutionalized Eastern European Adopted Children. Washington, DC; Joint Council for International Children's Services, 2002.

9. Aronson JE, Smith AM, Kothari V, et al. Elevated blood lead levels among internationally adopted children—United States, 1998. MMWR Morbid Mortal Wkly Rep 2000; 49:97–100.

10. Miller LC, Hendrie NW. Health of children adopted from China. Pediatrics 2000; 105:E76.

11. Rubin CH, Esteban E, Reissman DB, et al. Lead poisoning among young children in Russia: concurrent evaluation of childhood lead exposure in Ekaterinburg, Krasnouralsk, and Volgograd. Environ Health Perspect 2002; 110:559–62.

12. Geltman PL, Brown MJ, Cochran J. Lead poisoning among refugee children resettled in Massachusetts, 1995 to 1999. Pediatrics 2001; 108:158–62.

13. Wright RO, Tsaih S-W, Schwartz J, Wright RJ, Hu H. Association between iron deficiency and blood lead level in a longitudinal analysis of children followed in an urban primary care clinic. J Pediatr 2003; 142:9–14.

14. McGeehin MA. Getting the lead out: can iron help? J Pediatr 2003; 142:3–4.

15. Baghurst PA, McMichael AJ, Wigg NR, et al. Environmental exposure to lead and children's intelligence at the age of seven years. The Port Pirie Cohort Study. N Engl J Med 1992; 327:1279–84.

16. Bellinger DC, Stiles KM, Needleman HL. Low-level lead exposure, intelligence and academic achievement: a long-term follow-up study. Pediatrics 1992; 90:855–61.

17. Needleman HL, Bellinger D, Leviton A. Does lead at low dose affect intelligence in children? Pediatrics 1981; 68:894–6.

18. Needleman HL. The neurobehavioral consequences of low lead exposure in childhood. Neurobehav Toxicol Teratol 1982; 4:729–32.

19. Needleman HL. Lead exposure and children's IQ. Int J Epidemiol 1987; 16:485.

20. Needleman HL, Gatsonis CA. Low-level lead exposure and the IQ of children. A meta-analysis of modern studies. JAMA 1990; 263:673–8.

21. Needleman HL. Environmental lead and children's intelligence. Studies included in the meta-analysis are not representative. BMJ 1995; 310:1408; discussion 1409.

22. Schwartz J. Low-level lead exposure and children's IQ: a meta-analysis and search for a threshold. Environ Res 1994; 65:42–55.

23. Rogan WJ, Ware JH. Exposure to lead in children—how low is low enough? N Engl J Med 2003; 348:1515–16.

24. Canfield RL, Henderson CR, Cory-Slechta DA, Cox C, Jusko TA, Lanphear BP. Intellectual impairment in children with blood lead concentrations below 10 μg per deciliter. N Engl J Med 2003; 348:1517–26.

25. Lanphear BP, Dietrich K, Auinger P, Cox C. Cognitive deficits associated with blood lead concentrations <10 μg/dl in U.S. children and adolescents. Public Health Rep 2000; 115:521–9.

26. Binns HJ, Kim D, Campbell C. Targeted screening for elevated blood lead levels: populations at high risk. Pediatrics 2001; 108:1364–6.

27. Trope I, Lopez-Villegas D, Cecil KM, Lenkinski RE. Exposure to lead appears to selectively alter metabolism of cortical gray matter. Pediatrics 2001; 107:1437–42.

28. Liu X, Dietrich K, Radcliffe J, Ragan NB, Rhoads GG, Rogan WJ. Do children with falling blood levels have improved cognition? Pediatrics 2002; 110:787–91.

29. Recknor JC, Reigart JR, Darden PM, Goyer RA, Olden K, Richardson MC. Prenatal care and infant lead exposure. J Pediatr 1997; 130:123–7.

30. Ballew C, Khan LK, Kaufmann R, Mokdad A, Miller DT, Gunter EW. Blood lead concentration and

children's anthropometric dimensions in the Third National Health and Nutrition Examination Survey (NHANES III), 1988–1994. J Pediatr 1999; 134:623–30.

31. Sanin LH, Gonzalez-Cossio T, Romieu I, et al. Effect of maternal lead burden on infant weight and weight gain at one month of age among breastfed infants. Pediatrics 2001; 107:1016–23.

32. Odland JO, Nieboer E, Romanova N, Thomassen Y, Lund E. Blood lead and cadmium and birth weight among sub-arctic and arctic populations of Norway and Russia. Acta Obstet Gynecol Scand 1999; 78:852–60.

33. Selevan SG, Rice DC, Hogan KA, Euling SY, Pfahles-Hutchens A, Bethel J. Blood lead concentration and delayed puberty in girls. N Engl J Med 2003; 348: 1527–36.

34. Needleman HL, Riess JA, Tobin MJ, Biesecker GE, Greenhouse JB. Bone lead levels and delinquent behavior. JAMA 1996; 275:363–9.

35. Burns JM, Baghurst PA, Sawyer MG, McMichael AJ, Tong SL. Lifetime low-level exposure to environmental lead and children's emotional and behavioral development at ages 11–13 years. The Port Pirie Cohort Study. Am J Epidemiol 1999; 149:740–9.

36. Mendelsohn AL, Dreyer BP, Fierman AH, et al. Low-level lead exposure and behavior in early childhood. Pediatrics 1998; 101:E10.

37. Tuthill RW. Hair lead levels related to children's classroom attention-deficit behavior. Arch Environ Health 1996; 51:214–20.

38. Needleman HL, McFarland C, Ness RB, Fienberg SE, Tobin MJ. Bone lead levels in adjudicated delinquents: a case control study. Neurotoxicol Teratol 2002; 24:711–17.

39. Minder B, Das-Smaal EA, Brand EF, Orlebeke JF. Exposure to lead and specific attentional problems in schoolchildren. J Learn Disabil 1994; 27:393–9.

40. Bellinger D, Hu H, Titlebaum L, Needleman HL. Attentional correlates of dentin and bone lead levels in adolescents. Arch Environ Health 1994; 49:98–105.

41. Campbell TF, Needleman HL, Riess JA, Tobin MJ. Bone lead levels and language processing performance. Dev Neuropsychol 2000; 18:171–86.

42. Needleman HL. What can the study of lead teach us about other toxicants? Environ Health Perspect 1990; 86:183–9.

43. Needleman HL, Schell A, Bellinger D, Leviton A, Allred EN. The long-term effects of exposure to low doses of lead in childhood. An 11-year follow-up report. N Engl J Med 1990; 322:83–8.

44. Needleman HL. The current status of childhood low-level lead toxicity. Neurotoxicology 1993; 14:161–6.

45. Bellinger D, Sloman J, Leviton A, Rabinowitz M, Needleman HL, Waternaux C. Low-level lead exposure and children's cognitive function in the preschool years. Pediatrics 1991; 87:219–27.

46. Sovcikova E., Wsolova L. Effect of low-level body burdens of lead on the somatic development of children. Presented at ECOHSE Symposium, Kaunas, Lithuania, 2000. Available at: http://www.gla.ac.uk/ecohse/2000papers/sovcikova.pdf.

47. Hall P, Holm LE. Radiation-associated thyroid cancer—facts and fiction. Acta Oncol 1998; 37:325–30.

48. Pacini F, Vorontsova T, Molinaro E, et al. Thyroid consequences of the Chernobyl nuclear accident. Acta Paediatr Suppl 1999; 88:23–7.

49. Leenhardt L, Aurengo A. Post-Chernobyl thyroid carcinoma in children. Baillieres Best Pract Res Clin Endocrinol Metab 2000; 14:667–77.

50. Jacob P, Kenigsberg Y, Goulko G, et al. Thyroid cancer risk in Belarus after the Chernobyl accident: comparison with external exposures. Radiat Environ Biophys 2000; 39:25–31.

51. Jacob P, Kenigsberg Y, Zvonova I, et al. Childhood exposure due to the Chernobyl accident and thyroid cancer risk in contaminated areas of Belarus and Russia. Br J Cancer 1999; 80:1461–9.

52. Cotterill SJ, Pearce MS, Parker L. Thyroid cancer in children and young adults in the North of England. Is increasing incidence related to the Chernobyl accident? Eur J Cancer 2001; 37:1020–6.

53. Santoro M, Thomas GA, Vecchio G, et al. Gene rearrangement and Chernobyl-related thyroid cancers. Br J Cancer 2000; 82:315–22.

54. Kordysh EA, Emerit I, Goldsmith JR, et al. Dietary and clastogenic factors in children who immigrated to Israel from regions contaminated by the Chernobyl accident. Arch Environ Health 2001; 56:320–6.

55. Parizkova J. Dietary habits and nutritional status in adolescents in Central and Eastern Europe. Eur J Clin Nutr 2000; 54:S36–40.

56. Lomat L, Galburt G, Quastel MR, Polyakov S, Okeanov A, Rozin S. Incidence of childhood disease in Belarus associated with the Chernobyl accident. Environ Health Perspect 1997; 105:1529–32.

57. Chernobyl children-health consequences and psychosocial rehabilitation. 4th International Conference. Kiev, Ukraine. Available at: http://www.chernobyl.info/files/doc/Resolution-eng_draft.pdf.

58. Zetterstrom R. Child health and environmental pollution in the Aral Sea region in Kazakhstan. Acta Paediatr Suppl 1999; 429:49–54.

59. Kaneko K, Chiba M, Hashizume M, et al. Extremely high prevalence of hypercalciuria in children living in the Aral Sea region. Acta Paediatr Suppl 2002; 91: 1116–20.

60. Carpenter DO, Chew FT, Damstra T, et al. Environmental threats to the health of children: the Asian perspective. Environ Health Perspect 2000; 108:989–92.

25

RICKETS

Nutritional rickets, once common in industrialized and polluted northern cities of Western Europe and the United States,[1] is infrequently encountered in most general pediatrics populations in these regions. However, its re-emergence has recently been documented among some inner-city children in the United States.[2,3] In contrast, rickets is common among international adoptees, especially those arriving from northern latitudes. A history of "rachitis" (an old term for rickets) is found on many pre-adoptive medical records. In actuality, few children have obvious or severe rickets on arrival to the United States. However, subtle manifestations of rickets may be overlooked unless specifically sought on physical examination. On arrival, radiographs and laboratory test results may be atypical or inconclusive:[4] improved diet and sun exposure provided by adoptive parents during the brief interval between adoption and arrival in the United States may partially ameliorate this condition. In severe malnutrition or growth arrest, clinical expression of rickets may not develop despite inadequate intake of vitamin D and/or calcium.

Genetic forms of rickets are rare, these are discussed in standard pediatric texts.

Etiology

Rickets is a disorder of bone mineralization. Bone matrix is produced but not mineralized; unmineralized matrix therefore accumulates. Nutritional rickets is primarily due to deficiency of vitamin D, but it may also be caused by calcium or phosphorus deficiency. Inadequate exposure to sunlight also contributes to the development of rickets.[5,6] Children living in orphanages often lack one or more of these elements. Diets in some orphanages are notably deficient in dairy products or other calcium sources. High-fiber diets (especially phytates,[6] found in cereals and grains) may inhibit calcium absorption (as well as iron and zinc). Such diets, common in Asia, are often calcium deficient. Chronic diarrhea (due to enteric pathogens, lactase deficiency) may interfere with absorption of dietary calcium. Vitamin D–enriched cow's milk and other foods are unavailable in many parts of the world. Unfortified cow's milk contains only about 0.3–4 IU/100 ml of vitamin D.[7] Vitamin D supplements are expensive and rarely administered to orphanage residents.

Sunlight is necessary for the conversion of vitamin D precursors to cholecaliferol (vitamin D_3, found in skin); further activation takes place in the liver and kidneys. Children, especially those residing in northern latitudes, may have little exposure to sunlight during long, dark winters. For example, the Kola peninsula of Russia and polar regions of Siberia receive 0–2 hours of sunlight during the winter months, a significant risk for rickets. Institutionalized children in northern climates may be confined indoors with minimal sun exposure, especially during wintertime. Children with borderline calcium/vitamin D status are at high risk to develop rickets under these conditions. However, children in other climates may also develop rickets, even children residing near the equator.[8,9] Dark skin decreases vitamin D activation by ultraviolet light, and impoverished children everywhere may lack adequate dietary calcium.

Other risk factors for the development of rickets are listed in Table 25–1. In Romania, most institutionalized children receive regular injections of various vitamin D preparations; this is usually listed on pre-adoptive medical records as "vitaminization." Theoretically, this practice may lead to hypervitaminosis D, and may not prevent rickets unless adequate dietary calcium is also provided. Rickets often occurs in conjunction with other micronutrient deficiencies (see Chapter 11).

Diagnosis

Severe rickets presents with the typical bony deformities associated with poor mineralization of growing bone (Table 25–2, Fig. 25–1). Bowing of the legs, considered a classic feature of rickets, is not seen until weight-bearing and

Table 25–1 Risk factors for development of rickets

Dietary deficiency of calcium

Inadequate intake of vitamin D

Excessive intake of phytates (interferes with calcium absorption)

Inadequate sun exposure

Prematurity (reduces total body calcium stores at birth)

Dark skin (melanin reduces formation of vitamin D by ultraviolet light)

Genetic variation in calcium absorption[6]

Severe maternal vitamin D deficiency (rare)

Table 25–2 Signs of rickets

Skeleton

Thickened wrists

Genu varum or valgum

Thickened epiphyses especially noticeable at wrists and ankles

Anterior tibial bowing

Craniotabes

Frontal bossing

Delayed closure of anterior fontanelle

Bulging anterior fontanelle[10]

Flaring of lower ribs (Fig. 25–4)

Humeral bowing

Kyphosis and scoliosis

Beading of the ribs (rachitic rosary)

Pectus carinatum

Dentition

Dental enamel hypoplasia (especially distal); extensive caries

Delayed and out-of-sequence eruption of primary dentition

Other

Increased sweating especially around the head

Growth failure

Hypotonia

Increased incidence of pneumonia, even after adjustment for all confounding factors[6]

Source: Adapted from Chesney[7] and Thacher et al.[9]

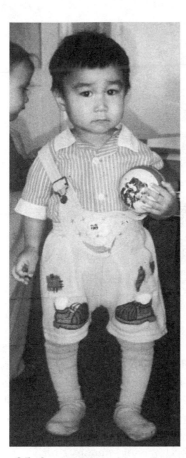

Figure 25–1 *Typical appearance of rickets in child residing in an orphanage in Kazakhstan.*

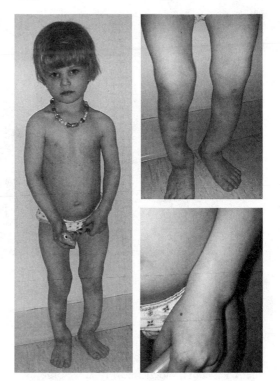

Figure 25–2 *Unusual appearance of tibial rickets in a 4½-year-old girl adopted from Russia (With permission). The distal tibial bowing has been attributed to the posteromedial angulation of the distal tibial growth plate by the lower leg muscles in children with delayed weight bearing.[4] Wrist shows typical rickets.*

walking are established. Young children from institutional care, with motor delays and minimal weight bearing, may have bowing of the distal rather than mid-tibiae[4] (Fig. 25–2). Alternatively, genu valgus may be seen. Short stature, hypotonia, weakness, delayed motor development, frequent falls, leg pain with or without ambulation, and history of fractures may also accompany clinical rickets.[9]

Radiographic changes in rickets are distinctive[7] (Fig. 25–3). Irregular epiphyses with cupping (or in advanced cases, angulation of bones), coarsened trabeculae, and subperiosteal collection of poorly mineralized matrix are common findings. Skeletal radiographs of internationally adopted children usually demonstrate "healing rickets." In these children, several weeks may have passed since adoptive

parents have assumed the care of the child, and have provided a multivitamin containing vitamin D, calcium-fortified foods, unlimited dairy products, and sun exposure. Radiographs are helpful at baseline to document the degree of changes. Few entities will be confused with full-blown clinical rickets; however, radiographs may be helpful in the child with isolated genu varus to exclude Blount's disease or other possibilities.

Biochemical analysis of a blood sample is important in the diagnosis and management of rickets. Typically, decreased calcium, phosphorus, and 25-OH D_3 levels are found, accompanied by an elevated (sometimes markedly so) alkaline phosphatase. However, dietary changes post-adoption may have resulted in normalization of some or all biochemical markers, along

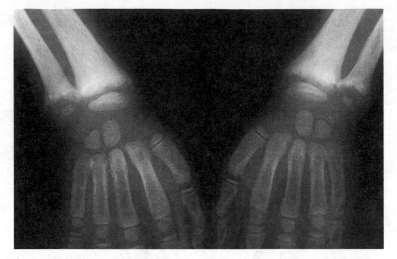

Figure 25–3 *Irregularities in the provisional zones of calcification of distal radii and ulnae; widening of the distal metaphyses.*

with elevation of $1,25(OH)_2D_3$ levels.[4] In our clinic, isolated elevation of alkaline phosphatase is the most common abnormality seen, likely reflecting residual biochemical rickets combined with an active growth spurt.

Treatment

Most children with mild (biochemical) rickets do not require treatment other than a vitamin D–containing multivitamin preparation, adequate dietary calcium, and sun exposure. The few children with skeletal deformities may benefit from supplemental vitamin D. The daily requirement for infants and children is 400 IU per day of vitamin D as ergocalciferol (D_2), or cholecalciferol (D_3). Rickets can be treated with 1–2000 IU/day of vitamin D for 1–2 months. Children with severe hypocalcemia should be treated carefully to prevent tetany. Diet should be carefully reviewed. Some misguided parents

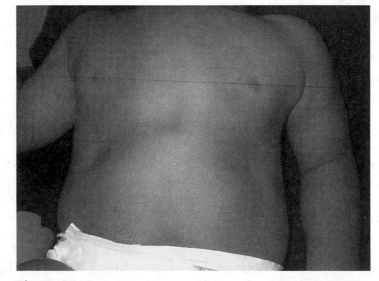

Figure 25–4 *Pechis carinatum and flaring of lower rib margins in rickets.*

Martha arrived at age 24 months of age from India. Her problem list at arrival included growth below the third percentile for all three measurements, developmental delay of 8–9 months, lead level 37 μg/dl, iron deficiency anemia (Hct 26%), parasites (Ascaris, Giardia, and B. hominis), and rickets (alkaline phosphatase 950, phosphorus 5.2, calcium 8.1). The rickets was managed with 2000 IU/day of vitamin D (Drisdol) for 6 months. Three years later, she is a delightful, verbal kindergartener who is slightly small (fifth to tenth percentile) and otherwise completely well.

select various soy or rice "milks" which are not specifically formulated for rapidly growing children; such preparations may lack adequate vitamin D or calcium unless specifically fortified. Extensive bony remodeling of even severe rickets usually occurs within 1–2 years. Orthopedic consultation may provide some advice about shoes or temporary orthotics. For most children, there is little or no role for surgical intervention.

Key Points for Internationally Adopted Children

- Rickets is common in international adoptees, especially those from countries in northern latitudes.
- Rickets has diverse skeletal and dental manifestations.
- Most children do not require specific treatment beyond good diet and multivitamins.
- Of those affected, most have "healing" rickets within weeks after adoption.

FAQs

Q. Four-year-old Dina was adopted from Kazakhstan. She has enormously bowed legs and frontal bossing. Her radiographs show "healing rickets" and all her blood biochemistry tests, including 25-OH-D levels, were normal. Her mom had started her on a daily multivitamin with 400 IU of vitamin D several weeks before leaving Kazakhstan. She's drinking nearly a quart of milk a day! Should she receive any special vitamin D or calcium supplementation now?

A. Continue the 400 IU of vitamin D daily. She is receiving adequate calcium in her diet.

Q. Nineteen-month-old Nina just came from Russia. Her alkaline phosphatase is over 2000! What do I do now? She doesn't seem to have obvious rickets on exam.

A. She probably has biochemical rickets that is already improving. It would be good to obtain serum calcium and phosphorus levels if not already done, and a 25-(OH)D as well. Radiographs are not absolutely necessary but might be helpful to document progress. Be sure she has adequate calcium and vitamin intake in her diet. Keep in mind that rickets is not the only explanation for the elevated alkaline phosphatase level. Does she have liver disease? (check liver transaminases, bilirubin, alkaline phosphatase isoenzymes) an occult fracture? (careful physical examination; consider radiographs) an *Entamoeba histolytica* hepatic abscess (see Chapter 17)? (check for hepatomegaly and tender right upper quadrant—consider liver ultrasound). Or Is this a massive growth spurt? Close clinical and laboratory follow-up should reveal the answers.

References

1. Rajakumar K. Vitamin D, cod-liver oil, sunlight, and rickets: a historical perspective. Pediatrics 2003; 112: e119–31.

2. Tomashek KM, Nesby S, Scanlon KS, et al. Nutritional rickets in Georgia. Pediatrics 2001; 107:E45.

3. Kreiter SR, Schwartz RP, Kirkman HN Jr, Charlton PA, Calikoglu AS, Davenport ML. Nutritional rickets in African American breast-fed infants. J Pediatr 2000; 137: 153–7.

4. Reeves GD, Bachrach S, Carpenter TO, Mackenzie WG. Vitamin D-deficiency rickets in adopted children from the former Soviet Union: an uncommon problem with unusual clinical and biochemical features. Pediatrics 2000; 106:1484–8.

5. Welch TR, Bergstrom WH, Tsang RC. Vitamin D–deficient rickets: the reemergence of a once-conquered disease. J Pediatr 2000; 137:143–5.

6. Bishop N. Rickets today—children still need milk and sunshine. N Engl J Med 1999; 341:602–4.

7. Chesney RW. Metabolic bone disease: bone structure, growth, and hormonal regulation. In: Behrman RE, Kliegman RM, Jenson HB, eds. Nelson's Textbook of Pediatrics. Philadelphia: W.B. Saunders, 2000: 2132–4.

8. Pfitzner MA, Thacher TD, Pettifor JM, et al. Absence of vitamin D deficiency in young Nigerian children. J Pediatr 1998; 133:740–4.

9. Thacher TD, Fischer PR, Pettifor JM, Lawson JO, Isichei CO, Chan GM. Case–control study of factors associated with nutritional rickets in Nigerian children. J Pediatr 2000; 137:367–73.

10. DeJong AR, Callahan CA, Weiss J. Pseudotumor cerebri and nutritional rickets. Eur J Pediatr 1985; 143: 219–20.

26

UNCERTAIN AGE

Correct age is often uncertain for internationally adopted children. Age is seldom known with certainty for Chinese children; many children from other countries also have uncertain ages. The most common reason for uncertain age is discrepant documents, e.g., discordant dates are found on different records. Often, this is due to transcription or translation errors, or misinterpretation of month/date format (09/03 being alternately translated as September 3 or March 9). Many sending countries in Eastern Europe use the convention of Roman numerals for the month and Arabic numerals for the day (e.g., 4 X is October 4). These puzzles are relatively easy to unravel, and generally a satisfactory interpretation of the child's actual birthdate may be formed.

However, some children truly have uncertain dates of birth. In others, the assigned date of birth is clearly incorrect. This section discusses the circumstances of uncertain age,

reviews methodologic considerations for dental and bone age determinations, and provides guidelines for the pediatrician to assign a reasonable date of birth for the child if necessary.

Circumstances of Uncertain Age

There are many reasons for a child's actual age not being known. Most commonly, the child is a true foundling—that is, found after abandonment. Unlike abandonment in the hospital or maternity home, no records accompany the child. Infants without identifying information are sometimes found in public settings such as parks, markets, bus stations, government buildings, or hospitals. Older children may be found wandering on the street, with no information— or with misinformation—about themselves and their families. In other cases, legal and medical documents are lost, often during multiple transfers among institutions. Further problems occur because of cultural differences. In some cultures, birth is recorded using non–Western methods (e.g., lunar calendar, or "born during the rice planting") difficult to translate into Western terms. Unfamiliar systems of age classification for older children ("big enough to herd goats" or "capable of carrying a younger sibling") are not readily translated into Western terms.[1] Whatever the situation, children with uncertain age are assigned a date of birth on entry into supervised care. Newborns with affixed umbilical cords do not present difficulties; however, errors may occur with older infants and children. Prematurity, malnutrition, and failure to thrive due to neglect all contribute to mistaken age assignments. However, nearly all age assignments given in the birth country are acceptable. It is unusual for the assigned age, even if known to be inaccurate, to be substantively incorrect. Assigned ages thus are appropriate to maintain for nearly all children.

Special Considerations: China

Virtually all Chinese children placed for adoption (with the exception of some special needs children) are foundlings. Information about the circumstances of the child's discovery is sometimes included in the referral packet provided to adoptive parents ("Found on the bridge/in front of police station"). Most are abandoned as newborns or very young infants; occasionally a child is abandoned at 11 or 12 months of age, possibly after the birth of a younger brother. Older children are sometimes abandoned after medical problems are detected—for example, a boy with acyanotic tetralogy of Fallot found in the train station at age 3 years, probably soon after this diagnosis was made in rural China. Sometimes, a note is pinned to a garment, giving the child's date of birth (see Chapter 3). More often, the age is assigned by the caregivers. Infants present fewer difficulties in accurate age assignment than older children, and any errors become proportionally less the older the child grows. Occasionally, bureaucratic

procedures dictate that a group of children within a particular orphanage are all given the same age assignment. Usually this becomes apparent when traveling parents discover multiple children in the group with identical birthdays (often the first day of the same month).

When to Be Suspicious

Appraisal of the adequacy of age assignment is part of the initial and follow-up evaluations of all newly arrived children. Because most new arrivals have growth and developmental delays, this assessment may be difficult. Extreme discrepancies between objective observations and age assignment should be carefully monitored; disparities of a few months are usually not cause for concern. It is worthwhile to ask parents at the initial visit if they suspect that age is uncertain for any reason. Strong parental misgivings about the age assignment should be addressed. Inaccuracies in age assignments may be either direction—too young or too old. Both are problematic for the child and the parents. Parents are often very anxious about age uncertainty—roughly analogous to the feelings of parents whose newborn has ambiguous genitalia. The second most common question new adoptive parents are asked (after the child's gender) is the new child's age. Age uncertainty affects school entry, eligibility for rehabilitative programs (e.g., Early Intervention), and sibling and peer relationships.

Practical Management

Comparison of the child's growth and development to age standards allows determination of the child's functional age. As a baseline, the child's growth measurements should be plotted on the same chart with any available growth information from the birth country. Arrival measurements should also be recorded as height age, weight age, and head circumference age (e.g., the ages for which the child's measurements are at the 50th percentile). Physical examination should include inspection and documentation of dentition. Older children should be closely examined for signs of incipient puberty. Bone age and dental radiographs may be useful especially if followed serially (see below). A detailed developmental assessment at arrival is essential to document skills at entry and to serve as a baseline for follow–up evaluations.

Age reassignment must be carefully approached, especially in the dynamic early post–adoption period (see Chapters 10, and 13). Although parents are anxious to "finalize" their child's age, they must be instructed that haste leads to problems—usually several years in the future. A period of observation is often warranted before a decision to reassign age is reached. Most children should be observed for a minimum of 4–6 months before age reassignment is undertaken. The usual rapid recovery of growth and developmental delays within this period often obviate the "need" to reassign age, or make the correct age very obvious. Dynamic changes in dental age and skeletal maturity during this observation period are useful in planning age reassignments, if needed. Age determination methods have been a recent subject of congressional debate.[2]

Dental Age

Dental age is determined clinically or radiologically. Most simply, dental age is estimated by counting erupted teeth. The tooth is erupted when its crown appears. The Bailey Formula is useful as a rough guide to dental age during the first 24 months of life (age in months = number of erupted teeth + 6).[3] This relationship becomes markedly asymptotic once 20 teeth have erupted,[4] and is less valuable for children over 24–30 months of age.[5] Skeletal maturation correlates poorly with deciduous tooth eruption in normal children.[5–8]

Clinical dental age has been extensively investigated as a proxy for chronologic age in young children. Field studies in the developing world rely on accurate age assessments to evaluate anthropometric data and disease prevalence. Accurate records of chronologic age are seldom available, however. Eruption of primary teeth has been compared in many racial and ethnic groups (Table 26–1) (see entire issue *Journal of Tropical Pediatrics and Environmental Child Health*, June 1973, for fascinating discussion). The timing of dental eruption is amazingly similar among healthy children of many racial and ethnic groups, although there is considerable individual variation[9] that impedes its usefulness for precise age determinations.[4]

Delayed dental eruption occurs in hypothyroidism, hypoparathyroidism, Down syndrome, prematurity, and hypopituitarism.[6,9] Most other childhood illnesses have little effect on dental eruption, although rickets (see Chapter 25) is associated with delayed dentition (and enamel defects) if the disease is active in the early stages of tooth formation and mineralization.[6] Dental formation and eruption date are probably programmed during fetal life.[6,9]

Malnutrition delays bone age, weight gain, and linear growth (see Chapter 10). In contrast, dental development is somewhat spared,

Betsy arrived from Russia in 1998. At that time, she was said to be 4 years 1 month. Her parents were concerned from the beginning about the lack of information in her dossier for the first year of her life. No vaccinations were given until 19 months of age. Her evaluations at arrival and follow-up are listed in Table 26–2.

Her parents stated, "We have always thought that Betsy was 1 year younger—physically, emotionally, and developmentally—than her records indicated. She has always done better with kids one year younger than her assigned age." Accordingly, after 1 year of observation, Betsy's age was reassigned. At follow-up 7 years later, she was socially comfortable with her sixth-grade classmates, in the 75th percentile for height and weight and third percentile for head circumference, had Tanner III pubertal changes, and had ongoing language delays requiring speech therapy.

Table 26–1 Mean number of erupted teeth in different populations

Age (months)	USA	London	Paris	Zurich	Dakar	Gambia	Newcastle (U.K.)
6	0.4	0.4	0.4	0.4	—	0.3	0.9
9	3.1	2.8	2.9	2.5	2.7	2.2	3.7
12	5.9	6.1	5.8	5.4	4.7	4.5	6.7
18	12.4	12.9	12.3	12.2	11.4	10.9	13.7
24	16.7	16.3	16.4	16.3	16.4	17.4	16.9
36	19.9	20.0	—	—	—	20.0	19.9

Source: Data from Billewicz.[10]

Table 26–2 Changes in growth and development after arrival (see sidebar page 333)

Factor	Arrival	13-month Follow-up	Change (months)
Chronological age	4 years 1 months	5 years 2 months	+13
Bone age	3 years	3 years 6 months	+6
Dental eruption	20 teeth	20 teeth	0
Weight age (months)	22	39	+17
Height age (months)	23	42	+19
Head circumference age (months)	18	24	+6
Gross motor skills (months)	28	36	+8
Fine motor skills (months)	35	42	+7
Social/emotional (months)	36	48	+12
Activities of daily living (months)	36+	48	+12
Language (months)	20–27	36–40	+13–16

perhaps because of the "vital nutritional importance" of the teeth to the growing child.[6,9] Mild or moderate malnutrition generally has little effect on dental eruption.[11–14] However, impoverished Indian children with malnutrition had fewer erupted deciduous teeth.[15] In contrast, no such relationship was found in malnourished Guatemalan children[16]; paradoxically, these children had more erupted teeth than their well–nourished peers. Institutionalization may delay dental eruption, possibly reflecting adversities other than malnutrition. For example, poorly nourished Jewish orphans in New York had moderately delayed dental eruption in a 1927 study.[6]

Radiologic determination of dental age is considerably more involved than enumerating erupted teeth. Numerous methods are available to assess the maturity and mineralization of the teeth. Reliability and reproducibility among these methods are imperfect, especially in older children.[17,18] In a comparison of two radiologic methods of dental age determination in 44 non–European adoptees in Sweden,[19] large variations in dental age (>12 months) limited the utility of this technique for age assignment in nearly half of the children (Fig. 26–1). The children had been in Sweden for a mean of 53 months (range, 2–120 months) at the time of the survey; earlier evaluation may have been more enlightening.

Bone Age

Bone age is a useful adjunct to the evaluation of the child with uncertain age.[20] The Greulich and Pyle method is widely used in the United States; European physicians tend to prefer the Tanner-Whitehouse method.[20] Both methods rely on comparisons to historical series of radiographs from particular reference populations: upper–middle class American Caucasian children in the 1930s (Greulich-Pyle) or Scottish working class

Evelyn arrived from China with the information that she was a "small 13 year-old" with a "low IQ." Her weight was 21.5 kg (weight age 7 years 2 months), height 118 cm (height age 6 years 6 months), and head circumference 49 cm (head circumference age 3 years). She had 24 teeth, all permanent. She had a reactive tuberculin skin test and negative chest x–ray, mild anemia, and uncorrected strabismus with a blind right eye. She had received minimal education in China, but could read second grade–level books in Mandarin. Her Mandarin spoken language was ~9 years, her visuomotor and drawing skills tested at 8 years. Bone age was 8 years 2 months. Infectious disease, endocrine, and gastrointestinal evaluations did not reveal specific causes for her growth delay. Her experienced adoptive parents (8 children!) felt she functioned as a normal 8-year-old. During 1 year of observation, Evelyn's weight increased to 8 years 6 months, height to 9 years, and head circumference age to 7 years. Her cognitive skills advanced to 9 years, and her English language expressive language tested at 5 years 6 months. Her drawing and language skills reached third- to fourth-grade level (Fig. 26–2). She had Tanner II breast development. A follow-up bone age was 9 years 10 months. She had spent the intervening year in third grade, with some academic difficulties, but was bright and eager to learn. The school recommended that Evelyn repeat third grade. After discussions, including Evelyn, a decision was made to reassign her age to 9 years.

children in the 1960s (Tanner-Whitehouse).[21,22] The applicability of these standards to other populations is debatable. For example, the Greulich-Pyle method is valid in central European, Dutch Caucasian, and Malaysian children,[23–25] but difficulties in its suitability for African American, Turkish, Pakistani, and Nepali children have been reported.[26–30] Japanese and Korean investigators established their own standards for bone age assessment;[31,32] Japanese children have advanced skeletal maturation compared to European, American, and Chinese peers.

Acutely, malnutrition delays bone age. However, bone age recovers after nutritional repletion in most (but not all) studies from Asia, Africa, and Europe (reviewed in Briers et al.[33]). Skeletal maturity was assessed in 71 Asian chil-

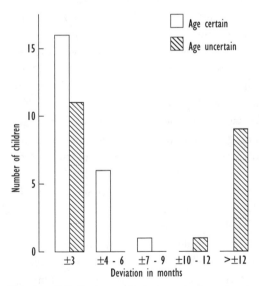

Figure 26–1 Two radiologic methods used to determine dental age in 44 non-European adoptees in Sweden[19] revealed large variations in dental age (>12 months), limiting the utility of this technique for age assignment. (With permission from Crossner CG, Mansfeld L. Determination of dental age in adopted non-European children. Swed Dent J 1983; 7:1–10.)

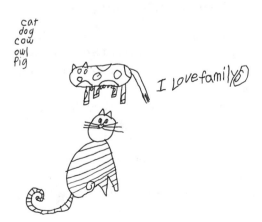

Figure 26–2 Drawing 1 year after arrival by girl adopted from China at age 13 years. All growth and developmental milestones suggested a much younger child (see sidebar, page 334).

Gustavo was found wandering alone in the garbage dumps of Manila by nuns who brought him to the orphanage to live. When asked his age, he emphatically stated that he was 7 years old. Within a few months, he was adopted by an American family. His parents, who had four other children, were convinced when they met Gustavo that he was much younger. Their pediatrician agreed, and after careful discussion and observation, felt an age reassignment was appropriate. However, Gustavo was a sensitive boy who was having some trouble with the enormous and rapid changes in his life. His parents decided not to take away one of the only pieces of identity he had from the Philippines. Instead, they celebrated his seventh birthday again the next year. It wasn't until his birthday 2 years after arrival that Gustavo "turned" 8.

dren (mostly Korean) adopted in Denmark.[34] Height, weight, and dental and skeletal ages were determined at arrival and 1 year later. Dental age increased appropriately given the time interval between the two examinations. Skeletal age accelerated for most children, especially in children >12 months of age at arrival. Height and weight velocities also exceeded those of the Danish–born controls.

When Not to Reassign Age

The decision to reassign age should not be undertaken lightly. The child's birth date, even if patently incorrect, is something that belongs to her, and was given to her by well-meaning caregivers in her birth country. Birth date is sometimes the only item retained after an international adoption—birth names, families, culture, language, and country are all lost by the child. Age should not be changed to satisfy parents' wishes that their child score well on developmental tests or to substitute for a proper evaluation of developmental problems or of growth delays in the "small" child. Age reassignments initiated for these reasons will likely be revealed as incorrect: after a brief period when

the child's developmental abilities are congruent to age peers, the child again falls behind. Sometimes, the child enters puberty far in advance of his age-peers, or, after rapid post-adoption catch-up growth, is suddenly the biggest child in the class. Age reassignment should therefore be carefully limited to children in whom (1) there is reason to believe that the assigned age is incorrect, and (2) the assigned age impedes the function and experience of the child by consigning him or her to an inappropriate peer group.

How to Reassign Age

After a period of observation (usually ~6 months), a complete reassessment should be performed and changes over time reviewed. Amount of progress in growth, dentition, skeletal maturity, and development should be calculated. For example, numbers of months of gain in height, weight, head circumference, dental, and skeletal age are tallied. Numbers of months of gain in gross and fine motor skills, cognition, language, and social–emotional development are counted. The child's functional fit with his present and proposed age cohort and his likely progress in the future are considered. The parents (and teachers, if appropriate) should indicate the ages of the child's preferred companions and playmates. If it appears that an age reassignment is warranted, a simple letter outlining the rationale for this recommendation is prepared. The adoptive parents may submit this letter to the judge who oversees the child's legal adoption in the United States. (see Chapter 1). This proceeding usually occurs about 6 months after the child arrives in the United States. This provides ample time for the pediatrician to observe the child on several occasions and make an informed opinion regarding an appropriate age assignment.

References

1. Jelliffe DB. Age assessment in field surveys of children of the tropics. J Pediatr 1966; 69:826–8.

2. Pierce WL. Debate over INS reorganization continues as care of child immigrants revives debate over estimating age. 2002. Available at: www.iavaan.org.

3. Bailey K. Dental development of New Guinean infants. J Pediatr 1963; 64:97.

4. Towlson KL, Peck D. Assessment of chronological age of third world children: can a simple tooth count help? Int Dent J 1990; 40:179–82.

5. Nystrom M, Peck L, Kleemola–Kujala E, Evalahti M, Kataja M. Age estimation in small children: reference values based on counts of deciduous teeth in Finns. Forensic Sci Int 2000; 110:179–88.

6. Robinow M. The eruption of the deciduous teeth. J Trop Pediatr Environ Child Health, 1973; 19:200–5.

7. Koshy S, Tandon S. Dental age assessment: the applicability of Demirjian's method in south Indian children. Forensic Sci Int 1998; 94:73–85.

8. Krailassiri S, Anuwongnukroh N, Dechkunakorn S. Relationships between dental calcification stages and skeletal maturity indicators in Thai individuals. Angle Orthod 2002; 72:155–66.

9. Jelliffe EF, Jelliffe DB. Deciduous dental eruption, nutrition and age assessment. J Trop Pediatr Environ Child Health 1973; 19:193–248.

10. Billewicz W. A note on estimation of calendar age on the basis of development of primary teeth. J Trop Pediatr Environ Child Health 1973; 19:243–6.

11. Korte R, Mndeme M. Dental development in shambaa children in Tanzania. J Trop Pediatr Environ Child Health 1973; 19:228–31.

12. Rao KV, Sushella TP, Swaminathan MC. Association of growth status and deciduous teeth eruption among rural Indian children. J Trop Pediatr Environ Child Health 1973; 19:223–7.

13. Truswell AS, Hansen JDL. Eruption of deciduous teeth in protein–calorie malnutrition. J Trop Pediatr Environ Child Health 1973; 19:214–6.

14. Neill J, Gurney J, Kuti O, Doherty D, Hanafy M, et al. Deciduous dental eruption time and protein–calorie malnutrition from different parts of the world. J Trop Pediatr Environ Child Health 1973; 19:217–22.

15. Mukherjee DK. Deciduous dental eruption in low income group Bengali Hindu children. J Trop Pediatr Environ Child Health 1973; 19:207–10.

16. Cifuentes E, Alvarado J. Assessment of deciduous dentition in Guatemalan children. J Trop Pediatr Environ Child Health 1973; 19:211–13.

17. Reventlid M, Mornstad H, Teivens AA. Intra– and inter–examiner variations in four dental methods for age estimation of children. Swed Dent J 1996; 20:133–9.

18. Davis PJ, Hagg U. The accuracy and precision of the "Demirjian system" when used for age determination in Chinese children. Swed Dent J 1994; 18:113–6.

19. Crossner CG, Mansfeld L. Determination of dental age in adopted non–European children. Swed Dent J 1983; 7:1–10.

20. Oestreich AE. Tanner–Whitehouse versus Greulich–Pyle in bone age determinations. J Pediatr 1997; 131:5–6.

21. Tanner J, Oshman D, Bahhage F, Healy M. Tanner–Whitehouse bone age references values for North American children. J Pediatr 1997; 131:34–40.

22. Cox LA. The biology of bone maturation and ageing. Acta Paediatr Suppl 1997; 423:107–8.

23. Groell R, Lindbichler F, Riepl T, Gherra L, Roposch A, Fotter R. The reliability of bone age determination in central European children using the Greulich and Pyle method. Br J Radiol 1999; 72:461–4.

24. van Rijn RR, Lequin MH, Robben SG, Hop WC, van Kuijk C. Is the Greulich and Pyle atlas still valid for Dutch Caucasian children today? Pediatr Radiol 2001; 31:748–52.

25. Chen ST, Jee FC, Mohamed TB. Bone age of Malaysian children aged 12 to 28 months. J Singapore Paediatr Soc 1990; 32:97–101.

26. Koc A, Karaoglanoglu M, Erdogan M, Kosecik M, Cesur Y. Assessment of bone ages: is the Greulich–Pyle method sufficient for Turkish boys? Pediatr Int 2001; 43:662–5.

27. Mora S, Boechat MI, Pietka E, Huang HK, Gilsanz V. Skeletal age determinations in children of European and African descent: applicability of the Greulich and Pyle standards. Pediatr Res 2001; 50:624–8.

28. Loder RT, Estle DT, Morrison K, et al. Applicability of the Greulich and Pyle skeletal age standards to black and white children of today. Am J Dis Child 1993; 147:1329–33.

29. Rikhasor RM, Qureshi AM, Rathi SL, Channa NA. Skeletal maturity in Pakistani children. J Anat 1999; 195:305–8.

30. Fleshman K. Bone age determination in a paediatric population as an indicator of nutritional status. Trop Doct 2000; 30:16–8.

31. Murata M. Population–specific reference values for bone age. Acta Paediatr Suppl 1997; 423:113–4.

32. Yeon KM. Standard bone–age of infants and children in Korea. J Korean Med Sci 1997; 12:9–16.

33. Briers PJ, Hoorweg J, Stanfield JP. The long–term effects of protein energy malnutrition in early childhood on bone age, bone cortical thickness and height. Acta Paediatr Scand 1975; 64:853–58.

34. Melsen B, Wenzel A, Miletic T, Andreasen J, Vagn–Hansen PL, Terp S. Dental and skeletal maturity in adoptive children: assessments at arrival and after one year in the admitting country. Ann Hum Biol 1986; 13:153–9.

27

PRECOCIOUS PUBERTY

In 1981, an abstract from Sweden reported a cluster of seven adopted Indian/Bangladeshi girls with early pubertal development.[1] Since then, a number of additional reports from Sweden, Belgium, France, and Italy indicate a surprising number of internationally adopted girls with precocious puberty.[2–8]

No clinical studies have yet precisely defined the prevalence of this condition; rather, reports originating from pediatric endocrine clinics suggest an apparent overrepresentation of internationally adopted girls with precocious puberty. For example, 8/32 girls with idiopathic central precocious puberty at a pediatric endocrine clinic in Belgium were adopted from (unspecified) developing countries.[3] A Swedish report describing specialized treatment of precocious puberty included 50 girls adopted from India, Sri Lanka, Indonesia, Colombia, and Peru.[7] Likewise, a Dutch report listed 27 girls and 3 boys with precocious puberty adopted

from Sri Lanka, India, Colombia, and South Korea.[6] Notably, only sporadic cases of internationally adopted boys with precocious puberty have been reported.

Do internationally adopted girls truly have an increased risk of precocious puberty? This section reviews the difficulties in defining this condition. The hypothetical basis for accelerated onset of puberty among internationally adopted girls is discussed, along with practical suggestions for the evaluation, treatment, and follow-up of such patients.

What Is Early Puberty?

The normal timing of puberty in American girls has been comprehensively reviewed recently[9–13] (Table 27–1). Tanner stage 2 development is achieved earlier than previously documented: 9.96 ±1.82 years in Caucasian girls and 8.87

Table 27–1 The prevalence of signs of puberty in young American girls

Finding/ethnicity	5.00–5.99	6.00–6.99	7.00–7.99	8.00–8.99	9.00–9.99
			Age (years)		
Breasts ≥Tanner 2					
White	1.6	2.9	5.0	10.5	32.1
African-American	2.4	6.4	15.4	37.8	62.6
Pubic Hair ≥Tanner 2					
White	0.4	1.4	2.8	7.7	20.0
African-American	3.4	9.5	17.7	34.3	62.6

Source: Data from Kaplowitz et al.[10]

±1.93 in African American girls for breast development, and 10.51 ±1.67 in Caucasian girls and 8.78 ±2.0 in African American girls for pubic hair development. The average age for menarche is about 12.88 years for Caucasian girls and 12.16 years for African American girls. This difference suggests that race, or some closely associated factor(s), affect the timing of puberty.

Other factors are also important. Historically, most girls experience menarche at a mean weight of 46 kg; undernourished girls thus tend to have later menarche.[14] The degree of body fatness may initiate the hormonal events of puberty,[15] especially in Caucasian girls. Signs of puberty become more prominent as body mass index [weight in kg/(height in meters)^2] increases.[15] Both the absolute values and velocity of change in weight seem to be important factors.[15] Low birth weight is also linked to earlier menarche in Filipino and Spanish girls.[16,17] Social class, a surrogate measure of nutrition and access to medical care (as well as other less well-defined factors), also influences the onset of puberty.

Less than 10% of American girls start to menstruate before 11 years, 90% are menstruating by age 13.75 years.[13] The age at menarche in well-fed and privileged populations are relatively similar throughout the world:[7] skeletal maturity scores for well-off Indian girls are similar to those of British girls.[6] In contrast, age of menarche among girls in India varies from 12.8 years to 14.4 years (reviewed in Proos et al.[18]), depending on social class. Thus, racial/ethnic factors, birth weight, social class, and alterations in body mass influence the onset of puberty.

Unfortunately, detailed studies describing the normal age of puberty are not available from most international adoption sending countries. Most of the internationally adopted children described with this condition are of Asian origin, raising the possibility that perhaps parents and physicians in Western countries are unfamiliar with "norms" for these children. Several authors caution against assumptions that puberty occurs earlier in developing or tropical countries.[6,7] In Asia, for example, average age of menarche ranges from 12.4 (urban Thailand) to 16.2 years (high-altitude Nepal).[19] In Africa, average age at menarche ranges from 13.5 (urban Nigeria) to 16.1 years (Senegal).[19] Moreover, internationally adopted children are racially and ethnically diverse, making generalizations about timing of puberty difficult. Even children from the same country may represent different ethnic or racial groups.

Other factors may confuse the assessment of the child with possible early puberty. Predictions based on parental height are essentially impossible, as such information about parental height is virtually never available, except from Russia (occasionally) and Korea; the nutritional and health status of the birth parents, espe-

> Rita was adopted from the Philippines at age 6 years 3 months. She had resided in an orphanage until 6 months prior to the adoption when she was transferred to foster care. She reportedly thrived and grew quickly while in foster care. On arrival to the United States, Rita was at the 50th percentiles for height, weight, and head circumference. One month after arrival, breast development puberty began, and subsequently progressed. She developed some body odor. Baseline thyroid studies were normal. Eight months after arrival, breast development was Tanner IV, vaginal mucosa was purplish and dull. luteinizing hormone was 1.5, follicle-stimulating hormone was 2.6, and estradiol was 88. Pelvic ultrasound showed very early maturation of the ovaries and uterus; bone age was 6 years 9 months. A CT scan of the hypothalamic–pituitary region was normal. Growth measurements were at the 90th percentile for age. Treatment with LHRH was begun, and over the next year no further progression of puberty occurred. Linear growth also slowed; her height was at the 75th percentile.

cially during early life, is never provided. Furthermore, use of European or American bone age charts to predict final height may not be appropriate, but no sensible alternatives exist. Some have suggested the use of the "segmented Greulich and Pyle bone age" to improve precision and accuracy.[6] In this method, the seven regions of the hand and wrist are scored separately (radius, ulna, carpals, metacarpals, proximal, medial and distal phalanges), and the accumulated score is divided by 7. Finally, in some children, age assignment is uncertain (see Chapter 26). Regardless of ethnic background, girls with signs of puberty (breast and/or pubic hair development with concomitant growth spurt) appearing before age 6–8 should be investigated for endocrine pathology.[20]

Precocious Puberty and Internationally Adopted Girls

Do internationally adopted girls truly have an increased incidence of precocious puberty? This has been addressed in studies from Sweden,[18,21] France,[2] the Netherlands, and Belgium. The first study surveyed the families of all Indian girls born in 1971 or earlier who were adopted in Sweden. This group of 107 girls had a median menarcheal age of 11.6 years, considerably less than the Swedish norm of 13 years (Table 27–2). Among the adopted children, later age at arrival was associated with earlier menarche and with faster growth recovery (especially if only those who arrived <7 years were included: $p < 0.001$, $r = -0.39$). Five of the girls had menarche before 9 years. In this group, lower initial height predicted lower final height: 8% of the girls were <145 cm final height.

In the French survey of 99 adoptive families,[2] precocious puberty was reported in 45% of girls and ~9% of boys. The 13 proband children with precocious puberty had very high rates of growth for the period from time of adoption to the onset of puberty: mean height increased from −1.3 to +1.5 standard deviation score (SDS) and the mean weight-for-height factor increased from +1.2 to 1.9 SDS. Early puberty was reported most frequently for children born in Africa and Central or South America (57% affected), followed by Asia (45%) and Eastern Europe (29%). Both the Swedish and French studies were questionnaire surveys and relied on parental determinations of the onset of puberty.

Mean menarcheal age of 446 internationally adopted girls in the Netherlands was 12.0, significantly less than that for Dutch girls.[19] In

Table 27–2 Median age at menarche in different populations

Population	Median age at menarche (years)
Study population (Indian girls adopted in Sweden)	11.6
Indian girls, Madras, urban, privileged	12.8
Swedish girls, multicenter study	13.0
Indian girls, all India, urban	13.7
Indian girls, Madras, rural	14.2
Indian girls, all India, rural	14.4

Source: Data from Proos et al.[18]

Belgium, calculations suggest that 0.8%–1.8% of adopted children have precocious puberty.[19,22]

Theoretical Explanations

Many reasons have been suggested to explain the apparent increase in precocious puberty among internationally adopted girls (Table 27–3). Most relate to the hypothesis that rapid growth recovery after malnutrition or undernutrition activates neuroendocrine triggers of puberty. Although these speculations remain unproven in children, studies in rats have demonstrated that food restriction followed by refeeding during critical periods can advance the timing of puberty.[3] In these carefully done studies, increased growth rate resulting from unrestricted feeding after nutritional deprivation was associated with accelerated hypothalamic and testicular maturity. However, these effects were only observed before weaning, indicating that hypothalamic maturation was sensitive to changes in nutritional conditions only during critical periods before the onset of puberty. Animal experiments suggest that specific

Table 27–3 Possible reasons for precocious puberty among internationally adopted girls

Increases in fat and lean mass primes hypothalamic–pituitary activity or the hypothalamic control of LH release[6,8]

Dietary changes (low-protein, low-energy vegetarian to balanced enriched diet) may increase IGF-1 (stimulates ovarian follicle maturation, production of estrogen and LHRH)[8,26]

Pre-adoption exposure to endocrine disruptors[19] such as dietary phytoestrogens or pesticides[22]

Refeeding, which increases insulin production (inhibits neuropeptide Y secretion—more LHRH activity)[8]

Psychologic factors (girls feel more secure)[8,27]

Increase in leptin secretion and IGF-1 levels (due to increase in body mass)[6,2,26]

Rapid weight-for-height recovery rate[2]

IGF-1, insulin-like growth factor 1; LH, luteinizing hormone; LHRH, luteinizing hormone–releasing hormone.

dietary exposures (such as soy protein) during infancy may accelerate pubertal changes[23]; evidence for this effect in human children has been controversial.[24,25]

Older age at adoption appears to be a risk factor for precocious puberty in internationally adopted children in some but not all studies. Early studies suggested that girls adopted after age 3 years were more likely to have precocious puberty.[1,18,21] In more recent studies, however, age at arrival varied widely. Of 30 children with precocious puberty adopted in the Netherlands, median arrival age was 4.5 months (range 1–84 months).[6] In contrast, of 19 children with this condition adopted in Italy, average arrival age was 4 years (range 0.33–8 years).[8] Nutritional condition on arrival is also a likely factor contributing to the development of early puberty. However, in other populations, such as South African children who recovered from early kwashiorkor, the timing of pubertal growth spurts was normal.[28] Some authors have suggested that velocity of growth recovery may increase the risk of precocious puberty,[2,8,21] but comparisons to growth velocity of children without precocious puberty have not been fully explored. It remains a curiosity to be explained that virtually all internationally adopted children reported with precocious puberty are from Asian or Latin countries, even though the nutritional condition of many children adopted from Eastern Europe are equally or more severely compromised.

Treatment of Precocious Puberty in Internationally Adopted Children

Should internationally adopted children with precocious puberty be treated? Social, behavioral, and psychological consequences of untreated precocious puberty may influence the adjustment to the adoptive family,[27] and individual treatment decisions must be made.[19] A psychological study of 30 internationally adopted children with precocious puberty who were participating in a treatment protocol failed to find any increase in behavioral or emotional problems either before or during treatment.[29] Children scored in the normal range for self-perception, and after treatment recorded high scores for acceptance by peers. Family stress was generally low. Concerns about short final height are difficult to address; some have argued that a short final height could impede the child's integration into her new culture and society.[8,27] Among American girls the mean increase in stature after menarche is 7.4 cm, but this figure is higher (~10 cm) for girls with early menarche.[10] Thus, concern that girls with borderline early puberty (between 6 and 8 years of age) will become very short adults if they don't have treatment may be overstated.[10] Whether this reasoning can and should be applied to this specialized population is not known.

Several studies report the outcome of internationally adopted girls with precocious puberty (Table 27–4) in Italy, Sweden, and the Netherlands.[6–8]

Premature Thelarche

Precocious puberty must be differentiated from isolated premature thelarche (development of breast tissue). Thelarche is the most reliable physical sign of pituitary–gonadal activation, but may occur without other clinical signs of sexual maturity. This condition, occasionally found in girls less than 2 years of age, is defined as a small amount of unilateral or bilateral breast tissue, no enlargement of the areola, normal linear growth, and no other signs of puberty[10] (Fig. 27–1). Usually considered a benign normal variant, premature thelarche may also reflect exposure to exogenous estrogens or estrogen-like compounds. Such exposure may have occurred prior to adoption, including medications or foods (e.g., phytoestrogens). Exposure to phthalates, a compound added to plastic to soften it and allow moulding and often present in pacifiers and other baby toys, has also been recognized as a possible factor in premature thelarche[30] (see Chapter 24). An internationally adopted child with breast bud devel-

Table 27–4 Responses of internationally adopted children with precocious puberty to treatment

Country	Patient Population	Study	Results	Comments
Italy[8]	19 girls referred to endocrine clinic (15 from India)	GnRH or no treatment (assignment based on clinical criteria)	5/7 untreated girls did not achieve predicted heights (~4 cm below predicted). 12 treated children did well.	Those adopted later (>5 years) had greater weight deficits and more delayed bone ages.
Sweden[7]	46 girls with precocious puberty from India, Sri Lanka, Indonesia, Colombia, and Peru	Open, randomized GH ± GnRH	Mean growth in GH+GnRH–treated girls was 14.6 cm vs. 10.9 cm in control group.	Combined treatment resulted in higher predicted final height.
Netherlands[6]	30 children (27 F:3 M) from India, Sri Lanka, and S. Korea Mean age at arrival was 4.5 months	Open, randomized GH ± GnRH	Height velocity was greater in combined treatment group.	Combined treatment resulted in higher predicted final height.

GH, growth hormone; GnRH, gonadotropin-releasing hormone.

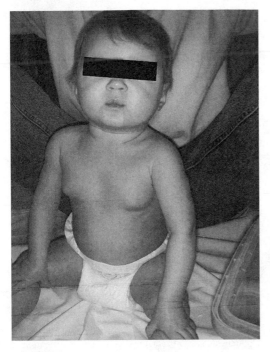

Figure 27–1 *Premature thelarche in 10-month-old from Russia. (With permission.)*

opment should be carefully monitored for signs of pubertal progression.[31,32] Serum estradiol, luteinizing hormone (LH), and follicle-stimulating hormone (FSH) levels identify the rare child with endogenous estrogen secretion who should be evaluated more completely (although some girls with premature thelarche have elevated estradiol levels).[33] Accelerating growth due to advancing puberty may be difficult to differentiate from catch-up growth after undernutrition. Because most growth-delayed international adoptees have delayed bone age, an advanced (or even normal) bone age should prompt further investigation and endocrinological consultation.

References

1. Adolfsson S, Westphal O. Early pubertal development in girls adopted from Far-Eastern countries. Pediatr Res 1981; 15:82.

2. Baron S, Battin J, David A, Limal JM. Precocious puberty in children adopted from foreign countries [in French]. Arch Pediatr 2000; 7:809–16.

3. Bourguignon JP, Gerard A, Alvarez Gonzalez ML, Fawe L, Franchimont P. Effects of changes in nutritional conditions on timing of puberty: clinical evidence from adopted children and experimental studies in the male rat. Horm Res 1992; 38:97–105.

4. Bureau JJ, Maurage C, Bremond M, Despert F, Rolland JC. Children of foreign origin adopted in France. Analysis of 68 cases during 12 years at the University Hospital Center of Tours [in French]. Arch Pediatr 1999; 6:1053–8.

5. de Monleon JV, Geneste B, Huet F. Precocious puberty in adopted children, a risk not to be forgotten [in French]. Arch Pediatr 1999; 6:589–90.

6. Mul D, Oostdijk W, Waelkens JJ, Schulpen TW, Drop SL. Gonadotrophin releasing hormone agonist treatment with or without recombinant human GH in adopted children with early puberty. Clin Endocrinol (Oxf) 2001; 55:121–9.

7. Tuvemo T, Gustafsson J, Proos LA. Growth hormone treatment during suppression of early puberty in adopted girls. Swedish Growth Hormone Advisory Group. Acta Paediatr 1999; 88:928–32.

8. Virdis R, Street ME, Zampolli M, et al. Precocious puberty in girls adopted from developing countries. Arch Dis Child 1998; 78:152–4.

9. Herman-Giddens ME, Bourdony C, Slora EJ, Wasserman RC. Secondary sexual characteristics and menses in young girls seen in office practice: a study from the Pediatric Research and Office Settings Network. Pediatrics 1997; 99:505–12.

10. Kaplowitz PB, Oberfield SE. Reexamination of the age limit for defining when puberty is precocious in girls in the United States: implications for evaluation and treatment. Drug and Therapeutics and Executive Committee of the Lawson Wilkins Pediatric Endocrine Society. Pediatrics 1999; 104:936–41.

11. Wu T, Mendola P, Buck GM. Ethnic differences in the presence of secondary sex characteristics and menarche among US girls: the third national health and nutrition examination survey 1988–1994. Pediatrics 2002; 110:752–7.

12. Freedman DS, Khan LK, Serdula MK, Dietz W, Srinivasan SR, Berenson GS. Relation of age at menarche to race, time period, and anthropometric dimensions: the Bogalusa heart study. Pediatrics 2002; 110:e43.

13. Chumlea WC, Schubert CM, Roche AF, et al. Age at menarche and racial comparisons in US girls. Pediatrics 2003; 111:110–3.

14. Frisch RE. Weight at menarche: similarity for well-nourished and undernourished girls at differing ages, and evidene for historical constancy. Pediatrics 1972; 50:445–30.

15. Kaplowitz PB, Slora EJ, Wasserman RC, Pedlow SE, Herman-Giddens ME. Earlier onset of puberty in girls: relation to increased body mass index and race. Pediatrics 2001; 108:347–53.

16. Adair LS. Size at birth predicts age at menarche. Pediatrics 2001; 107:E59.

17. Ibanez L, Ferrer A, Marcos MV, Hierro F, de Zegher F. Early puberty: rapid progression and reduced final height in girls with low birth weight. Pediatrics 2000; 106:E72.

18. Proos LA, Hofvander Y, Tuvemo T. Menarcheal age and growth pattern of Indian girls adopted in Sweden. Acta Paediatr Scand 1991; 80:852–8.

19. Mul D, Oostdijk W, Drop SL. Early puberty in adopted children. Horm Res 2002; 57:1–9.

20. Midyett LK, Moore WV, Jacobson JD. Are pubertal changes in girls before age 8 benign? Pediatrics 2003; 111:47–51.

21. Proos LA, Hofvander Y, Tuvemo T. Menarcheal age and growth pattern of Indian girls adopted in Sweden. II. Catch-up growth and final height. Indian J Pediatr 1991; 58:105–14.

22. Krstevsk-Konstatinova M, Charlier C, Craen M, DuCaju M, Heinrichs C, deBeaufort C. Sexual precocity after immigration from developing countries to Belgium: evidence of previous exposure to organochlorine pesticides. Hum Reprod 2001; 16:1020–6.

23. Badger TM, Ronis MJ, Hakkak R. Developmental effects and health aspects of soy protein isolate, casein, and whey in male and female rats. Int J Toxicol 2001; 20:165–74.

24. Klein KO. Isoflavones, soy-based infant formulas, and relevance to endocrine function. Nutr Rev 1998; 56:193–204.

25. Freni-Titulaer LW, Cordero JF, Haddock L, Lebron G, Martinez R, Mills JL. Premature thelarche in Puerto Rico. A search for environmental factors. Am J Dis Child 1986; 140:1263–7.

26. De Monleon JV. Foreign adopted children growth follow-up [in French]. Ann Endocrinol (Paris) 2001; 62:458–60.

27. Bona G, Marinello D. Precocious puberty in immigrant children: indications for treatment. J Pediatr Endocrinol Metab 2000; 13:831–4.

28. Cameron N, Jones PRM, Moodie A, et al. Timing and magnitude of adolescent growth in height and weight in Cape Coloured children after kwashiorkor. J Pediatr 1986; 109:548–55.

29. Mul D, Versluis-den Bieman HJ, Slijper FM, Oostdijk W, Waelkens JJ, Drop SL. Psychological assessments before and after treatment of early puberty in adopted children. Acta Paediatr 2001; 90:965–71.

30. Colon I, Caro D, Bourdony CJ, Rosario O. Identification of phthalate esters in the serum of young Puerto Rican girls with premature breast development. Environ Health Perspect 2000; 108:895–900.

31. Della Manna T SN, Damiani D, Kuperman H, Dichtchekenian V. Premature thelarche: identification of clinical and laboratory data for the diagnosis of precocious puberty. Rev Hosp Clin Fac Med Sao Paulo 2002; 57:49–54.

32. Pasquino AM, Pucarelli I, Passeri F, Segni M, Mancini MA, Municchi G. Progression of premature thelarche to central precocious puberty. J Pediatr 1995; 126: 11–4.

33. Klein KO, Mericq V, Brown-Dawson JM, Larmore KA, Cabezas P, Cortinez A. Estrogen levels in girls with premature thelarche compared with normal prepubertal girls as determined by an ultrasensitive recombinant cell bioassay. J Pediatr 1999; 134:190–2.

28

LACTOSE INTOLERANCE

Lactose intolerance is often blamed—incorrectly—for intestinal symptoms in internationally adopted children. Lactose intolerance, or the inability to digest and absorb the milk sugar lactose, results from deficiency of the enzyme, lactase, or more precisely, lactase-phlorizin hydrolase. Although many children come from ethnic groups with high prevalence of acquired lactose intolerance (Table 28–1), this condition is rare in infants and young children. Except under pathologic conditions, lactase remains active during the first few years of life to enable children to absorb and digest breast milk.

Cultures that practice animal-milk production tend to have a low incidence of adult lactose intolerance. Dairying is less common in cultures with a high incidence of adult lactose intolerance. It is not known whether people from dairying cultures adapted biologically to absorb lactose, or whether dairying became established in ethnic groups in which lactase activity persists to adulthood. Generally, individuals of Aryan or European descent have lower likelihood of genetically acquired lactase deficiency. Lactase deficiency is also unusual among pastoralist herders who maintain dairy animals. These include ethnic groups from northern India, Pakistan, Afghanistan, and Africa (Hima and Tussi tribes).[1] Lactose intolerance is frequent among adult Asian, African, Native American, and Mediterranean populations.

Clinical Features

Symptoms of lactose intolerance usually include abdominal pain, cramps, distention, nausea, flatulence, diarrhea, and vomiting, with the latter being one of the more common symptoms in young children.[2] These symptoms may be episodic. Lactose intolerance may occur temporarily in association with enteric infection

Table 28–1 Frequency of lactose intolerance in adults from various ethnic groups

Ethnic Group	Lactose Intolerance (%)
Aborigines (Australia)[2]	67
African Americans[2]	81
American Indians (Oklahoma)[2]	95
Asian Americans[3]	90
Asian Americans [2]	100
China[4]	
Han Chinese	92
Mongols	88
Kazakhs	76
Danes[2]	3
Dutch[2]	0
Greeks[2]	53
Hungary[5]	
General population	37
Roma	56
India[1]	
South India	67
North India	27
Italians[2]	71
Mexican Americans[2]	56
Nigerians (Ibo, Yoruba)[2]	89
Russia[6]	
General population	12
Byelorussians	13
Ukrainians	6
Russia (northern)[7]	
Kildin Saami	48
Komi-Izhem	63
Northern Mansi	71
Northern Khanty	72
West Siberian Nenets	78
Slav/Russian	40–49
Permian Finns	50–59
Russia—various ethnic groups[8]	
Khant	94
Mari	81
Western Russians	57
Vietnamese-Americans[9]	100
White Americans[2]	24

Not all studies are directly comparable because of wide variations in methodologies and definitions of lactose intolerance. These figures are shown to give a rough idea of statistical comparisons.

(bacterial, parasitic, or viral [especially rotavirus]) when mucosal cells are injured. Although genetic factors definitely play a role in the susceptibility to lactose intolerance, envi-

Table 28–2 Lactose intolerance in Thai orphanage or village children

Age	Orphanage (%)	Village (%)	P
6 months to			
1 year	41	14	<0.02
1 to 2 years	75	30	<0.002
>2 years	87	87	NS

NS, not significant.

Source: Data from Keusch et al.[10]

ronmental factors are also important. A study of 172 children in Thailand[10] living either in orphanages or with their families showed that the orphanage children developed lactose intolerance at a much earlier age than the village children (Table 28–2). Recurrent episodes of diarrhea common among the orphanage children were thought to contribute to their earlier onset of lactose intolerance. Notably, some children were lactose tolerant when tested again several weeks later, emphasizing the intermittent nature of this condition.

Age of Onset of Symptoms

The age of onset of symptoms varies considerably. Generally, even in populations with frequent lactose intolerance in adults, some lactase activity persists to approximately 5–7 years of age.[2] However, the number of lactose malabsorbers in susceptible populations usually increases greatly after 1 year of age (Table 28–3). From an evolutionary perspective, lactase insufficiency develops to relieve the mother of the burden of lactation and to encourage weaning.

Differential Diagnosis

Bacterial and parasitic enteric infection should be ruled out in internationally adopted children with signs of lactase deficiency (see Chap-

Table 28–3 Age of onset of lactose intolerance in various ethnic groups

Ethnic Group/Country	Children with Lactose Intolerance (%)
African American[11]	29% of 13- to 59-month-olds
American Indians[12]	20%–40% before age 5 years

Australia[13]	By 5–12 years:
	    Asians 93%
	    Greek 56%
	    Mediterranean/Middle East 41%

Baganda of East Africa[12]	27% 1 week to 5 months
Bangladesh[12]	20% of healthy 7- to 18-month-olds
China[14]	< 2 years old—few
China[15]	<15% of preschoolers 45% of young school-age children 60% of older school-age children 70% of adolescents
China[16]	12% of 3- to 5-year-olds 31% of 7- to 8-year-olds
Finland[12]	None before age 7 years, most 10–20 years
Hong Kong Chinese[17]	3% age 8 years 27% age 18 years—biggest increase between 14 and 15 years
Israel[12]	None before age 6 1/2 years
Jamaica[18]	56%, but 21% had normal lactose tolerance when retested 7–8 months later 17% of malabsorbers were still being breast fed
Japanese[19]	< 2 years—none 30% age 3 years 36% age 4 years 58% age 5 years 86% age 6 years 85% school-age, 90% of adults
Mexican American children[20]	37% (vs. 8% of Anglo-Americans) age 2–14 years
Nigeria[12]	29% < 1 year, 27% 1–2 years, 94% 2–4 years
Pacific Islands[21]	41%–60% Samoan schoolchildren
South Africa[22]	Black 50% (with earlier onset: 32% intolerant before age 5 years) Indians 22% (late onset: only 6% before 8 years)
Thailand (northern)[23]	7/13 children <4 years old were lactose intolerant all 24 children >4 years old were lactose intolerant
Thailand[24]	33% soon after birth; percentage increases with age—by age 4 years all were lactose intolerant
Thailand[12]	34% of 1- to 12-month-olds; 59% of 1- to 2-year-olds

Studies are not entirely comparable in terms of definitions of lactose intolerance or test methods used.

ter 17). Previously screened children should be retested, as pathogenic parasites can be missed. Viral gastroenteritis (rotavirus) and other enteric infections may be complicated by temporary lactase deficiency. Celiac disease, *Giardia* infection, severe protein malnutrition, and cystic fibrosis may cause lactase deficiency. Other forms of food intolerance, including milk allergy or other forms of carbohydrate intolerance, can masquerade as lactose intolerance. Dietary history should be obtained, including amount and type of juice ingested, as excess juice can contribute to toddler's diarrhea.

Clinical suspicion of lactose intolerance is confirmed by response to withdrawal of lactose from the diet. Hydrogen breath tests are useful to corroborate the diagnosis. Intestinal biopsies or lactose tolerance tests are rarely necessary.[2]

Management

Withdrawal of lactose is necessary in children with lactose intolerance, even if this is a temporary condition. Infants should be given non–lactose-containing formulas, and other dairy products should be withheld. Yogurt is sometimes well tolerated (as it contains endogenous β-galactosidase)[2] and can provide needed calcium and calories. Older lactose-intolerant children may "self-treat" by selecting foods that they can tolerate. These children may have ongoing symptoms, however, as many hidden sources of lactose are present in the American food supply. Parents must be educated to read labels. Referral to a nutritionist is recommended to ascertain that the child receives adequate dietary calcium and vitamin D. Many families mistakenly assume that substitution of rice milk or soy milk from health food stores contains adequate calcium and vitamin D for growing children.

Newly arrived international adoptees should be carefully screened for intestinal parasites or bacterial pathogens before lactose intolerance is used as an explanation of intestinal symptoms. Children who have been home for a period of time should be retested for enteric pathogens if new symptoms suggestive of lactose intolerance develop. Occasionally a child will be identified with late presentation of parasites (see Chapter 17).

Key Points for Internationally Adopted Children

- Lactose intolerance is common in many ethnic groups of internationally adopted children.
- Primary lactose intolerance is unusual during early childhood.

- Other causes of intestinal problems should be investigated in young children with symptoms of lactose intolerance, regardless of ethnic background.

Resources

National Digestive Diseases Information Clearing house (NDDIC). Detailed review of the management of lactose intolerance. Available at: http://www.niddk.nih.gov/ddiseases/pubs/lactoseintolerance/index.htm.

References

1. Tandon RK, Joshi YK, Singh DS, Narendranathan M, Balakrishnan V, Lal K. Lactose intolerance in North and South Indians. Am J Clin Nutr 1981; 34:943–6.

2. Buller HA, Grand RJ. Lactose intolerance. Annu Rev Med 1990; 41:141–8.

3. National Digestive Diseases Information Clearing house (NDDIC). Lactose Intolerance. Available at: http://www.niddk.nih.gov/ddiseases/pubs/lactoseintolerance/index.htm.

4. Wang YG, Yan YS, Xu JJ, et al. Prevalence of primary adult lactose malabsorption in three populations of northern China. Hum Genet 1984; 67:103–6.

5. Czeizel A, Flatz G, Flatz SD. Prevalence of primary adult lactose malabsorption in Hungary. Hum Genet 1983; 64:398–401.

6. Valenkevich LN. Current problems of lactase deficiency [in Russian]. Vopr Pitan 1987:31–4.

7. Kozlov AI. Hypolactasia in the indigenous populations of northern Russia. Int J Circumpolar Health 1998; 57:18–21.

8. Lember M, Tamm A, Piirsoo A, et al. Lactose malabsorption in Khants in western Siberia. Scand J Gastroenterol 1995; 30:225–7.

9. Anh NT, Thuc TK, Welsh JD. Lactose malabsorption in adult Vietnamese. Am J Clin Nutr 1977; 30:468–9.

10. Keusch GT, Troncale FJ, Miller LH, Promadhat V, Anderson PR. Acquired lactose malabsorption in Thai children. Pediatrics 1969; 43:540–5.

11. Paige DM, Bayless TM, Mellitis ED, Davis L. Lactose malabsorption in preschool black children. Am J Clin Nutr 1977; 30:1018–22.

12. Simoons FJ. Age of onset of lactose malabsorption. Pediatrics 1980; 66:646–8.

13. Brand JC, Darnton-Hill I. Lactase deficiency in Australian school children. Med J Aust 1986; 145:318–22.

14. Chang MH, Hsu HY, Chen CJ, Lee CH, Hsu JY. Lactose malabsorption and small-intestinal lactase in normal Chinese children. J Pediatr Gastroenterol Nutr 1987; 6:369–72.

15. Ting CW, Hwang B, Wu TC. Developmental changes of lactose malabsorption in normal Chinese children: a study using breath hydrogen test with a physiological dose of lactose. J Pediatr Gastroenterol Nutr 1988; 7:848–51.

16. Yang Y, He M, Cui H, Bian L, Wang Z. The prevalence of lactase deficiency and lactose intolerance in Chinese children of different ages. Chin Med J (Engl) 2000; 113:1129–32.

17. Tadesse K, Yuen RC, Leung DT. Late-onset hypolactasia in Hong Kong school children. Ann Trop Paediatr 1991; 11:289–92.

18. Stoopler M, Frayer W, Alderman MH. Prevalence and persistence of lactose malabsorption among young Jamaican children. Am J Clin Nutr 1974; 27:728–32.

19. Nose O, Iida Y, Kai H, Harada T, Ogawa M, Yabuuchi H. Breath hydrogen test for detecting lactose malabsorption in infants and children. Prevalence of lactose malabsorption in Japanese children and adults. Arch Dis Child 1979; 54:436–40.

20. Woteki CE, Weser E, Young EA. Lactose malabsorption in Mexican-American children. Am J Clin Nutr 1976; 29:19–24.

21. Seakins JM, Elliott RB, Quested CM, Matatumua A. Lactose malabsorption in Polynesian and white children in the South West Pacific studied by breath hydrogen technique. Br Med J (Clin Res Ed) 1987; 295:876–8.

22. Wittenberg DF, Moosa A. Lactose maldigestion—age-specific prevalence in black and Indian children. S Afr Med J 1990; 78:470–2.

23. Flatz G, Saengudom C, Sanguanbhokhai T. Lactose intolerance in Thailand. Nature 1969; 221:758–9.

24. Varavithya W, Valyasevi A, Manu P, Kittikool J. Lactose malabsorption in Thai infants and children: effect of prolonged milk feeding. Southeast Asian J Trop Med Public Health 1976; 7:591–5.

VII

NEUROCOGNITIVE AND BEHAVIORAL ISSUES

29

ATTACHMENT

A child forsaken, waking suddenly,
Whose gaze afeared on all things round doth rove,
And seeth only that it cannot see
The meeting eyes of love.

George Eliot (quoted in Bowlby[1])

Attachment is the reciprocal affectionate relationship that binds two people deeply together, or, more simply, love. Attachment is also the process by which infants internalize emotional connections to others—that is, learn to love. Attachment influences all aspects of child development and becomes the basis by which the child relates to the world, learns, and forms relationships throughout life.[2] The life experiences of most internationally adopted children prior to placement conspire to interfere with this process. Although no statistics are available, disordered attachment undoubtably occurs more frequently among international adoptees, who are virtually all placed after 6 months of age, than among adoptees

placed as newborns. Disordered attachment profoundly affects the well-being of the child and family. Through the publicizing of several cases of international adoptees with severe attachment disorder in the popular media, awareness of attachment issues for internationally adopted children has greatly increased.

The pediatrician's advice about attachment may be sought at several times: before the adoption (to assess the risk that a particular child will have disordered attachment), during the process (to confirm that attachment is progressing as expected), and after the adoption (when the reality of the child's adjustment to the family becomes apparent). The pediatrician caring for the internationally adopted child must recognize and screen for signs of attachment problems. In this section, normal and abnormal attachment will be reviewed from a pediatric perspective. The clinical manifestations and diagnosis of attachment disorder, differential diagnosis, attachment and the internationally adopted child, basic strategies to promote attachment in adoptive families, and the concepts involved in treatment will be discussed. Although most pediatricians will not be called upon to provide treatment for children with severe attachment disorder, it is helpful to be aware of the current literature and approaches to this complex problem.

Attachment: What Is It?

Attachment is the reciprocal, affectionate enduring emotional bond between individuals.[3] The child's first attachment to his or her primary caregiver is the model for all later attachments in life. Surprisingly, most pediatric textbooks offer limited information about attachment, even though this is a fundamental developmental task for all human infants.

The early psychiatric literature about attachment was based on observations of children left without parental care in institutions or hospitals. Lessons learned from children with obvious and severe attachment disorders have been applied to children who have experienced abuse, neglect, multiple foster care placements, or other disruptions in normal family life (including day care).[4,5] The classic works by Bowlby and Spitz[1,6–8] are excellent overviews of basic attachment theory; Karen,[9] Keck,[10,11] and Hughes[12] provide accessible introductions to attachment. Experimental work of Harry Harlow and others on primate models of emotional and social deprivation provides a theoretical framework for attachment disorder.[13–40]

Attachment is the basis for many human relationships, including spouses, siblings, and extended family. The attachment of child to parent, however, is the most primal form of attachment, and the type of most importance in adoption.

Cross-cultural research in Africa, China, Japan, Israel, Puerto Rico, and the United States demonstrates that each society has different standards for attachment. The person (or persons) to whom the infant is expected to attach and the behaviors that express attachment vary greatly.

Sleep patterns, age of weaning, and demonstration of independence are very culture-specific. Each culture's attachment process prepares the child for adulthood in that culture, and regardless of differences, most children become securely attached to their caregivers.[41]

Development of Attachment

The normal experiences of an infant in a loving family naturally promote attachment (Fig. 29–1).[11] The child feels a "need," such as hunger, thirst, discomfort, or fear. He fusses, cries, vocalizes, or in some way expresses this need, and becomes progressively more "aroused." The parents respond with attention and attempts to satisfy the need (feeding, changing diaper, rocking, touching, making eye contact, vocal soothing). The infant's gratification results in trust that his needs will be fulfilled, that his parents will protect and care for him, and that he will be loved and nurtured. This process has been described as "attunement,"[42] as the parent and child synchronize their emotions. Some physiologic processes, such as heart rate, also become

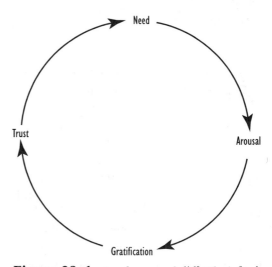

Figure 29–1 Attachment cycle.[11,65] The infant's needs (hunger, wet, desire to be held) create arousal (cries, angry, upset). When the needs are met, the infant is gratified and develops trust. When the needs are not met consistently, the cycle is interrupted.

attuned.[43] In normal family life, this cycle is repeated countless times during infancy and childhood. Through these patterns, the child learns what kind of person he is and what kind of responses to expect from people around him; these internal models are carried into adulthood.[3] The child learns to accept a range of emotions and behaviors in his parents and in himself.[42]

Early social responses develop in concert with the normal stages of attachment. Children exhibit a nonspecific smiling response at ~3 months, followed by specific social smiling that differentiates among individuals. Reactions to strangers (carefully examines, frowns, cries at unknown face) evolve; by 6–12 months separation and stranger anxiety emerge.[44] Children begin to protest a caregiver's departure, eagerly greet the caregiver on return, cling when frightened, and follow the caregiver when able.[3,9] By 8–10 months of age, a preferred relationship with one (or a few) caregiver(s) has been established; this relationship solidifies by 18 months of age.

Disordered Attachment

Abnormal attachment may occur if these normal cycles are disrupted, disordered, or never established. For example, as described by Keck and Kupecky, the child born into a neglectful or abusive environment learns very different lessons compared with the situation in a loving home. For these children, "need" stimulates "arousal," but when the "need" is not met, "arousal" escalates to "high arousal."[11] If still not gratified, the infant becomes exhausted or may develop self-gratification techniques (for example, rocking or head banging). The infant thus learns self-reliance and suspicion of the ability of others to meet her needs. In an abusive environment, "high arousal" may be met with injury or physical silencing, which after a time may be experienced as a pathologic form of gratification. The parent's strong emotion creates an intense but unsatisfying connection. The child does not learn to trust and also loses the sense of logical

consequences.[11] These experiences, if repeated, become ingrained into the child's most fundamental behaviors and psyche.

The first 2 years of life are the most vulnerable period for the development of attachment problems. Formation of attachment by institutionalized children may be impaired by many factors[2] (Table 29–1).

Children removed from loving caretakers display a predictable succession of symptoms if not permitted to form new attachments. René Spitz[6] described the successive stages of "emotional deprivation syndrome" of children in these circumstances. Most children sequentially exhibit weepiness, demanding attitude, loss of appetite and weight, arrest and regression of developmental quotient (Table 29–2 and Fig. 29–2), withdrawal, and insomnia. If the loved one does not reappear, children display decreased movement, irreversible regression of developmental quotient, susceptibility to infection, facial rigidity, and atypical finger movements. According to Spitz, children suffering from these symptoms show increased morbidity and "spectacular mortality."

Bowlby similarly describes the predictable responses of a secure 15- to 30-month-old child[1] removed from his mother. The infant first exhibits "protest," which may last hours to a week

Table 29–1 Factors interfering with attachment of institutionalized children to their caregivers

- Sudden or traumatic separation from primary caretaker (through death, illness, hospitalization of caretaker, or removal of child)
- Physical, emotional, or sexual abuse
- Neglect (of physical or emotional needs)
- Illness or pain which cannot be or is not alleviated by caretaker
- Frequent moves and/or placements
- Inconsistent or inadequate care (holding, talking, nurturing, as well as meeting basic physical needs)
- Chronic depression of primary caretaker
- Neurological problem in child which interferes with perception of or ability to receive nurturing (i.e., babies exposed to crack cocaine in utero)

Source: Data from http://www.attach.org.[2]

Table 29–2 Influence of reunion with mother on Developmental Quotient

Duration of Separation	Increase in DQ Points after Reunion
<3 months	+25
3–4 months	+13
4–5 months	+12
Over 5 months	–4

Source: Data from Spitz.[6]

or more. The child "appears acutely distressed, cries loudly, shakes his cot, throws himself about, looks eagerly towards any sight or sound which might prove to be his missing mother." This stage is followed by "despair," in which the behavior suggests increasing hopelessness. The infant's active physical movements diminish, crying is monotonous or intermittent, and the child becomes withdrawn, inactive, makes no demands on people, and appears to be in deep mourning. This stage is followed by "detachment," commonly misconstrued as a sign of recovery. The child accepts his caregivers, may even smile and be sociable. However, if his mother visits, he is listless and apathetic, and seems to have lost all interest in her. He begins to act as if neither mothering nor contact with humans has much significance for him.

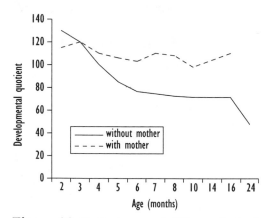

Figure 29–2 *Environmental differences in development. Developmental quotient (y-axis) of children raised with or without their mothers are compared at different ages (x-axis). (Adapted from The First Year of Life, by RA Spitz. By permission of International Universities Press, Inc. Copyright 1965 by IUP.)*

Characteristics of Attachment Disorder

Although some children may recover from a single loss of this magnitude, others unfortunately suffer recurrent psychic losses. Some children gradually commit themselves less and less to succeeding parent figures and eventually no longer attach to anyone. Such children may appear cheerful, easy-going, and unafraid, and may be described as affectionate and charming. However, this sociability is superficial and closer inspection reveals a child who is indiscriminately friendly (see below). Such behaviors mask inner feelings of insecurity and self-hate.[42] Deep down, the child no longer cares for anyone.

Children with attachment issues have little or no understanding of family bonds, the depth of parental commitment, or the desires a parent has in acting for the child's best interests. The unattached child determines what is best for himself; it does not occur to him that adults would try to understand what is best for him and to help him. The child has little desire for relationships with adults except as a means to fulfill wishes. There is little empathy or concern for parents or the rest of the family.[42] These children have difficulties with reciprocal relationships, accepting responsibilities, and developing a conscience.[11] A variety of behavioral problems are common among children with disordered attachment (Table 29–3).

Reactive Attachment Disorder

Attachment disorders comprise a spectrum. The most severe form is reactive attachment disorder (RAD) (see diagnostic criteria in Appendix 29–3). These children have severe, lifelong problems if not treated. Their problems extend beyond the individual and family as described by Spitz in psychoanalytic terms:

From the societal aspect, disturbed object relations in the first year of life, be they deviant, improper, or insufficient, have consequences which imperil the very foundation of society. Without a template, the

Table 29–3 Characteristics of attachment disorder

Superficially engaging and "charming" behavior
Indiscriminate affection toward strangers
Lack of affection with parents on their terms (not cuddly)
Little eye contact with parents
Persistent nonsense questions and incessant chatter
Inappropriate demanding and clingy behavior
Lying about the obvious ("crazy lying")
Stealing
Low self-esteem
Destructive behavior to self, to others, and to material things ("accident prone")
Abnormal eating patterns
No impulse control (may be misdiagnosed as ADHD)
Lags in learning
Abnormal speech patterns
Poor peer relationships
Lack of cause-and-effect thinking, difficulty learning from mistakes
Lack of a conscience
Cruelty to animals
Preoccupation with fire, blood, gore

Source: Adapted from refs. 2, 4, and 11.

Kevin was adopted from Russia at 8 months. One night four years later, his mom offered to read him a story about Russia. Kevin said "NO! I don't want to hear it! I don't like Russia!" When his mom gently asked why, Kevin said, "I cried when I was there. They were bad to me. They tied me to my back. They stuck a pointy spoon in my mouth." His mom was amazed, as she had seen the children in his group fed in exactly this way—restrained in a supine position, with large spoons full of food offered to the children so rapidly that most of them choked while swallowing. When she later asked if he had any good memories of Russia, he said, "They put cream on my back"—probably referring to the infant massage that is common in many orphanages.

victims of disturbed object relations subsequently will themselves lack the capacity to relate. They are not equipped for the more advanced, more complex forms of personal and social interchange without which we as a species would be unable to survive. They cannot adapt to society. They are emotional cripples. . . . Their capacity for normal human and social relations is deficient. . . . Even their capacity for transference is impaired, so that they are handicapped in profiting from therapy.[6]

At the milder end of the spectrum are children with attachment issues who do not fulfill

diagnostic criteria for RAD. This includes many international adoptees, who may have signs of disordered attachment, usually of the insecure or anxious type. This may also result in social, behavioral, cognitive, and emotional problems (Table 29–4). Common findings are lack of awareness of social boundaries, social cues, and differentiation in responses to adults. Some children readily go off with a stranger, fail to check back with the parent, and develop distress without coming to the parent for comfort.

Attachment and Institutionalization

The early life experiences of many internationally adopted children greatly increase the

Table 29–4 Spectrum of attachment

Securely Attached	Insecurely Attached	Poorly Attached
Confident, high functioning	Gives up when frustrated	Lacks empathy
Strong sense of self-worth	Collapses when stressed	Lacks conscience
Highly developed empathy	Overcontrol of emotions, aggressive	Unable to relate to others except as objects to meet their needs
Able to engage in healthy, mutually enhancing relationships in and out of the family	Doesn't seek comfort when distressed	Dissociates

Source: Adapted from Beck et al.[45]

likelihood of attachment problems. Prenatal exposure to stress may influence the hormonal regulation of attachment (see Chapter 8). After birth, few children (with the exception of most Korean and some Guatemalan children) go directly from the maternity hospital to loving, consistent foster care until adoption. Most children experience institutionalization for months or years. The orphanage experience may be one of impersonal, inattentive care with few caregivers, so that the children experience deprivation and neglect. (This was the situation in Romania, about which much of the recent research on attachment after adoption is based.) Other orphanage environments may have adequate staff numbers, but the structure and staffing arrangements expose the children to inconsistent caregivers. Caregivers work rotating shifts, and children must adjust to various personal styles of caregiving at different hours and different days. Staff turnover may be high. Children are often moved to new groups as they age, leaving beloved caregivers (and peers) behind. The lack of a consistent caregiver is the most common experience in the institution. In one study, it was estimated that by the age of 2 years, the child in a well-staffed orphanage has encountered 20 different caregivers; by 4 years, 40 caregivers, and by 8 years, 80 different caregivers.[46–48]

Although many children attach to their caregivers, these attachments are frequently disrupted and do not have the same depth or quality as attachments developed in a loving family. Thus it is not surprising that after adoption some post-institutionalized children display behaviors characteristic of attachment disorder. These behaviors overlap with many other entities common in post-institutionalized children (Table 29–5).[45] Such behaviors are expected in the first days and weeks after adoption. In most cases, they do not indicate permanent attachment problems but reflect the extraordinary psychic adjustments to adoption. Conversely, many behaviors seen after adoption may be rooted in insecure attachment (Appendix 29–1).

Table 29–5 Differential diagnosis of abnormal attachment in post-institutionalized children

Grief
Adjustment reaction
Post-traumatic stress disorder
Sensory integration disorder
Language delay
Developmental delay
Learning disabilities

Attachment after Adoption

Although considerable research has addressed the effects of institutionalization on attachment, relatively little has been reported about the effects of adoption after institutionalization. Early research suggested that children were incapable of developing a first attachment after infancy.[49,50] More recently, others have found no relationship to age at placement and attachment security,[48,51] although differences in attachment quality among children adopted after 6–10 months of age[52] or those adopted interracially[51] have been cited. In one study of 13- to 18-month-old infants adopted between 3 and 10 months of age,[51] no relationship was found between the infant's developmental quotient, number of foster homes, and age at adoption and the quality of mother–infant attachment. However, clinginess, attention seeking, difficulties establishing deep social attachments, and indiscriminate friendliness may persist for years after adoption[9,51] as "minor" signs of disturbed attachment. The experience of the child during the transition to the new adoptive family also affects attachment. Hughes,[12] Keck and Kupecky,[10–11] and Gray[52a] discuss attachment after adoption in their accessible and comprehensive books.

Indiscriminate Friendliness

Indiscriminate friendliness is common among post-institutionalized children.[53,54] Indiscriminate friendliness must be differentiated from sociability or gregariousness, also common in post-institutionalized children. Indiscriminately friendly children respond to any adult as long as their needs and wishes are met[55]: one person can easily replace another. For children living in institutional care, indiscriminate friendliness has adaptive advantages. Indiscriminate friendliness may occur regardless of whether the child has a preferred attachment figure.[55] After adoption, it is problematic. Evaluation of 14 institutionalized children who entered foster care at age 18 to 24 months found that these children initially displayed fear at separation from their foster parents, but several months later they displayed indiscriminate friendliness to all adults.[48,53,55] In a longer follow-up study of children adopted from institutions at age 2 years, indiscriminate friendliness continued for several years, but was gone by age 8 years in most children.[48]

Attachment and International Adoption

The incidence of attachment issues among internationally adopted children is unknown, as is the outcome of children with these problems. Attachment research on international adoptees to date has focused on a specific group of children: those adopted from Romania in the late 1980s to early 1990s.[53,54,56,57] These children came from institutions where they suffered extreme neglect and deprivation. These studies on attachment address the ability of children to develop a first attachment after infancy.

In a comparison of Canadian-born children with Romanian children adopted to Canada after either >8 or <4 months of institutionalization, several important findings emerged.[53,54] Not surprisingly, the longer-institutionalized children had lower attachment security and more indiscriminate friendliness, but there was no relation between these two behaviors. Some of the characteristics that differentiated each group are shown in the Tables 29–6 and 29–7. Interestingly, parent attachment scores correlated with the security of attachment in the longer-institutionalized Romanian children.

> Ramona was adopted from loving foster care in Korea at 5 months of age. Her adoptive father traveled to Korea to receive her, and had a great time meeting her foster family. Ramona did well on the trip home, "a great traveler and an easy baby," said her dad. Her mom had stayed home with their elder son, age 4. When dad and Ramona returned, mom was anxious about her ability to care for the baby and her older son too. The first night, Ramona wouldn't sleep, but cried inconsolably for hours. She arched her back, wouldn't snuggle at all, and refused to look at her mother. She cried when she was given a bottle (too hot? too cold? wrong nipple? wrong formula? her mother wondered), when she was bathed or changed. Only Ramona's father could comfort her, but he had to return to work as he had taken time off for the travel. Ramona and her mom were both in tears each night the first three weeks after adoption when dad returned home. "I can't figure out how to make her happy," said her mom. "She just doesn't want me."

When the same children were reevaluated 3 years later, attachment had improved, and the longer-institutionalized children did not differ in attachment security compared to the other two groups. However, more of the longer-institutionalized children had insecure or atypical attachment patterns (a risk for development of psychopathology). Those with insecure attachment were more likely to have lower IQs, behavior problems, and more stressed parents. These families also had lower socioeconomic status than those of children with more secure attachments. The author speculates that this subgroup of children with more problems had families with more problems. This resulted in a "vicious cycle" in which the neediest children required the most support from families with the fewest resources (emotional and otherwise).

Indiscriminate friendliness was also reevaluated at the 3-year follow-up. The longer-institutionalized children still displayed more signs of indiscriminate friendliness, even some of those with secure attachments. Seventy-one percent of parents of longer-institutionalized

Table 29–6 Differences in attachment security

More Typical of Longer-institutionalized Children

Wants to be put down, then fusses and wants to be picked right back up

Is demanding and impatient

Easily becomes angry at parent

When upset tends to stay where he or she is and cries

Plays roughly with parent: bumps, scratches, or bites

Is quick to greet parent when parent enters a room

More Typical of Non-adopted Controls

When picked up puts arms around parent

More Typical of Shorter-institutionalized Children

Shows a pattern of using parent as a secure base from which to explore

Follows parent when asked to do so

Recovers quickly from crying if held

Source: Adapted from Chisolm et al.[53,54]

children described them as overly friendly; 90% reported little or no improvement in this behavior with time. It is possible that this behavior may have been reinforced by both parents and strangers early after the adoption. Children with more signs of indiscriminate friendliness were more likely to have been favorites in the orphanage, which suggests the adaptive nature of this behavior. Only the extreme measures of indiscriminate friendliness (Table 29–7) differentiated children with secure and insecure attachment. Indiscriminate friendliness was not a sign of RAD.

In another long-term follow-up study of Romanian adoptees (to the United Kingdom),[56,57] 21% had attachment problems compared with 3.8% of matched domestic adoptees. Among the Romanian adoptees, a "dose–response" between duration of deprivation and severity of attachment disorder behaviors was found at age 6 years. However, there was substantial variability in the duration of deprivation among those with severe attachment disturbance. Interestingly, 70% of children exposed to profound deprivation for more than 2 years did not exhibit severe attachment disorder, leading the authors to comment that "our understanding of the causal mechanism is limited." In contrast, some children had significant difficulties even when the deprivation was limited to the early months of life. Attachment disorder behaviors often occurred along with attentional and conduct problems. Little improvement in attachment behaviors was noted over 2 years of observation in most of children; however, improvements in attachment soon after adoption would not have been reflected in the study.

The conclusion of these investigations (and others) is that most post-institutionalized children are capable of forming attachments to their parents. This includes even those children exposed to extreme institutional conditions. However, compared to children raised in families, these children have less secure attachments.[54,58]

Table 29–7 Measures of indiscriminate friendliness in Romanian children adopted in Canada

Child's Behavior	Those with behavior (%)	
	>8 months in institution	<4 months in institution
Wanders away and is not distressed at being separated from parent[a]	43	24
Is very friendly with all new adults	65	45
Is never shy with new adults	42	14
Typically approaches new adults, begins talking, ask questions	61	34
Would be willing to go home with a stranger[a]	52	28

[a]Most extreme measures of indiscriminate friendliness.

Source: Data from Chisolm et al.[53,54]

Attachment: Practical Aspects

Research supports the clinical impression that most internationally adopted children form attachment to their parents. However, it is apparent that many children have attachment issues. After adoption, some post-institutionalized children fail to exhibit normal pre-attachment behaviors, such as eye contact, smiling, and making their needs known. Some children do not signal their parents when then waken, do not show that they are in pain, or come to their parents when distressed. These are behaviors that a child normally uses to foster attachment, but they were never learned or reinforced during institutional life. These uncommunicative behaviors of the child make it more difficult for their parents to recognize their child's need for attachment and to respond in ways to promote attachment.[54] If the child does display attachment-seeking behaviors, the parent may perceive these as "immature" rather than appropriate—for example, clingy, not cuddly, or demanding, not needy. Likewise, indiscriminate friendliness is usually not perceived as a particular problem by most parents shortly after adoption.[54] Over time, however, many parents become alarmed about their child's safety, and disappointed that their own relationship with the child has not grown deeper over time. Sleep behaviors are also an important area related to attachment. Parents who expect newly adopted infants to sleep through the night in their own rooms may be misguided. In her book, *Toddler Adoption: The Weaver's Craft*, Mary Hopkins-Best[59] states:

Always assume that a request for parental contact and comforting represents a need for a toddler struggling to develop attachment. Meet that need on demand, day or night. Parents need to reframe their thoughts about getting up at night with a new toddler as a wonderful opportunity to build attachment, rather than a dreaded chore. Do NOT leave an adopted toddler [or infant] alone crying at night as often recommended by many parent discipline specialists. The techniques of temporary segregation and isolation are for children who are securely attached,

not for toddlers [and infants] learning to trust that their parents will meet their needs in a loving and responsive manner.

Little scholarly work has addressed the parent's attachment to the child. Clearly, the parent's own emotional makeup, along with his or her expectations about the child, are crucial to this vital process (see Chapter 35).

Screening for Attachment Disorder

Adoptive parents are usually reluctant to mention concerns about attachment, or may not be able to verbalize their feelings that something is awry with the post-adoption adjustment. The pediatrician should be aware that this area may be a major concern of adoptive parents. It is helpful to ask specific questions, such as whether the child prefers the parent(s) to others, prefers one parent greatly over the other, or seems overfriendly to strangers; how the child reacts to separations from the parents (even at bedtime); and the range of emotions expressed by the child. Children with attachment issues may not enjoy close and playful interactions, show shame over misbehaviors, grief over loss, or sadness over the consequences of misbehaviors (but may show rage over perceived unfairness).[42]

The parent's own attachment to the child should also be assessed. Adoptive parents may not attach to the child as readily as imagined. The realities of parenthood, as well as specific behaviors, physical characteristics, or idiosyncrasies of the child, may interfere with the parent's attachment to the child. Parents should be asked if their feelings for the child are what they imagined and hoped for. Reassurances that "love at first sight" is not the rule in adoption, and that parenting is hard work may be very welcome to the new adoptive parent.

Techniques to Promote Attachment

Information, preparation, and support before and after adoption assists parents to deepen their emotional bonds to the child.[42] Understanding the barriers to attachment experienced by their child may help parents make decisions about child care, returning to work, and other practical matters. The parent's *direct* involvement in caregiving is the *critical* foundation for building attachment. Extraneous caregivers, day care providers, and well-meaning assistants should be minimized as much as is practical, especially in the early months after adoption. Several sources at the end of this chapter list some lighthearted activities that may promote attachment (Appendix 29–2). (These are *not* remedies for severe attachment disorder.) Additional suggestions can be found on various Web sites (see Resources).

Treatment of Attachment Disorder

The treatment of RAD is arduous and complex. Treatment of less severe attachment problems is also difficult and challenging. The goal is to increase empathy and attunement.[42] Although traditional therapy presupposes that the child had the readiness and ability to form a therapeutic relationship that may be used to resolve past trauma, children with attachment problems are not likely to enter into a relationship with a therapist. Most theories of treatment attempt to replicate normal attachment sequences at some level. In the "developmental attachment" model, children must develop a relationship with their primary caregivers who then provide a secure base from which to resolve their earlier trauma. As described by Hughes,[12,42] this is promoted by "playful, engaging interactions that provide the attunement essential to forming a relationship and help the child come to terms with experiences that have left him feeling shame and isolation." "Theraplay" is attachment-based play that purports to help with anger, aggression, depression, attentional difficulties, and developmental delays.[60,61] "Holding therapy" has also been espoused as a treatment for attachment disorder. In this therapy, the child is physically restrained in the hope that she will learn to feel safe and tolerate "affective intensity" that is generated during the therapy session. Responsible practitioners elicit the child's consent and explain the intervention to the child, and only do this in the presence of the parents. This technique should be used only by highly trained, experienced practitioners. Overall, mild attachment problems may respond within 6–9 months, but more often 18–24 months may be required. Sadly, some children do not respond to therapeutic interventions.

Severe Attachment Disorder

Attachment disorder and international adoption have been linked in the news on several tragic occasions over the past 10 years. At least two Russian adoptees said to have RAD have been killed.[62] In both cases, the adoptive parents were accused and/or convicted of the crimes (see Chapter 35). The defense claimed that the children had severe RAD and that their injuries were self-inflicted. In addition to these two tragedies, many more children with severe behavioral disturbances have been adopted by American families. Many have been removed from the adoptive homes and placed in specialized foster care, juvenile detention facilities, or psychiatric facilities. No statistics are kept that reveal the scope of this problem. However, between 1994 and 2001, one agency that arranges adoptions of special-needs youngsters (Tressler Lutheran Services, Baltimore, MD) placed 105 Eastern European children who were unable to remain with their original adopting families, often due to RAD. Some children had to be placed with three or even four different families. Many of the children had been neglected and sexually abused in Russia; after adoption some displayed severely aggressive behaviors, molesting others and even attempting murder. The tragedy for these children and their parents is enormous.

Key Points for Internationally Adopted Children

- Orphanage life conspires to produce disordered attachment.
- There is a spectrum of disordered attachment.
- Many internationally adopted children have some disordered attachment behaviors.
- Most international adoptees develop good attachment to their families.
- A small minority have severe reactive attachment disorder.
- Treatment of reactive attachment disorder is complex and arduous.

Appendix 29–1 Common Behaviors from an Attachment Perspective

- When we got Carly, she attached to us instantly. She clung to me and wouldn't let go for hours. She insisted that she sleep next to me while we were in China, and in fact, she still does.

Comment: "Instant" attachment does not occur. It's not surprising for a child to respond in this way early after adoption. How terrifying it must be to suddenly lose all familiar people, places, language, foods, and things! Co-sleeping can be very helpful during this difficult transition.

- Natalia wouldn't look at us for 3 days after we got her. She reluctantly took food we offered, and listlessly played with toys in the hotel room. On the fourth morning, she was sitting silently on the floor in front of some toys, and I noticed huge tears rolling down her cheeks. When I tried to comfort her, she looked away, then started to sob loudly and inconsolably for over an hour. Alex screamed and cried inconsolably for 4 days after we got him. It was a horror show. Everywhere we went, people were staring at us. While we were waiting at the embassy, we couldn't believe that other parents who had also just gotten their children were able to play, talk, and interact with them. He just didn't stop screaming unless he exhausted himself and fell asleep. On the fifth day,

"My daughter was adopted at age 4 from Romania. The last 9 years have been a nightmare. She never connected with us or with her two older brothers (also adopted). She's been threatening to kill us. She defecates and urinates in her room and refuses to bathe. She wrung the neck of our 10-year-old cat. Most recently, she was arrested for assault and placed in a foster home. The foster mother was afraid to go to sleep at night because L. was out of control. She was arrested again and sent to juvenile detention. She was there for 60 days. Eight different group homes or residential treatment centers refused to accept her after reviewing the 94 incidents in her 60 days in detention. Finally, I found a group home in another state that would accept her. The doctor there put her on Risperdal, Tegretol, Doxepin, Depakote, Zoloft, and Thorazine. She's been diagnosed with severe reactive attachment disorder, bipolar disorder, intermittent explosive disorder, and posttraumatic stress disorder. They say she will be sent home as they can't manage her. I'm terrified. The only place that will take her is the state mental facility—but I have to disrupt the adoption and make her a ward of the state for this to happen. In spite of everything, I don't want my daughter to feel like I have abandoned her. Could she be acting out because she knows the only place she can go is home?"[63]

he woke from a deep sleep, looked me deep in the eyes, and then started to accept our care.

Comment: Not unusual beginnings at all. It sounds like both children were deeply attached to their caregivers. Their reactions are exactly what Spitz and Bowlby described. You stuck with Alex, and he started to trust you. Natalia will probably start to come around soon. However, don't forget what major losses these children suffered.

- Reba is the most social baby! She loves everyone. She's such a flirt—when I took her to my office, everyone had such a good time holding her. I was actually able to work at my desk for over 2 hours while everyone else played with her.

Comment: This could be one of those lovely gregarious babies, or is she indiscriminately friendly? Careful observation of her behaviors with others and her parents could help differentiate these two possibilities. Two hours is a long time to go without checking in with mom. Some more detailed questions, review of child care arrangements and expectations, and careful follow-up are in order.

- I'm amazed how much work I've been able to get done in the mornings—everyone said this would be difficult with a 10-month-old! After Alison wakes up at 6 AM, I just give her a bottle and she plays by herself in her crib until 11 AM. She's so good!

    Comment: First-time parents may not realize how abnormal this behavior is. Alison has learned during institutional life to entertain herself and not to expect any interaction from her caregivers. It will be great when Allison starts to protest being left alone, but meanwhile Mom needs to be with Alison, interrupt her solitude, and engage her in activities and interactive games.

- Tyler never seems to notice when I come to get him at day care. I have to go up to him and interrupt him at whatever he is doing. He willingly leaves with me, but if I didn't show up one day, I don't think he'd care.

    Comment: This could be a child who has difficulty with transitions. If the quality of interaction with the parent is solid, the coming and going behaviors may not be so worrisome. Would he really not care if you didn't come? This is worth exploring in more detail.

- Evie gets hysterical if I leave the room for just a minute. She clings to me desperately, and hides her face if we go out in a crowd. I haven't had a minute alone since she came home 2 months ago. I'm not sure what's going to happen when I go back to work next month.

    Comment: Evie is especially needy. She obviously is desperate for your focused care and love. She needs some specialized reassurance for her anxiety (which is totally understandable, given her early life experiences). Telling her "she's a big girl and doesn't need Mama" is definitely NOT advisable. Some quiet "together time" several times a day that she can count on might help. Think about your work plans carefully—if you must leave, strongly consider a loving attentive nanny rather than group day care.

- I'm a single father, and it really bothers me that Maxim goes up to any woman he sees and tries to climb on her lap. He seems happier with a woman he doesn't even know than with me—and he's been home for almost 6 months now.

    Comment: Men sometimes have it rough when adopting post-institutionalized children. Most of these kids have seen few if any men, and may be terrified of them. Others have "learned" that women are more reliable providers of comfort and care. Look at your parenting style and see if you are providing the physical affection that Maxim needs. Careful follow-up is indicated.

- I'm so terrified that 5-year-old Mike will go off with a stranger. He just doesn't "get it" that I'm his mom. I know that he'd go with anyone who offered him an ice cream cone. I've explained about "bad people" until I'm blue in the face, but just don't know what to do anymore.

- I thought that Kira bonded to me instantly when she took my hand in the orphanage and gave me a big smile. She didn't look back for a minute as we walked out. Now I see she behaves like that with any new person. She seems to be thinking, "maybe you're going to take care of me now." She doesn't understand what it means to be in a family.

    Comment: These children both have signs of indiscriminate friendliness. Depending on how recent the adoptions were, and other qualities of the parent-child relationship, you may wish to consider expert advice.

- At bedtime, Erica packed her suitcase every night for a year and stood by the door for almost an hour. When she finally got enough English, she told us she was waiting for her "real mother" to come and get her. We later learned that her birth mother had visited in her in the orphanage shortly before the adoption, and told Erica, then 7 years old, that she'd come to get her some day. I think deep down Erica is still waiting.

    Comment: Many complicated issues may impede attachment in older children. Erica's understanding of adoption is limited by her age. Reframing the story of Erica's adoption for her may help her cope.

Appendix 29–2A Activities to promote healthy attachment

1. Wear infant in chest carrier, all day if possible.
2. Mom should initially be the only person meeting her needs. Baby needs to build a bond with one person first, then she can branch out to others.
3. Bathe together, to promote skin-to-skin contact. Baby and Mom wear the same lotion; baby associates scent with Mom.
4. When child gets a shot, Mom shouldn't be the person to hold her. Ask nurse to hold her, and then have Mom be the one to comfort her.
5. Laminate loving family pictures of you together and put around her crib and other places.
6. Outline her body, as well as your own, on huge sheets of newsprint. Color them. Tape the "portraits" to her ceiling.
7. When feeding her something she particularly likes, tell her you are a good mommy or daddy. Telling her with words that you are a good mommy is important—otherwise, how would she know?
8. If you use cologne (or if you don't, use your shampoo), place a tiny bit on her arm so she has your smell with her at all times.
9. Play with dolls to act out how parents always return after the child goes to day care, babysitter, bed, etc.
10. Limit choices. At first, parents should make all decisions, including foods, toys, and clothes. This helps the child feel safe. Then as the child becomes accustomed to the new family, limited choices can be offered.

Source: Reprinted with permission from Attach-China, www.attach-china.org.[45]

Appendix 29–2B Activities to promote attachments in toddlers

1. Bottle feed your toddler, no matter what the age. Encourage eye contact by gently touching her cheek. *Do not* let her hold the bottle. Nourishment has to come from parent(s); be sure to hold her when feeding.
2. If she turns away (avoiding eye contact) try placing a large mirror across from you. That way, when she turns away, she will see herself in your embrace.
3. Continue to hold her in your gaze. It may take a long time for her to glance at you. When she finally does, be ready with a warm, loving, approving smile. This sounds little but is really big and pays big rewards in our experience.
4. Encourage eye contact by gently tapping the bridge of her nose and yours as a hand signal to look at you.
5. Play peek-a-boo.
6. Have the baby pull a sticker off your nose—and put it back.
7. Hold the baby in your arms and dance with her—a very synchronous activity.
8. Swim together.
9. Paint each other's faces with paint, powder, or just pretend.
10. Play musical nose—sing a song and let your child pinch your nose so you sound very silly. You stop singing if she breaks eye contact.
11. Play musical swing—put child in a baby swing. Face her as you push. Encourage eye contact by singing a song, and stop if she looks away.
12. Fill your cheeks with air. Have child "pop" them.
13. Put lotion on each other.
14. Ask her to feed you. This works great with raisins, Cheerios, or popcorn.
15. Give Eskimo kisses—rub noses and stare into each other's eyes.
16. Play in front of a mirror. Make faces, painting Mommy's face, trace each other's faces on the mirror with washable marker, finger paint, shaving cream. Let your child be your puppet and make her dance. Make dolls dance. Any kind of game that gets your child to relax and meet your eyes in the mirror will likely get her relaxed enough to meet your eyes directly.
17. Instead of using an actual mirror, take turns being each other's mirror. Sit face to face, and have your child imitate every facial movement you make, and vice versa. Then try it with your whole body, mirroring each other's movements.
18. For an older child, try lipreading with each other. While you're not really getting eye contact, you're at least looking at each other's faces.
19. Play a memory game with a more personal touch. Have your child look you over carefully. Then leave the room and return after you've changed something about yourself. See if she can figure out what is different. It could be something really obvious for younger kids, like taking off a sweater, but for older kids you could do something more challenging like buttoning one more button on the sweater.[45]

These are listed as suggestions only; children with attachment disorder require professional help.

Source: Reprinted with permission from Attach-China, www.attach-china.org

Appendix 29–3 Reactive attachment disorder of infancy and early childhood

A. Markedly disturbed and developmentally inappropriate social relatedness in most contexts, beginning before age 5 years, as evidenced by either (1) or (2):

    1. Persistent failure to initiate or respond in a developmentally appropriate fashion to most social interactions, as manifest by excessively inhibited, hypervigilant, or highly ambivalent and contradictory responses (e.g., the child may respond to caregivers with a mixture of approach, avoidance, and resistance to comforting, or may exhibit frozen watchfulness).

    2. Diffuse attachment as manifest by indiscriminate sociability with marked inability to exhibit appropriate selective attachments (e.g., excessive familiarity with relative strangers or lack of selectivity in choice of attachment figures).

B. The disturbance in Criterion A is not accounted for solely by developmental delay (as in mental retardation) and does not meet criteria for pervasive developmental disorder.

C. Pathogenic care as evidenced by at least one of the following:

    1. Persistent disregard for the child's basic emotional needs for comfort, stimulation, and affection

    2. Persistent disregard for the child's basic physical needs

    3. Repeated changes of primary caregiver that prevent formation of stable attachments (e.g., frequent changes in foster care)

D. There is a presumption that the care in Criterion C is responsible for the disturbed behavior in Criterion A (e.g., the disturbances in Criterion A began following the pathogenic care in Criterion C).

Specify type: Inhibited type: if Criterion A1 predominates in the clinical presentation
                 Disinhibited type: if Criterion A2 predominates in the clinical presentation

Reprinted with permission from the *Diagnostic and Statistical Manual of Mental Disorders, 4th edition, Text Revision*. Washington, DC: American Psychiatric Association, 2000.[64]

Resources

Federici R. Help for the Hopeless Child. Alexandria, VA: Dr. Ronald Federici and Associates, 1998 (400 South Washington St., Alexandria, VA 22314, 703-548-0721, fax 703-836-8995).

Gray DD. Attaching in Adoption. Indianapolis: Perspectives Press, 2002.

Hopkins-Best M. Toddler Adoption: The Weaver's Craft. Indianapolis: Perspectives Press, 1997.

Hughes DA. Building the Bonds of Attachment. Northvale, NJ: Jason Aronson, Inc., 1998.

Jernberg A, Booth PB. Theraplay: Helping Parents and Children Build Better Relationships Through Attachment-based Play. San Francisco: Jossey-Bass, 1999.

Keck GC, Kupecky RM. Adopting the Hurt Child. Colorado Springs: Pinon Press, 1995.

Keck GC, Kupecky RM. Parenting the Hurt Child. Colorado Springs: Pinon Press, 2002.

Practical Attachment. Available at: http://home.att.net/~PracticalAttachment/index.html.

Association for Treatment and Training of in the Attachment of Children (ATTACH). Available at: http://www.attach.org.

References

1. Bowlby J. Attachment. Attachment and Loss, Vol. I. New York: Basic Books, 1982.

2. Association for treatment and training in the attachment of children (ATTACH). Available at: http://www.attach.org.

3. Booth PB, Wark L. The nature of attachment relationships. Am Assoc Marriage Fam Ther J 2001; 3:1–7.

4. Magid K, McKelvey CA. High Risk: Children Without a Conscience. New York: Bantam, 1987.

5. Vaughan BE, Gove FL, Egeland B. The relationship between out of home care and the quality of infant–mother attachment in an economically disadvantaged population. Child Dev 1980; 51:1203–14.

6. Spitz RA. The First Year of Life. New York: International Universities Press, Inc., 1965.

7. Bowlby J. Separation, Vol. II. New York: Basic Books, 1973.

8. Bowlby J. Loss: Sadness and Depression, Vol. III. New York: Basic Books, 1980.

9. Karen R. Becoming Attached. New York: Warner Books, 1994.

10. Keck GC, Kupecky RM. Parenting the Hurt Child. Colorado Springs: Pinon Press, 2002.

11. Keck GC, Kupecky RM. Adopting the Hurt child. Colorado Springs: Pinon Press, 1995.

12. Hughes DA. Building the Bonds of Attachment. Northvale, NJ: Jason Aronson, Inc., 1998.

13. Arling GL, Harlow HF. Effects of social deprivation on maternal behavior of rhesus monkeys. J Comp Physiol Psychol 1967; 64:371–7.

14. Griffin GA, Harlow HF. Effects of three months of total social deprivation on social adjustment and learning in the rhesus monkey. Child Dev 1966; 37:533–47.

15. Hansen EW, Harlow HF, Dodsworth RO. Reactions of rhesus monkeys to familiar and unfamiliar peers. J Comp Physiol Psychol 1966; 61:274–9.

16. Harlow HF, Dodsworth RO, Harlow MK. Total social isolation in monkeys. Proc Natl Acad Sci USA 1965; 54:90–7.

17. Harlow HF, Harlow M. Learning to love. Am Sci 1966; 54:244–72.

18. Harlow HF. The primate socialization motives. Trans Stud Coll Physicians Phila 1966; 33:224–37.

19. Harlow HF, Mc Kinney WT, Jr. Nonhuman primates and psychoses. J Autism Child Schizophr 1971; 1:368–75.

20. Harlow HF, Suomi SJ. Social recovery by isolation-reared monkeys. Proc Natl Acad Sci USA 1971; 68:1534–8.

21. Harlow HF, Suomi SJ. Production of depressive behaviors in young monkeys. J Autism Child Schizophr 1971; 1:246–55.

22. Harlow HF, Plubell PE, Baysinger CM. Induction of psychological death in rhesus monkeys. J Autism Child Schizophr 1973; 3:299–307.

23. Harlow HF, Suomi SJ. Induced depression in monkeys. Behav Biol 1974; 12:273–96.

24. Kerr GR, Chamove AS, Harlow HF. Environmental deprivation: its effect on the growth of infant monkeys. J Pediatr 1969; 75:833–7.

25. McKinney WT Jr, Suomi SJ, Harlow HF. Depression in primates. Am J Psychiatry 1971; 127:1313–20.

26. McKinney WT Jr, Suomi SJ, Harlow HF. Repetitive peer separations of juvenile-age rhesus monkeys. Arch Gen Psychiatry 1972; 27:200–3.

27. McKinney WT Jr, Suomi SJ, Harlow HF. Vertical-chamber confinement of juvenile-age rhesus monkeys. A study in experimental psychopathology. Arch Gen Psychiatry 1972; 26:223–8.

28. Mears CE, Harlow HF. Play: early and eternal. Proc Natl Acad Sci USA 1975; 72:1878–82.

29. Meyer JS, Novak MA, Bowman RE, Harlow HF. Behavioral and hormonal effects of attachment object separation in surrogate-peer-reared and mother-reared infant rhesus monkeys. Dev Psychobiol 1975; 8:425–35.

30. Ruppenthal GC, Harlow MK, Eisele CD, Harlow HF, Suomi SJ. Development of peer interactions of monkeys reared in a nuclear-family environment. Child Dev 1974; 45:670–82.

31. Ruppenthal GC, Arling GL, Harlow HF, Sackett GP, Suomi SJ. A 10-year perspective of motherless-mother monkey behavior. J Abnorm Psychol 1976; 85: 341–9.

32. Seay B, Harlow HF. Maternal separation in the rhesus monkey. J Nerv Ment Dis 1965; 140:434–41.

33. Suomi SJ, Harlow HF, Domek CJ. Effect of repetitive infant–infant separation of young monkeys. J Abnorm Psychol 1970; 76:161–72.

34. Suomi SJ, Harlow HF. Depressive behavior in young monkeys subjected to vertical chamber confinement. J Comp Physiol Psychol 1972; 80:11–8.

35. Suomi SJ, Harlow HF, McKinney WT Jr. Monkey psychiatrists. Am J Psychiatry 1972; 128:927–32.

36. Suomi SJ, Eisele CD, Grady SA, Harlow HF. Depressive behavior in adult monkeys following separation from family environment. J Abnorm Psychol 1975; 84:576–8.

37. Suomi SJ, Harlow HF. Effects of differential removal from group on social development of Rhesus monkeys. J Child Psychol Psychiatry 1975; 16:149–64.

38. Suomi SJ, Delizio R, Harlow HF. Social rehabilitation of separation-induced depressive disorders in monkeys. Am J Psychiatry 1976; 133:1279–85.

39. Suomi SJ, Collins ML, Harlow HF, Ruppenthal GC. Effects of maternal and peer separations on young monkeys. J Child Psychol Psychiatry 1976; 17:101–12.

40. Young LD, Suomi SS, Harlow HF, McKinney WT Jr. Early stress and later response to separation in rhesus monkeys. Am J Psychiatry 1973; 130:400–5.

41. Rothbaum F, Weisz J, Pott M, Miyake K, Morelli G. Attachment and culture. Am Psychol 2000; 55:1093–1104.

42. Hughes DA. Adopting children with attachment problems. Child Welfare 1999; 78:541–60.

43. Field T. Attachment and separation in young children. Annu Rev Psychol 1996; 47:541–61.

44. Parens H. Indices of the child's earliest attachment to his mother, applicable in routine pediatric examination. Pediatrics 1972; 49:600–3.

45. Beck L, D'Antonio N, Lyon L. Why Chinese children are at risk for RAD. FCC Metro Detroit Newsletter, 2000:4–19. Available at: Attach-China. http://www.attach-china.org.

46. Hodges J, Tizard B. IQ and behavioral adjustment of ex-institutional adolescents. J Child Psychol Psychiatry 1989; 30:53–75.

47. Hodges J, Tizard B. Social and family relationship of ex-institutional adolescents. J Child Psychol Psychiatry 1989; 3:77–97.

48. Tizard B, Hodges J. The effect of early institu-

tional rearing on the development of eight-year-old children. J Child Psychol Psychiatry 1978; 19:99–118.

49. Goldfarb W. Effects of psychological deprivation in infancy and subsequent stimulation. Am J Psychiatry 1945; 102:18–33.

50. Goldfarb W. Psychological privation in infancy and subsequent adjustment. Am J Orthopsychiatry 1945; 14:247–55.

51. Singer LM, Brodzinsky DM, Ramsay D, Steir M, Waters E. Mother–infant attachment in adoptive families. Child Dev 1985; 56:1543–51.

52. Yarrow LJ, Goodwin MS. The immediate impact of separation: reactions of infants to a change in mother figure. In: Stone LJ, Smith HT, Murphy LB, eds. The Competent Infant. New York: Basic, 1973: 1032–40.

52a. Gray DD. Attaching in Adoption. Indianapolis: Perspective Press, 1997.

53. Chisholm K, Carter MC, Ames EW, Morison SJ. Attachment security and indiscriminately friendly behavior in children adopted from Romanian orphanages. Dev Psychopathol 1995; 7:283–94.

54. Chisholm K. A three-year follow-up of attachment and indiscriminate friendliness in children adopted from Romanian orphanages. Child Dev 1998; 69:1092–106.

55. Provence S, Lipton RC. Infants in Institutions. New York: International Universities Press, 1962.

56. Rutter M, Kreppner JM, O'Connor TG. Specificity and heterogeneity in children's responses to profound institutional privation. Br J Psychiatry 2001; 179:97–103.

57. O'Connor TG, Rutter M. Attachment disorder behavior following early severe deprivation: extension and longitudinal follow-up. English and Romanian Adoptees Study Team. J Am Acad Child Adolesc Psychiatry 2000; 39:703–12.

58. Zeanah CH. Disturbances of attachment in young children adopted from institutions. J Dev Behav Pediatr 2000; 21:230–6.

59. Hopkins-Best M. Toddler Adoption: The Weaver's Craft. Indianapolis: Perspectives Press, 1997. Used with permission.

60. Jernberg A. Theraplay: A New Treatment Using Structured Play for Problem Children and Their Families. San Francisco: Jossey-Bass, 1979.

61. Jernberg A, Booth PB. Theraplay: Helping Parents and Children Build Better Relationships Through Attachment-based Play. San Francisco: Jossey-Bass, 1999.

62. Hastings D. Adopted Russian children killed in the United States, 2001.

63. Anonymous. L's story. With permission: Parent Network for the Post-Institutionalized Child, November 14, 2001 [modified to protect privacy].

64. First MB, Frances A, Pincus HA. DSM-IV-TR Handbook of Differential Diagnosis. Washington, DC: American Psychiatric Press, 2002.

65. Cline FW, Fay J. Parenting with Love and Logic. Colorado Springs: Pinon Press, 1990.

66. Lach C. Overwhelmed families dissolve adoptions. Pittsburgh Post-Gazette, August 14, 2000. Available at: http://www.post-gazette.com/headlines/2000814 russiatodaytwo1.asp

30

BEHAVIORAL AND MENTAL DISORDERS

In 1960, child psychiatrist Marshall D. Schechter reported a hundredfold increase of adopted patients in his practice compared with what would be expected in the general population.[1] This claim (based on a small group of children seen by one psychiatrist), though reportedly based on a misinterpretation of the published adoption literature,[2] received widespread publicity, reinforcing the notion that adoptees frequently have mental and psychiatric disturbances. Adoptees are overrepresented among mental health care recipients: about 8%–10% of children receiving in-patient or out-patient psychiatric services are adopted (range 2.4%–25%).[2–5] However, the reasons for this are complex. Adoptive families may be more likely to seek help for problems because of their relative maturity, socioeconomic status, and familiarity with social service availability.[6] Indeed, adoptees are underrepresented in juvenile court populations, possibly because adoptive parents seek psychiatric care if their child demonstrates delinquent or undesirable behaviors.[3] Similarly, adoptees may be underrepresented among adult mental health populations,[7] perhaps because psychological issues are addressed during the teenage years.

Nonetheless, professionals and parents may wonder if adopted children, especially those adopted internationally, are at increased risk for behavioral and mental disorders. Genetic factors, separation from birth parents, environmental exposures (both pre- and postnatal), some facets of adoption itself, and the adoptive home environment all potentially increase the likelihood of these disorders. This chapter is divided into four sections. The first reviews the links between genetics and mental health disorders (schizophrenia, affective disorder, and antisocial personality disorder). In the second, the relationship between adoption and behavior problems, as well as the difficulties interpreting research in this area, are discussed. The third section explores the risks of mental health disorders in international adoption and the relationship between behaviors observed in the orphanage and after adoption (see Chapters 4, 9, and 29). Finally, the fourth section examines the long-term mental health outcome of adoptees. Post-traumatic stress disorder and depression are also discussed in Chapter 8.

Genetics, Adoption, and Mental Health Disorders

The genetic components of various mental disorders have been investigated in hundreds of twin, family aggregation, and adoption studies.[8] Possible or likely genetic factors have been identified for a number of psychiatric conditions, including schizophrenia, affective disorders, antisocial behavior, conduct disorder, autism, dyslexia, attention-deficit hyperactivity disorder, conduct disorder, Tourette syndrome, and obsessive-compulsive disorder.[9] To date, only the adult forms of schizophrenia, affective disorder, and obsessive-compulsive disorder have been linked to such factors. Attempts to identify single susceptibility loci for mental diseases have been largely unsuccessful.[10,11] Several recent reviews summarize the biologic bases of psychiatric disorders.[8,12–15]

In this section, the links between mental disorders and adoption are reviewed. It is prudent to interpret these data with caution, as many factors contribute to the development of such problems. Adoption studies may be biased by variations in age at adoption, pre-adoptive placement, age at evaluation, and experiences in the adoptive home. For example, adoptive families may themselves have increased incidence of mental disorders and stress. Accurate and complete information about birth families may also be lacking, especially about birth fathers. Moreover, adoptive placements may be biased by "inadvertent"[16] or deliberate matching of the adoptive and biologic families for shared characteristics that influence the development of

mental illness. Finally, intrafamilial and extrafamilial adoption are not distinguished in some studies.

Schizophrenia and Adoption

Numerous adoption studies support current hypotheses of a genetic basis for schizophrenia.[17] Adopted-away children of schizophrenic mothers have three- to fourfold risk of developing schizophrenia compared with adopted-away children of mothers without this diagnosis.[18–21] The risks of disease expression are increased if the adoptive home is unstable.[22–24] Mental illness is more common among biologic relatives of schizophrenic adoptees.[25–28] The heritability of schizophrenia may be as high as ~70%;[29] higher risks are associated with closer genetic ties.

Affective Disorders and Adoption

Genetic susceptibility contributes to the expression of depression and bipolar disorders.[9,29–31] Adoption studies support this conclusion.[32,33] However, investigators agree that environmental factors are crucial in modulating disease expression. Heritability of major depression is estimated in the range of 31%–42%,[29] although certain subtypes may be higher.[34,35] Inherited variations in regional brain volume and shape increase susceptibility to depression,[36] although this is not certain.[37] Other factors, such as prenatal alcohol exposure[38] (possibly mediated via postnatal exposure to maternal depression) or early adverse life events[39] (possibly mediated via altered hypothalamic–pituitary axis responsiveness[40]), also contribute to disease expression. Genetic evidence links affective disorders to autism spectrum disorders,[41] conduct disorder,[42] and hyperactivity.[9]

Antisocial Behaviors and Adoption

Several studies show that children adopted at birth from "antisocial biologic backgrounds" exhibit increased antisocial behaviors.[43–45]

Cadoret and Cain[43] evaluated 246 adoptees separated at birth from their biologic parents. One or both birth parents of nearly half the children had a psychiatric condition. Children were evaluated after age 10 years (84/246 were >18 years). Having an antisocial or alcoholic birth parent predicted antisocial behavior in the adoptee at adolescence. Environmental factors, including a psychiatrically ill adoptive family member, divorced adoptive parents, or exposure to multiple foster mothers, also significantly correlated with antisocial behavior among the adoptees. In addition, mental retardation in the biologic family of the female adoptees predicted increased antisocial behavior.

In a follow-up study,[46] multiple regression analysis differentiated genetic and environmental effects among 197 adult adoptees whose biologic parents had antisocial personality disorder and/or alcoholism. Again, an adverse biologic background predicted adolescent aggression and conduct disorder, as well as antisocial behaviors in adulthood. These difficulties were augmented in children raised in unfavorable adoptive home environments. Genetic influences accounted for about 50% of the variance in aggressive, externalizing behaviors in a survey of siblings adopted together.[47]

Similarly, adopted adolescents with oppositional defiant disorder were more likely to have birth parents with antisocial personalities (often with drug or alcohol abuse).[48,49] Criminal behaviors in adult adoptees were more common in those with criminal birth parents in one study but not another.[43,50]

Adoption and Behavior

Do adopted children exhibit more behavioral problems than their non-adopted peers? Adoption itself is a risk factor for mental health disorders. Adoption undoubtably influences the family's responses to the child. Unresolved issues related to infertility, adoption, or beliefs about the child's heritage may alter parental availability, affection, or involvement.[4,46] The adoptive family may have psychopathology, and the adopted child may experience disruptions, stresses, and trauma in that environment.[7] Few studies account for variation in the child's age at adoption, the care received prior to adoption, the composition of the adoptive family, and how the adoption was handled in the family (kept secret, celebrated, etc.).[44] The acceptance of the adoption and the adopted child by grandparents and other relatives also affects the family dynamics. The experience of institutionalization also contributes to the likelihood of behavioral problems[51,52] (see also Chapter 2). Mismatch of temperament is more likely to occur in adoption, and this may contribute to mental health disorders.[53] Furthermore, mental conditions may be overdiagnosed among adoptees; "normative crises" and adjustment reactions of adoption may be misconstrued.[46,54] Well-meaning but misinformed mental health professionals may make things worse for the adoptive family in crisis, by their failure to recognize and support existing bonds at times of family stress, as pointed out by adoption expert and child psychiatrist, Steven L. Nickman.[55] Finally, many studies compare the mental health of adopted children with that of their birth parents. However, the sources and accuracy of information regarding diagnoses in birth parents may be questionable. At the time medical history is obtained (often at relinquishment), birth parents may be young, and mental disorders may not have fully emerged or been properly diagnosed or recorded. Little or no information is usually available about birth fathers. Most studies evaluate a narrow age range of children: some behaviors may improve, while others may not have yet emerged.

A survey of adopted teens found that most had positive self-concepts, warm relationships with their parents, and psychological health, comparable to non-adopted teens.[56] Although one-third received counseling or psychotherapy, most of those reported good mental health. Positive adoption outcomes likely are underreported.[57]

Nonetheless, certain behavior problems appear more commonly in adoptees than in non-adopted children. Numerous studies indicate that adoptees in clinical settings more frequently have externalizing aggressive behaviors than non-adopted children.[2–5,7,58–62] In nonclinical samples of children, more frequent problem behavior is reported by parents and teachers among adopted than nonadopted children. In Sweden, maladjustment was more common among 579 adopted 11-year-olds than among controls. However, by ages 15, 18, and 22 years, the differences from non-adopted peers decreased.[63] In Britain, more maladjusted behavior occurred among 108 adopted 7-year-old boys than among controls; in girls, frequency of behavior problems was unrelated to adoption.[64] Adoptees in the United States had reduced social competence and school achievement.[65] In Ontario, all 104 adopted children in the province were surveyed to investigate the association between adoptive status, psychiatric morbidity, school achievement, and substance abuse.[58,59] Adopted children did not differ from non-adopted children in educational achievement or substance abuse. However, adopted boys had more psychiatric disorders, especially if school performance was poor. In a New Zealand study, adopted children were more likely to abuse drugs or have antisocial personality or conduct disorder than control children.[53] Adopted children complained more often of somatic disorders in another study.[66] Finally, although adolescent adoptees more commonly attempted suicide than their non-adopted peers, the great majority of adoptees do not attempt suicide and do not differ in other aspects of emotional and behavioral health from non-adoptees.[67]

Behavior Problems and Internationally Adopted Children

Additional components may influence the behavior of international adoptees compared with that of domestically adopted children. Many international adoptees are transracially adopted. They appear physically different from their parents and perhaps from their siblings. They may belong to a racial minority in their communities. Within the family and community, these children are "visibly" adopted. The effects of this visible adoption has not yet been fully evaluated. Results may differ in various receiving countries. For example, the Scandinavian countries receive many internationally adopted children from Asia and Latin America. These countries are relatively homogeneous; adopted children may be mistaken for immigrants and assumptions made about socioeconomic class, education, and background (see Chapter 34). Even in more heterogeneous societies, such as the Netherlands, internationally adopted children may stand out compared to their Dutch-born peers. About 30% of 7-year-old internationally children in the Netherlands scored in the clinical range on the Child Behavior Check List, compared to 10% of controls.[68] When biologically related and unrelated international adoptees were compared, genetic contributions were identified as important to attention problems and externalizing behaviors.[68a] In a larger study, Verhulst investigated behavior issues among 2,148 international adoptees in the Netherlands.[63,69,70] The children were adopted from Korea (32%), Colombia (14.6%), India (9.5%), Indonesia (7.9%), Bangladesh (6.7%), Lebanon (4.9%), Austria (5%), and other countries (19.4%) (a different distribution of birth countries than that for children adopted by American parents). The majority of adopted children had scores similar to non-adopted Dutch children on the Achenbach Child Behavior Checklist. However, nearly four times more 12- to 15-year-old adopted boys had delinquent behaviors ("steals outside the home," "steals at home," "hangs around children who get into trouble," "vandalism," "lying and cheating," "truancy") and other misconduct, and more than three times more scored in the deviant range on the Hyperactive scale. About three times more adopted 12- to 15-year-old girls scored high on the Schizoid scale ("hears things that are not there," "stares blankly," "strange ideas," "daydreams or gets lost in her thoughts," "strange behavior," and others). Notably, the adopted children scored better than non-adopted children in sports and non-sports activities. More adopted than non-adopted children were attending special schools (13.2% vs. 4.4%). Adopted children from lower socioeconomic adoptive homes showed better academic performance, fewer school problems, and higher total competence scores than children from higher socioeconomic homes.

The authors further determined that, in general, the older the child at placement the greater the risk of "delinquent and uncommunicative syndromes" in boys and "cruel, depressed, and schizoid" syndromes in girls, although the relationship of problems to age at adoption was complex and nonlinear.[70] No country-specific differences were noted, although boys from Colombia, Lebanon, and some European countries had higher problem scores. A follow-up study of the same cohort found psychiatric diagnoses in 28% of 14-year-old international adoptees (22% for girls, 36% for boys), somewhat higher than for the general population.[69] Conduct disorders, antisocial behaviors, and mood disorders were most common. About 20% of adolescents had deviant behaviors by self- or parent-report.[71] The authors caution against the application of their results to all internationally adopted children because of the variations in age at adoption and experiences prior to adoption. Nonetheless, this series suggests that adopted children are more likely to have behavioral issues in adolescence than their non-adopted peers.

In Sweden, 125 adolescent adoptees had similar health and family life styles as non-adopted controls.[72] However, the adopted girls had more suicidal thoughts, school truancy, and risk behaviors (not using safety belts, sexual intercourse, unpleasant sexual encounters, and contact with illicit drugs). In contrast, the emotional health of Indonesian adoptees living in Australian families was similar to that of adolescents residing in the community with their birth families. Both groups had significantly better emotional and behavioral health than adolescents referred to mental health clinics.[72a]

Risk of Mental Disorders in International Adoption

Pre-adoptive Medical Records

Family medical history, especially mental health history, is rarely if ever available for internationally adopted children (see Chapter 4). If available, interpretation of psychiatric diagnoses from culturally different medical systems is difficult. For example, a birth mother reported to have "depression" may have the expected emotional responses to her difficult circumstances which require that she relinquish her child, rather than major depressive or bipolar disorder. A recent small survey suggests that most relinquishing birth mothers in Russia are clinically depressed.[73] "Antisocial personality" may refer

---

The Smith family received a referral of a beautiful 14-month-old baby girl from Russia. Everything looked favorable, except the maternal grandmother of the child had been diagnosed with "schizophrenia." The Smiths were told that several Russian families had rejected the referral on this basis. After medical consultation, the Smiths decided to proceed with the adoption. They became very friendly with the caregiver in the baby's room at the orphanage, and over several days, with the help of the interpreter, learned that the child's grandmother was a kindergarten teacher, frequently came to visit, and often brought toys for all the children in the group. When asked about the diagnosis of schizophrenia, the caregiver stated that the grandmother was "nervous" and went to a health spa once a year for treatment.

to a parent who has engaged in minor or major criminal activity, or simply to a young woman who has become pregnant out of wedlock. Parents may be incarcerated for reasons that might or might not be valid in the United States. "Oligophrenia" is seen occasionally on pre-adoptive records from Eastern Europe. This has been variously translated as mental retardation, depression, and schizophrenia. These examples highlight the difficulties in understanding noso-logic categories of neuropsychiatric illnesses from another culture.

Lack of information about family mental health disorders should not be construed to mean that no problems exist. Little information is available about birth fathers. However, birth mothers with mental retardation, mental illness, antisocial behaviors, and/or substance abuse likely favor birth fathers with similar qualities (assortative mating).[43,44] Thus, some children inherit a double dose of unfavorable genes.

Finally, fabricated or exaggerated psychi-atric diagnoses are occasionally included on pre-adoptive medical records for "legal reasons" (e.g., to expedite the adoption of the child). It is usually impossible to differentiate among these various situations, but a request to the adoption agency or intermediary for further information is often warranted.

Mental and Behavioral Disorders at Adoption

Children residing in institutional care often ex-hibit abnormal behaviors. These behaviors are usually adaptations to an abnormal, underre-sponsive environment (see Chapter 2). Such behaviors often persist in the early post-adoptive period. These behaviors must be dif-ferentiated from intrinsic behavior problems that may persist after adjustment to the adoption. In this section, the manifestations of depres-sion, autistic-like behavior, and aggression in the orphanage and after adoption are discussed. Because of the frequency of questions about

these problems, diagnostic criteria are listed in Appendix 30–1.

Depression

In the orphanage. Depression is probably the most underdiagnosed condition among institu-tionalized children. The earliest clinical descrip-tions of childhood depression derive from ob-servations of institutionalized children[74,75] (see Chapter 29). "Anaclitic depression" describes the behavior of infants left without maternal care: characteristics include "withdrawal, weight loss, insomnia, weeping, and developmental re-tardation." Less dramatic symptoms of depres-sion may be readily observed among children in most orphanages, and clearly relate to the lack of a consistent primary caregiver.

After adoption. Some children display symp-toms of depression after adoption. Withdrawal, anhedonia, anorexia, lack of eye contact, limited motor activity, and limited language production are normal reactions to the drastic change in environment experienced by the children (see Chapter 9). Parents must be prepared for this reaction and accept that their children may grieve for lost caregivers and the loss of the fa-miliar environment. Sleep disturbances and feed-ing difficulties are common. While such behav-iors are generally transient, some symptoms of depression may persist. In some children, symp-toms may emerge some time after the adoption, even if the initial adjustment was smooth. Mem-ories of lost friends, caregivers, and places may be triggered by comments, books, movies, school projects, or other events in the child's life (see Chapter 34). Months and years after adop-tion the child's interpretation of this experience may lead to depression, shame, and sense of worthlessness ("if I had been good, my birth mother would have kept me"). These issues are explored fully and sensitively in many books (for example, Pavao[54]). Exposure to newborns and young infants, arrival of a new sibling (by birth or adoption), and passage through typical developmental stages (graduations or other achievements, dating, intimacy, marriage, parenthood) may all amplify a sense of loss associated with adoption. Pediatricians and adoptive parents must be sensitive and aware of possible triggers of depression at various lifestages.

In one study, depression in childhood was associated with increased adult body mass index.[76]

"Autistic" Behavior

In the orphanage. The autism spectrum disorders (see Appendix 30–1 for diagnostic criteria) are a heterogeneous group of conditions that share the characteristics of lack of eye contact, aloofness, failure to orient to name, failure to use gestures to point or show, lack of interactive play, lack of interest in peers, and language delays. Many of these characteristics are common in institutionalized children. Biologically, this "quasi-autism" (or acquired institutional autism) may result from prolonged hypercortisolemia, combined with severe sensory and social deprivation (see Chapter 8). The resulting hippocampal damage impairs memory and social and communication skills. Malnutrition, prenatal exposures, and prematurity contribute further complications. Social factors may also play a role. For example, gestures and interactive play may not have been rewarded or encouraged in the orphanage environment. Children may have been forbidden to point or ask for things, forbidden to explore, and never engaged or taught peek-a-boo or pretend play. Some children may have sensory dysfunction that interferes with enjoyment of physical experiences (see Chapter 33).

Parents traveling to collect their child sometimes observe autistic-like behaviors. Care must be taken to distinguish these from the normal adaptive behaviors of a child removed from a familiar environment and placed in the care of well-meaning but frightening strangers. Withdrawal, lack of interactive communication, and lack of eye contact are typical responses of a child

> Randy, a 4-year-old from Romania, left the orphanage with his new parents a few hours after meeting them for the first time. The first week he spent with them in a hotel room in Bucharest, he repetitively lined up blocks for hours. He made poor eye contact, refused to offer affection, and made few vocalizations. Well-meaning relatives in the United States suggested to his worried parents that he might be autistic. Within a month, ritualistic behavior diminished significantly. Excellent social and cognitive skills emerged, and Randy became a source of delight to his family.

in the first hours or days after placement. Lack of response to the child's name sometimes results from (unintentional) mispronunciation by the parents, unfamiliarity with the new name, or an undiagnosed hearing problem. Many parents describe their child as "shut down," or "completely passive and withdrawn" during the first hours and days after placement. Observation over time is perhaps the best means to differentiate these adjustment behaviors from the more serious conditions "acquired institutional autism" and "true autism." The Checklist for Autism in Toddlers[77,78] and the Diagnostic and Statistical Manual of Mental Disorders criteria for autism/pervasive developmental delay[79] (see Appendix 30–1) are useful tools to highlight problem areas, but may not be accurate in the early days after placement (see also the Web site for the Autism Society of America[80]).

After adoption. Some children continue to display autistic-like behaviors for a considerable period of time after adoption. These children have significant impairment of social and communication skills, but in contrast to typical autism, this "quasi-autism" (or acquired institutional autism) tends to improve to some extent by age 6 years.[81] Furthermore, although some children have severe mental impairment at arrival, many have dramatic improvement in IQ (~20 points) in the first several years after adoption. In contrast to typical autism, these children usually have

Gustavo, a 12-month-old from Guatemala, had been in foster care prior to adoption. When his family received him, they were disturbed to note that he didn't make eye contact. He seemed happiest in his crib facing a wall, where he would roll from side to side for hours if left alone. He screamed when picked up and didn't seem to "mold" to his parents' embraces. If they provided direct eye contact, he'd scream, or roll his eyes. His only interaction with toys was to throw or bang them. His parents gently and quietly continued to provide contact and staged stimulation, and to respond to his slightest overtures with extravagant praise. Three months after arrival, he started to show some eye contact and would laugh if they made silly faces. One year later, although severely language delayed, he would engage in interactive play with his parents and 5-year-old cousin, had good eye contact with his parents and strangers, and used gestures frequently (pointing, pulling mom by the hand). His parents felt that he was continuing to show many signs of progress in social skills.

(or achieve) a normal head circumference, and unlike the male preponderance in typical autism, boys and girls are affected equally.

Aggression

In the orphanage. Some children may display aggressive, violent behaviors when first encountered in the orphanage. In poorly supervised environments, normal childhood aggression may not be controlled. Some children may hit, bite, scratch, and push as a matter of course in order to have access to food, water, toys, and caregivers. In some situations, extreme corporal punishment may be used.

After adoption. Aggression appears after adoption for several reasons. In some children, violent behavior has been a way of life, and no other ways to interact or solve problems have ever been explored. In other children, fear provokes aggressive acts. The child may not understand the realities of adoption (leaving

behind friends, caregivers, all that is familiar) for a complete change in environment, culture, and language. Others may fear that they have now been removed beyond the reach of birth family, and that misbehavior is necessary so that they can return "home." For some children from abusive backgrounds, placement in an adoptive family creates anxiety that the abuse will recur, whereas in the orphanage, some sense of safety was garnered from the presence of the other children. Inability to communicate, fright, fantasy, and poor preparation for adoption may all contribute to aggressive behaviors. Severe aggression may signal reactive attachment disorder (see Chapter 29).

Mental Health of Adult Adoptees

What is the long-term mental health outcome of adopted children as adults? Psychiatric theory indicates that developmental, genetic, and loss issues may predispose adult adoptees to poor psychological adjustment.[82] Despite these prevalent theories, surprisingly little research has been reported. Indeed, in contrast to the data suggesting an overrepresentation of child adoptees receiving mental health services, several studies suggest adult adoptees may be underrepresented in the mental health clinical population.[5,7] Among 716 adult adoptees recruited from various sources (most from adoptee-based Internet sites), anger, symptom, and depression scores were above-normal ranges, but below levels typical of out-patient mental health populations. Adults who had never searched for birth relatives reported the least maladjustment, compared to those who had actively searched or been reunited[82] (see Chapter 34). In a psychiatric epidemiologic survey in New Zealand,[53] 24 adult adoptees were compared with 1212 individuals raised by their birth families. Psychiatric conditions were more common among the adoptees (drug abuse or dependence, conduct disorder, antisocial personality disorder in males, major depression, alcohol abuse or dependence, or conduct disorder in females). However, adults raised by biological relatives after disruption of their birth families had similar or even higher incidence of alcohol abuse and conduct disorder. Separation of the child from both parents for more than 1 month prior to age 15 years appeared as a distinct risk factor. Thus, family disruption and separation from parents rather than adoption itself appeared to contribute to poor outcome.[6] Similarly, a cohort of 2215 adoptees in Sweden were tracked as adults. "Reactive neurotic depression" was more common in children placed between 6 and 12 months of age; otherwise no relation was detected between early life experiences and psychiatric and social outcomes.[83]

In the only large outcome study of adult internationally adopted children to date,[84] the mental health and social adjustment of 11,320 adult adoptees in Sweden was compared to that of the general population, their Swedish-born siblings, and age-matched immigrants. Death from suicide, attempted suicide, admission for psychiatric disorder, drug abuse, alcohol abuse, and criminal behavior were all more common among the intercountry adoptees (odds ratios 3.6, 3.6, 3.2, 5.2, 2.6, and 1.6, respectively). Siblings in adoptive homes had lower odds ratios for most outcomes than did adoptees, whereas adoptees and immigrant children had similar odds ratios. The authors concluded that adoptees in Sweden have a high risk for severe mental health problems and social maladjustment in adolescence and young adulthood. They speculate that difficulty integrating into a physically homogeneous society and early attitudes and secrecy about adoption may have contributed to problems for some of the children. Notably, however, 92% of the girls and 85% of the boys had no mental health or social adjustment difficulties.

Similar comprehensive studies from the United States are awaited with interest.

The R family accepted a referral of two beautiful sisters from Russia, age 3 and 5. After months of waiting (and decorating rooms, buying clothes, and showing off the girls' pictures), they were told to travel to receive their children. When they arrived, they were stunned to learn that the girls had been adopted by a Russian family the week before. Their adoption agency encouraged them to look at some other children, rather than return home "empty-handed." They were shown two unrelated boys, ages 4 and 6 years, whom they decided to adopt. A few days after their return to the United States, "all hell broke loose." The elder boy, Thomas, screamed incessantly, destroyed furniture, scratched and bit the younger child and his parents, and shouted that he wanted to return to Russia. He threw his food, smashed plates, defecated in the living room, peeled wallpaper off the walls, and could not be controlled. He would often waken in a fugue state: unaware of his surroundings, disoriented, confused, and frightened. Desperate, his parents arranged a psychiatric emergency admission for Thomas. A Russian-speaking therapist elicited a convincing history of horrific physical and sexual abuse, both in the orphanage and with his birth family. After trials of several different medications, Risperidone was given. Thomas calmed down considerably and entered kindergarten, where he performed well. Temper tantrums at home gradually decreased in frequency and intensity. Seven months after adoption, the family was able to take an enjoyable holiday trip to the beach.

Key Points for Internationally Adopted Children

- Genetic susceptibility contributes to mental disorders in adopted children.
- Unstable adoptive environment increases the likelihood of expression of mental disorders.
- Adoptees generally have more behavioral and mental health disorders during childhood and adolescence than non-adopted peers.
- Symptoms of mental health disorders are common at adoption and immediately thereafter as children adjust; many of these symptoms are transient.
- Mental health disorders are more common in adopted adults, but most individuals have good mental and social adjustment.

Appendix 30–1 Checklists for autism and pervasive developmental disorders

Checklist for Autism in Toddlers (CHAT)—18 Months[77,78]

Section A: Ask Parent

1. Does your child enjoy being swung, bounced on your knee, etc.?
2. Does your child take an interest in other children?
3. Does your child like climbing on things, such as up stairs?
4. Does your child enjoy playing peek-a-boo or hide-and-seek?
5. Does your child ever *pretend*, for example, to make a cup of tea using a toy cup and teapot, or pretend other things?
6. Does your child ever use his or her index finger to point, to *ask* for something?
7. Does your child ever use his or her index finger to point, to indicate *interest* in something?
8. Can your child play properly with small toys (e.g., cars or bricks) without just mouthing, fiddling with, or dropping them?
9. Does your child ever bring objects over to you (parent) to *show* you something?

Section B: Observation

i.   During the appointment, has the child made eye contact with you?
ii. Get child's attention, then point across the room at an interesting object and say, "Oh look! There's a (name of toy!)." Watch child's face. Does the child look across to see what you are pointing at?
iii. Get the child's attention, then give child a miniature toy cup and teapot and say, "Can you make a cup of tea?". Does the child pretend to pour out tea, drink it, etc.?
iv. Say to the child, "Where's the light?" or "Show me the light." Does the child *point* with the index finger at the light?
v.   Can the child build a tower of bricks? (If so how many?) (Number of bricks:_____)

Scoring: Five key items: A5 (pretend play), A7 (protodeclarative pointing), Bii (following a point), Biii (pretending), and Biv (producing a point). If a child fails all five key items, they have a high risk of developing autism. Children who fail items A7 and Biv have a medium risk of developing autism.

Pervasive Developmental Disorders; Autistic Disorder[79]

A. A total of six (or more) items from (1), (2), and (3), with at least two from (1), and one each from (2) and (3):

1. Qualitative impairment in social interaction, as manifested by at least two of the following:
   a. Marked impairment in the use of multiple nonverbal behaviors such as eye-to-eye gaze, facial expression, body postures, and gestures to regulate social interaction
   b. Failure to develop peer relationships appropriate to developmental level
   c. Lack of spontaneous seeking to share enjoyment, interests, or achievements with other people (e.g., by a lack of showing, bringing, or pointing out objects of interest)
   d. Lack of social or emotional reciprocity

2. Qualitative impairments in communication as manifested by at least one of the following:
   a. Delay in, or total lack of, the development of spoken language (not accompanied by an attempt to compensate through alternative modes of communication such as gestures or mime)
   b. In individuals with adequate speech, marked impairment in the ability to initiate or sustain a conversation with others
   c. Stereotyped and repetitive use of language or idiosyncratic language
   d. Lack of varied, spontaneous make-believe play or social imitative play appropriate to developmental level

3. Restricted repetitive and stereotyped patterns of behavior, interests, and activities, as manifested by at least one of the following:
   a. Encompassing preoccupation with one or more stereotyped patterns of interest that is abnormal either in intensity or focus
   b. Apparently inflexible adherence to specific, nonfunctional routines or rituals
   c. Stereotyped and repetitive motor mannerisms (e.g., hand or finger flapping or twisting, or complex whole-body movements)
   d. Persistent preoccupation with parts of objects

B. Delays or abnormal functioning in at least one of the following areas, with onset prior to age 3 years: *(1)* social interaction, *(2)* language as used in social communication, or *(3)* symbolic or imaginative play.

C. The disturbance is not better accounted for by Rett's or childhood disintegrative disorder.

Source for Pervasive Developmental Disorders: Reprinted with permission from the *Diagnostic and Statistical Manual of Mental Disorders, 4th edition, Text Revision.* Washington, DC: American Psychiatric Association, 2000.

References

1. Schechter MD. Observations on adopted children. Arch Gen Psychiatry 1960; 3:21–32.

2. Kirk D, Jonassohn K, Fish AD. Are adopted children especially vulnerable to stress? A critique of some recent assertions. Arch Gen Psychiatry 1966; 14:291–8.

3. Kim WJ, Davenport C, Joseph J, Zrull J, Woolford E. Psychiatric disorder and juvenile delinquency in adopted children and adolescents. J Am Acad Child Adolesc Psychiatry 1988; 27:111–5.

4. Offord DR, Aponte JF, Cross LA. Presenting symptomatology of adopted children. Arch Gen Psychiatry 1969; 20:110–6.

5. Rogeness GA, Hoppe SK, Macedo CA, Fischer C, Harris WR. Psychopathology in hospitalized, adopted children. J Am Acad Child Adolesc Psychiatry 1988; 27:628–31.

6. Dickson LR, Heffron WM, Parker C. Children from disrupted and adoptive homes on an inpatient unit. Am J Orthopsychiatry 1990; 60:594–602.

7. Brinich PM, Brinich EB. Adoption and adaptation. J Nerv Ment Dis 1982; 170:489–93.

8. Folstein S. Twin and adoption studies in child and adolescent psychiatric disorders. Curr Opin Pediatr 1996; 8:339–47.

9. Lombroso PJ, Pauls DL, Leckman JF. Genetic mechanisms in childhood psychiatric disorders. J Am Acad Child Adolesc Psychiatry 1994; 33:921–38.

10. Feng J, Zheng J, Gelernter J, et al. An in-frame deletion in the alpha(2C) adrenergic receptor is common in African Americans. Mol Psychiatry 2001; 6:168–72.

11. Vincent JB, Kovacs M, Krol R, Barr CL, Kennedy JL. Intergenerational CAG repeat expansion at ERDA1 in a family with childhood-onset depression, schizoaffective disorder, and recurrent major depression. Am J Med Genet 1999; 88:79–82.

12. Rutter M. Implications of genetic research for child psychiatry. Can J Psychiatry 1997; 42:569–76.

13. Rutter M, Silberg J, O'Connor T, Simonoff E. Genetics and child psychiatry: I Advances in quantitative and molecular genetics. J Child Psychol Psychiatry 1999; 40:3–18.

14. Reiss D, Neiderhiser JM. The interplay of genetic influences and social processes in developmental theory: specific mechanisms are coming into view. Dev Psychopathol 2000; 12:357–74.

15. Gershon ES. Bipolar illness and schizophrenia as oligogenic diseases: implications for the future. Biol Psychiatry 2000; 47:240–4.

16. Clerget-Darpoux F, Goldin LR, Gershon ES. Clinical methods in psychiatric genetics. III. Environmental stratification may simulate a genetic effect in adoption studies. Acta Psychiatr Scand 1986; 74:305–11.

17. Kringlen E. Adoption studies in functional psychosis. Eur Arch Psychiatry Clin Neurosci 1991; 240: 307–13.

18. Tienari P, Sorri A, Lahti I, et al. Interaction of genetic and psychosocial factors in schizophrenia. Acta Psychiatr Scand Suppl 1985; 319:19–30.

19. Tienari P, Lahti I, Sorri A, et al. The Finnish adoptive family study of schizophrenia. J Psychiatr Res 1987; 21:437–45.

20. Tienari P, Wynne LC, Moring J, et al. Finnish adoptive family study: sample selection and adoptee DSM-III-R diagnoses. Acta Psychiatr Scand 2000; 101:433–43.

21. Tienari P. Interaction between genetic vulnerability and family environment: the Finnish adoptive family study of schizophrenia. Acta Psychiatr Scand 1991; 84:460–5.

22. Tienari P, Sorri A, Lahti I, et al. Genetic and psychosocial factors in schizophrenia: the Finnish Adoptive Family Study. Schizophr Bull 1987; 13:477–84.

23. Tienari P, Sorri A, Lahti I, et al. The Finnish adoptive family study of schizophrenia. Yale J Biol Med 1985; 58:227–37.

24. Wahlberg KE, Wynne LC, Oja H, et al. Thought disorder index of Finnish adoptees and communication deviance of their adoptive parents. Psychol Med 2000; 30:127–36.

25. Kety SS. Schizophrenic illness in the families of schizophrenic adoptees: findings from the Danish national sample. Schizophr Bull 1988; 14:217–22.

26. Tienari PJ, Wynne LC. Adoption studies of schizophrenia. Ann Med 1994; 26:233–7.

27. Kendler KS, Gruenberg AM. An independent analysis of the Danish Adoption Study of Schizophrenia. VI. The relationship between psychiatric disorders as defined by DSM-III in the relatives and adoptees. Arch Gen Psychiatry 1984; 41:555–64.

28. Kendler KS, Gruenberg AM, Kinney DK. Independent diagnoses of adoptees and relatives as defined by DSM-III in the provincial and national samples of the Danish Adoption Study of Schizophrenia. Arch Gen Psychiatry 1994; 51:456–68.

29. Sullivan PF, Neale MC, Kendler KS. Genetic epidemiology of major depression: review and meta-analysis. Am J Psychiatry 2000; 157:1552–62.

30. Kovacs M, Devlin B, Pollock M, Richards C, Mukerji P. A controlled family history study of childhood-onset depressive disorder. Arch Gen Psychiatry 1997; 54:613–23.

31. Kovacs M, Gatsonis C, Paulauskas SL, Richards C. Depressive disorders in childhood. IV. A longitudinal study of comorbidity with and risk for anxiety disorders. Arch Gen Psychiatry 1989; 46:776–82.

32. Wender PH, Kety SS, Rosenthal D, Schulsinger F, Ortmann J, Lunde I. Psychiatric disorders in the biologic and adoptive families of adopted individuals with affective disorders. Arch Gen Psychiatry 1986; 43:923–29.

33. Cadoret RJ. Evidence for genetic inheritance of primary affective disorder in adoptees. Am J Psychiatry 1978; 135:463–6.

34. Wickramaratne PJ, Warner V, Weissman MM. Selecting early onset MDD probands for genetic studies: results from a longitudinal high-risk study. Am J Med Genet 2000; 96:93–101.

35. Thapar A, McGuffin P. A twin study of depressive symptoms in childhood. Br J Psychiatry 1994; 165:259–65.

36. Todd RD, Botteron KN. Family, genetic, and imaging studies of early-onset depression. Child Adolesc Psychiatry Clin North Am 2001; 10:375–90.

37. Nolan CL, Moore GJ, Madden R, et al. Prefrontal cortical volume in childhood-onset major depression: preliminary findings. Arch Gen Psychiatry 2002; 59:173–9.

38. O'Connor MJ, Kasari C. Prenatal alcohol exposure and depressive features in children. Alcohol Clin Exp Res 2000; 24:1084–92.

39. Hallstrom T. Major depression, parental mental disorder and early family relationships. Acta Psychiatr Scand 1987; 75:259–63.

40. Heim C, Newport DJ, Bonsall R, Miller AH, Nemeroff CB. Altered pituitary-adrenal axis responses to provocative challenge tests in adult survivors of childhood abuse. Am J Psychiatry 2001; 158:575–81.

41. DeLong R. Children with autistic spectrum disorder and a family history of affective disorder. Dev Med Child Neurol 1994; 36:674–87.

42. Wozniak J, Biederman J, Faraone SV, Blier H, Monuteaux MC. Heterogeneity of childhood conduct disorder: further evidence of a subtype of conduct disorder linked to bipolar disorder. J Affect Disord 2001; 64:121–31.

43. Cadoret RJ, Cain C. Sex differences in predictors of antisocial behavior in adoptees. Arch Gen Psychiatry 1980; 37:1171–75.

44. Crowe RR. An adoption study of antisocial personality. Arch Gen Psychiatry 1974; 31:785–91.

45. Cunningham L, Cadoret RJ, Loftus R, Edwards JE. Studies of adoptees from psychiatrically disturbed biological parents: psychiatric conditions in childhood and adolescence. Br J Psychiatry 1975; 126.

46. Cadoret RJ, Yates WR, Troughton E, Woodworth G, Stewart MA. Adoption study demonstrating two genetic pathways to drug abuse. Arch Gen Psychiatry 1995; 52:42–52.

47. van der Valk JC, Verhulst FC, Neale MC, Boomsma DI. Longitudinal genetic analysis of problem behaviors in biologically related and unrelated adoptees. Behav Genet 1998; 28:365–80.

48. Langbehn DR, Cadoret RJ. The adult antisocial syndrome with and without antecedent conduct disorder: comparisons from an adoption study. Compr Psychiatry 2001; 42:272–82.

49. Langbehn DR, Cadoret RJ, Yates WR, Troughton EP, Stewart MA. Distinct contributions of conduct and oppositional defiant symptoms to adult antisocial behavior: evidence from an adoption study. Arch Gen Psychiatry 1998; 55:821–9.

50. Bohman M. Some genetic aspects of alcoholism and criminality. A population of adoptees. Arch Gen Psychiatry 1978; 35:269–76.

51. Fisher L, Ames EW, Chisholm K, Savoie L. Problems reported by parents of Romanian children adopted to British Columbia. Int J Behav Dev 1997; 20:67–82.

52. Marcovitch S, Goldberg S, Gold A, et al. Determinants of behavioural problems in Romanian children adopted in Ontario. Int J Behav Dev 1997; 20:17–31.

53. Sullivan PF, Wells JE, Bushnell JA. Adoption as a risk factor for mental disorders. Acta Psychiatr Scand 1995; 92:119–24.

54. Pavao JM. The Family of Adoption. Boston: Beacon Press, 1998.

55. Nickman SL, Lewis RG. Adoptive families and professionals: when the experts make things worse. J Am Acad Child Adolesc Psychiatry 1994; 33:753–55.

56. Sharma AR, McGue MK, Benson PL. The psychological adjustment of United States adopted adolescents and their nonadopted siblings. Child Dev 1998; 69:791–802.

57. Bower B. Adapting to adoption: adopted kids generate scientific optimism and clinical caution. Sci News 1994; 146:104–7.

58. Lipman EL, Offord DR, Racine YA, Boyle MH. Psychiatric disorders in adopted children: a profile from the Ontario Child Health Study. Can J Psychiatry 1992; 37:627–33.

59. Lipman EL, Offord DR, Boyle MH, Racine YA. Follow-up of psychiatric and educational morbidity among adopted children. J Am Acad Child Adolesc Psychiatry 1993; 32:1007–12.

60. Miller BC, Fan X, Grotevant HD, Christensen M, Coyl D, van Dulmen M. Adopted adolescents' overrepresentation in mental health counseling: adoptees' problems or parents' lower threshold for referral? J Am Acad Child Adolesc Psychiatry 2000; 39:1504–11.

61. Schechter MD, Holter FR. Adopted children in their adoptive families. Pediatr Clin North Am 1975; 22:663–61.

62. Schwartz EM. Problems after adoption: some guidelines for pediatrician involvement. J Pediatr 1975; 87:991–4.

63. Verhulst FC, Althaus M, Versluis-den Bieman HJ. Problem behavior in international adoptees: I. An epidemiological study. J Am Acad Child Adolesc Psychiatry 1990; 29:94–103.

64. Seglow J, Kellmer Pringle M, Wedge P. Growing up Adopted. Windsor, England: National Foundation for Educational Research in England and Wales, 1972.

65. Brodzinsky DM, Schechter DE, Braff AM, Singer LM. Psychological and academic adjustment in adopted children. J Consult Clin Psychol 1984; 52:582–90.

66. Cadoret RJ, Cunningham L, Loftus R, Edwards J. Studies of adoptees from psychiatrically disturbed biological parents. III. Medical symptoms and illnesses in childhood and adolescence. Am J Psychiatry 1976; 133:1316–8.

67. Slap G, Goodman E, Huang B. Adoption as a risk factor for attempted suicide during adolescence. Pediatrics 2001; 108:E30.

68. Stams GJ, Juffer R, Rispens J, Hoksbergen RA. The development and adjustment of 7-year-old children adopted in infancy. J Child Psychol Psychiatry 2000; 41:1025–37.

68a. Van den Oord EJCG, Moomsam DI, Verhulst FC. A study of problem behaviors in 10- to 15-year-old biologically related and unrelated international adoptees. Behav Genetics 1994; 24:193–205.

69. Verhulst FC, Versluis-den Bieman H, van der Ende J, Berden GF, Sanders-Woudstra JA. Problem behavior in international adoptees: III. Diagnosis of child psychiatric disorders. J Am Acad Child Adolesc Psychiatry 1990; 29:420–8.

70. Verhulst FC, Althaus M, Versluis-den Bieman HJ. Problem behavior in international adoptees: II. Age at placement. J Am Acad Child Adolesc Psychiatry 1990; 29:104–11.

71. Versluis-den Bieman HJ, Verhulst FC. Self-reported and parent reported problems in adolescent international adoptees. J Child Psychol Psychiatry 1995; 36:1411–28.

72. Berg-Kelly K, Eriksson J. Adaptation of adopted foreign children at mid-adolescence as indicated by aspects of health and risk-taking. Eur Child Adolesc Psychiatry 1997; 6:199–206.

72a. Goldney RD, Donald M, Sawyer MG, et al. Emotional health of Indonesian adoptees living in Australian families. Aust N Zealand J Psych 1996; 30:534–9.

73. Shaginian N. The Influence of Psychological and Social Factors on Pregnancy and Abandoned Newborns. Washington, DC: Joint Council for International Children's Services, 2002.

74. Bowlby J. Separation, Vol. II. New York: Basic Books, 1973.

75. Spitz RA. The First Year of Life. New York: International Universities Press, Inc., 1965.

76. Pine DS, Goldstein RB, Wolk S, Weissman MM. The association between childhood depression and adulthood body mass index. Pediatrics 2001; 107:1049–56.

77. Robins DL, Fein D, Barton ML, Green JA. The Modified Checklist for Autism in Toddlers: an initial study investigating the early detection of autism and pervasive developmental disorders. J Autism Dev Disord 2001; 31:131–44.

78. Baron-Cohen S, Allen J, Gillberg C. Can autism be detected at 18 months? The needle, the haystack, and the CHAT. Br J Psychiatry 1992; 161:839–43.

79. American Psychiatric Association. Diagnostic and Statistical Manual of Mental Disorders (DSM-IV). Washington, DC: American Psychiatric Association, 1994.

80. Autism Society of America. Available at: http://www.autism-society.org.

81. Rutter M, Andersen-Wood L, Beckett C, et al. Quasi-autistic patterns following severe global deprivation. J Child Psychol Psychiatry 1999; 40:537–49.

82. Cubito DS, Brandon KO. Psychological adjustment in adult adoptees: assessment of distress, depression, and anger. Am J Orthopsychiatry 2000; 70:408–13.

83. von Knorring AL, Cloninger CR, Bohman M, Sigvardsson S. An adoption study of depressive disorders and substance abuse. Arch Gen Psychiatry 1983; 40:943–50.

84. Hjern A, Lindblad F, Vinnerljung B. Suicide, psychiatric illness, and social maladjustment in intercountry adoptees in Sweden: a cohort study. Lancet 2002; 360:443–8.

31

LANGUAGE COMPETENCE

Many newly arrived international adoptees have delayed speech in their primary languages (Table 31–1) (see Chapter 13). These delays may not be obvious after immersion in a new language milieu. Inexperienced parents may overlook the important delays in pre-speech development common among young children. Published studies also likely underestimate the prevalence of language delays.

Language acquisition and mastery are key factors for acceptance in a new country. Fluency is linked to learning, as well as cognitive, social and emotional development,[1] adjustment, and outcome.

Although some children catch up quickly and develop English fluency in a surprisingly short time, others struggle to acquire adequate communication skills. No comprehensive surveys have yet described the sequence and timing of acquisition of language competence in this complex group of children. Lessons about re-

covery after delayed language acquisition may be gleaned from other populations of children, such as those with hearing impairment (including persistent otitis media/effusion), deaf parents (lack of verbal inputs), neglect (adverse environmental influences), English as a second language (need to learn new language), and "late talking" (isolated delays in expressive language). Most of these children eventually recover from early language delays (with some notable exceptions), although subtle language processing deficits persist in some. Internationally adopted children differ from these other groups of children in several important ways. The linguistic experiences of international adoptees are unique. A typical child in an orphanage experiences multiple pre- and postnatal risk factors for language delays (Table 31–2) and a paucity of language input during institutionalization, followed by placement in an enriched family environment in which a new language is used.

Table 31–1 Prevalence of language delays in internationally adopted children

Country of Origin (N)	Adoptees with Language Delays[a] (%)
Russia and Eastern Europe (105)[2]	56
Russia and Eastern Europe (56)[3]	59
Various countries (129)[4]	18
Romania (46)[5]	57 (100% when parents first met child in orphanage)
Romania (22)[6]	Mean developmental quotient for language was 79[b]
China (192)[7]	43

[a]Different methods were used to test language competence and to define delay.
[b]% delayed not specified.

In this chapter, the factors contributing to language delays in internationally adopted children will be reviewed, along with recommendations for assessment and remediation. The associated problem of auditory processing disorder is also reviewed.

Reasons for Language Delays in Internationally Adopted Children

Many factors contribute to language delays in post-institutionalized children (Table 31–2).

For the individual child, many of these elements are unknown; complete information about pre-adoptive circumstances is rarely available. In addition to possible prenatal exposures, paucity of language exposure in the institutional environment undoubtably is the major cause of poor language development. In contrast to a home, where children are encouraged and rewarded for their vocalizations, institutionalized children receive few or inconsistent responses to their efforts. A family child's needs, wants, and relationships to other family members are paramount, while the orphanage child is a passive

Table 31–2 Possible factors in language delays in post-institutionalized children

Family history
Prematurity
Prenatal exposures (see Chapters 5–7)
   Alcohol
   Drugs
   Tobacco[8]
   Others
Prenatal infections
   Syphilis
   Cytomegalovirus
   Rubella
   HIV (language delay may be the presenting sign of HIV encephalopathy)
Postnatal drug exposures
Lead
Paucity of language exposure in institutional environment
Recurrent otitis media with effusion, perhaps undiagnosed or untreated
Other hearing impairment
Possible cortical damage from auditory deprivation
Auditory hypersensitivity and inattention (possibly due to diminished auditory exposures during early life)
Global developmental delays
Environmental toxins
Deprived oral sensorimotor experiences and delayed oral-motor function (see Chapter 9)
Other

Nap-time is over. Of the 12 toddlers, all about 18 months old, 7 are awake. One is crying softly, one is cooing quietly to himself, and the rest wait silently in their cribs. They know that they must be quiet until the lights are turned back on and they are back in their playroom. The nanny starts at one end of the room, and picks each child up and puts him in a chair at a low table in the playroom. One by one, the children are moved from their cribs to their chairs. Sitting in their chairs, some begin to vocalize and hum. When all are seated, a plate of food appears before each child, and the caregiver and her assistant circulate around the room assisting the few children who cannot feed themselves. The room is perfectly quiet as the children eat, except for the scattered conversation between the caregivers about their weekend plans. After the children finish their food, the plates are wisked away. Each child is carried to his potty chair, and all sit on their potties for 30 minutes while the food is cleared away. Afterward, the children are permitted to get up, and those who "produced" get a word of praise; those who didn't, stay on their potty chairs for another 30 minutes or so. As each child finishes, he wanders over to the play area. Most simply wander aimlessly, a few grab toys and bang or throw them. The caregivers, who are still cleaning the potty chairs, sorting laundry, and washing dishes, usually intervene when a child falls down, cries, or hurts another child. Occasionally, the caregiver speaks directly to the child: "Don't do that!" or "What are you trying to do?" After 2 hours, the children are brought back to their cribs for another rest. Not one word is spoken directly to the children as individuals during the morning, except for Alexei, who was told "Stop that!" when he hit Anton.

Beth, 18 months old, wakens from her nap and after stretching a minute, calls out "Mama, Mama!" Her mother, listening on the baby monitor, comes up to Beth's room. "Hello, sweetie, did you have a nice nap?" Beth, all smiles and giggles, snuggles into her mother's arms and says "Mama, play!" This is her signal for her mother to make funny noises into Beth's neck. Beth laughs and tries to imitate the raspberries, clicks, and other funny sounds that her mom makes. Every sound Beth makes, Mom makes back. The doorbell rings. "Who do you think it is, Beth?" asks Mom. "Dada" says Beth. "No, Beth, Daddy has a key—he doesn't ring the doorbell. Should we go see who it is?" "Yes, go," says Beth. When they get to the door, they see a package has been left. "Wow, a package," says Mom. "What do you think is inside?" "Cookies," says Beth joyfully. "Open, Mama." "Looks like it is a surprise from Grandma," says Mom. "Surprise, surprise," says Beth, a new word for her that day. Later when Dad comes home, Beth runs to him and says "Surprise!" Daddy scoops her up and praises her for her new big word.

recipient of the rote daily schedule, routine, and activities. Institutional life elicits little need to vocalize: the daily schedule unfolds as a matter of course, without regard to individual responses or needs. Thus, the functions of early language and preverbal communication (Table 31–3) are ineffectual to motivate speech development in the orphanage child. Not surprisingly, a survey conducted by Russian educators and psychologists found that only 14% of 2-year-olds residing in Moscow orphanages spoke in two-word phrases.[9]

Aspects of Language Development

Oral-Motor Function

The stages of normal language development are familiar to the pediatrician. Assessment of oral-motor function is not as familiar a task. Correct oral-motor function is a necessary foundation for speech and language development. Delayed oral-motor milestones, sometimes complicated by oral hypersensitivity (see Chap-

Table 31–3 Early functions of language

Type of Function	Function
Instrumental	To satisfy child's needs or wants (I want, I need)
Regulatory	To order behavior of others (Stop!)
Interactional	To establish and maintain contact with others (you and me)
Personal	To establish awareness of self (Here I am)
Heuristic	To seek information (Why?)
Imaginative	To play act (Let's pretend)
Informative	To give information or share knowledge about an event (Let me tell you something)

Source: Data from Kusko.[10]

ter 33), also contribute to language delays in orphanage residents. Children who miss the opportunities to develop orofacial muscle tone and dexterity by exposure to various food textures often have associated expressive language and pre-speech delays (see Chapter 9). Orphanage feeding practices limit the opportunity to suck (bottle propping, large holes cut in nipples to speed feeding) (Fig. 31–1) and chew (diet limited to pureed foods and liquids), resulting in hypotonicity and decreased sensory awareness of orofacial muscles (Fig. 31–2). Excessive drooling, delayed dentition, and limited experience mouthing toys are also frequent among institutionalized children and may interfere with proper speech mechanics. Speech and occupational therapists and multidisciplinary feeding teams can assist with diagnosis and treatment of these problems.

Receptive Language

Receptive language precedes expressive language. Assessment of receptive language usually relies on observation of behavioral responses, which may be difficult in the office setting. New parents may not yet be comfortable with or completely familiar with their child's responses. Assessing the child's receptive skills in a new language shortly after arrival does not provide

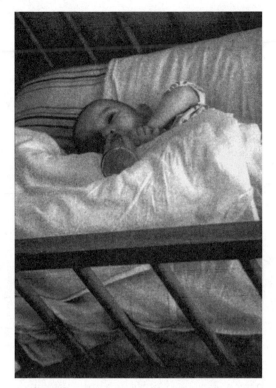

Figure 31–1 *Bottle propping is a common method of feeding in orphanages.*

accurate information about true abilities or potential. An interpreter may assist, although some children react negatively to hearing their birth language after the adoption (see Chapter 9).

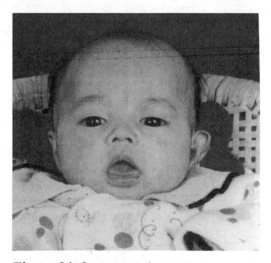

Figure 31–2 *Hypotonic facies with open mouth in Chinese adoptee. (With permission.)*

Moreover, the child must be able to attend to the directed task. Because most evaluation tools for language skills in young children are relatively simplistic, some youngsters with normal receptive language scores later present with complex problems in expressive language, auditory processing, or auditory memory.

Expressive Language

Expressive language may be assessed more objectively. Pre-speech vocalizations transition from cooing (usually long drawn-out vowel sounds emitted during pleasure) to babbling with consonants between 4 and 6 months of age. Babbling has been described as "soundplay for its own sake."[10] Jabbering or jargoning follow, with the production of the first word at about 12 months of age. By 18 months of age, the child typically has a vocabulary of 50 words, not all of which are readily understandable by strangers. After a vocabulary of 50–75 words is acquired, there is a sudden rapid acceleration in language production, with 4–6 new words each day and combining words into phrases. Two- to three-word phrases suggest a language ability of at least 24 months. Expressive language delays should be differentiated from disorders of articulation or oral-motor planning (dyspraxia).[11] Identification of expressive language delays in older children is complicated by the need to learn a new language. Children usually lose expressive ability in their primary language within the first few months after arrival in the United States.[2]

Language and Hearing Assessments

Accurate assessment of language abilities in an internationally adopted child is best accomplished in the child's birth country prior to departure. Parents should procure any available information about speech and language assessments that have been done on their child. Most regions in Russia and Kazakhstan mandate regular assessments of orphanage residents by staff speech therapists (logopedists). If no formal evaluations have been performed, it is desirable for parents to obtain as much explicit information as possible from their child's caregivers. Assistance of a skilled translator is invaluable. At a minimum, a translator should assist the parents in determining the child's basic language skills before the child is removed from her familiar environment and caregivers. Such information is highly useful after adoption to determine the degree of primary language delay and as a baseline to measure progress.

After arrival in the United States, children should undergo a complete developmental assessment (see Chapter 13). Language should be assessed along with other developmental and sensory processing domains. Multiple screening tools are available to assess language in young children; most pediatricians rely on the Denver Developmental Screening Test. However, this tool will not identify subtle difficulties, especially in the first 18 months of life. The Mullen Scales of Early Learning[12] is one example of an easy-to-administer, reliable, informative language assessment tool for children from birth to 72 months. General language and articulation milestones from birth to age 5 years are listed in Appendix 31–1.

Language assessment should be performed shortly after arrival in the United States, especially if no assessment from the birth country is available. A qualified bilingual language specialist is best able to provide accurate information. If such a person is not available, the examiner should be assisted by a qualified interpreter. Surprisingly often, international adoptees (especially those under 5 years of age) become frightened and tearful when hearing their birth language some days or weeks after adoption. In these cases, it is best to proceed in English and monitor closely.

A formal hearing assessment should be obtained in all new arrivals, and is particularly urgent in any child with severe language delays (Table 31–4). Children may respond to a clap, bell, squeak toy, or their names, but still lack adequate reception of normal speaking tones.[11] Hearing must be within 30 dB of normal throughout the frequency range of 500–40000

Table 31–4 Risks for hearing loss

Neonatal intensive care >48 hours

Genetic syndromes

Family history

Any visible abnormality of the head or face, including
    even mild deformity of ear

History of congenital infection: rubella, herpes,
    toxoplasmosis, cytomegalovirus

Postnatal infection such as meningitis

Severe jaundice, oxygen administration, or ventilator

Head trauma

Repeated or chronic ear infection with fluid in middle
    ear for >3 months

Source: Reprinted with permission of Simon & Schuster Adult
    Publishing Group from *When the Brain Can't Hear:
    Unraveling the Mystery of Auditory Processing Disorder* by
    Teri James Bellis, Ph.D.. Copyright © 2002.

Hz. Even mild conductive or unilateral hearing loss may interfere with expressive language development.

Language cannot be assessed in isolation. A full developmental assessment is necessary to determine if language delays are isolated or part of global developmental delays. While international adoptees often have global delays, disproportionate language delays should be carefully monitored. Assumptions that the delay is due to the need to learn a new language should be frequently reassessed. Children who are persistent toe-walkers may be at higher risk for ongoing language delays.[14,15]

The Internationally Adopted Child with Language Delay

Children in a new language milieu quickly lose their birth language, making precise determination of language abilities difficult in the early weeks and months after adoption.[2] After arrival, most internationally adopted children have significant delays in both expressive and receptive language, not surprising for a child who has recently been removed from his or her birth language and expected to function in a new language. The speed with which most young children acquire good receptive English, however, is truly impressive. Clinical experience suggests that by 3–4 months after adoption, most children <36 months of age are within 6–9 months of age level for receptive language in English. Deficits greater than this should be carefully explored.[16] Good receptive language effectively rules out mental retardation, autism, severe auditory processing disorder, and significant hearing loss, even in the child with marked expressive language delays.[17] Communicative, meaningful gestures, response to commands, vocal imitation, and symbolic play all suggest good capacity for language processing. Many international adoptees quickly become excellent communicators, so much so that the "language façade dazzles."[1] However, decontextualized language is weaker; this usually becomes evident when language ability is challenged by school demands.

Many adoptees are between 2 and 3 years of age. This is a particularly ambiguous time to assess language competence, because about 10%–15% of normal children show substantial language delays during this period.[16] However, only ~4–5% remain delayed beyond 3 years of age. The challenge among international adoptees is to identify those at higher risk of protracted language delays who would benefit from Early Intervention and speech remediation.[18] Language researchers Glennen and Masters evaluated 130 children adopted from Eastern Europe by parent survey.[19] No relation was found between pre-adoption medical risk factors and eventual language development for most children, possibly reflecting incomplete or inaccurate pre-adoptive medical information. Not surprisingly, the time to development of English language milestones varied with the age of adoption. Most children adopted before 12 months of age developed English language milestones comparable to their English-speaking non-adopted peers. Children adopted at 13–18 months rapidly acquired expressive English language, with more than 16 English words within 3–5 months, and normal expressive language skills by 24 months (50 word vocabulary, 2-word phrases). Children adopted at 19–24 months had at least 50 English words and 2-word phrases by 28 months. Those adopted at

Alison arrived from China at 12 months, with no words in Mandarin and limited pre-speech vocalizations. Her single mom, a Spanish teacher, decided to speak only Spanish to her. She soon returned to work full-time. The loving nanny who was hired happened to be Russian, and spoke English poorly and with a heavy accent. Seven months later, Alison's expressive abilities in any language remained limited, although she had good Spanish and fair English receptive skills.

25–30 months had 79 words and 2-word phrases by 31 months. The investigators suggest that children who do not achieve these milestones should be considered language-delayed, and speech-language services should be provided.[19]

Older children usually arrive monolingual in their primary language, then become monolingual in English within several months.[2] Mastery of conversational English does not guarantee proficiency in more complex language functions, however.

Bilingualism

Many parents wonder if older adopted children with well-established fluency in their birth language can become bilingual. International adoptees only rarely reside with adoptive parents who are fluent in the child's birth language, the only situation in which true bilingualism is possible. Children raised from birth in a truly bilingual environment initially have slight delays in expressive language output in both languages; however, by age 3 years, children usually have age-appropriate expressive skills in both lan-

Alexa was adopted from Ukraine at age 4. She had moderate language delays in Russian. Her French-English bilingual family was eager for her to learn both new languages. However, because of her delays in her primary language, they spoke only English for the first year she was home. They then spent the summer in France, and all spoke French. She returned to the United States completely bilingual.

guages. It is only in such circumstances that the child may truly become bilingual. Under unusual circumstances, older children with well-established fluency in the birth language may add a second language (English) while maintaining the first language, if given the opportunity to practice and advance their first language. Some parents arrange this by enrolling the child in specialized language schools, hiring a fluent speaker of the birth language to spend time with the child as a sitter or "cultural big brother or sister," or arranging play dates with native speakers (see Chapter 34). Children must be exposed to fluent adults to advance their birth language skills. When older fluent siblings are adopted together, they often maintain their birth language as a "secret way" to communicate without the parents. Without exposure to more advanced speech, however, their language skills will not progress. Young children without well-established fluency in the primary language are unable to maintain it. But if they are continually exposed to two (new) languages in the home, these children may become truly bilingual.

Treatment

Little is known about the best ways to promote recovery from language delays in post-institutionalized children. Immersion in the family environment is vital. In contrast to the language-poor orphanage, the new environment is language-rich. The adoptive family uses language to communicate, to label everyday events, to express ideas and feelings, and to elicit verbal responses from the child.[17] Speech and language specialists and Early Intervention educators also help children recover from language delays. Some mistakenly ascribe language delays to the need to learn a new language, even in infants with clearly delayed or disordered pre-speech skills. Older children may be enrolled in English as a Second Language (ESL) programs in the school system. Although sometimes helpful, these programs are usually designed for children fluent in their first language who continue to speak it at home—definitely not the situation for most international adoptees. Participation in such groups may mask more subtle and pervasive difficulties with speech. Fortunately, most children acquire functional, age-appropriate language skills without specific therapies within 6–8 months after adoption. Those with more persistent delays and those with more profound delays at entry should definitely receive vigorous supportive services to identify specific language disorders and to promote language development. For example, rarities such as selective mutism sometimes occur.

Outcome

Language proficiency emerges in several stages. Virtually all internationally adopted children develop useful "communicative language fluency," or conversational English.[2,18,20] This level of language ability includes practical daily communication skills, using fundamental pronunciation, vocabulary, and grammar, and, in older children, elementary reading and writing. Communicative language fluency is context based. More advanced language skills are designated "cognitive language mastery," and are not necessarily achieved by all children with good conversational skills.[2] This higher function allows advanced cognitive and academic language use[2,18] and becomes increasingly important as children progress through school. In contrast to communicative language fluency, this level of language function is context-free (reading a text, writing an essay, discussing hypothetical situations). Some experts suggest that a 9-year-old child (fluent in her birth language) achieves communicative language fluency within 2 years after introduction to a new language, but that cognitive language mastery is not achieved for 5–7 years.[18] No studies have yet investigated the time required to achieve cognitive language mastery by internationally adopted children. Delays in this area may account for poor school performance in some children. Some children have difficulties with the verbal or written expression of thoughts and emotions.

Rebecca came back to the International Adoption Clinic after an absence of 3 years. She'd grown into a healthy, beautiful 4½-year-old. Her mother was concerned because Rebecca refused to talk outside of the home. By report, she chatted non-stop at home with her parents and sisters. She had mastered complex vocabulary and syntax and had good articulation. Her parents were mystified when the preschool teachers told them that Rebecca never spoke at school. She gladly nodded, gestured, and indicated wants, but never used her expressive language. She interacted minimally with the other children, but seemed content to do puzzles or color alone. Her mom described her as extremely anxious with any changes in routine, but there were no obsessive behaviors noted. Upon arrival from China at age 18 months, Rebecca had typical growth and developmental delays that seemed to recover quickly. A diagnosis of selective mutism was made, and cognitive/behavioral therapy begun.

Early Language Delays and Other School Problems

Is early language delay a risk factor for other neurocognitive deficits? Frustratingly little is known about the possible contributions of early language delays and development of later learning and reading disabilities. The applicability of the few studies in this area to internationally adopted children is limited. Compared to children living with birth families, international adoptees have different reasons for delayed language, and their language environment dramatically improves after adoption. Nonetheless, several studies suggest that early language delays may presage later learning disabilities.[11] In a follow-up study of 2- to 3-year-olds with isolated speech delay (defined as expressive vocabulary <10 words in the absence of other developmental problems or understimulating environment), nearly half the children had articulation problems 2–4 years later, although nearly all had appropriate language skills.[21] In another study, 40% of 63 preschoolers with language delays had persistent problems or other learning disorders when evaluated 4–5 years later.[22] Children with early language delays may be prone to reading problems, particularly if their language skills do not catch up.[23–25] Such problems may persist to adolescence and beyond.[26,27]

Auditory Processing Disorder

Some language delays result from auditory processing disorder (also known as central auditory processing disorder). *Auditory processing disorder* is a disability in handling auditory information in the absence of impaired peripheral hearing.[13] Auditory processing disorders are probably more common than hearing loss in contributing to language delay. Internationally adopted children may be at high risk for auditory processing disorders because of the complexities of their early life. Early auditory deprivation may result in permanent cortical changes.[28] Auditory perception is a complex process that involves focus, attention, tracking, sorting, scanning, comparing, retrieving, and sequencing. Defects in any of these areas may result in difficulties managing auditory information. Auditory processing disorders become more apparent when the sound signal is in any way degraded, i.e., by competing noise, distance, or muffled speech. Children with this disorder have reduced ability to discriminate, identify, or comprehend auditory stimuli in complex listening situations. Some children have difficulty attending to auditory information; others appear hypersensitive to sounds and are readily distracted by the hum of neon lights, airplanes flying overhead, or voices from the playground (see Chapter 33). Such children are unable to filter out these extraneous sounds from the voice of the teacher giving the homework assignment. Difficulty with multistep instructions and verbal directions are most characteristic of this problem. Children may be mistakenly labeled with behavioral problems, attention-deficit disorder, or cognitive delay (Table 31–5). The occasional child with auditory processing disorder exhibits extreme discomfort around loud sounds (sirens, firecrackers, thunder). Unless specific testing is done, such problems are overlooked as conventional

Table 31–5 Differential diagnosis of auditory processing disorder

Hearing impairment
Behavior problems
Attention deficit hyperactivity disorder
Autism
Neurocognitive delays (especially disordered executive function {memory and planning})
Nonverbal learning disability

Source: In part from Bellis.[13] Reprinted with permission of Simon & Schuster Adult Publishing Group from *When the Brain Can't Hear: Unraveling the Mystery of Auditory Processing Disorder* by Teri James Bellis, Ph.D.. Copyright © 2002.

hearing screens are normal. Auditory processing disorders may coexist with mild conductive or unilateral hearing loss.

In some children, auditory processing disorder is linked to nonverbal learning disability[13] (see Chapter 13). These children have difficulty understanding intent (e.g., tone of voice) rather than content. They have problems with nonverbal tasks (such as math calculation or visual–spatial problems) and allocation of attention. Because of their poor ability to appreciate sarcasm or humor, they may experience social difficulties or depression. These problems may reflect trauma to or inefficiency of the right brain hemisphere, or white-matter abnormalities common in former premature infants.[29]

Some helpful questions to screen school-age children for auditory processing problems are listed in Table 31–6. Delayed milestones in

Table 31–6 Screening questions for auditory processing disorder and language delays

Does the child have a speech problem? Has he had speech therapy?
Does the child use appropriate sentence structure?
Does the child understand what is said to him?
Can the child follow multistage commands?
Does the child have difficulty expressing himself verbally?
Does the child confuse words that sound similar?
Does the child have difficulty reproducing the melody and rhythm of music?
Is the child distracted by auditory stimuli?
Does the child complain that loud noise(s) in the classroom bother him?

Source: Extracted from Page.[28]

language or articulation (Appendix 31–1 and 31–2) should prompt consideration of auditory processing disorder. A full assessment for auditory processing disorders should be done by a qualified audiologist or speech-language pathologist.

Key Points for Internationally Adopted Children

- Language delays are common among internationally adopted children.
- Functional communication language usually catches up quickly.
- Achievement of language mastery is more prolonged.

- Few children are able to become bilingual unless reared in a bilingual environment.
- Auditory processing disorders complicate language development in some internationally adopted children.

Appendix 31–1 Articulation milestones

Age (years)	Mastery of Sounds
3	m, n, ng, p, f, h, w
3.5	y (as in yes)
4	k, b, d, g, r
4.5	s, sh, ch
6	t, v, l, th
7	z, zh, th, j

Source: Reprinted with permission of Simon & Schuster Adult Publishing Group from *When the Brain Can't Hear: Unraveling the Mystery of Auditory Processing Disorder* by Teri James Bellis, Ph.D. Copyright © 2002.

Appendix 31–2 Language milestones for young children

Birth
Startles to loud noises
Cries when uncomfortable, hungry, or wet
May calm to a familiar, comforting voice
May cease behavior when child hears a new sound

6 months
Makes many different sounds, including laughing, gurgling, cooing
Reacts to tone of voice, especially if loud or angry
Turns in the direction of new sounds
Enjoys toys that make noise, such as rattles or squeakers, musical toys, being sung to
Babbles to get attention, using consonants such as p, b, and m
Smiles when spoken to
Indicates that he or she wants something through sound or gesture

8 months
Responds to his or her name
Says at least four or more different, distinct sounds
Uses syllables such as da, ba, ka
Listens to his or her own voice and others' voices
Tries to imitate some sounds
Responds to "No"
Enjoys participating in games such as peekaboo and pat-a-cake

10 months
Mama or Dada (nonspecific)
Shouts, squeals, or makes other vocal non-crying sound to attract attention
Uses connected syllables that sound like real speech in intonation and consonant–vowel makeup, including both long and short groups of sounds
Repeats certain syllables or sequences of sounds over and over

12 months
Recognizes his or her name and turns to look when name is called
Says "Mama" and "Dada" and may have two or three additional words
Imitates familiar words and animal sounds
Understands simple instructions ("Give me" or "Come here")
Waves and understands "bye-bye"
Makes appropriate eye contact and shows affection for familiar people
Responds to sounds such as doorbell ringing or the dog barking
Understands that words are symbols for objects
Understands "No" (but does not always agree with it)

(Continues)

Appendix 31–2 Continued

18 months

Uses at least 5–10 words, including names of people and familiar things

Uses some words to express wants or needs ("More"), but also often points or gestures to the desired object

Begins to combine two words

Points to familiar body parts

Recognizes pictures of familiar things and people

Gets a familiar object upon request, even if it is in another room

Imitates sounds and words more accurately

Hums or sings simple tunes

Hears and responds to quiet speech

24 months

Uses two- to three-word sentences, including negatives ("No want", "No go")

Has a vocabulary of 200–300 words, uses at least 50–100 words regularly

Expresses simple desires or needs for familiar things or actions through speaking rather than pointing

Refers to self by name rather than "me" or "I"

Asks "wh" questions ("What that?", "Where kitty?")

Understands simple questions and commands

Names familiar pictures

30 months

Has a 400-word vocabulary and can name familiar objects and pictures

Says his or her first name and holds up fingers to show age

Says "no" but may mean "yes"

Refers to self as "me" rather than by name

Answers "where" questions

Uses short sentences regularly, such as "Me do it"

Uses past tense and plurals, although not always correctly

Talks to other children and adults

Can match at least three colors

Knows "big" and "little"

36 months

Should be intelligible to strangers, even though many articulation errors occur

Has a vocabulary of nearly 1000 words and speaks in three- to four-word sentences

Names at least one color, can match all primary colors

Knows concepts such as night/day, boy/girl, big/little, in/on, up/down, go/stop

Follows two-step requests such as "Get the toy and put it in the box"

Can sing familiar songs

Talks a lot (to self and others)

Expresses abstract thoughts, ideas, and concepts verbally and can tell a short story

Asks "what" and "why" questions

Can hear his or her name when called from another room

Can hear the television or radio at the same level as others in the family

4 years

Has a vocabulary of 1500 words

Uses four- to five-word sentences

Begins to use more complex sentences

Uses plurals, contractions, and past tense

Asks many questions, including "Why?"

Understands simple "who," "what," and "where" questions

Can follow commands and directions, even if the target object is not present

Can identify some basic shapes (circle, square)

Can identify primary colors

Can talk about concepts in the abstract and imaginary conditions

Begins to copy patterns on a page (lines, circles)

Pays attention to a short story and may be able to answer questions about it

Hears and understands most of what is said at home and at school

Relates incidents that happened at school or at home

5 years

Has a vocabulary of 2000 words

Uses five- to six-word sentences

Produces most speech sounds correctly

Uses all types of sentences, including complex ones that describe cause–effect or temporal relations and different verb tenses

Can count to 10

Can tell what objects are used for and made of and knows spatial relations

Knows opposite concepts (hard/soft, long/short, same/different)

Asks questions for the purpose of gaining new information

Knows right and left on self, not necessarily on others

Can express feelings, dreams, wishes, and other abstract thoughts

Can copy basic capital letters when shown a model, may be able to write name, can draw rudimentary pictures

Hears and understands most of what is said at home and at school

Source: Reprinted with permission of Simon & Schuster Adult Publishing Group from *When the Brain Can't Hear: Unraveling the Mystery of Auditory Processing Disorder* by Teri James Bellis, Ph.D. Copyright © 2002.

References

1. Rygvold A-L. Intercountry adopted children's language and academic skills. In: Rygvold A-L, Dalen M, Saetersdal B, eds. Mine–yours–ours and theirs. Oslo: University of Oslo, 1999: 221–9.

2. McGuinness T, McGuinness J. Speech and language problems in international adoptees. Am Fam Physician 1999; 60:1322–3.

3. Albers LH, Johnson DE, Hostetter MK, Iverson S, Miller LC. Health of children adopted from the former Soviet Union and Eastern Europe. Comparison with preadoptive medical records. JAMA 1997; 278:922–4.

4. Miller LC, Kiernan MT, Mathers MI, Klein-Gitelman M. Developmental and nutritional status of internationally adopted children. Arch Pediatr Adolesc Med 1995; 149:40–4.

5. Ames EW. The development of Romanian children adopted to Canada. Burnaby, B.C. Canada: National Welfare Grants Program, 1997.

6. Benoit TC, Jocelyn LJ, Moddemann DM, Embree JE. Romanian adoption. The Manitoba experience. Arch Pediatr Adolesc Med 1996; 150:1278–82.

7. Miller LC, Hendrie NW. Health of children adopted from China. Pediatrics 2000; 105:E76.

8. McCartney JS, Fried PA, Watkinson B. Central auditory processing in school-age children prenatally exposed to cigarette smoke. Neurotoxicol Teratol 1994; 16;269–76.

9. Dubrovina I, et al. Psychological Development of Children in Orphanages. Moscow: Prosveschenie Press, 1991.

10. Kusko CW. Language and linguistic development. Otolaryngol Clin North Am 1985; 18:315–22.

11. Whitman RL, Schwartz ER. The pediatrician's approach to the preschool child with language delay. Clin Pediatr (Phila) 1985; 24:26–31.

12. Mullen EM. Mullen Scales of Early Learning, AGS edition. Circle Pines, MN: AGS, 1995.

13. Bellis TJ. When the Brain Can't Hear. New York: Pocket Books, 2002.

14. Accardo P. On one's toes about developmental language disorders. J Pediatr 1997; 130:509–10.

15. Shulman LH, Sala DA, Chu ML, McCaul PR, Sandler BJ. Developmental implications of idiopathic toe walking. J Pediatr 1997; 130:541–6.

16. Glennen S. Language development and delay in internationally adopted infants and toddlers: a review. Amer J Speech-Lang Pathol 2002; 11:339–9.

17. Stein MI, Parker S, Coplan J, Feldman H. Expressive language delay in a toddler. Pediatrics (Suppl) 2001; 197:905–9.

18. Gindis B. Language-related issues for international adoptees and adoptive families. In: Tepper T, Hannon L, Sandstrom D, eds. International Adoption: Challenges and Opportunities. Meadow Lands, PA: PNPIC, 1998: 98–108.

19. Glennen S, Masters MG. Typical and atypical language development in infants and toddlers adopted from Eastern Europe. Amer J Speech-Lang Pathol 2002; 11: 417–33.

20. Gindis B. Language-related issues for international adoptees and adoptive families. Available at: http://www.bgcenter.com/language.htm.

21. McRae KM, Vickar E. Simple developmental speech delay: a follow-up study. Dev Med Child Neurol 1991; 33:868–74.

22. Aram DM, Nation JE. Preschool language disorders and subsequent language and academic difficulties. J Commun Disord 1980; 13:159–70.

23. Scarborough HS. Very early language deficits in dyslexic children. Child Dev 1990; 61:1728–43.

24. Scarborough HS, Dobrich W. Development of children with early language delay. J Speech Hear Res 1990; 33:70–83.

25. Bishop DV, Adams C. A prospective study of the relationship between specific language impairment, phonological disorders and reading retardation. J Child Psychol Psychiatry 1990; 31:1027–50.

26. Snowling M, Bishop DV, Stothard SE. Is preschool language impairment a risk factor for dyslexia in adolescence? J Child Psychol Psychiatry 2000; 41:587–600.

27. Aram DM, Ekelman BL, Nation JE. Preschoolers with language disorders: 10 years later. J Speech Hear Res 1984; 27:232–44.

28. Page JM. Central auditory processing disorders in children. Otolaryngol Clin North Am 1985; 18:323–35.

29. Rourke BP, Ahmad SA, Collins DW, Hayman-Abello BA, Hayman-Abello SE, Warriner EM. Child clinical/pediatric neuropsychology: some recent advances. Annu Rev Psychol 2002; 53:309–39.

32

SCHOOL ISSUES

The prevalence of school problems among internationally adopted children is unknown. Most clinicians suspect an increased incidence of learning disabilities, behavior problems (such as attention–deficit hyperactivity disorder), language delays, auditory processing disorder (see Chapter 31), and other problems that impede school performance in this population of children. Genetic predisposition may contribute to these problems, exacerbated by pre- or postnatal exposures, stress, malnutrition, micronutrient deficiencies, toxic exposures, and other factors (see Chapters 5–8, 10–13, 24). Although some learning and behavior problems may appear prior to the school years, these issues are generally recognized after school entry. This chapter reviews the genetics of learning disabilities, intelligence, attentional regulation, and other factors that affect school competence and performance in internationally adopted children.

School Difficulties in Adopted Children

Learning disabilities are defined as problems with reading, memory, language, or mathematic computation that reduce academic achievement below what is expected from general intellectual potential.[1] About 5% of American children manifest learning disabilities. The diagnosis of learning disabilities depends on local school system standards, parental vigilance, and other factors.

Adopted children are considerably more likely to have school problems than their non-adopted peers. Adoption expert David Brodzinsky states that adoptees are about four times as likely to be diagnosed with learning disabilities than non-adoptees.[2,3] Joyce Maguire Pavao reports that in any population of learning-disabled children, about 28% will be adopted—far out of proportion to their numbers in the population. These statistics reflect a combination of biologic and psychologic factors. Some speculate that personality traits associated with learning disabilities, including impulsivity, poor judgement, and immaturity, may result in unplanned and unwanted pregnancy.[2] These birth mothers (and birth fathers, through assortative mating) may be more likely to be learning disabled themselves and pass on the genetic predisposition. In addition, infants placed for adoption may have experienced adverse prenatal exposures (including a stressful intrauterine environment) (see Chapters 5–8) and perinatal complications which increase the likelihood of learning disabilities.

The frequency of learning disabilities among post-institutionalized, internationally adopted children is suspected to be considerably greater than that for domestic adoptees, but this has not yet been definitively determined. Many internationally adopted children have the additional risk factors of malnutrition, micronutrient deficiencies, microcephaly, and environmental deprivation, all of which contribute to the likelihood of learning disabilities. Some children have significant memory problems, possible due to stress-induced hippocampal damage in early life (see Chapter 8).

Poor self-esteem often occurs with learning disabilities, compounding the adopted child's sense of being different.[2] Behavioral issues in children sometimes serve to distract attention from cognitive or learning disabilities. Academic demands may provoke anxiety; children then resort to hyperactive, clowning, or aggressive behavior to conceal cognitive difficulties.

Genetics and Intelligence

Some learning disabilities and aspects of intelligence are genetically determined. Genetics strongly influence cognitive ability and school performance.[4–7] Mild mental retardation tends to run in families (severe mental retardation is usually caused by birth complications, head injuries, novel genetic mutations[8]). Twin and adoption studies confirm that verbal and spatial abilities are largely inherited[8,9]: test scores of do-

Martin arrived from Russia at age 8 years. He'd been abused and molested prior to entering the orphanage 7 months before adoption. After arrival in the United States, he entered second grade. It rapidly became obvious to his parents and teacher that he had extreme anxiety in class. Even with a bilingual aide, Martin was unable to sit or concentrate. He cried every morning before boarding the school bus, was unable to make friends, and started to lose weight. Many different approaches were tried. Over the course of the school year, he became reasonably fluent in English, but still seemed unable to adjust to the classroom. The school became frustrated at their inability to understand Martin's problems, but continued to offer support services in reading and math. Eventually, Martin's parents chose to home school him. After 2 years of home school, his mother says, "I'm just beginning to appreciate the severity of his anxiety. Despite medication, counseling, and all the love and support we have tried to provide, Martin still becomes so anxious with demands for performance that he has trouble learning. He's made a lot of progress, so we're going to try again with school this year."

mestically adopted children resemble those of their birth parents, not their adoptive parents. This becomes more prominent as children grow up: at age 3 years, the correlation between verbal or spatial abilities of adopted children and their birth parents is about 0.1, but by age 16, this correlation increases to about 0.3 (Fig. 32–1). In other analyses, verbal, spatial, perceptual speed, and visual memory heritability estimates range from 0.26 to 0.53, indicating that approximately half of the phenotypic correlations are due to genetic effects.[10] Similar results are found in studies of heritability of verbal IQ: parents' scores correlate with those of their birth children (~0.36 to 0.41) but not their adopted children (~0.16 to 0.18).[11] A moderate genetic influence on reading performance is found at ages 7, 12, and 16 years.[12]

Genes appear to exert increasing influence on IQ over time.[10,13–15] Although other maternal factors ("womb" and "home" environments) strongly influence cognitive ability, genetic

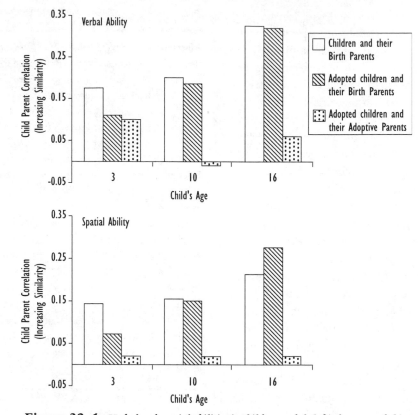

Figure 32–1 *Verbal and spatial abilities in children and their birth parents (white bars), adopted children and their birth parents (cross-hatched bars), and adopted children and their adoptive parents (spotted bars). Adopted children come to resemble their birth parents as much as children raised by their birth parents do. In contrast, adopted children do not end up resembling their adoptive parents. The results imply that most of the family resemblance in cognitive skills is caused by genetic factors, not environment. (Adapted from "The genetics of cognitive abilities and disabilities," Plomin R, DeFries J. Copyright © 1998 by Scientific American, Inc. All rights reserved.)*

effects on IQ become more apparent as the individual ages.[16] Genetic influences on cortical brain structure, particularly Broca's and Wernicke's language areas and frontal brain regions, suggest a structural basis for the inheritance of cognitive abilities.[17]

Genetics, Learning Disabilities, and Attention-Deficit Hyperactivity Disorder

The common types of learning disabilities include dyslexia, dysgraphia, dyscalculia, dyski-

nesia, dysphasia, and nonverbal learning disabilities. Attentional problems (ADHD) are the most common reason for school difficulties. Genetic factors may contribute to each of these. Evidence for the heritability of dyslexia and ADHD are discussed below.

Dyslexias

Reading disabilities (dyslexias) are highly heritable,[18–23] although not all investigators[24] agree with this finding. Specific genetic loci (6p21.3, 2p12, 15, 18p11.2, and 1p, among others) mediate various forms of dyslexia in some families.

Reading disabilities are often associated with behavioral disturbances (internalizing and externalizing), disorders of attentional regulation, and other learning disabilities. A common genetic link may explain the coexistence of these diverse abnormalities.[20] No studies have yet focused on the prevalence of dyslexia among internationally adopted children.

Attention-Deficit Hyperactivity Disorder

Attention-deficit hyperactivity disorder (ADHD) is the most common neurobehavioral disorder of childhood, affecting between 4% and 12% of American elementary school age children.[25] Few studies outside the United States and parts of Europe have been reported: a survey in Germany found ADHD symptom prevalence in 17.8% of 1077 school children.[26] Symptom prevalence was estimated at 19.8% of 600 10- to 12-year-olds residing near the Chernobyl reactor in Ukraine.[27] The diagnosis of ADHD relies on the observations of parents (or other family members) and teachers (see Table 32–2 for diagnostic criteria). By definition, the behavioral symptoms are pervasive, affect function in two or more settings (home, school, among peers), present before the age of 7 years, and cause "clinically significant social, academic, or occupational impairment."[28–30] Symptoms tend to worsen as environmental demands increase. Children with ADHD may be shorter than nonaffected controls (possibly because of treatment with stimulant medications), although these height deficits normalize in late adolescence.[31]

Studies of twins and adoptees support the notion that ADHD is inherited.[32–38] Although exact associations have not been defined, considerable evidence suggests that the dopamine *DRD-4* receptor gene and dopamine transporter gene (*DAT1*) are linked to ADHD susceptibility. However, not all studies confirm this.[39] Some studies suggest that birth relatives of children with ADHD more frequently have psychiatric problems including conduct disorder, depression, anxiety, and learning disorders (reviewed in Thepar et al.[38]). Different suscep-

tibility clusters may be inherited separately (i.e., ADHD/conduct disorder and ADHD/depression). It appears that genes linked to hyperactivity overlap with genes that influence conduct disorder symptoms and reading disabilities,[33] although this is not universally accepted.[40] An association has been reported between "activity-limiting" maternal mental health disturbances including depression, anxiety, or emotional problems and ADHD in their children.[41]

Some investigators have speculated that ADHD is more common among internationally adopted children,[2,42–44] although this has not yet been definitively proven. The differential diagnosis of ADHD-type symptoms is broad in internationally adopted children (Table 32–1). This diagnosis should not be made without careful consideration of the time interval since adoption: many recent arrivals show impulsive, inattentive, distractible behavior in the early months in their new homes and schools as they adjust to the new, stimulating, and rich environments. Frequent comorbid problems such as learning disabilities (at least 25% of children with ADHD[29]), anxiety, disorders of memory, cognition, language, and mood, may exacerbate the symptoms of ADHD and must be addressed separately.[29] Adoption expert Joyce Maguire Pavao points out that the extra emotional work necessary for adopted children influences their learning styles and may be mistaken for learning disabilities or attentional problems.[42] She describes a child who said "I can't do subtraction. As soon as they say 'take away', it makes me feel really sad." Adopted children are rightfully distracted, she says, because something is missing from their lives. Day-dreaming is frequent among adopted children and may be misinterpreted as poor attention.

Internationally adopted children have additional risk factors for attentional problems. Inattention and overactivity may follow institutional deprivation.[45–47] For example, 152 Romanian children who experienced severe deprivation and were then adopted by British families were compared at age 6 years with 52 within-U.K. adoptees who did not experience

Table 32-1 Differential diagnosis of attention–deficit hyperactivity disorder in internationally adopted children

Developmental Differences
Recently arrived child (responding to "overstimulating" new environment")
Language disorder (including child frustrated with communication difficulties in new language environment)
Learning disabilities
Cognitive impairments
Perceptual or processing disorders and disorders of sensory modulation (see Chapter 33)

Emotional and Behavioral Disorders
Anxiety disorders (including separation anxiety) (see Chapter 29)
Depression or mood disorders
Post-traumatic stress disorder (see Chapter 8)
Oppositional defiant disorder
Conduct disorder
Adjustment disorder
Disturbed sleep[52] (see Chapter 9)

Environmental Disorders
Child abuse or neglect
Stressful home environment
Sociocultural differences
Parental issues
Inappropriate school setting

Medical Disorders
Sensory impairments (hearing or visual loss)
Fetal alcohol syndrome (see Chapter 5)
Lead poisoning (see Chapter 24)
Malnutrition (see Chapter 10)
Iron deficiency anemia (see Chapter 11)
Substance abuse
Thyroid disorder (see Chapter 11)
Tourette syndrome

Source: Adapted from refs. 28–30.

deprivation.[45] The Romanian children adopted after age 6 months had more inattention and overactivity as rated by parents and teachers. About 40% of the Romanian children adopted after age 2 years and about 33% of those adopted between 6 and 24 months showed signs of inattention or overactivity. The duration of depri-

vation correlated with inattention or overactivity, but not with the presence of conduct or emotional disturbances. In contrast to ADHD occurring in other populations, post-institutional attention problems affected boys and girls equally and was (somewhat) unrelated to cognitive impairment. The children with ADHD, furthermore, were more likely to have signs of impaired attachment. The long-term outcome of children with ADHD as a consequence of institutionalization is unknown; between age 4 and 6 years, these behaviors tend to become more persistent. A behavioral rating survey of 45 adopted children from China detected normal overall scores, but abnormal subscale scores for hyperactivity, aggression, conduct problems, and attention problems. Hyperactivity and aggression were more commonly endorsed among those children who were older at adoption.[48]

Two recent studies address the incidence of ADHD in post-institutionalized children after adoption.[49,50] A higher incidence of inattention, distractibility, impulsivity, and hyperactivity was found among post-institutionalized children. Fifty percent of longer-institutionalized adopted children met criteria for ADHD, according to the Conners Rating Scale, an average of 3 years post-adoption.

Diagnostic criteria for ADHD are shown in Table 32–2. Treatment guidelines for ADHD have recently been reviewed by the American Academy of Pediatrics Subcommittee on Attention-Deficit Hyperactivity Disorder.[51]

School Competence

Little is known about overall school performance of international adoptees. Verhulst et al reviewed the academic performance of 2148 internationally adopted children in the Netherlands (32% from Korea) and compared these children with 2076 Dutch children from the general population.[54] The non-adopted children scored better as a group on measures of academic performance (Table 32–3).

Table 32–2 Diagnosis of attention–deficit hyperactivity disorder

Inattention

Six or more for at least 6 months to a degree that is maladaptive and inconsistent with the patient's developmental level

- Fails to give close attention to details
- Has difficulty sustaining attention in activities
- Does not listen when spoken to directly
- Does not follow through on instructions
- Has difficulty organizing tasks
- Avoids engaging in tasks that require sustained mental effort
- Loses things necessary for activities
- Is easily distracted by extraneous stimuli
- Is forgetful on a daily basis

Hyperactivity and Impulsivity

Six or more for at least 6 months to a degree that is maladaptive and inconsistent with the patient's developmental level

Hyperactivity

- Is fidgety
- Leaves seat when expected to remain seated
- Runs about in situations in which it is inappropriate
- Has difficulty playing quietly
- Acts as if "driven by a motor"
- Talks excessively

Impulsivity

- Blurts out answers before questions have been completed
- Has difficulty taking turns
- Interrupts or intrudes on others

Reprinted with permission from the *Diagnostic and Statistical Manual of Mental Disorders, 4th edition, Text Revision.* ©2000 American Psychiatric Association.[53]

Adopted children from lower socioeconomic status adoptive homes showed better academic performance, were less often referred to special classes, and had fewer school problems than adopted children from higher socioeconomic status homes. One possible explanation is that these adoptive parents were less demanding of their children's academic performance. Overall, 23% of adopted 12- to 15-year-old boys scored in the problem range of behavior, compared to 10.3% of non-adopted boys.[55] Clustered behavior problems included poor school work, poor motivation, problems with teacher, expulsion from school, truancy, difficulty with directions, and poor relations with other pupils.

In Norway, adoptive parents were far more supportive of their child's school situation than the parents of birth children (according to several surveys, quoted in Dalen[44]). Examples cited include the adoptive parents' increased involvement in supervision of homework and school activities. As in the Netherlands, international adoptees in families with high social status have more school-related problems and worse school performance than those in lower social status families—the opposite of findings for non-adopted children. Moreover, teenagers of working class adoptive parents more often choose to study theoretical or general subjects while those with academic parents choose vocational subjects. The former group is more likely to complete their secondary education than the latter group. Possible explanations include unrealistic expectations and pressure from the "academic"

Table 32–3 Academic performance of international adoptees (*n* = 2148) compared with non-adopted children (*n* = 2076)

School History	Non-adopted (%)	Adopted (%)		
		Boys	Girls	Total
Attended special schools	4.4[a]	17.1	9.6	13.2
Ever repeated a grade	20.4	27.3	21.7	24.4
Other school problems	22.5[a]	45.7	31.3	38.2

[a]*p* < 0.01 (non-adopted compared with total adopted).

Source: Data from Verhulst et al.[54]

> *Ronni's mom reports, "We had to move to a new school district to get our daughter's educational needs met. She doesn't fit any neat category—she has language-processing delays, dyslexia, and behavioral problems. The new district is great and is willing to meet with me every 3 months to update her Individualized Educational Plan. She is improving so fast now that she is in a supportive environment."*

adoptive parents, or broader acceptance of differences by adoptive parents (see Chapter 34).

Lipman and colleagues[56] reviewed the educational achievements of 104 domestically adopted children in Ontario, Canada in 1983 and again in 1987. School performance was no different from that for non-adopted children. However, children with psychiatric difficulties identified in the initial survey were more likely to have impaired school performance 4 years later. The proportion of boys with poor school performance decreased from 33.3% to 25.8% over the 4 years. The data further suggest that these differences decrease over time.

Similarly, 71% of 8- to 12-year-olds adopted from Eastern Europe[43] were at or within 1 year of expected grade level, and general measures of social competence were good 4.5 years after adoption.

Overall, family attitudes are likely to be more important than adoptive status in determining school performance and later achievements.[57] School performance and achievement relates directly to the individual characteristics of the child, including genetics, prenatal exposures, and early life experiences, rather than simply age at adoption.

Complex Neurobehavioral Disorder

A large cohort of post-institutionalized children (mostly from Eastern Europe) was adopted in the past 5–9 years. As this group of children ages, an unusual constellation of problems has emerged with surprising frequency. Although the prevalence has not been established, a subgroup of these children have a complex neurobehavioral disorder, consisting of learning disabilities, behavior problems, and mental health disorders. Poor school performance, impaired family and peer relationships, and anxiety, depression, and post-traumatic stress disorder are common features. Such children have extreme difficulties participating in school. Many have associated cognitive delays and ADHD. Other troublesome behaviors also occur. For example, in a survey of 81 adopted Eastern European 8- to 12-year-olds,[43] 36% had learning disabilities, and 45% had multiple complex diagnoses, including 38% with ADHD, 32% with post-traumatic stress disorder, 19% with depression, 19% with anxiety, 16% with reactive attachment disorder, and 5% with obsessive compulsive disorder (see Chapters 13 and 30).

Pre-adoption risk factors (malnutrition, prenatal alcohol exposure, prematurity, physical or social neglect, abuse, and >6 months of institutionalization) have been linked to both internalizing and externalizing behavior problems.[58] Other factors are also likely to contribute to individual variation in response to adverse environmental exposures. For example, variants in the monoamine oxidase gene determine the likelihood of antisocial behaviors in individuals abused in childhood. Thus genotypes moderate children's sensitivity to environmental insults.[59]

Some children demonstrate improvement in these symptoms over time. In others, problems appear to worsen, likely associated with increasing academic and social demands. Many children who appear to be developing well in the early preschool and school-age years begin to have significant difficulty in third grade as the demands increase for more abstract thought. Designing appropriate school placements and support programs for such children is difficult, as traditional diagnostic categories do not apply. Pediatricians must work closely with the school and parents to find suitable services for these children.

Special School Challenges for Adopted Children

School presents many specific challenges to the adopted child.[42] Teachers and classmates may be uninformed about adoption, unintentionally leading to insensitive, hurtful remarks. Thoughtless school assignments may be difficult for adopted children. Considerable information is available for parents and teachers to avert these problems[60,61] (Table 32–4). School systems may benefit from guidance from parents or physicians. Such suggestions aid children from other diverse types of families (step-children, children of gay or lesbian parents, children of single parents, etc.) as well.

The Pediatrician and the School

Adoptive parents may request assistance from the pediatrician in communicating with the school. The pediatrician can reassure parents that the adjustment to classroom expectations, English language, and the daily school routine take time. Children should be carefully observed in the early days after school placement to ascertain that an appropriate grade assignment was made. Children who seem to be struggling should be supported and reassigned if necessary. The pediatrician will also be a resource for parents whose children receive an Individualized Educational Plan (IEP) (see Resources). Review of the IEP with the parents prior to their acceptance of this document may be quite helpful. Physicians and parents unfamiliar with the IEP process may find helpful guidelines on the Internet. Participation in Early Intervention or other supportive programs prior to school entry can smooth the adjustment of post-institutionalized children into the classroom.

FAQs

Q. Ethan was just adopted at age 6 from Russia. His Russian expressive language is nearly age-appropriate, and he is bright and inquisitive. However, he obviously has had little experience with pre-academic skills (doesn't know colors, can't tell a story from pictures, can't match shapes, immature drawing skills, unable to use scissors). On the other hand, his social skills are good, and he clearly wants to be with other kids. Should he enter kindergarten?

A. These are always hard choices. The expectations of the school and the parents should be reviewed. The school's willingness to accommodate Ethan is critical. If they are willing to accept his delays and work closely with him in the first 6

Table 32–4 Suggested responses to school-related problems for adoptive families

Problem	Suggested Responses
Should teacher be informed about the adopted child's status?	Yes. This is not an issue for visible adoptions. Other adoptions should be disclosed to the teacher so that the child will be supported if a difficult situation arises. The teacher can also introduce adoption informally in the classroom.
How should the child respond to questions?	Children should help decide what information they wish to disclose. Role-play may help the child prepare to answer questions.
Problematic assignments	Suggest alternative choices to make more inclusive such assignments as "bring in a baby picture," "draw your family tree," "describe your family history," "write your autobiography," "study your genetic inheritance from your parents," etc. Talk to the teacher in advance to see if these activities are part of the curriculum.
Transracial or transcultural adoption	Prepare the child for thoughtless or negative comments, prepare for possible changes in relationships once dating begins

Source: From Rogers,[60] reprinted with permission.

months, he may do well. School and parents should be prepared for 2 years in kindergarten for Ethan if his pre-academic skills don't recover as quickly as anticipated.

Q. What about a child with similar skills who is 7 years old? Should he enter first grade?

A. Kindergarten is probably a better choice unless the child has been home long enough to get a sense of the trajectory of his developmental progress. A child like this who rapidly learns new skills and seems to crave challenges may succeed in a supportive first-grade class.

Q. How do I differentiate ADHD from some of the other concerns mentioned? It seems that most of my internationally adopted patients meet criteria for ADHD diagnosis.

A. Probably some of them do have true ADHD, and would benefit from a comprehensive treatment plan addressing behavior and possible stimulant medications. A poor response to treatment or an atypical presentation (e.g., concurrent anxiety, depression, learning disabilities, sensory processing dysfunction, or other disorders) should trigger a more comprehensive investigation. Also, ADHD, particularly in post-institutionalized children, occurs with other disorders, thus a multifaceted approach to treatment is needed. Medication alone is rarely adequate.

Resources

Directory of State Departments of Education. Available at: Yellow pages for kids with disabilities. http://www.yellowpagesforkids.com/help/seas.htm.

The Association for Retarded Citizens. Available at: http://www.thearclink.org.

The Federation for Children with Special Needs. Available at: http://www.fcsn.org.

Families Adopting in Response (FAIR). Available at: http://www.fairfamilies.org.

Wood L, Ng NS. Adoption and the Schools. Available at: FAIR, P.O. Box 51436 Palo Alto, CA 94303.

References

1. Blasco P. Early developmental indicators of intellectual deficit. Pediatr Rounds 1993; 2:1–3.

2. Brodzinsky DM, Schecter MD, Henig RM. Being Adopted. New York: Anchor Books, 1993.

3. Brodzinsky DM, Steiger C. Prevalence of adoptees among special education populations. J Learn Disabil 1991; 24:484–9.

4. Bartels M, Rietveld MJ, Van Baal GC, Boomsma DI. Genetic and environmental influences on the development of intelligence. Behav Genet 2002; 32:237–49.

5. Wadsworth SJ, DeFries JC, Fulker DW, Plomin R. Cognitive ability and academic achievement in the Colorado Adoption Project: a multivariate genetic analysis of parent-offspring and sibling data. Behav Genet 1995; 25:1–15.

6. Petrill SA, Thompson LA. The phenotypic and genetic relationships among measures of cognitive ability, temperament, and scholastic achievement. Behav Genet 1993; 23:511–8.

7. Rowe DC, Jacobson KC, Van den Oord EJ. Genetic and environmental influences on vocabulary IQ: parental education level as moderator. Child Dev 1999; 70:1151–62.

8. Plomin R, DeFries JC. The genetics of cognitive abilities and disabilities. Sci Am 1998; 278:62–9.

9. Bouchard TJ, Jr., Segal NL, Lykken DT. Genetic and environmental influences on special mental abilities in a sample of twins reared apart. Acta Genet Med Gemellol (Roma) 1990; 39:193–206.

10. Alarcon M, Plomin R, Fulker DW, Corley R, DeFries JC. Multivariate path analysis of specific cognitive abilities data at 12 years of age in the Colorado Adoption Project. Behav Genet 1998; 28:255–64.

11. Neiss M, Rowe DC. Parental education and child's verbal IQ in adoptive and biological families in the National Longitudinal Study of Adolescent Health. Behav Genet 2000; 30:487–95.

12. Wadsworth SJ, Corley RP, Hewitt JK, Defries JC. Stability of genetic and environmental influences on reading performance at 7, 12, and 16 years of age in the Colorado Adoption Project. Behav Genet 2001; 31:353–9.

13. Loehlin JC. Using EQS for a simple analysis of the Colorado Adoption Project data on height and intelligence. Behav Genet 1992; 22:239–45.

14. Phillips K, Fulker DW. Quantitative genetic analysis of longitudinal trends in adoption designs with application to IQ in the Colorado Adoption Project. Behav Genet 1989; 19:621–58.

15. Baker LA, DeFries JC, Fulker DW. Longitudinal stability of cognitive ability in the Colorado Adoption Project. Child Dev 1983; 54:290–7.

16. Devlin B, Daniels M, Roeder K. The heritability of IQ. Nature 1997; 388:468–71.

17. Thompson PM, Cannon TD, Narr KL, et al. Genetic influences on brain structure. Nat Neurosci 2001; 4:1253–8.

18. Pennington BF. Genetics of learning disabilities. J Child Neurol 1995; 10:S69–77.

19. Flint J. The genetic basis of cognition. Brain 1999; 122:2015–32.

20. Grigorenko EL. Developmental dyslexia: an update on genes, brains, and environments. J Child Psychol Psychiatry 2001; 42:91–125.

21. Plomin R. Genetic factors contributing to learning and language delays and disabilities. Child Adolesc Psychiatr Clin North Am 2001; 10:259–77, viii.

22. Shalev RS, Gross-Tsur V. Developmental dyscalculia. Pediatr Neurol 2001; 24:337–42.

23. Olson RK. Dyslexia: nature and nurture. Dyslexia 2002; 8:143–59.

24. Jennekens-Schinkel A. Sense and nonsense with respect to the gene for dyslexia [in Dutch]. Ned Tijdschr Geneeskd 1998; 142:2445–7.

25. Brown RT, Freeman WS, Perrin JM, et al. Prevalence and assessment of attention-deficit/hyperactivity disorder in primary care settings. Pediatrics 2001; 107:e43.

26. Baumgaertel MD, Wolraich ML, Dietrich M. Comparison of diagnostic criteria for attention deficit disorders in a German elementary school sample. J Am Acad Child Adolesc Psychiatry 1995; 34:629–638.

27. Gadow KD, Nolan EE, Litcher L, et al. Comparison of attention-deficit/hyperactivity disorder symptom subtypes in Ukrainian schoolchildren. J Am Acad Child Adolesc Psychiatry 2000; 39:1520–1527.

28. American Academy of Pediatrics. Committee on Quality Improvement. Clinical Practice Guideline: diagnosis and evaluation of the child with attention-deficit/hyperactivity disorder. Pediatrics 2000; 105:1158–70.

29. Miller KJ, Castellanos FX. Attention deficit/hyperactivity disorders. Pediatr Rev 1998; 19:373–384.

30. Zametkin AJ, Ernst M. Problems in the management of attention-deficit-hyperactivity disorder. New Engl J Med 1999; 340:40–46.

31. Spencer T, Biederman J, Wilens TE. Growth deficits in children with attention deficit hyperactivity disorder. Pediatrics 1998; 102:501–6.

32. Alberts-Corush J, Firestone P, Goodman JT. Attention and impulsivity characteristics of the biological and adoptive parents of hyperactive and normal control children. Am J Orthopsychiatry 1986; 56:413–23.

33. Cadoret RJ, Stewart MA. An adoption study of attention deficit/hyperactivity/aggression and their relationship to adult antisocial personality. Compr Psychiatry 1991; 32:73–82.

34. Faraone SV, Doyle AE. Genetic influences on attention deficit hyperactivity disorder. Curr Psychiatry Rep 2000; 2:143–6.

35. Faraone SV, Doyle AE. The nature and heritability of attention-deficit/hyperactivity disorder. Child Adolesc Psychiatr Clin North Am 2001; 10:299–316, viii–ix.

36. Huessy H. ADD, genetics, and adoptees' behavior. J Am Acad Child Adolesc Psychiatry 1987; 26:113.

37. Roman T, Schmitz M, Polanczyk G, Eizirik M, Rohde LA, Hutz MH. Attention-deficit hyperactivity disorder: a study of association with both the dopamine transporter gene and the dopamine D4 receptor gene. Am J Med Genet 2001; 105:471–8.

38. Thapar A, Holmes J, Poulton K, Harrington R. Genetic basis of attention deficit and hyperactivity. Br J Psychiatry 1999; 174:105–11.

39. Castellanos FX, Lau E, Tayebi N, et al. Lack of an association between a dopamine-4 receptor polymorphism and attention-deficit/hyperactivity disorder: genetic and brain morphometric analyses. Mol Psychiatry 1998; 3:431–4.

40. Lahey BB, Piacentini JC, McBurnett K. Psychopathology in the parents of children with conduct disorder and hyperactivity. J Am Acad Child Adolesc Psychiatry 1988; 27:163–70.

41. Lesesne CA, Visser SN, White CP. Attention-deficit/hyperactivity disorder in school-aged children: association with maternal mental health and use of health care resources. Pediatrics 2003; 111:1232–7.

42. Pavao JM. The Family of Adoption. Boston: Beacon Press, 1998.

43. Tirella LG, Miller LC. Educational achievements of 8- to 12-year-old children adopted from Eastern Europe. Joint Council for International Children's Services. Washington, DC. April 10, 2002.

44. Dalen M. The status of knowledge of foreign adoptions. Oslo: Department of Special Needs Education, Faculty of Education, 1999.

45. Kreppner JM, O'Connor T, Rutter M. Can inattention/overactivity be an institutional deprivation syndrome? J Abnorm Child Psychol 2001; 29:513–28.

46. Morison SJ, Ames EW, Chisholm K. The development of children adopted from Romanian orphanages. Merrill-Palmer Q 1995; 41:411–30.

47. Tizard B, Hodges J. The effect of early institutional rearing on the development of eight-year-old children. J Child Psychol Psychiatry 1978; 19:99–118.

48. Rojewski JW, Shapiro MS, Shapiro M. Parental assessment of behavior in Chinese adoptees during early childhood. Child Psychiatry Hum Dev 2000; 31:79–96.

49. Kadlec MB, Cermak S. Activity level, organization, and social-emotional behaviors in post-institutionalized children. Adopt Q 2002; 6:43–57.

50. Lin SH. Sensory Integration, Growth, and Emotional and Behavioral Regulation in Adopted Post-Institutionalized Children. Doctoral dissertation. Sargent College of Health and Rehabilitation Sciences. Boston: Boston University, 2003:133.

51. American Academy of Pediatrics Subcommittee on Attention-Deficit/Hyperactivity Disorder. Clinical prac-

tice guideline: treatment of the school-aged child with attention-deficit/hyperactivity disorder. Pediatrics 2001; 108:1033–44.

52. O'Brien LM, Holbrook CR, Mervis CB, et al. Sleep and neurobehavioral characteristics of 5- to 7-year old children with parenterally reported symptoms of attention-deficit/hyperactivity disorder. Pediatrics 2003; 111:554–63.

53. American Psychiatric Association. Diagnostic and Statistical Manual of Mental Disorders, 4th ed. (DSM-IV). Washington, DC: American Psychiatric Association, 2000.

54. Verhulst FC, Althaus M, Versluis-Den Bieman HJM. Problem behavior in international adoptees: an epidemiologic study. J Am Acad Child Adolesc Psychiatry 1990; 29:94–103.

55. Verhulst FC, Versluis-Den Bieman HJM, Van der Ende J, Berden GFMG, Sanders-Woudstra JAR. Problem behavior in international adoptees: III. Diagnosis of child psychiatric disorders. J Am Acad Child Adolesc Psychiatry 1990; 29:420–8.

56. Lipman EL, Offord DR, Boyle MH, Racine YA. Follow-up of psychiatric and educational morbidity among adopted children. J Am Acad Child Adolesc Psychiatry 1993; 32:1007–12.

57. Scarr S, Weinberg RA. Educational and occupational achievements of brothers and sisters in adoptive and biologically related families. Behav Genet 1994; 24:301–25.

58. Johnson D. International adoptee follow-up studies: what have we learned from families and how should this information change adoption practice? Washington, DC: Joint Council on International Children's Services, April 9, 2003.

59. Caspi A, McClay J, Moffitt TE, et al. Role of genotype in the cycle of violence in maltreated children. Science 2002; 297:851–4.

60. Rogers CR. Adoption and school issues: challenges for the adoptive family and ways to address them. Personal communication, Boston, MA, 2003.

61. Wood L, Ng N. Adoption and the Schools: Resources for Parents and Teachers. Palo Alto, CA: FAIR (Families adopting in response) Available at: http://www.fairfamilies.org. 2001.

33

DYSFUNCTION OF SENSORY INTEGRATION

"[A]ll that a mammal does is fundamentally dependent on his perception, past or present"

D.O. Hebb, 1953 (quoted in Casler[1])

Children in institutional care experience many forms of sensory deprivation. Crib confinement and swaddling limit tactile experience, motor activity, vestibular and proprioceptive stimulation, and visual input. Quiet orphanage rooms reduce auditory exposures. Liquid and puréed diets diminish oral-motor stimulation. When sensory experiences are disturbed, children may develop disorders of sensory integration (DSI). This disorder is not discussed in many general pediatric textbooks, yet has gained increasing recognition as a theoretical and practical explanation for many behavioral and developmental problems in young children. Disorders of sensory integration are discussed in books on autism and in some developmental pediatric books. Developed by occupational therapist and psychologist A. Jean Ayres in the 1960s and 1970s,[2,3] sensory integration theory provides a logical framework for the diagnosis and treatment of some of the difficulties experienced by institutionalized and post-institutionalized children. Because this subject is unfamiliar to most pediatricians, this chapter briefly reviews sensory integration theory. The effects of institutional life on sensory development, the clinical features, and differential diagnosis of sensory integration dysfunction seen in some internationally adopted children after arrival in the United States are also discussed.

What Is Sensory Integration?

Sensory integration is the coordination and interpretation of visual, auditory, tactile, kinesthetic, vestibular, and proprioceptive information. Sensory information is processed at four levels: *registration* (detection of stimuli from the body or the environment), *modulation* (matching

405

Jack was adopted at age 12 months from Russia. He was withdrawn, frequently rocked, and "bopped" his head. He bit, kicked, and scratched his parents, who often had to forcibly restrain him to prevent injury. Language and cognition scored at 4–5 months. By age 6, he was age-appropriate for language but showed immature behavior. He was able to attend school with the assistance of a part-time aide. He covered his ears when he heard the loud noises of laundry carts bumping the other side of the exam room wall (no one else noticed the sound). At one point during the visit, he yelled, "Those lights are hurting my ears," bringing our attention to the soft humming noise of the fluorescent lights in the exam room. On physical examination, his gastrocnemius muscles were notably overdeveloped. His mother offered, "Oh, could that be from all the jumping that Joey is doing? He usually spends about 1 hour a day jumping on a trampoline. It really calms him down, and he knows now that if he gets upset that he'll feel better if he jumps."

arousal, attention, and activity level to the demands of the environment without being distracted by irrelevant sensory input), *discrimination* (identification of the temporal and spatial characteristics of sensory information and recognition of their meaning, as in stereognosis), and *praxis* (developing and carrying out a motor plan for interaction with the environment).[4] Difficulties with any of the stages may result in a disorder of sensory integration.

Disorders of sensory integration present with a wide range of symptoms, including hyperactivity, distractibility, feeding problems (see Chapter 35, first sidebar), behavior problems (irritability, inability to share, inability to recognize needs of others, overly sensitive, difficulty coping with everyday stress), or low muscle tone and difficulty with coordination or motor planning, and may result in poor self-esteem (Table 33–1). Sensory defensiveness, the easiest category to recognize, occurs when certain types of normal sensory inputs are experienced as uncomfortable or threatening (Table 33–2). Not all professionals accept the existence of sensory integration disorder. Neurologist Peter Rosenberger, quoted in the *Boston Globe*, states that the prevalence of sensory integration disorder is greatly exaggerated, and that "there is a broad range of normalcy when it comes to sensory sensitivity and motor skill deficits like clumsiness." However, sensory integration theory provides a useful construct to understand and address a wide range of problems.

Normal sensory function depends on receipt of normal sensory inputs during infancy. Children residing in orphanages often lack these experiences. The most pervasive form of sen-

Jacqueline was adopted from China at age 19 months. She had never taken solid foods, but had subsisted on formula. Her mother tried everything to persuade her to eat, but the slightest texture was spit out, and the effort ended with mom and baby both crying. Jacqueline refused toothbrushing or any physical contact with her mouth. To make things worse, Jacqueline was significantly malnourished with all measurements below the third percentile. Except for feeding, Jacqueline was a happy and rewarding baby. She quickly caught up developmentally and grew well on a complete formula. Her language skills blossomed. Her mother continued to try to introduce solids. The pediatrician said, "Don't worry, when she is hungry she will eat," and advised her mom to stop the liquid feeds and wait. With the assistance of an occupational therapist specializing in oral motor dysfunction, Jacqueline gradually learned to tolerate touch on her mouth. This was followed by a gradual acceptance of some yogurt added to her feeds to provide slight texture and thickening. After several months of slow, steady work, Jacqueline one day accepted, chewed, and swallowed a half of a Cheerio. Six months later, she was eating yogurt, pudding, Cheerios (four at a time), soup, and small bites of grilled cheese sandwich.

Table 33–1 Signs of sensory integration dysfunction

Dysfunction	*Behavior*
Sensory defensive	Withdraws when touched, avoids textures, certain clothes, foods. Fearful reaction to ordinary movement activities such as playground play; sensitive to loud noises; distractible
Underreactive to sensory stimulation	May seek out intense sensory experiences such as body whirling, falling, and crashing into objects, or may appear oblivious to pain or to body position; fluctuates between under- and overresponsiveness
Coordination problems	May have poor balance and great difficulty learning new motor tasks such as tying shoes; does not have a good sense of where body is in space, appears awkward, clumsy
Delays in pre-academic or academic achievement or activities of daily living	May have problems in handwriting, scissors use, and buttoning and zipping clothes; may have problems in academic areas despite normal or above-normal intelligence
Poor organization of behavior	May be impulsive, distractible, and disorganized in approach to tasks; does not anticipate results of actions. Has difficulty adjusting to a new situation or following directions, difficulty with transitions; frustrated, aggressive, or withdrawn

Adapted from Cermak and Groza.[6] Reprinted with permission from Kluwer Academic/Plenum Publishers.

sory deprivation for children residing in orphanages is the lack of nurturing physical contact (see Chapter 2). Even in well-staffed American orphanages in the 1960s and early 1970s, children were held, "petted," and rocked only ~18% as much as family children.[7] In another study, family children received 7–13 times more tactile stimulation than orphanage children.[8] Auditory and language exposure is greatly reduced in orphanages compared with families: during 4 hours of observation time, orphanage children were spoken to for 13.2 minutes vs. 166.2 minutes for family children.[7] Crib confinement and swaddling thwart the child's natural instincts to explore and master successive sensorimotor tasks. Crying, thumbsucking, rocking, head banging, and other "self-stimulatory" behaviors may be viewed as the child's attempt to satisfy these kinesthetic and vestibular needs (see Chapters 2 and 8).

Some authors suggest that sensory or perceptual deprivation rather than the lack of parental love is the chief adverse effect of institutionalization.[1] A survey of 22 infants living in a Romanian orphanage revealed poor oculomotor control and responses to tactile deep pressure, which improved after 6 months of "enhanced caregiving."[9] However, attempts to remediate the adverse effects of institutionalization with sensory enrichment alone are only partially successful.[7,10,11] Clearly, a loving parent is the best provider of sensory stimulation to the

Table 33–2 Types of sensory defensiveness

Type of Defensiveness	*Behavior*
Tactile defensiveness	Dislikes (light) touch, crowds, hair wash or cut, certain clothing. Often also hyperactive, poor social relations
Oral defensiveness	Avoids certain textures of food, dislikes toothbrushing
Gravitational insecurity	Fearful of changes in position—moving head backwards (washing head in tub, diaper change)
Auditory defensive	Sensitive to loud noises, especially high-pitched ones
Visual defensiveness	Oversensitive to light, visual distraction, gaze avoidance, difficulty focusing with background movement
Olfactory defensiveness	Oversensitive to smells (school cafeteria, certain foods)

Adapted from Cermak and Groza.[6] Reprinted with permission from Kluwer Academic/Plenum Publishers.

Wilma, an active and busy 5-year-old, arrived from China at 3 years of age. For the first year after her arrival, she was unable to sleep through the night in her own bed. The entire household was disrupted by her restlessness and crying. She would start her night in her own bed, but woke nightly around midnight agitated and upset. As her language emerged, she was able to explain to her parents: "I need to spin!" They realized that 15 minutes on her "sit-and-spin" toy at midnight somehow soothed her and allowed her to sleep peacefully the remainder of the night.

Table 33–3 Screening questions for sensory integration disorder in new arrivals

- Does the baby like to be held? Does she mold her body into yours comfortably? *(tactile)*
- Is the baby comfortable being moved (or moving herself from one position to another)? Does she seem upset when laid back for a diaper change or to be dressed? *(proprioception)*
- Does the baby avoid interactions with others? *(adaptive motor)*
- Does she initiate play? Does she touch and explore toys? Does she avoid certain types of toys (fluffy, slippery, noisy)? *(adaptive motor, tactile)*
- Does she mouth toys or avoid mouthing toys? *(tactile)*
- Does she use only her fingertips to manipulate a toy? *(tactile)* (Fig. 33–1)
- Does she tolerate walking on different textures (carpet, grass, wood floor)? *(tactile)*
- Does she use both hands together and work across her midline? *(adaptive motor)*
- Does she tolerate textured foods? Does she chew? *(tactile)*
- Does she "tune out" if more than one stimulus is presented? *(regulatory)*
- Does she sleep through the night? Does she have trouble soothing herself at night or after being upset? *(regulatory)*

Source: Adapted from Schaaf et al.[15]

infant (see Chapter 29). Sensory integration theory also emphasizes the importance of the therapist–child interactions as critical to the therapeutic process and does not see sensory input in isolation as being effective.[12]

Sensory integration problems are not limited to children who have been institutionalized or physically deprived in other ways. Sensory integration difficulties may be exacerbated by other factors common among this population, including prenatal toxic exposures (alcohol, drugs, nicotine) (see Chapters 5–7) and lack of prenatal care with resultant increases in prematurity, low birth weight, and birth complications. Prenatal stress impairs sensory processing via altered regulation of stress hormones (see Chapter 8). Hereditary factors may also contribute to sensory integration disorders.

Therefore, post-institutionalized children are particularly vulnerable to sensory integration problems. Amidst the excitement that accompanies the arrival of a new child, such problems may not be apparent immediately after adoption. Growth delays and medical concerns may be paramount. However, identification of sensory integration problems in new arrivals (Table 33–3) allows interventions that smooth the transition to the new adoptive home and may prevent future problems.

As shown by Cermak and others, difficulty in sensory integration may not be noted until environmental demands increase, months or years after the child's arrival. Compared with age-matched American-born family children, 73 children adopted from Romania had more problems with touch, movement, vision, and audition as assessed by parent report when assessed 42 months

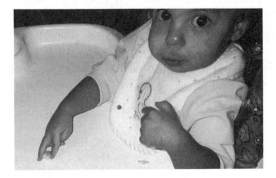

Figure 33–1 *Tactile defensiveness may be a sign of dysfunction of sensory integration. This child refuses to use pincer or palmar grasp, but rather explores objects using her index and middle finger tips. (With permission.)*

(±7.4) after adoption.[13] In addition, the Romanian children had more problems with activity level, feeding, organization, and social–emotional behaviors (see Appendix 33–1). Severity and prevalence of sensory dysfunction in children assessed after adoption increase with duration of prior institutionalization.[14]

Evaluation of the Child

Evaluation of the child with possible sensory dysfunction is accomplished by two methods. First, a parent (and possibly teacher) questionnaire identifies possible problem areas in sensory processing. Sample items are shown in Table 33–4. (A more complete sample questionnaire is included in Appendix 33–2; it is worth reviewing to see the wide range of problems that may be addressed with occupational therapy incorporating sensory integration principles). Standardized assessments include The Sensory Profile[16] for children ages 3–10 and The Infant/Toddler Sensory Profile[17] for children from birth to 3 years. Although alternative explanations exist for poor performance on individual items, the overall pattern of difficulties may be extremely useful to direct therapy for the child.

Table 33–4 Short sensory profile

Subtest	Sample Item
Tactile sensitivity	Responds emotionally or aggressively to touch
Taste and smell sensitivity	Picky eater regarding textures
Underresponsive or seeks sensation	Seeks all kinds of movement; this interferes with daily routines
Auditory filtering	Is distracted or has trouble functioning if there is a lot of background noise
Visual and auditory sensitivity	Responds negatively to unexpected or loud noises (i.e., vacuum, dog barking, hairdryer)
Low energy or weak	Poor endurance, tires easily
Movement sensitivity	Becomes anxious or distressed when feet leave the ground

Source: Adapted from Miller et al.[18]

Second, in addition to assessing sensory processing, an evaluation of sensory integration is undertaken by an occupational therapist with specialized training in this area. A commonly used tool is the Sensory Integration and Praxis Test (SIPT),[19] but other methods are also available. The SIPT is comprised of 17 subtests arranged in four categories (tactile, visual, kinesthetic perception, and motor performance). The child's score for each subtest is compared with the normative sample.

Third, the child is observed in a natural context, either in his or her preschool or school, and, for younger children, within the family context. Play observations, observation of the child in gym class or playground, are important to identify the child's strengths and challenges.

The therapist then designs a program of treatment that addresses problem areas.[2,3] Although the efficacy of such treatment has not been tested in large controlled trials, it is nonetheless very successful in some children. Even those with multiple complex diagnoses may benefit. The psychological benefits of understanding the etiology of the child's problems may also be important. Alternative therapies are sometimes sought by families or recommended by some practitioners. (An up-to-date review of some of these complementary therapies is provided in Wilberger and Wilberger).[20]

Differential Diagnosis of Dysfunction of Sensory Integration

The differential diagnosis of sensory integration disorder is extensive. Many "look-alikes" mimic sensory integration disorder; some of these disorders may coexist. Special consideration should be given to attention-deficit hyperactivity disorder, learning disabilities, developmental delays, reactive attachment disorder, bipolar disorder, post-traumatic stress disorder, autism, and various neuromuscular conditions, all of which share signs and symptoms with sensory integration disorder. Sensory-based treatment may benefit some of these other conditions as well.

Appendix 33–1 Interpretation of behaviors within a sensory-processing framework

Behavior	Interpretation	Comments
Oral Defensiveness		
It was a heartrending shock to see that my newly adopted son would not put a cracker to his mouth and gagged at the sight of any food he could not drink.	These behaviors may all be understood as manifestations of oral defensiveness. This is a very common description in post-institutionalized children and can be explained in part by the feeding practices and lack of play opportunities. In many of the orphanages, children are only fed from a bottle until they are almost 2 years old. Pacifiers are not used. There are few toys for the children to play with and mouth. As a result, children are not used to having things in their mouths. Their mouths become overly sensitive and food and other objects produce an uncomfortable feeling.	It is interesting to note that premature infants who have been tube fed show a similar response when a bottle is introduced and have marked difficulty with beginning feeding. Because of this, current practice has been to provide the infant with non-nutritive sucking while being tube fed.
He doesn't like to eat. At age 2½ he couldn't tolerate a Cheerio. He still gagged on some food at age 4. He eats only when he is starving or else made to eat. He sucks on his fingers, coat, and shirts. He used to suck his tongue when anxious, and mouthed toys until age 5.	Since many children from the institutions are already poorly nourished, feeding can be a major issue and the child's refusal to eat may present major stress to the family.	
She screamed and cried at getting her teeth brushed or having anything of size or texture in her mouth (she spit out all food that required chewing).	For some children, oral defensiveness subsides with patience and slowly introducing different foods and textures. For other children for whom the problem persists, more active intervention is recommended.	
Tactile Defensiveness		
She disliked being bathed but, as with other behaviors, we felt it was because she wasn't used to it.	Discomfort with bathing, with having fingernails and toenails cut, and with having tags on clothing are all examples of tactile defensiveness.	
She does not like to be hugged or kissed—it is still not natural to her. She screeched at any attempt of a sibling to touch her. She had an aversion to children.	It is possible that this child is showing tactile defensiveness. Her "screeching" at siblings and "aversion to children" may reflect her awareness that light touch is "hurtful" to her; it may be her way of avoiding having this happening. Unexpected touch is more likely to produce a defensive response than is expected touch. Children are more unpredictable in their behaviors than adults.	

Appendix 33–1 Continued

Behavior	*Interpretation*	*Comments*
She likes to "bump" people with her head, almost like a defense mechanism to keep from other physical contact such as hugging.	Liking to bump people with her head may be interpreted as seeking strong proprioceptive input. Many children with tactile defensiveness seem to "seek" firm touch and deep pressure. This seems to be calming or organizing to the nervous system.	
He gets "like a board" at times when hugged but other times loves to be cuddled and loves massage.	This child is showing a problem in modulation, i.e., staying in the middle range. He is swinging between showing overarousal (sensory defensiveness) and underarousal. His enjoyment of being massaged may reflect the fact that deep touch pressure is calming to the nervous system.	

Auditory Defensiveness

He was terrified of vacuum cleaners until this past year or so. We supposed that he's remembering some archaic medical equipment from the orphanage.	It is possible that, rather than remembering medical equipment from the orphanage, this child was showing auditory defensiveness and was bothered by the high-pitched noise of the vacuum cleaner.	

Reduced Sensory Awareness

The only problem I see with L. is that she pockets her food in her mouth—she won't swallow. She used to stuff her mouth so full of bread that she couldn't chew it and had to take it back out.	This child may be showing an undersensitivity or a problem in discrimination. Only when she stuffs her mouth (and stretches the receptors in her cheeks) does she register that there is food in her mouth.	An alternative explanation would be that the child is storing food because she doesn't know where her next meal is coming from.
He had never had solid food, and whenever anything (i.e., cracker crumbs, bread) touched his lips, he would gag and throw up. This lasted a couple or 3 weeks. When he did finally start eating, he would stuff his cheek with food and keep it there for hours. We'd have to clean out his mouth when we put him to bed.	Sometimes, when sensory defensiveness subsides and the child begins to tolerate food, he will show a reduced ability to discriminate and will need to "stretch" the sensory receptors to be aware of the food.	
My daughter was adopted at age 4½ from an orphanage where she lived since birth. She did not cry for the first 3 months, even when having stitches or blood tests.	Lack of response to pain has been a very common description from parents who have adopted institutionalized children. These examples reflect an underreaction to sensory input.	An alternative explanation is that in the orphanage, no one responded when the child was uncomfortable and so the child "learned" not to show a response to pain.

(Continues)

Appendix 33–1 Continued

Behavior	Interpretation	Comments
She barely cried after she arrived even though she put her tooth through her lower lip.		

Sensation-Seeking Behavior

Behavior	Interpretation	Comments
He thinks it's funny to fall off the bed at full speed; he also likes to crash into other unsuspecting people.	Many children seek a lot of deep pressure as a way of organizing their nervous systems.	
She wants to be pushed on the swing 1–2 hours a day; she wanted to jump on the rebound up to 700 jumps at a time.	Some other children seem to crave sensory input and need more than other children; they do not seem to register it in a typical way.	

Rocking

Behavior	Interpretation	Comments
Our child displayed almost "autistic" characteristics when we got her a week before her third birthday. She could not speak any language, could barely walk, and could not perform any activities. She preferred to sit and rock and play with her hands and feet.	There are a variety of interpretations as to why institutionalized children show stereotypical movements, including rocking and head banging. One interpretation is that these movements provide vestibular stimulation that is lacking in the child's environment. This movement is a way of stimulating the nervous system. Another interpretation is that rhythmic stimulation is calming.	From the early 1900s, self-stimulation and stereotypic movements have been described as clinical manifestations of deprivation and neglect. This was more fully documented by Spitz[23] and Provence and Lipton.[24] During a recent survey of adoptive parents of Romanian orphans, the persistence of repetitive stereotypic movement was a major concern of parents.[25]
Our daughter rocked if not held, would not make eye contact, and showed no facial expression when we adopted her. We felt compelled to hold, hug, dance with, and bounce her, and make contact in any way we could to keep her from rocking when we put her down. She did not know how to walk and had never had solid food at 18 months of age. We felt she was at least 12 months behind in all skills, including language. (The mother later reported that within 6 months her daughter had reached normal age–level abilities and continues at or above age level in all skills, physical, social, and intellectual.)		
At first she needed a lot of self-stimulation. She rocked and banged her head and was obsessed with small objects. My husband and I were thrilled when she could fall asleep without rocking.		

Appendix 33–1 Continued

Behavior	Interpretation	Comments
She rocks in her bed if she wakes at night until she goes back to sleep—1 to 15 times per night. She rocks back and forth when she is riding in a car and makes humming or repetitive noises. She rocks from foot to foot when she hears music.		

Source: From Cermak and Groza,[6] reprinted with permission from Kluwer Academic/Plenum Publishers.

Appendix 33–2 Evaluation of Sensory Processing Questionnaire[a]

Auditory System

1. Does your child have trouble understanding what other people mean when they say something?
2. Is your child bothered by any household or ordinary sounds, such as the vacuum, hair dryer, or toilet flushing?
3. Does your child respond negatively to loud noises as in running away, crying, or holding hands over ears?
4. Does your child appear to not hear certain sounds?
5. Is your child distracted by sounds not usually noticed by other people?
6. Is your child frightened of sounds that do not usually convey alarm to other children the same age?
7. Does your child seem to underreact to loud noises?
8. Does your child have difficulty interpreting the meaning of simple or common words?
9. Is your child easily distracted by irrelevant noises such as a lawn mower outside, children talking in the back of the room, crinkling paper, an air conditioner, a refrigerator, or fluorescent lights?
10. Does your child seem too sensitive to sounds?

Olfactory System

1. Does your child gag, vomit, or complain of nausea when smelling odors such as soap, perfume, or cleaning products?
2. Does your child complain that foods are too bland or refuse to eat bland foods?
3. Does your child prefer very salty foods?
4. Does your child like to taste non-food items such as glue or paint?
5. Does your child gag when anticipating an unappealing food?

Proprioception System

1. Does your child grasp objects so tightly that it is difficult to use the object?
2. Does your child grind his or her teeth?
3. Does your child seem driven to seek activities such as pushing, pulling, dragging, lifting, and jumping?
4. Does your child seem unsure of how far to raise or lower his or her body during movement such as sitting down or stepping over an object?
5. Does your child grasp objects so loosely that it is difficult to use the object?
6. Does your child seem to exert too much pressure for a task, such as walking heavily, slamming doors, or pressing too hard when using pencils or crayons?
7. Does your child jump a lot?
8. Does your child have difficulties playing with animals appropriately, such as petting them with too much force?
9. Does your child have difficulty positioning him- or herself in a chair?
10. Does your child bump or push other children?
11. Does your child seem generally weak?
12. Does your child chew on toys, clothes, or other objects more than other children do?

Tactile System

1. Does your child pull away from being touched lightly?
2. Does your child seem to lack the normal awareness of being touched?
3. Does your child react negatively to the feel of new clothes?
4. Does your child show an unusual dislike for having his or her hair combed, brushed, or styled?
5. Does your child prefer to touch rather than be touched?
6. Does your child seem driven to touch different textures?
7. Does your child refuse to wear hats, sunglasses, or other accessories?
8. Does it bother your child to have his or her finger or toe nails cut?

(Continues)

Appendix 33–2 Continued

9. Does your child struggle against being held?
10. Does your child have a tendency to touch things constantly?
11. Does your child avoid or dislike playing with gritty things?
12. Does your child prefer certain textures of clothing or particular fabrics?
13. Does it bother your child to have his or her face touched?
14. Does it bother your child to have his or her face washed?
15. Does your child resist or dislike wearing short-sleeved shirts or short pants?
16. Does your child dislike eating messy foods with his or her hands?
17. Does your child avoid foods of certain textures?
18. Does your child mind getting his or her hands in finger paint, paste, sand, clay, mud, glue, or other messy things?
19. Does it bother your child to have his or her hair cut?
20. Does your child overreact to minor injuries?
21. Does your child have an unusually high tolerance to pain?

Vestibular System

1. Does your child seem excessively fearful of movement, as in going up or down stairs or riding swings, teeter totters, slides, or other playground equipment?
2. Does your child demonstrate distress when he or she is moved or riding on moving equipment?
3. Does your child have good balance?
4. Does your child balance in activities such as walking on curbs or on uneven ground?
5. Does your child like fast, spinning carnival rides, such as merry-go-rounds?
6. When your child shifts his or her body, does he or she fall out of the chair?
7. Is your child unable to catch him- or herself when falling?
8. Does your child seem to not get dizzy when others usually do?
9. Does your child seem generally weak?
10. Does your child spin and whirl his or her body more than other children?
11. Does your child rock him- or herself when stressed?
12. Does your child like to be inverted or tipped upside down or enjoy doing activities that involve inversion,

such as hanging upside down or doing somersaults?
13. Was your child fearful of swinging or bouncing as an infant?
14. Compared with other children the same age, does your child seem to ride longer or harder on certain playground equipment, such as a swing or merry-go-round?
15. Does your child demonstrate distress when his or her head is in any other position than upright or vertical, such as having the head tilted backward or upside down?

Visual System

1. Does your child have trouble telling the difference between printed figures that appear similar, for example, differentiating between b an p or + and x?
2. Is your child sensitive to or bothered by light, especially bright light (blinks, squints, cries, or closes eyes)?
3. When looking at pictures, does your child focus on patterns or details instead of the main picture?
4. Does your child have difficulty keeping his or her eyes on the task or activity at hand?
5. Does your child become easily distracted by visual stimuli?
6. Does your child have trouble finding an object when it is amid a group of other things?
7. Does your child close one eye or tip his or her head back when looking at something or someone?
8. Does your child have difficulty with unusual visual environments such as a bright, colorful room or a dimly lit room?
9. Does your child have difficulty controlling eye movement when following objects like a ball with his or her eyes?
10. Does your child have difficulty naming, discriminating, or matching colors, shapes, or sizes?

For Children Older Than 6 Years

1. Did your child make reversals in words or letters when writing or copying or read words backwards (such as reading saw for was) after the first grade?
2. Does your child lose his or her place on a page while reading, copying, solving problems, or performing manipulations?
3. In school, does your child have difficulty shifting gaze from the board to the paper when copying from the board?

---

[a]Other resources include the Sensory Profile,[16] which describes standardized assessments for children age 3–10 years, and the Infant Toddler Sensory Profile,[17] for children birth to 3 years.

Source: From Clinical observations of neuromotor performance, evaluation of sensory processing, and touch inventory for elementary school children. In: Bundy AC, Lane SJ, Murray EA, eds. Sensory Integration. Philadelphia: F.A. Davis Co., 2002: 194–6.

Resources

Sensory Integration International. Available at: http://www.sensoryint.com.

American Occupational Therapy Association. Available at: http://www.aota.org.

Communication/Therapy Skill Builders, 555 Academic Court, San Antonio, TX 78204-2498. Tel: 800-228-0752.

Occupational Therapy Associates of Watertown, P.C. 124 Watertown Street, Watertown MA, 02472. Tel: 617-923-4410. Available at: http://www.otawatertown.com.

Pediatric Therapy Network. Available at: http://www.pediatrictherapy.com.

Kranowitz C. The Out-of-Sync Child. New York: Perigee, 1998.

Williams MS, Shellenberger S. How Does Your Engine Run? Leader's Guide to the Alert Program for Self-Regulation. Albuquerque, NM: Therapy Works Inc., 1994.

Cermak S, Larkin D. Developmental Coordination Disorder. Stamford, CT: Singular Publishing, 2001.

References

1. Casler L. Perceptual deprivation in institutional settings. In: Newton G, Levine S, eds. Early Experience and Behavior. Springfield, IL: Charles C. Thomas, 1968: 573–626.

2. Ayres AJ. Sensory Integration and the Child. Los Angeles: Western Psychological Services, 1979.

3. Ayres AJ. Sensory Integration and Learning Disorders. Los Angeles: Western Psychological Services, 1980.

4. Spitzer S, Roley SS. Sensory integration revisited. In: Roley SS, Blanche EI, Schaaf RC, eds. Understanding the Nature of Sensory Integration with Diverse Populations: Therapy Skill Builders. San Antonio, TX: Harcourt Health Sciences, 2001: 3–27.

5. Giordano A. Sensory overload. Boston Globe. Boston, 2001: April 24, C1.

6. Cermak S, Groza V. Sensory processing problems in post-institutionalized children: implications for social workers. Child Adolesc Soc Work J 1998; 15:5–37.

7. Casler L. Supplementary auditory and vestibular stimulation: effects on institutionalized infants. J Exp Child Psychol 1975; 19:456–63.

8. Rheingold HL. The measurement of maternal care. Child Dev 1960; 31:565–75.

9. Haradon G, Bascom B, Dragomir C, Scripcaru V. Sensory functions of institutionalized Romanian infants: a pilot study. Occupat Ther Int 1994; 1:250–60.

10. Casler L. The effects of extra tactile stimulation on a group of institutionalized infants. Genet Psychol Monogr 1965; 71:137–75.

11. Casler L. The effects of supplementary verbal stimulation on a group of institutionalized infants. J Child Psychol Psychiatry 1965; 6:19–27.

12. Bundy AC, Koomar J. Orchestrating intervention: the art of practice. In: Bundy AC, Lane SJ, Murray EA, eds. Sensory Integration: Theory and Practice. Philadelphia: F.A. Davis Co., 2002: 242–60.

13. Cermak SA, Daunhauer LA. Sensory processing in the post-institutionalized child. Am J Occup Ther 1997; 51:500–7.

14. Lin S. Sensory Integration in Post-institutionalized Eastern European Children. Dissertation. Department of Occupational Therapy. Boston: Boston University, 2002.

15. Schaaf RC, Anzalone M, Burke J. The sensory integration observation guide. In: Roley SS, Blanche EI, Schaaf RC, eds. Understanding the Nature of Sensory Integration with Diverse Populations: Therapy Skill Builders. San Antonio, TX: Harcourt Health Sciences, 2001: 307–11.

16. Dunn W. Sensory Profile User's Manual. San Antonio, TX: Psychological Corporation, 1997.

17. Dunn W. Infant-Toddler Sensory Profile User's Manual. San Antonio, TX: Psychological Corporation, 2002.

18. Miller LJ, Reisman JE, McIntosh DN, Simon J. An ecological model of sensory modulation. In: Roley SS, Blanche EI, Schaaf RC, eds. Understanding the Nature of Sensory Integration with Diverse Populations: Therapy Skill Builders. San Antonio, TX: Harcourt Health Sciences Co., 2001: 57–82.

19. Ayres AJ. Sensory Integration and Praxis Test. Los Angeles, CA: Western Psychological Services, 1989.

20. Wilberger J, Wilberger P. Alternative and complementary programs for intervention. In: Bundy AC, Lane SJ, Murray EA, eds. Sensory Integration. Philadelphia: F.A. Davis Co., 2002: 335–341.

21. Bundy AC. Clinical observations of neuromotor performance, evaluation of sensory processing, and touch inventory for elementary school children. In: Bundy AC, Lane SJ, Murray EA, eds. Sensory Integration. Philadelphia: F.A. Davis Co., 2002: Appendix 7–1. 194–6.

22. Cermak S, Larkin D, Larkin D. Developmental Coordination Disorder. Stamford, CT: Singular Publishing, 2001.

23. Spitz RA. Hospitalism: an inquiry into the genesis of psychiatric conditions in early childhood. The psychoanalytic study of the child. Vol. 1. New York: International Universities Press, 1945: 53–74.

24. Provence S, Lipton RC. Infants in Institutions. New York: International Universities Press, 1962.

25. Mainemer H, Gilman L. The experience of Canadian parents adopting children from Romanian orphanages. Symposium on development of Romanian children adopted to Canada. Proceedings. Quebec City: Canadian Psychological Assoc., 1992: 21–30.

34

CULTURE AND IDENTITY

doption issues emerge repeatedly during various life stages of the child and the adoptive family. The issues differ at different times. This chapter reviews some diverse topics that may arise for adoptive family members, including culture, race, identity, and searching for the birth family. Cultural issues only occasionally arise in domestic adoption. The latter three topics, however, have been extensively investigated in relation to domestic adoption; much less is known about these subjects for internationally adopted children. In this chapter, a brief overview of these subjects is provided to assist the pediatrician caring for the internationally adopted child. Several excellent texts and reviews address these topics individually;[1–11] the interested reader is referred to these and other resources for more complete explorations of these complex topics.

Cultural Issues for Internationally Adopted Children

The importance of cultural identity is increasingly recognized as a part of international adoption. Occasionally the child's country of origin is part of the family's heritage. In these situations, the shared culture strengthens the ties between parent and child ("we chose a child from Ukraine because my grandparents emigrated to the United States from Ukraine," "I've always been interested in Central America since studying Spanish in school," or "I wanted a child from China because I am Chinese-American, and grew up speaking Cantonese at home"). More commonly the internationally adopted child brings a new culture to the adoptive family. As discussed in Chapter 3, the large cohort of Korean children adopted by Americans in the 1950s–70s were pioneers of "visible" adoption.

The existence of adoptive families with children who did not resemble their parents exposed many cultural issues and identity assumptions inherent in adoption practices at the time. The secrecy that permeated many aspects of adoption could no longer be maintained (see Chapter 1). Adoption professionals and parents gradually realized that recognition and celebration of the child's cultural heritage was healthier and more psychologically appropriate than the pretense that the child was "just like the parents" and that "adoption didn't matter." That these attitudes seem so odd today is a tribute to the shift in perspective over the past few decades.[1–3,7–8]

Today, cultural identity is considered a vital part of the individuality of the internationally adopted child. Most adoptive parents embrace the opportunity to provide their child with a connection to his country of origin. Exposure to toys, clothing, songs, special foods, and books from the child's country are routine. Parents excitedly recount their own adventures during their own journey to receive their child. An unexpected benefit of the "two-trip system" in Russia and Vietnam has been to allow parents to gain more familiarity with their child's birth country. Parents who adopt from Kazakhstan (and in previous years from Peru) often spend many weeks in the country for legal procedures. Many report that this experience enhances their connection with the country, allows time to establish friendships with local citizens, and promotes fuller appreciation of the culture.

Magazines for adoptive parents are replete with information about different cultural activities for internationally adopted children from specific countries (e.g., special recipes for typical foods, pictures or even sewing patterns for traditional garments, descriptions of particular celebrations). Many adoptive family support groups are culturally based (e.g., Families for Russian and Ukrainian Adoption, Families with Children from China). These organizations offer adoptive families the chance to meet others whose children came from the same country.

Social events may be planned around themes such as Russian Christmas or Chinese New Year. Families and children learn about important cultural traditions and incorporate the child's cultural heritage into their own traditions. Other events such as special dance lessons (India, Cambodia, Thailand), language lessons, or even a special week at a "culture camp" (e.g., Korean Culture Camp) offer wonderful opportunities for the child to incorporate some parts of his or her heritage into daily life. Such activities provide children the opportunity to see other families that look like theirs (e.g., Asian child with white parents).[12] Birth siblings may also benefit (e.g., white sister and Indian brother).

Many adoption agencies have regular gatherings for previous clients. Families who met before, during, or after the adoption process have the opportunity to reconnect. Since many agencies work with a limited number of orphanages, this may also offer children the chance to meet with previous "group-mates" or at least children from the same orphanage ("Marla, come meet Kelly. She came from your orphanage!").

Children respond differently to these cultural activities, in part depending on developmental stage and understanding of adoption. Some whole-heartedly join the fun. For others, especially new arrivals grappling with transition issues, these events may be terrifying. For children at some stages, exposure to the birth country language, culture, restaurants, and activities raises terrifying or disquieting questions: Is my birth mother here? Will I meet her? Could that man be my birth father? Am I going to be sent back to the orphanage?[1,7,8]

The existence of these activities, programs, and groups represents a dramatic shift in the way adoption, culture, and identity are viewed. No formal studies have been done to evaluate the long-term effects of incorporating such activities and exposures into the child's life. It will be of great interest to compare the identity formation of these children as they enter adolescence and adulthood with that of children raised in a climate of secrecy about adoption and family origins. The widening acceptance of multiracial, multicultural families is reflected in recent media and advertising images. This transformation in adoption is thus mirrored in society at large.[8]

Race

Many international adoptions are also transracial adoptions. This adds another layer of complexity to the adoption. The distinction between racial and cultural identity is unclear in most adoption outcome studies.[10] Visible adoption affects the whole family; the family loses its privacy and becomes a transracial family.[7,10,13] The child may have the stressful experience of "double consciousness"—identification with two cultures simultaneously but alienation from both.[14] Depending on the makeup of the surrounding community, the child may be stigmatized within the daily environment.[15] This may be subtle and insidious; adoptive parents are sometimes unaware of their child's experience of covert racism.

The negative experiences of some transracial adoptees in Scandinavian countries likely reflects the homogeneity of the society.[16,17] Children in many communities in America could have similar experiences. For example, international adoptees in Sweden may be mistaken for refugees, with assumptions about socioeconomic status and background.[18] One woman states, "I can't walk in town without people looking strange at me. They talk English with me and treat me as . . . I don't know how. It feels terrible. I am Swedish! Sometimes I would like to scream."[18] Another states, "In such situations, I answer them in the typical local dialect that I am Swedish, and then it is okay."[18] The authors of a large cohort study of internationally adopted children in Sweden speculate that racial differences contribute to the social maladjustment and poor mental health outcomes of some of the children.[16] Lack of ethnic pride in international adoptees interferes with ability to respond to racism and discrimination as adults.[19]

Transracial adoption or transcultural adoption accounted for 14% of all domestic adoptions in the United States in 1994;[10] adjustment was deemed successful in 70%–90%. Some question whether good adjustment comes at the cost of sacrifice of heritage. This concern is the basis for the current practice supported by most social work organizations of transracial placement only after the possibility of same-race placement is exhausted.[9]

Experts on transracial adoption recommend that parents cultivate special awareness of the roles of race, ethnicity, and culture in the lives of their children.[10,15] They must become sensitized to racism and discrimination, and create opportunities for their child to learn about and participate in his or her culture of birth, beyond attending the occasional ethnic festival. This is best accomplished by finding role models for their children within their birth culture. Finally, parents must provide their child with survival skills to cope successfully with racism. A survey of transracial adoptive parents generated 39 recommendations for prospective parents considering this type of adoption (see Appendix 34–1).[10] The pediatrician called upon to advise such families will find this list useful.

Identity Issues for Adopted Children

Pediatricians are familiar with the stages of identity formation in children and have a privileged overview of these normal transitions in the lives of patients. From the toddler's first declarations of "No!" and "Mine!" through the teenager's struggles with individuality to the young adult's formation of independent identity, the stages are familiar and predictable. The adopted child must also progress through these stages; however, this journey is complicated by the additional psychic tasks imposed by adoption. The adopted child's progress through these stages necessarily differs from that of a non-adopted peer. Professionals must be prepared and knowledgeable about these differences to support the child and family through these transitions. Because the psychological tasks for the adoptee at each stage differ from that of the non-adoptee, the adopted child's behavior and emotional responses may be misinterpreted as "abnormal." Renowned adoption expert Joyce Maguire Pavao relabels these stages as "normative crises": necessary and important steps in identity formation for the adopted child. In her acclaimed work on adoption, she advises professionals and parents to broaden their awareness of the developmental tasks of the adopted child. Her book, *The Family of Adoption*,[7] is a readable, insightful, and comprehensive description and analysis of these stages.

Another useful tool is provided by Brodzinsky, Schecter, and Henig.[2] Using Erik Erikson's developmental stages for identify formation as a template, these authors add the necessary adoption-related tasks at each level (Table 34–1). Each psychosocial stage is complicated by adoption; the adopted child must reconcile these issues to progress to the next psychological level. In every stage of life, except infancy, toddlerhood, and old age, "coping with adoption-related loss" is necessary. This means different challenges arise at different times in life. Adjusting to the fact of adoption is not something that happens once, but must be processed again and again.

Understanding Adoption

Young children have little understanding of adoption, although most can parrot their adoption stories and readily declare that they are adopted. It is not until school age that most children realize that adoption started with a loss— the loss of their birth family. Brodzinsky and co-authors[2] suggest that ages 6–18 years are the most difficult for adoptees. The complexities of understanding adoption and its meaning res-

onate deeply for many children in this age group. For some school-age children, adoption itself is a risk factor for low self-esteem, academic problems, rebellious behavior (aggression, lying, hyperactivity, oppositional behavior, stealing, running away). This constellation of symptoms was defined in early 1980s as "adopted child syndrome." In 1994, the *Diagnostic and Standard Manual IV* introduced a code for "identity problem" (code 313.82).[15]

The frequency of these behaviors may account for the overrepresentation of adopted school-age children who require mental health support services (see Chapter 30). However, as Dr. Pavao suggests, struggles with adoption issues at this age is normal and should be supported.[7] In *Being Adopted*,[2] the authors state, "Adoption loss is more pervasive, less socially recognized, and more profound than other losses." They compare losses associated with adoption with those due to divorce and death (Table 34–2). Internationally adopted children face additional psychological tasks. For these children, the toll of adoption also includes the loss of language, culture, and heritage. The psychological burden of adjustment to these losses has not yet been fully evaluated. Child psychiatrist and adoption expert Steven Nickman states that "relatively few parents are equipped to help their kids face the depths of sadness they feel regarding their losses."[20]

Belonging in Adoptive Families

The formation of a family requires time and adjustment for everyone (Fig. 34–1). Perceived similarities and differences between parents and children are an important facet of this adjustment. Biologic families search for similarities in appearance, temperament, intelligence, interests, and behavior. Identification of these traits promote bonding and closeness between parent and child. In adoptive families, the meaning of similarity and difference between parent and child is more complex.[21] Various terms have been applied to these patterns, including matching/

Table 34–1 Adaptation of Erikson's pathways of building tasks for identity

Age Period	Erikson's Psychosocial Tasks	Adoption-related Tasks
Infancy	Trust vs. mistrust	Adjusting to transition to a new home
		Developing secure attachments, especially in cases of delayed placement
Toddlerhood and preschool years	Autonomy vs. shame and doubt; initiative vs. guilt	Learning about birth and reproduction
		Adjusting to initial information about adoption
		Recognizing differences in physical appearance, especially in interracial and intercountry adoption
Middle childhood	Industry vs. inferiority	Understanding the meaning and implications of being adopted
		Searching for answers regarding one's origin and the reasons for relinquishment
		Coping with physical differences from family members
		Coping with the stigma associated with adoption
		Coping with peer reactions to adoption
		Coping with adoption-related loss[a]
Adolescence	Ego identity vs. identity confusion	Further exploration of the meaning and implications of being adopted
		Connecting adoption to one's sense of identity
		Coping with racial identity in cases of interracial adoption
		Coping with physical differences from family members
		Resolving the family romance fantasy
		Coping with adoption-related loss,[a] especially as it relates to the sense of self
Young adulthood	Intimacy vs. isolation	Further exploration of the implications of adoption as it relates to the growth of self and the development of intimacy
		Further considerations of searching; beginning the search
		Adjusting to parenthood in light of the history of one's relinquishment
		Facing one's unknown genetic history in the context of the birth of children
		Coping with adoption-related loss[a]
Middle adulthood	Generativity vs. stagnation	Further exploration of the implications of adoption as it relates to the aging self
		Reconciling the creation of a psychological legacy with one's unknown past
		Further consideration of searching
		Coping with adoption-related loss[a]
Late adulthood	Ego integrity vs. despair	Final resolution of the implications of adoption in the context of a life review
		Final considerations regarding searching for surviving biological family

[a]Necessary at every stage of life.

From *Being Adopted, the Lifelong Search for Self*, by Dr. David Brodzinsky, M. Schechter and R. Henig, copyright ©1992 by David M. Brodzinsky, Marshall D. Schechter, and Robin Marantz Henig. Used with permission of Doubleday, a division of Random House, Inc.

Table 34–2 Comparison of losses: divorce, death, adoption

	Divorce	*Death*	*Adoption*
Universality	Not universal, but common	Universal, but not always death of a parent	Uncommon, may lead to feelings of isolation and "differentness"
Permanence	At least potentially reversible, if the parents remarry; the noncustodial parent is often visited; reunion fantasies are common among children of divorce	Permanent, irreversible	Seems potentially reversible, since the birth parents may be alive; reunion fantasies are common among adopted children
Relationship with the lost parent	A long history of a relationship before divorce affords the child a store of memories, which may help the child come to terms with the loss	A long history of a relationship before death affords the child a store of memories, which may help the child come to terms with the loss	No history of a relationship with the birth parents, little information about them provided by the adoptive parents; the lost parents often linger as "ghosts" in the adoptees' mental and emotional life, making it hard to come to terms with the loss
Voluntary vs. involuntary circumstances	A voluntary decision on the part of at least one parent, fostering anger toward the parents and guilt and self-blame for the child	Involuntary, no one to blame	A voluntary decision on the part of at least one parent, fostering anger toward the parents and guilt and self-blame for the child
Extent of the loss	Partial loss of a single parent	Permanent loss of a single parent	Loss of both birth parents and of extended birth family; loss of cultural and genealogical heritage; sometimes loss of a sense of permanence, sense of connectedness to adoptive family, sense of self, social status
Social recognition of loss	Loss rarely recognized; few rituals or support systems exist to help the child get through the loss	Universally recognized; rituals and support systems are plentiful to help the child get through the loss	Loss rarely recognized; few rituals or support systems exist to help the child get through the loss

From *Being Adopted, the Lifelong Search for Self*, by Dr. David Brodzinsky, M. Schechter and R. Henig, copyright ©1992 by David M. Brodzinsky, Marshall D. Schechter, and Robin Marantz Henig. Used with permission of Doubleday, a division of Random House, Inc.

mismatch, rejection/acceptance of differences, goodness of fit, mold, "elbow babies," or perceived incompatibility.[21] These qualities mirror the parent's expectations of the child and parental ability to handle the child's behavior. Renowned Norwegian adoption researcher Monica Dalen studied the effects of similarity and belonging on the styles of interaction of adoptive families.[21] She describes five behavior patterns in adopted children related to the degree of similarity and

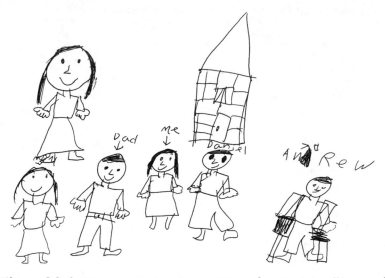

Figure 34–1 *Five-year-old adopted at age 4.5 years from Russia is well integrated into her adoptive family (including two birth brothers; brother Andrew is on crutches). (With permission.)*

acceptance between the family and the child (Table 34–3). These patterns are intertwined with the quality of family relationships.

Considerable literature supports the notion that adoptive parents have higher expectations and more satisfying experiences in parenting than biologic parents, and offer significantly more warmth, affection, and acceptance of their child.[2,11,22] Parenting quality is often superior to that of birth parents, which suggests that genetic ties are less important for family function than strong desire for parenthood. Adoptive parents tend to be highly functional individuals, less inclined to live vicariously, and more tolerant or sensitive of differences.

Pertman quotes Ellen Goodman, syndicated columnist for the *Boston Globe*, describing the family interactions of her friends who adopted a son.[8] In contrast to her own parenting style, she writes,

My friends started out in the parenting business one step ahead of the rest of us. Those of us who give our genes as well as our love to our children set out to reproduce ourselves. We deliver unconscious expectations in the birthing room. We think we know them. Because they are "ours." . . . Only later, sometimes much later, are we forced to get to know our children as they are, to stop assuming and start listening or watching . . . What I have learned from my friends and their son is that our children may be our own but we can't claim ownership . . . we must learn . . . to share them with themselves.

Table 34–3 Behavior patterns of adopted children in relation to degree of similarity and acceptance in family

Child's pattern of function in family	Similarity	Acceptance	Increasing Level of Family Conflict
Well-adjusted	High	High	
Creative	Low	High	
Ethnically different	Low	Moderate	
Satellite	Moderate	Moderate	
Fighter	Very low	Very low	

Source: From Dalen.[21]

Adoption Issues for Children and Teenagers

Adoption issues are raised at many different times during childhood.[2,7] Birthdays bring thoughts of birth parents and questions about why the adoption took place. School assignments (drawing the family tree, describing the family, bringing in baby pictures) place the adopted child in a predicament (see Chapter 32). Teasing or taunting on the playground and unthinking remarks by others may particularly resonate with the adopted child. Many stories, cartoons, and movies have parental loss and adoption themes (most recently, the Harry Potter series), and bring up questions or concerns for the child.

Worries about physical appearance become more common in pre-teens and teens. Adopted children may have particular anxiety about not resembling family members, and not knowing what to expect. One adopted teen stated, "I couldn't take it for granted that I looked like my parents. My non-adopted sister can look at our mother and see what she will look like when she grows up. I wish I could look ahead like that."[2]

Children may feel embarrassment or shame about unknowns in their medical history. During the teen years as they explore sexuality, some common themes emerge. Thoughts that "my birth mother got into trouble, I will too" may lead to sexual acting out as a form of identification with the birth mother. Some children, especially girls, resolve the wish for a blood relative by having a baby, and reason that keeping that child in some way rectifies the mistakes made by the birth mother.[2]

Nonetheless, in a large survey of teens adopted as infants, most had positive self-concepts, warm relationships with their parents, and psychological health comparable to non-adopted teens.[23] The survey included 881 adopted adolescents and their 78 non-adopted siblings from 715 families; 289 were adopted transracially, most from Korea. Nearly 75% of the teens had good mental health, although one-third had received counseling or mental health services. Two-thirds of the teens were interested in searching for their birth parents. The children had stronger involvement in churches and volunteer community organizations than non-adopted peers; the investigators concluded that these activities were emphasized by the adoptive families. The authors caution that such findings may not be applicable to all adopted children; the families that participated in this survey were notable in that there were few divorces or separations.

In a Swedish longitudinal study of nearly 600 adopted children,[24] about 20% had emotional and behavioral problems at age 11 years, significantly more than the non-adopted control group—possibly as children tested the commitment of the adoptive family. However, by age 15 years, few differences were found between the two groups of children. A Finnish study compared the adjustment of internationally adopted children and their Finnish-born classmates and found few differences although the former had "somewhat more problematic" adolescence.[17] In a larger version of the study, the international adoptees had more memory deficits, hyperactivity, school problems, and concentration difficulties, and higher scores on defiance and suspicion scales. However, these differences were considered relatively slight (see Chapter 30).

Searching for Birth Parents

Adoption records in most states in the United States are sealed. Domestically adopted children are issued a "new" birth certificate at the time of adoption, and have no legal right to the information on their original birth certificate. In the past decade, many adopted people have viewed this as an abrogation of their civil rights. Individually and in groups, adopted people have tried to break down some of the legal barriers that separate them from information about themselves. In many ways, such efforts have succeeded, and more importantly, these efforts have raised awareness about the need for adopted people to have access to this information for their medical and psychological well-being. Many adoptees conduct searches for their birth parents, often wanting simply to "see a face that looks like mine." Depending on age and individual circumstances, most adoptees are "not looking for a relationship, but for a relation."[2]

The authors of *Being Adopted* respond to the question, "What percent of adoptees search for their birth parents?" with the answer "100%."[2] The Internet has greatly facilitated the ability to search. The typical searcher is a female in her late 20s, usually married. The search is often triggered by a significant life event such as having a child, or death or divorce of an adoptive parent. Experts concur that for most children, a major consequence of search is the clarification of the adoptive parents' dominant position in the adoptee's life.[11] A survey of Danish-born adoptees, now adults, who met with their birthparents found that most subjects concurred with social anthropologist David Schneider's statement that "kinship is socially constructed not biologically inscribed."[25] These young adults all emphasized to the researchers that "when I said my real mother of course I meant my adoptive mother."

Although the psychological benefits of a search (and of many, but not all, reunions) have been carefully studied for domestic adoptees,[2,7,8] this area remains murky for international adoptees. The practical difficulties of a search in another country are considerable. The legal records provided at the time of the adoption are often scanty and incomplete (see Chapter 4). In Eastern Europe, it is common to have the name and date of birth of one or both parents, and some additional identifying information (ethnic background, occasionally address). Number of siblings may also be listed (sometimes with first names and ages). However, in some cases, these records have been deliberately falsified by birth mothers who do not wish to be identified or traced. Records of infants placed from Guatemala include DNA testing of the relinquishing birth mother, her name, national identity card number, and other facts. In China, the unusual circumstances of child abandonment forestall identification of the birth parents. In other countries, information is variable.

Searching for roots raises complex identity issues for international adoptees: the child may not feel fully a part of his new culture, but finds upon return to his birth country that he does not have a common cultural understanding or language despite the physical resemblance.[12] The usual terminology applied to adoption, that the child "comes home," implies that he finally arrived at where he was meant to be all along. This diminishes the biologic processes and transforms the birth parents and birth country into temporary caretakers.[12]

A Swedish study of 181 adoptees ages 13–27 years found that most had good mental health and self-esteem.[18] Nonetheless, 70% thought of their biologic families and imagined many things about them. Few variables predicted which children were in this group—age at adoption, for example, did not relate to thoughts of the biologic family. Seven percent of the group were intensively preoccupied by thoughts of their birth families. Many of the children imagined a return to their birth country—most were more interested in an "ethnic search" (to learn more about the country) than actually finding their birth families.

Adoption researchers agree that some children may benefit from such a search. With the adoptive parents, the child (usually an older teen or young adult) may wish to travel to his or her country of origin. "Homeland tours" are increasing in popularity (some travel agents advertise such group tours in adoption magazines). The child may visit his town of birth, possibly visit the orphanage where he resided, and even perhaps meet some of his early caretakers. It is particularly poignant to realize that the child would likely need an interpreter to talk with any birth relatives. Regardless of these limitations, this type of search offers the opportunity for the child to reconnect with his culture of origin, and may dramatically reveal the stark contrasts in his life as it would have been had he not been adopted. Such tours may benefit family members who feel a special purpose and meaning while traveling together with others who have had similar experiences in adoption.[12] These visits, however, must not be undertaken without careful consideration of the child's wishes and his present developmental stage and needs. Expert consultation may be advisable before endorsing a plan for such a trip.

Key Points for Internationally Adopted Children

- International adoptions must recognize and respect differences in culture and race between children and parents.
- Adopted children must process their identity throughout life.
- Adoptive families should prepare for "normative crises" as children progress through different life stages.[7]
- Identity problems for internationally adopted children may include racial and cultural differences.
- Openness in international adoption is logistically problematic, but efforts should be made to maintain a connection with the country of origin.

Appendix 34–1 Checklist for awareness by prospective transracial adoptive parents

Racial Awareness

1. I understand how my own cultural background influences the way I think, act, and speak.
2. I am able to recognize my own racial prejudice.
3. I am aware of stereotypes and preconceived notions that I may hold toward other racial and ethnic minority groups.
4. I have examined my feelings and attitudes about the birth culture and race of my children.
5. I make ongoing efforts to change my own prejudiced attitudes.
6. I have thoroughly examined my motivation for adopting a child of a different race or culture than myself.
7. I am knowledgeable of and continue to develop respect for the history and culture of my children's racial heritage.
8. I understand the unique needs of my child related to his or her racial or cultural status.
9. I know that transracial—cultural adoptive parenting involves extra responsibilities over and above those of in-racial parenting.
10. I have examined my feelings about interracial dating and marriage.
11. I know that others may view my family as "different."
12. I know that my children may be treated unkindly or unfairly because of racism.

Multicultural Planning

1. I include regular contact with people of other races and cultures in my life.
2. I place my children in multicultural schools.
3. I place my children with teachers who are racially aware and skilled with children of my child's race.
4. I understand how my choices about where to live affect my child.
5. I have developed friendships with families and individuals of color who are good role models for my children.
6. I purchase books, toys, and dolls that are like my child.
7. I include traditions from my child's birth culture in my family.
8. I provide my children with opportunities to establish relationships with adults from their birth country.
9. I provide my children with the opportunity to learn the language of their birth culture.

(Continues)

Appendix 34–1 Continued

Multicultural Planning

10. I provide my children with the opportunity to appreciate the music of their birth culture.
11. I have visited the country or community of my child's birth.
12. I have demonstrated the ability for sustained contact with members of my child's racial or ethnic group.
13. I seek services and personal contacts in the community that will support my child's ethnicity.
14. I live in a community that provides my child with same-race adult and peer role models on an ongoing basis.

Survival Skills

1. I educate my children about the realities of racism and discrimination.
2. I help my children cope with racism through open and honest discussion in our home about race and oppression.
3. I am aware of the attitudes of friends and family members toward my child's racial and cultural differences.
4. I am aware of a variety of strategies that can be used to help my child cope with acts of prejudice or racism.
5. I know how to handle unique situations, such as my child's attempts to alter his or her physical appearance to look more like family members or friends.
6. I help my children recognize racism.
7. I help my children develop pride in themselves.
8. I tolerate no biased remarks about any group of people.
9. I seek peer support to counter frustration resulting from overt and covert acts of racism toward my children, my family, or me.
10. I seek support and guidance from others who have a personal understanding of racism, particularly those from my child's race or birth culture.
11. I have acquired practical information about how to deal with insensitive questions from strangers.
12. I help my children understand that being discriminated against does not reflect personal shortcomings.
13. I am able to validate my children's feelings, including anger and hurt related to racism or discrimination.

From Vonk,[10] with permission. Copyright 2001, National Association of Social Workers, Inc., Social Work.

References

1. Bartholet E. Family Bonds: Adoption, Infertility, and the New World of Child Production. Boston: Beacon Press, 1993.
2. Brodzinsky DM, Schecter MD, Henig RM. Being Adopted. New York: Anchor Books, 1993.
3. Eldridge S. Twenty Things Adopted Kids Wish Their Adoptive Parents Knew. New York: Dell Trade Paperback, 1999.
4. Kirk HD. Shared Fate. Glencoe, IL: Free Press, 1964.
5. Lifton BJ. Lost and Found: The Adoption Experience. New York: Dial Press, 1979.
6. Paton JM. Orphan Voyage. New York: Vantage Press, 1968.
7. Pavao JM. The Family of Adoption. Boston: Beacon Press, 1998.
8. Pertman A. Adoption Nation: How the Adoption Revolution Is Transforming America. New York: Basic Books, 2000.
9. Vonk ME. Political and personal aspects of inter-country adoption of Chinese children in the United States. J Contemp Hum Serv 1999; 80:496.

10. Vonk ME. Cultural competence for transracial adoptive parents. Social Work 2001; 46:246.
11. Leon IG. Adoption losses: naturally occurring or socially constructed? Child Dev 2002; 73:652.
12. Howell S. Biologizing and de-biologizing kinship. In: Rygvold A-L, Dalen M, Saetersdal B, eds. Mine—Yours—Ours and Theirs. Oslo: University of Oslo, 1999: 32–51.
13. Register C. Are Those Kids Yours? American Families with Children Adopted from Other Countries. New York: Free Press, 1991.
14. Friedlander ML. Ethnic identity development of internationally adopted children and adolescents: implications for family therapists. J Marital Fam Therapy 1999; 25:43–60.
15. Grotevant HD. New kinship patterns, new issues. In: Rygvold A-L, Dalen M, Saetersdal B, eds. Mine—Yours—Ours and Theirs. Oslo: University of Oslo, 1999: 101–117.
16. Hjern A, Lindblad F, Vinnerljung B. Suicide, psychiatric illness, and social maladjustment in intercountry adoptees in Sweden: a cohort study. Lancet 2002; 360:443–8.

17. Forsten-Lindman A. Teenage psychosocial adjustment of child adoptees in Finland. In: Rygvold A-L, Dalen M, Saetersdal B, eds. Mine—Yours—Ours and Theirs. Oslo: University of Oslo, 1999: 156–170.

18. Irhammar M. Meaning of biological and ethnic origin in adoptees born abroad. In: Rygvold A-L, Dalen M, Saetersdal B, eds. Mine—Yours—Ours and Theirs. Oslo: University of Oslo, 1999: 171–188.

19. Saetersdal B, Dalen M. Norway: Intercountry adoptions in a homogeneous country. In: Alstein H, Simon RJ, eds. Intercountry Adoption: A Multinational Perspective. New York: Praeger, 1991: 83–108.

20. Nickman S. The Adoption Experience. New York: Julian Messner, 1985.

21. Dalen M. Interaction in adoptive families. In: Rygvold A-L, Dalen M, Saetersdal B, eds. Mine—Yours—Ours and Theirs. Oslo: University of Oslo, 1999: 82–100.

22. Hoopes JL. Prediction in Child Development: A Longitudinal Study of Adoptive and Non-Adoptive Families. New York: Child Welfare League of America, 1982.

23. Bower B. Adapting to adoption: adopted kids generate scientific optimism and clinical caution. Sci News 1994; 146:104.

24. Bohmann MS, Sigvardsson S. A prospective, longitudinal study of children registered for adoption. Acta Psychiatr Scand 1980; 61:339–55.

25. Cristensen IB. Is blood thicker than water? In: Rygvold A-L, Dalen M, Saetersdal B, eds. Mine—Yours—Ours and Theirs. Oslo: University of Oslo, 1999: 147–155.

35

AFTER THE ADOPTION: UNSPOKEN PROBLEMS

Most internationally adopted children are a source of immense joy to families. However, some families have unexpectedly difficult experiences during the adoption process or afterward. These problems related to international adoption are rarely addressed or only reported in sensational media stories. Moreover, adoptive families are not immune to troublesome issues which affect birth families. Adoption adds an extra dimension of complexity to these situations. In this section, some of these unspoken topics—parent stress, severely disturbed children, adoption disruption and dissolution, and post-adoption child abuse—will be discussed.

Parent Stress

International adoptions take place after a long, deliberate process initiated and pursued by parents. The adoption usually takes months or years to complete. In addition to the predictable difficulties associated with this prolonged and laborious process, unexpected challenges may arise. Referrals may be withdrawn, even at the "last minute," sometimes without explanation. Waiting parents may be told that their expected child was adopted by a local family, that a birth relative was unexpectedly located and the child's legal status must be reviewed, that the child developed new medical problems, or even that the child died. Losing the expected child in these ways is akin to experiencing a miscarriage, stillbirth, or death, and should be respected as such by pediatricians and other professionals.

In other circumstances, parents decide to reject the referral of a specific child offered for adoption. This decision is deeply fraught with emotional difficulties for adopting parents, especially if they have met and spent time with the child (as is the case recently for many adoptions in Ukraine, Russia, and Vietnam). Guilt for abandoning the child and hopelessness at ever achieving a successful adoption may be anguishing for prospective adoptive parents.

One mother writes (quoted in Cermak):[13] "I thought completing a Romanian adoption was hard—it was nothing compared to living with Andrea. Andrea has many problems, the most difficult being sensory integration. Currently our main issue is getting Andrea to eat. She is now 17 months old and still will not put anything in her mouth. She would rather starve herself to death than eat a piece of food. Andrea is a very unhappy child. It is hard for me to understand how such a young baby could be so discontented. She whines and cries constantly. I never know if she is sick, cold, hot, hungry, or what her problem could be; I just never know with Andrea because nothing really makes her happy. She does not like to be held for comfort—she is not a cuddly baby; she is more like a 17-month-old loner. Everyone told us "Andrea will outgrow this; love and attention is all she needs." I don't see an end in sight and I feel as if my family life as I once knew it is over. No one ever told us about the damaging effects orphanage life causes."

Parent stress also occurs after adoption. Some parents feel despondent and depressed after the adoption, comparable to postpartum depression. Post-adoption depression is widely underrecognized by professionals. Depression and anxiety strike new adoptive parents even when children arrive healthy, progress well developmentally, and adjust well to their new surroundings. It may be difficult for parents to verbalize or accept these feelings. As with postpartum depression, these symptoms occur at a time new parents expect feelings of joy and happiness. After working so hard to achieve the adoption, parents may be ashamed to confess negative or ambivalent feelings to relatives and friends. For some parents, these feelings begin the moment they receive their child. Contrary to the popular myth of "instant bonding," many adoptive parents describe apprehension and anxiety as their initial feelings at the moment of meeting their child. Such feelings are rarely shared or discussed. Many worry that these initial feelings are abnormal and foretell future problems with the adoption. Clearly, such anxieties may multiply if not addressed appropriately. Parents should be reassured that physical proximity over time is necessary to develop meaningful attachment and bonding.[1]

Much has been written about the bonding process of children to parents (see Chapter 29). Less is known about the process by which adoptive parents bond to their new children. The reasons for the adoption, such as primary infertility, secondary infertility, or altruism, influence the parent's ability to bond with the child.[2] Parental age,[3] marital status and duration, and expectations also affect family adjustment, although these factors have not been comprehensively evaluated. In international adoption, this process is complicated by the age of the chil-

Ms. H. traveled to Vietnam to adopt her 4-month-old daughter, about whom she had one page of information and a single tiny photo. "I fell head over heels in love with her the moment I met her. She was beautiful and everything I imagined," she stated. "But then I learned she had hepatitis B. Friends in the United States whom I called told me that I shouldn't adopt her under any circumstances. It was heart-breaking to leave her there. I returned a month later when my agency said another baby girl was available. It was a totally different experience. The baby was floppy and didn't make eye contact. She threw up every time I fed her. She felt like skin and bones when I held her. Now I have to decide whether to accept her or not. I know I'm still grieving for the first baby, but my agency says if I don't take this baby, it will be a long wait until I receive another referral. My documents are about to expire and I'll have to start the whole process over again. If it takes more than 6 months, I'll be too old to adopt."

dren: none are newborns. Parents responding to a survey conducted by their adoption agency provided the following comments about the post-adoptive period:[4]

- "Be patient, it's more like a courtship than a birth or a newborn child."
- "We were prepared that our daughter might not be receptive to her mother, but not to such an extent."
- "We did not anticipate the emotional stress and physical exhaustion involved in traveling to Russia to complete the adoption. Nor did we anticipate our daughter's depression."
- "Parents tell you what it is like to have no privacy or quiet, but it is not real until you have experienced it."
- "I was naive to the difficulty the children would have in terms of adjustment. To my mind we offered so much that was so much better, I thought it would be easy for them."
- "It has been more of a challenge than we have been able to handle at times."
- "No one is really prepared to go from being childless to with child in 1 day."
- "Patience, patience, patience."
- "Be ready and willing to redefine 'normal.' "

Parents whose adopted children display difficult and challenging behaviors or unexpected medical issues sometimes have more severe emotional problems after adoption.[5] In one of the few studies of internationally adopting families, parenting stress was linked to the adopted child's attachment security and number of problem behaviors.[6] Other factors, including the mother's age, income, and number of children adopted, also contributed to parental stress.[6] In another study of Canadian families who adopted from Romania, highest parental stress scores were found in those parents whose children were insecurely attached, had lower IQ scores, and more problem behaviors.[7]

Stress derives from several sources. Child characteristics, parent–child interactions, family cohesion, parental adjustment, and adoptions service issues all contribute to stress.[8] Marital stresses are common after adoption (or the birth) of a child with emotional and behavioral issues or with severe developmental disabilities. Both parents may not have been equally committed to the adoption, even before problems were recognized. After adoption, the realities of parenting a behaviorally challenging child may augment marital discord, and in some cases result in divorce. Parental satisfaction with adoption is worse than expected if the child has emotional and behavioral problems or a history of sexual abuse.[9]

Adoptive parents whose children require unexpected hospitalization shortly after adoption may experience extreme stress. Parents have cited their own lack of knowledge of the child's medical history, concerns about attachment, and lack of awareness of adoption issues on the part of the medical staff as factors contributing to the stress.[10] In contrast, parents whose children arrive with known physical disabilities generally adjust well.[9,11]

Pediatricians are poor at recognizing depressive symptoms in parents.[12] Physicians caring for internationally adopted children should be especially alert to signs of parental depression or anxiety. Open-ended questions ("Is the adoption everything you thought it would it be?" "Was it hard the first few days when you couldn't comfort her?" "Do you sometimes wish you hadn't adopted?") may reveal parental issues that should be directly addressed.

Mr. and Mrs. Q. adopted a sibling group of 3 children, ages 3, 5, and 7 years. The children were loud, rambunctious, active, and energetic. They had no conception of table manners, but wildly stuffed all food into their mouths. They broke toys, furniture, windows, and mirrors with their wild running, throwing, and playing in the house. They spoke Russian together and seemed to be laughing at their adoptive parents behind their backs. They refused to use even one word of English. "Why did we ever think we wanted to do this?" sobbed Mrs. Q. "I can't believe what I've done to my life."

Severely Disturbed Children

Sadly, some children placed for international adoption are profoundly disturbed (see Chapter 30). Severe early deprivation and abuse, perhaps coupled with genetic factors and prenatal exposures, damage some children irreparably. Adoptive parents of these children describe horrific behaviors, such as animal cruelty, fire-setting, molestation of other children, and even attempted murder.[14] Most have reactive attachment disorder (See Chapter 29), often complicated by other psychiatric conditions. Such children usually are placed in long-term psychiatric hospital settings, a tragic outcome for all concerned. Exact figures for the numbers of these children are not maintained. Anecdotal but compelling information comes from Thais Tepper and Lois Hannon, co-founders of the Parent Network for the Post-Institutionalized Child, who report enormous increases in calls from parents seeking information about their severely disturbed children (T. Tepper and L. Hannon, personal communication).

> An informal support group for parents of older internationally adopted children met on a regular basis. One week a parent asked how many other members were taking medication for anxiety or depression since their children had been adopted. There was laughter mixed with tears as all other 12 parents attending the meeting raised their hands.

> The S family was delighted with their adoption of 3-year-old Robbie. A year later, they adopted Max, "so that Robbie wouldn't be an only child". They later learned that Max, age 4 on arrival, had been brutally molested in his birth home for the first 3 years of his life. "He never seemed to settle in with the family," said Mrs. S. "My husband and I started to argue all the time about how to handle Max. We even fought about whether we should have adopted him. My husband said we should dissolve the adoption, but I felt we owed it to Max to try our best to help him. My husband said that if I felt that way, he would leave the family. Now it's just me and the two boys. I can't believe what happened in my family the last few years."

Adoption Disruption and Dissolution

One of the unspoken realities of adoption is that sometimes disruptions or dissolutions occur. Unlike other life choices such as a house, job, or even marriage,[15] adoption is viewed as an extraordinarily stronger, more permanent commitment. Yet the unhappy fact is that some adoptions do not succeed. The term *disruption* is incorrectly used to describe adoption termination at any time.[9] Legally, this term indicates adoptions that end after the child is placed in the family but before the adoption is legalized. Disruptions are usually handled by the placing agency without court involvement. *Dissolution* is the termination of an adoption any time after it has been legalized. Most internationally adopted children arrive in the country after legal adoption in their birth countries; therefore, a legal dissolution is required to terminate the adoption. The adoption agency usually tries to identify a new placement for the child, but occasionally the child enters state care.

Exact figures for the numbers of international adoptions that disrupt or dissolve are not maintained by any central authority (although this may change once the Hague Convention is implemented). Tressler Lutheran Services finds homes in Pennsylvania, Delaware, and Maryland for children with special needs, including troubled children. In its first 22 years, the agency was not asked to take a single internationally adopted child. Between 1994 and 2000, Tressler placed 105 Eastern European adoptees with a second set of American parents (or sometimes a third or fourth).[14]

Surveys of domestic adoption disruptions or dissolutions suggest that about 10%–14% of special-needs placements are terminated.[9] Risk factors related to the parents and the child have been identified. Child risk factors include age

The first day the A Family met their Russian daughter-to-be, she repetitively lined up blocks in a row, and refused eye contact. Mr. A. felt sure that she was autistic. After returning home with her, they noted that she exhibited this behavior frequently, especially when stressed. Medical evaluations did not confirm autism, but the family felt that the girl's behavior was adversely affecting their birth son, and chose to dissolve the adoption.

The D family excitedly traveled to Thailand to receive their 9-month-old son, after gazing lovingly at a single tiny photo of him for 5 months. When they received him, both parents felt immediately that the child in their arms was not the child in the photo. They were told by the local facilitator and orphanage workers that this was impossible. Even after returning home with him, they strongly felt that this was "the wrong child." They visited three pediatricians, two child neurologists, and a developmental specialist to seek confirmation of their belief that this was a different child, and moreover, that "something was wrong with him." Not surprisingly, the boy cried constantly, and appeared hypertonic and tense. After several weeks, they decided to dissolve the adoption.

(older children, especially those who have been in neglectful or abusive situations for longer periods) and behavior problems (violation of family norms, cruelty, defiance, sexual acting out, physically harming or threatening others).[9]

Children with physical handicaps are less likely to experience adoption disruptions, possibly because families have more realistic expectations than parents who adopt children with less obvious cognitive or affective problems. Parents who terminate adoptive placements usually state that their child's behavior problems were more severe, pervasive, and incorrigible than they imagined or "were led to believe." Some parents may have the mistaken notion that by adopting from Eastern Europe, for example, they can avoid children with emotional issues found in many American children residing in foster care.[16]

Factors in the adoptive family are linked to the risk of disruption or dissolution.[9] Some studies of domestic adoption cite parental age as a factor, with younger (presumably less experienced) parents more likely to disrupt. Higher expectations and higher educational achievements of the adoptive parents (especially mothers) have been cited in some but not all studies of adoption disruptions. Sibling group adoptions were also more likely to disrupt in some but not all studies. Another risk factor that undoubtably also applies to many international adoptions is pre-adoptive information that seems "scanty or too favorable." Lack of opportunity for a "get-acquainted" period prior to adoptive placement may also increase the likelihood of disruptions, especially for older children (see Summer Programs in Chapter 3). Major themes in adoption disruptions are lack of post-placement services, family system strain and overload, lack of parental empathy, incomplete attachment, inadequate preparation, lack of family support and resources, and insurmountable obstacles.[9]

Some protective factors have been identified by adoption researchers.[9] Other children in the home, lower family income, and previous experience with adoption all seem to decrease the likelihood of adoption disruptions. Availability of post-adoption support further minimizes disruptions. Support groups, respite care, counseling, mental health services, and other

Erica, 12 months old from Korea, joined two older brothers from Korea in the Y family. She'd been adopted by the L family in Virginia at 8 months of age. Mrs. L had unexpectedly become pregnant during the wait for a referral. She delivered just a week before Erica arrived. The L family stated, "This just doesn't feel right," and dissolved the adoption.

Jacqueline and Robert, unrelated siblings, were brought to the International Adoption Clinic for evaluation. The children were healthy and happy, and the whole family seemed to be adjusting well to the adoption. At the scheduled 6-month follow-up, the parents appeared only with Robert. When queried, they stated that Jacqueline never settled into the family and they had become greatly alarmed that she had reactive attachment disorder. She was removed from the household and placed with a family in another state where they were told she was doing well as an only child.

programs may sustain the family through difficult times. Unfortunately, access to postplacement services may depend heavily on finances and health insurance. In some states, parents may need to relinquish the child to a state welfare agency to receive needed services. This misguided approach can exacerbate the child's emotional and behavioral issues.

Child Abuse and Worse

No one wants to imagine that adoptive parents abuse their children. The home study is carefully designed to screen adoptive parents. Trained social workers have interviewed them extensively about their personal lives, child-rearing beliefs, and psychological preparedness. The process of international adoption is spread over many months or even years, allowing adoption workers the opportunity to get to know their clients well and to observe their responses to stress, disappointment, and uncertainty. Postplacement visits are done to assess family function. Despite these safeguards, some parents abuse their internationally adopted children. One case was heavily covered in the media. Karen and Richard Thorne were found guilty of abusing their two just-adopted 4-year-old Russian girls after multiple witnesses observed them slapping and screaming at the children on the plane returning from Moscow to the United States.[16] The court ordered the Thornes to receive parental training and therapy. Nine months later, they were given custody of their daughters, who had meanwhile resided in five different foster homes.

Undoubtably, some children are abused abroad prior to adoptive placement. In newly arrived children with suspicious findings, ascertaining the timing of abuse may be extremely problematic. Suspect fractures found clinically or serendipitously (for example, on a routine chest x-ray) may prompt a distressing abuse investigation of the family, and even removal of the child from the adoptive home. Attachment and bonding may be profoundly and permanently

Rudy was diagnosed with fetal alcohol syndrome and severe microcephaly shortly after her adoption at age 6. She did well initially, but shortly after entering school had increasing behavioral problems. Rudy became violent and aggressive, and frequently ran away from home. By age 10, she had been in three different psychiatric hospitals. Her single mom, a special-needs school teacher, was devoted to Rudy, and made heroic efforts to address her daughter's needs. As a young teenager, Rudy became more and more difficult to control. She was kicked out of four special schools because of behavior problems, and spent 2 months in a locked psychiatric ward in a private facility. Her mother's insurance benefits for mental health services ran out and the facility scheduled her for discharge. Her mother felt strongly that her daughter was not ready to come home (the psychiatrists agreed), but her savings were exhausted. The state agreed to assume financial responsibility for Rudy's mental health care, but only if she was relinquished to the state. "How can anyone think that it is in Rudy's interest to be removed from her family?" said her mom. "She'll be discharged into foster care and they won't even tell me where she is or allow visitation. I know she will think I've abandoned her."

> *Eloise was adopted from Cambodia at age 18 months. Her adoptive mother became alarmed about Eloise's breathing after she'd been home for 10 days. A chest radiograph done in the emergency room revealed a recent fracture in her left proximal humerus and two rib fractures. A skeletal survey showed two other recent fractures. A child abuse investigation was undertaken, and Eloise was placed in foster care. When she was returned to her family 4 weeks later, she was passive and withdrawn. Her parents, though relieved to have her back, were distraught and emotionally exhausted. "What a terrible beginning to our life as a family," said her mother. "I don't know if any of us will ever get over this. If only we'd done the skeletal survey on the way home from the airport!"*

> *Seven-year-old Rebecca was adopted from Bulgaria. She had been sexually abused from age 1 until 5 years while living with her birth family. Upon arrival to the orphanage, she was a traumatized and unhappy little girl. After lots of love and support from the orphanage staff, she began to feel safe and secure. Two years later, she was thriving in first grade, and her sparkly personality delighted everyone. The orphanage staff was thrilled when Rebecca was chosen for adoption by an American couple. The parents had taken some special courses at their adoption agency about parenting children with prior sexual abuse. Rebecca happily embarked on her new life. Overall, Rebecca seemed to adjust well to school, friends, and neighbors. However, her mother always felt a bit disappointed that her relationship with her new daughter wasn't closer, and thought that Rebecca was underachieving in school. Rebecca attended several series of sessions with a child psychologist. The psychologist determined that Rebecca's problems related to her prior history of sexual abuse. Three years later, Rebecca's adoptive mother learned to her horror that her husband had been sexually abusing their daughter since her arrival in their home.*

disturbed for both the child and the parents. Yet child abuse is occasionally perpetrated by adoptive parents.[17]

Even more tragic is the story of David Polreis, a Russian adoptee who was beaten to death at 2 years of age, 8 months after adoption. His adoptive mother was convicted of child abuse and sentenced to 22 years in prison. Appallingly, as many as 12 other cases of suspected or proven murder by adoptive parents have occurred in the last decade.[18]

Physicians caring for the internationally adopted child must therefore be prepared to protect this child as any other. Improbable as it may seem, abuse of the internationally adopted child does occur. Legal requirements to report suspected abuse must not be ignored.

References

1. Leon IG. Adoption losses: naturally occurring or socially constructed? Child Dev 2002; 73:652.

2. Brodzinsky DM, Schechter MD, Henig RM. Being Adopted. New York: Anchor Books, 1993.

3. Schecter MD, Holter FR. Adopted children in their adoptive families. Ped Clin North Am 1975; 22:653–61.

4. MAPS International. Survey of post-adoptive parents. Portland, Maine: Maine Adoption Placement Service International, undated.

5. Groza V, Ryan SD. Pre-adoption stress and its association with child behavior in domestic special needs and international adoptions. Psychoneuroendocrinology 2002; 27:181–97.

6. Mainemer H, Gilman LC, Ames EW. Parenting stress in families adopting children from Romanian orphanages. J Fam Issues 1998; 19:164–180.

7. Chisholm K. A three-year follow-up of attachment and indiscriminate friendliness in children adopted from Romanian orphanages. Child Dev 1998; 69:1092–106.

8. McGlone K, Santos L, Kazama L, Fong R, Mueller C. Psychological stress in adoptive parents of special-needs children. Child Welfare 2002; 81:151–71.

9. Barth RP. Risks and rates of adoption disruption. In: Marshner C, Pierce WL, eds. Adoption Factbook III. Waite Park, MN: National Council for Adoption, 1999: 381–92.

10. Smit EM. Maternal stress during hospitalization of the adopted child. MCN Am J Matern Child Nurs 2000; 25:37–42.

11. Glidden LM, Johnson VE. Twelve years later: adjustment in families who adopted children with developmental disabilities. Ment Retard 1999; 37:16–24.

12. Heneghan AM, Silver EJ, Bauman LJ, Stein REK. Do pediatricians recognize mothers with depressive symptoms? Pediatrics 2000; 106:1367–73.

13. Cermak SA. The effects of deprivation on processing, play, and praxis. In: Roley S, Blanche E, Schaaf R, eds. Understanding the nature sensory integration with diverse populations. Therapy Skill Builders: San Antonio, TX, 2001.

14. Hastings D. Adopted Russian Children Killed in the United States. Associated Press. January 29, 2001.

15. Bartholet E. Family Bonds: Adoption, Infertility, and the New World of Child Production. Boston: Beacon Press, 1993.

16. Pertman A. Adoption Nation: How the Adoption Revolution Is Transforming America. New York: Basic Books, 2000.

17. www.kutv.com. Couple accused of starving two adopted children, 2002.

18. Working R, Madhani A. Parents often not ready for needy foreign kids. Chicago Tribune. January 5, 2004. Available at: http://www.sunherarld.com/mld/Sunherald/news/nation/7636493.htm.

36

RESOURCES

General Resources on Adoption

Child Welfare League of America
440 First Street, N.W.
Washington, D.C. 20001
202-638-2952
www.cwla.org

Congressional Coalition on Adoption
6723 Whittier Avenue, Suite 306
McLean, VA 22101
703-288-9700
http://www.ccainstitute.org

Evan B. Donaldson Adoption Institute
215 East 69th St.
New York, NY 10021
212-269-5080
http://www.adoptioninstitute.org

International Association of Voluntary
   Adoption Agencies and NGOs
1667 K Street, N.W., Suite 520

Washington, D.C. 20006
202-293-7979
http://www.iavaan.org

Joint Council for International
   Children's Services
7 Cheverly Circle
Cheverly, MD 20785
http://www.jcics.org

National Adoption Information
   Clearinghouse
P.O. Box 1182
Washington, D.C. 20013
888-251-0075
http://www.calib.com/naic

National Council for Adoption
1930 17th Street, NW
Washington, DC 20009
202-328-1200
http://www.ncfa-usa.org

North American Council on Adoptable
Children
970 Raymond Avenue
St. Paul, MN 55114
612-644-3036
http://www.nacac.org

Updated Medical Literature on Adoption

Medlineplus Adoption. Available at:
http://www.nlm.nih.gov/medlineplus/adoption.html

Clinical Trials for Adopted Persons

Clinical trials.gov-adoption. Available at:
http://www.clinicaltrials.gov/

Child Development and Special Needs

Interdisciplinary council on developmental and
learning disabilities. Available at: http://
www.icidl.com/ICDLguidelines/toc.htm
Parents Network for the Post-Institutionalized Child.
Available at: http://www.pnpic.org

Helpful Books

Infectious diseases
American Academy of Pediatrics. 2003 Red Book:
Report of the Committee on Infectious Diseases.
Pickering LK, ed. Elk Grove Village, IL: American
Academy of Pediatrics, 2003.

Adoption (an abbreviated selection)
1. Adoption Factbook III. Marshner C, Pierce WL,
eds. Waite Park, MN: National Council for Adoption,
1999.
2. Bartholet E. Family Bonds: Adoption, Infertility,
and the New World of Child Production. Boston: Beacon
Press, 1993.
3. Brodzinsky DM, Schechter MD, Henig RM. Being
Adopted. New York: Anchor Books, 1993.
4. Federici RS. Help for the Hopeless Child. Alexandria, VA: Dr. Ronald S. Federici and Associates, 1998.
5. Handbook of Infant Mental Health. Zeanah CH, ed.
New York: Guilford Press, 2000.
6. Hopkins-Best M. Toddler Adoption: The Weaver's
Craft. Indianapolis, IN: Perspectives Press, 1997.

7. Hughes DA. Building the Bonds of Attachment.
Northvale, N.J.: Jason Aronson, Inc., 1998.
8. Keck GC, Kupecky RM. Adopting the hurt child.
Colorado Springs: Pinon Press, 1995.
9. McKenzie RB (ed). Rethinking Orphanages for the
21st Century. Thousand Oaks, CA: Sage Publications,
Inc., 1999.
10. Pavao JM. The Family of Adoption. Boston:
Beacon Press, 1998.
11. Pertman A. Adoption Nation: how the adoption
revolution is transforming America. New York: Basic
Books, 2000.

Travel Information

Centers for Disease Control and Prevention, Travel
Medicine. Available at: http://www.cdc.gov/travel/
index.htm.
U.S. State Department Travel Advisories. Available at:
http://www.travel.state.gov.
World Health Organization. Available at: http://
www.who.int/home-page or http://www.who.int/csr/
don/en/ (emerging infections).

Vaccinations

Atkinson WL, Pickering LK, Schwartz B, Weniger BG,
Iskander JK, Watson JC. General Recommendations on
Immunization: Recommendations of the Advisory Committee on Immunization Practices (ACIP) and the American Academy of Family Physicians (AAFP). 51(RR02);
1–36. February 8, 2002. Available at: http://www.cdc.
gov/mmwr/preview/mmwrhtml/rr5102a1.htm.

Journal Articles (Reviews or Country-specific)

1. Albers LH, Johnson DE, Hostetter MK, Iverson S,
Miller LC. Health of children adopted from the former
Soviet Union and Eastern Europe. Comparison with
preadoptive medical records. JAMA 1997; 278:922–4.
2. Bureau JJ, Maurage C, Bremond M, Despert F, Rolland JC. Children of foreign origin adopted in France.
Analysis of 68 cases during 12 years at the University Hospital Center of Tours. [in French]. Arch Pediatr 1999;
6:1053–8.
3. Glennen S. Language development and delay in internationally adopted infants and toddlers: a review. Amer
J Speech—Lang Pathol 2002; 11:333–9.
4. Hostetter MK, Iverson S, Dole K, Johnson D. Unsuspected infectious diseases and other medical diagnoses

in the evaluation of internationally adopted children. Pediatrics 1989; 83:559–64.

5. Hostetter M, Johnson DE. International adoption. An introduction for physicians. Am J Dis Child 1989; 143:325–32.

6. Hostetter MK, Iverson S, Thomas W, McKenzie D, Dole K, Johnson DE. Medical evaluation of internationally adopted children. N Engl J Med 1991; 325:479–85.

7. Hostetter M. Infectious diseases in internationally adopted children: the past five years. Pediatr Infect Dis J 1998; 17:517–8.

8. Jenista JA, Chapman D. Medical problems of foreign-born adopted children. Am J Dis Child 1987; 141: 298–302.

9. Jenista JA, ed. International Adoption. Pediatr Ann 2000; 29(4). (entire issue)

10. Johnson DE, Miller LC, Iverson S, et al. The health of children adopted from Romania. JAMA 1992; 268: 3446–51.

11. Lange WR, Warnock-Eckhart E. Selected infectious disease risks in international adoptees. Pediatr Infect Dis J 1987; 6:447–50.

12. Miller LC, Kiernan MT, Mathers MI, Klein-Gitelman M. Developmental and nutritional status of internationally adopted children. Arch Pediatr Adolesc Med 1995; 149:40–4.

13. Miller LC, Hendrie NW. Health of children adopted from China. Pediatrics 2000; 105:E76.

14. Nicholson AJ, Francis BM, Mulholland EK, Moulden AL, Oberklaid F. Health screening of international adoptees. Evaluation of a hospital-based clinic. Med J Aust 1992; 156:377–9.

15. Proos LA, Hofvander Y, Wennqvist K, Tuvemo T. A longitudinal study on anthropometric and clinical development of Indian children adopted in Sweden. Ups J Med Sci 1992; 97:93–106.

16. Saiman L, Aronson JE, Zhou J, et al. Prevalence of infectious diseases among internationally adopted children. Pediatrics 2001; 108:608–12.

17. Smith-Garcia T, Brown JS. The health of children adopted from India. J Community Health 1989; 14: 227–41.

18. Staat MA. Infectious disease issues in internationally adopted children. Pediatr Infect Dis J 2002; 21: 257–8.

INDEX